THE ADULT KNEE

THE ADULT KNEE

Volume II

Editors

John J. Callaghan, M.D.
Lawrence and Marilyn Dorr Chair and Professor
Department of Orthopaedics and Bioengineering
University of Iowa College of Medicine
Iowa City, Iowa

Aaron G. Rosenberg, M.D.
Professor of Surgery
Rush Medical College of Rush University
Chicago, Illinois

Harry E. Rubash, M.D.
Edith M. Ashley Professor of Orthopaedic Surgery
Harvard Medical School
Chief
Department of Orthopaedic Surgery
Massachusetts General Hospital
Boston, Massachusetts

Peter T. Simonian, M.D.
Clinical Professor
Department of Orthopaedic Surgery
University of California, San Francisco, School of Medicine,
Fresno, California

Thomas L. Wickiewicz, M.D.
Professor of Clinical Orthopaedic Surgery
Department of Orthopaedics
Weill Medical College of Cornell University
Attending Orthopedic Surgeon and Chief
Department of Sports Medicine and Shoulder Service
Hospital for Special Surgery
New York, New York

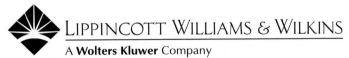

LIPPINCOTT WILLIAMS & WILKINS
A **Wolters Kluwer** Company
Philadelphia • Baltimore • New York • London
Buenos Aires • Hong Kong • Sydney • Tokyo

Acquisitions Editor: James Merritt
Developmental Editor: Anne Snyder
Supervising Editor: Mary Ann McLaughlin
Production Editor: Brooke Begin, Silverchair Science + Communications
Manufacturing Manager: Tim Reynolds
Cover Designer: QT Design
Compositor: Silverchair Science + Communications
Printer: Walsworth Publishing

© 2003 by LIPPINCOTT WILLIAMS & WILKINS
530 Walnut Street
Philadelphia, PA 19106 USA
LWW.com

Printed in the USA

Library of Congress Cataloging-in-Publication Data
The adult knee / editors, John J. Callaghan ... [et al.].
    p. ; cm.
  Includes bibliographical references and index.
  ISBN 0-7817-3247-6
  1. Knee--Surgery. 2. Arthroplasty. I. Callaghan, John J.
  [DNLM: 1. Joint Diseases--surgery. 2. Knee Joint--surgery. 3. Arthroplasty,
Replacement, Knee--methods. 4. Knee Injuries--surgery. 5. Knee Joint--physiology. WE
870 A244 2003]
  RD561 .A35 2003
  617.5'82059--dc21

                                        2002030014

10 9 8 7 6 5 4 3 2 1

To my wife, Kim,
and our children, Patrick and Katie,
for providing a balanced perspective on life
and for their unconditional love, friendship,
and never-ending support

—*J.J.C.*

To my wife, Iris,
without whose support my work would not be possible,
and to our children, AJ, Jessica, Becca, and Cody,
who serve as a constant source of inspiration and joy;
to my patients, whose faith in me has sustained my practice,
and my teachers, whose example focused my energy;
and to my parents, Murray and Beverly,
whose efforts set me on the path

—*A.G.R.*

To my wife, Kimberly,
for her love, support, and never-ending friendship;
to my wonderful children, Kristin, Bradley, and Steven,
for their strength, enthusiasm, and complexities;
to Dr. Jim Herndon for asking me to move to the
Massachusetts General Hospital in Boston;
and to Dr. Bill Harris for his years of mentoring

—*H.E.R.*

To my wife, Patricia;
our children, Lauren and Taylor;
and my parents, Gary and Elaine

—*P.T.S.*

To my wife, Catherine,
and children, Philip and Laura,
without whose support such endeavors
would be impossible

—*T.L.W.*

Contents

VOLUME I

SECTION I: HISTORICAL PERSPECTIVES

SECTION II: BASIC SCIENCE

Part A. Anatomy

Part B. Biomechanics

VOLUME II

SECTION VIII. PRIMARY TOTAL KNEE ARTHROPLASTY

SECTION IX. PERIOPERATIVE MANAGEMENT
IN TOTAL KNEE REPLACEMENT

SECTION X. COMPLICATIONS OF TOTAL KNEE REPLACEMENT

SECTION XI. REVISION TOTAL KNEE ARTHROPLASTY

Part A. Management of the Infected Total Knee Replacement

SECTION XII. FUTURE PERSPECTIVES

Contributing Authors

Amy E. Abbot, M.D., M.S.
Postdoctoral Residency Fellow
Orthopaedic Research Laboratory
Columbia University College of Physicians
*   and Surgeons*
New York Orthopaedic Hospital
New York, New York

Steven P. Arnoczky, D.V.M.
Director and Professor
Laboratory for Comparative Orthopaedic Research
Michigan State University
East Lansing, Michigan

Karen Atkinson, M.D., M.P.H.
Instructor in Medicine
Department of Medicine/Rheumatology
Massachusetts General Hospital
Boston, Massachusetts

David C. Ayers, M.D.
Associate Professor of Orthopaedic Surgery
Director of Joint Replacement Surgery
Department of Orthopaedic Surgery
State University of New York Upstate Medical
*   University*
Syracuse, New York

Bernard R. Bach, Jr., M.D.
Professor of Orthopedic Surgery
Department of Orthopedic Surgery
Rush Medical College of Rush University
Director, Sports Medicine Section
Rush-Presbyterian-St. Luke's Medical Center
Chicago, Illinois

Janet Baker, M.D.
Assistant Professor
Department of Orthopaedics and Rehabilitation
University of Miami School of Medicine
Miami, Florida

Robert L. Barrack, M.D.
Professor of Orthopaedic Surgery
Tulane University School of Medicine
New Orleans, Louisiana

Gene R. Barrett, M.D.
Mississippi Sports Medicine and Orthopaedic Center
Jackson, Mississippi

Richard A. Berger, M.D.
Midwest Orthopedics
Chicago, Illinois

John A. Bergfeld, M.D.
Director
Department of Orthopaedic Surgery
Cleveland Clinic Sports Health
The Cleveland Clinic Foundation
Cleveland, Ohio

Daniel J. Berry, M.D.
Professor of Orthopedics
Department of Orthopedic Surgery
Mayo Clinic
Rochester, Minnesota

Robert E. Booth, Jr., M.D.
Clinical Professor of Orthopaedic Surgery
University of Pennsylvania School of Medicine
Philadelphia, Pennsylvania

Mathias P. G. Bostrom, M.D.
Associate Professor
Department of Orthopaedic Surgery
Weill Medical College of Cornell University
New York, New York

Gino Bradica, B.S.
Doctoral Candidate in Biomedical Engineering
Department of Pathology and Laboratory
*   Medicine*
University of Medicine and Dentistry of New Jersey
*   Robert Wood Johnson Medical School*
Piscataway, New Jersey

Barry D. Brause, M.D.
Clinical Professor of Medicine
Weill Medical College of Cornell University
New York Presbyterian Hospital
Hospital for Special Surgery
New York, New York

Calvin R. Brown, Jr., M.D.
Associate Professor of Medicine
Section of Rheumatology
Rush Medical College of Rush University
Chicago, Illinois

Charles H. Brown, Jr., M.D.
Clinical Instructor of Orthopaedic Surgery
Harvard Medical School
Brigham and Women's Hospital
Boston, Massachusetts

Joseph A. Buckwalter, M.S., M.D.
Professor of Orthopaedics
Department of Orthopaedic Surgery
University of Iowa Hospitals
Iowa City, Iowa

Frederick F. Buechel, M.D.
Clinical Professor of Orthopaedic Surgery
Department of Orthopaedics
New Jersey Medical School
University of Medicine and Dentistry of New Jersey
Newark, New Jersey

Bennett S. Burns, M.D.
Private Practice
New England Orthopaedic Surgeons
Springfield, Massachusetts

E. Lyle Cain, Jr., M.D.
Clinical Instructor
American Sports Medicine Institute
Birmingham, Alabama

John J. Callaghan, M.D.
Lawrence and Marilyn Dorr Chair and Professor
Department of Orthopaedics and Bioengineering
University of Iowa College of Medicine
Iowa City, Iowa

Arnold I. Caplan, Ph.D.
Professor of Biology
Case Western Reserve University
Cleveland, Ohio

Creg A. Carpenter, M.D.
Major
Department of Orthopedic Surgery
United States Air Force Medical Corps
Wilford Hall Medical Center
Lackland AFB, Texas

Eric W. Carson, M.D.
Clinical Instructor
Emory University School of Medicine
Atlanta, Georgia

Thomas R. Carter, M.D.
Head of Orthopedic Surgery
Arizona State University Medical Center
Tempe, Arizona

John T. Cavanaugh, M.Ed., P.T., A.T.C.
Senior Physical Therapist
Department of Rehabilitation
Sports Medicine Center
Hospital for Special Surgery
New York, New York

William G. Clancy, Jr., M.D.
Orthopaedic Surgeon
Alabama Sports Medicine and Orthopaedic Center
Fellowship Director
American Sports Medicine Institute
Birmingham, Alabama

Mark Clatworthy, F.R.A.C.S.
Consultant Orthopaedic Surgeon
Department of Orthopaedics
Middlemore Hospital
Auckland, New Zealand

Brian J. Cole, M.D., M.B.A.
Associate Professor of Orthopedic Surgery
Department of Orthopedic Surgery
Rush-Presbyterian-St. Luke's Medical Center
Chicago, Illinois

Struan H. Coleman, M.D., Ph.D.
Assistant Attending of Orthopedic Surgery
Department of Orthopedics
Hospital for Special Surgery
New York, New York

William W. Colman, M.D.
Attending Physician
Department of Orthopedics
California Pacific Medical Center
San Francisco, California

T. Derek V. Cooke, M.A., M.B., B.Chir., F.R.C.S.(C.)
Professor of Surgery and Rehabilitation
Queen's University Faculty of Medicine
Kingston, Ontario, Canada
Department of Orthopedics
Sulaiman Al-Habib Medical Centre
Riyadh, Saudi Arabia

Daniel E. Cooper, M.D.
Department of Orthopaedics
W. B. Carrell Memorial Clinic
Dallas, Texas

James A. Cooper, Jr., M.S.
Graduate Fellow
Department of Chemical Engineering
Drexel University
Philadelphia, Pennyslvania

Henry R. Cowell, M.D., Ph.D.
Lecturer
Department of Orthopaedic Surgery
Harvard Medical School
Boston, Massachusetts

Fred D. Cushner, M.D.
Assistant Clinical Professor
Department of Surgery
Division of Orthopaedic Surgery
Albert Einstein College of Medicine of Yeshiva
*   University*
Beth Israel Medical Center
New York, New York

Craig J. Della Valle, M.D.
Assistant Professor
Department of Orthopedic Surgery
Rush-Presbyterian-St. Luke's Medical
*   Center*
Chicago, Illinois

Douglas A. Dennis, M.D.
Director of Clinical Research
Rocky Mountain Musculoskeletal Research
*   Laboratory*
Denver, Colorado

Regina F. Doherty, M.S., O.T.R./L.
Clinical Specialist
Department of Occupational Therapy
Massachusetts General Hospital
Boston, Massachusetts

Lawrence D. Dorr, M.D.
Arthritis Institute
Centinela Hospital Medical Center
Inglewood, California

Mark C. Drakos, B.A.
Department of Sports Medicine
Hospital for Special Surgery
New York, New York

Clive P. Duncan, M.D., F.R.C.S.C.
Professor and Chairman
Department of Orthopaedics
University of British Columbia Faculty of
*   Medicine*
Vancouver, British Columbia, Canada

Gerard A. Engh, M.D.
Director of Knee Research
Anderson Orthopaedic Research Institute
Inova Health Systems
Alexandria, Virginia

Jill A. Erickson, B.S., PA-C
Physician Assistant
Department of Orthopedics
University of Utah Medical Center
Salt Lake City, Utah

John David Evanich, M.D.
Total Joint Fellow
Department of Orthopedic Surgery
University of Utah
Salt Lake City, Utah

Deborah A. Faryniarz, B.S.
Previous Sports and Shoulder Fellow
Department of Sports Medicine and Shoulder Service
Hospital for Special Surgery
New York, New York

Stephen Fealy, M.D.
Assistant Attending Orthopedic Surgeon
Department of Sports Medicine and Shoulder Service
Hospital for Special Surgery
New York, New York

Anthony B. Fiorillo, M.D.
Assistant Professor of Clinical Medicine
Department of Internal Medicine
University of Pittsburgh School of Medicine
Pittsburgh, Pennsylvania

Rebecca Fishbein, P.T., O.C.S.
Outpatient Clinical Service Coordinator
Massachusetts General Hospital Physical Therapy
*   Services*
Massachusetts General Hospital
Boston, Massachusetts

Andrew A. Freiberg, M.D.
Arthroplasty Service Chief
Department of Orthopaedic Surgery
Massachusetts General Hospital
Boston, Massachusetts

Jorge O. Galante, M.D., D.M.Sc.
Professor of Orthopedic Surgery
Rush Medical College of Rush University
Chicago, Illinois

Timothy M. Ganey, Ph.D.
Tampa, Florida

Donald S. Garbuz, M.D., M.H.Sc., F.R.C.S.C.
Assistant Professor
Department of Orthopaedics
University of British Columbia Faculty of
*   Medicine*
Vancouver, British Columbia, Canada

Kevin L. Garvin, M.D.
Professor and Chair
Department of Orthopaedic Surgery and
*   Rehabilitation*
University of Nebraska Medical Center
Omaha, Nebraska

J. Robert Giffin, M.D., F.R.C.S.C.
Assistant Professor
Department of Surgery
Fowler Kennedy Sports Medicine Clinic
London Health Sciences Centre
University of Western Ontario
University Hospital
London, Ontario, Canada

Thomas J. Gill, M.D.
Assistant Professor
Department of Orthopaedic Surgery
Harvard Medical School
Massachusetts General Hospital
Boston, Massachusetts

Scott D. Gillogly, M.D.
Atlanta Sports Medicine and Orthopaedic
*   Center*
Atlanta, Georgia

Victor M. Goldberg, M.D.
Professor
Department of Orthopaedics
Case Western Reserve University
University Hospital
Cleveland, Ohio

Nelson V. Greidanus, M.D., M.P.H., F.R.C.S.C.
Assistant Professor
Department of Orthopaedic Surgery
University of British Columbia Faculty of
*   Medicine*
Vancouver, British Columbia, Canada

Ronald P. Grelsamer, M.D.
Chief of Hip and Knee Surgery
Orthopaedic Surgery
Maimonides Medical Center
Staff Orthopaedic Surgeon
Hospital for Joint Disease
New York, New York

Allan E. Gross, M.D., F.R.C.S.C.
Professor of Surgery
Department of Orthopaedic Surgery
University of Toronto Faculty of Medicine
Mount Sinai Hospital
Toronto, Ontario, Canada

Brian D. Haas, M.D.
Director of Clinical Research
Rocky Mountain Musculoskeletal Research
*   Laboratory*
Denver, Colorado

Scott A. Hacker, M.S., M.D.
Orthopaedic Fellow
Steadman Hawkins Clinic
Vail, Colorado

Nadim James Hallab, Ph.D., M.S.
Assistant Professor
Department of Orthopedic Surgery
Rush-Presbyterian-St. Luke's Medical
*   Center*
Chicago, Illinois

Timothy S. Hamby, M.D.
Fellow, Sports Medicine
Department of Orthopaedic Surgery
Atlanta Sports Medicine and Orthopaedic
*   Center*
Atlanta, Georgia

Arlen D. Hanssen, M.D.
Professor of Orthopedics
Mayo Clinic
Mayo Foundation
Rochester, Minnesota

Christopher D. Harner, M.D.
Professor
Department of Orthopedic Surgery
Center for Sports Medicine
University of Pittsburgh Medical Center
Pittsburgh, Pennsylvania

John H. Healey, M.D.
Professor
Department of Orthopaedic Surgery
Weill Medical College of Cornell
*   University*
Chief of Orthopedic Surgery
Memorial Sloan-Kettering Cancer Center
New York, New York

William L. Healy, M.D.
Professor of Orthopaedic Surgery
Boston University School of Medicine
Boston, Massachusetts
Chairman
Department of Orthopaedic Surgery
Lahey Clinic
Burlington, Massachusetts

Kevin T. Heaton, D.O.
Orthopedic Surgeon
Merle West Medical Center
Klamath Falls, Oregon

Diane M. Heislein, P.T., M.S., O.C.S.
Clinical Specialist
Department of Physical Therapy
Massachusetts General Hospital
Boston, Massachusetts

Laurence D. Higgins, M.D.
Assistant Professor of Surgery
Department of Surgery
Division of Orthopaedics
Duke University Medical Center
Durham, North Carolina

Daniel P. Hoeffel, M.D.
Orthopedic Surgeon
Summit Orthopedics, Ltd.
St. Paul, Minnesota

Aaron A. Hofmann, M.D.
Professor of Orthopedic Surgery
University of Utah School of Medicine
Salt Lake City, Utah

Douglas S. Holden, M.D.
Fellow, Adult Reconstruction, 2001
Lenox Hill Hospital
New York, New York

Timothy R. Hooper, M.D.
Radiology Fellow
Department of Radiology and Imaging
Hospital for Special Surgery
New York, New York

William J. Hozack, M.D.
Professor of Orthopaedic Surgery
Director of the Adult Reconstruction Service
Director of Clinical Research
Department of Orthopaedics
Rothman Institute
Jefferson Medical College of Thomas Jefferson
  University
Thomas Jefferson University Hospital
Philadelphia, Pennsylvania

Richard Iorio, M.D.
Assistant Professor of Orthopaedic Surgery
Boston University School of Medicine
Boston, Massachusetts
Lahey Clinic Medical Center
Burlington, Massachusetts

Douglas W. Jackson, M.D.
Orthopaedic Research Institute
Memorial Medical Center
Southern California Center for Sports
  Medicine
Long Beach, California

Joshua J. Jacobs, M.D.
Crown Family Professor
Department of Orthopedic Surgery
Rush Medical College at Rush University
Chicago, Illinois

Amir A. Jamali, M.D.
Attending Surgeon
Department of Orthopaedic Surgery
Palo Alto Veterans Administration Hospital
Palo Alto, California

Sanjiv Jari, B.Sc., M.B.Ch.B., F.R.C.S.(Eng.),
  F.R.C.S.(Tr. and Orth.)
Consultant Lower Limb
Orthopaedic Sports Medicine Surgeon
Department of Orthopaedic and Trauma
  Surgery
University of Manchester
Hope Hospital
Manchester, England, United Kingdom

Don H. Johnson, M.D., F.R.C.S.(C.)
Clinical Associate Professor of Orthopaedic
  Surgery
Department of Orthopaedic Surgery
University of Ottawa Faculty of Medicine
Ottawa, Ontario, Canada

Brian M. Katt, M.D.
Orthopaedic Resident
Department of Orthopaedic Surgery
University of Medicine and Dentistry of New Jersey
  Robert Wood Johnson Medical School
New Brunswick, New Jersey

Edward Michael Keating, M.D.
Orthopaedic Surgeon
Center for Hip and Knee Surgery
St. Francis-Mooresville Hospital
Mooresville, Indiana

Michael A. Kelly, M.D.
Director
Department of Orthopaedic Surgery
Insall Scott Kelly Institute for Orthopaedics and
    Sports Medicine
Singer Division
Beth Israel Hospital
New York, New York

J. G. Kennedy, M.D.
Memorial Sloan-Kettering Cancer Center
New York, New York

Axel R. W. Kentsch, M.D.
Facharzt Orthopaedie, Consultant
Department of Orthopaedics
Praxisklinik 2000
Freiburg, Germany

Imran A. Khan, M.D.
Resident in Orthopaedic Surgery
Department of Orthopaedics
McLaren Regional Medical Center
Flint, Michigan

Masashi Kobayashi, M.D.
Orthopaedic Surgeon
Department of Orthopaedic Surgery
Kyoto Prefectural University of Medicine
Kyoto, Japan

Richard D. Komistek, Ph.D.
President and Executive Director
Rocky Mountain Musculoskeletal Research
    Laboratory
Denver, Colorado

Paul F. Lachiewicz, M.D.
Professor of Orthopaedics
Department of Orthopaedics
University of North Carolina at Chapel Hill
Chapel Hill, North Carolina

Roger V. Larson, M.D.
Associate Professor of Orthopaedics and
    Sports Medicine
Department of Orthopaedics
University of Washington School of Medicine
Seattle, Washington

Richard S. Laskin, M.D.
Professor of Orthopaedic Surgery
Weill Medical College of Cornell University
Hospital for Special Surgery
New York, New York

Cato T. Laurencin, M.D., Ph.D.
Clinical Professor of Orthopaedic Surgery
Helen I. Moorehead Distinguished Professor of
    Orthopaedic Surgery
Department of Orthopaedic Surgery and Chemical
    Engineering
Drexel University College of Medicine
Philadelphia, Pennsylvania

Michael A. Lehmicke, B.S.M.E.
Student
Department of Biochemical Engineering
Drexel University
Philadelphia, Pennsylvania

Seth S. Leopold, M.D.
Associate Professor
Department of Orthopaedic Surgery and Sports
    Medicine
University of Washington Medical Center
Seattle, Washington

William N. Levine, M.D.
Assistant Professor
Department of Orthopedic Surgery
Columbia University College of Physicians and
    Surgeons
New York, New York

David G. Lewallen, M.D.
Professor of Orthopedic Surgery
Mayo Medical School
Chair, Division of Adult Reconstructive Surgery
Department of Orthopedic Surgery
Mayo Clinic
Rochester, Minnesota

Guoan Li, Ph.D.
Assistant Professor of Orthopaedic Surgery and
    Bioengineering
Harvard Medical School
Massachusetts General Hospital
Boston, Massachusetts

Jay R. Lieberman, M.D.
Department of Orthopaedic Surgery
University of California, Los Angeles,
    UCLA School of Medicine
Los Angeles, California

Jianhao Lin, M.D.
Assistant Professor of Orthopaedic Surgery
Department of Orthopaedic Surgery
People's Hospital, Peking University
Beijing, People's Republic of China

Adolph V. Lombardi, Jr., M.D., F.A.C.S.
Clinical Assistant Professor
Department of Orthopaedic Surgery
Department of Biomedical Engineering
Ohio State University
Columbus, Ohio

Jess H. Lonner, M.D.
Attending Orthopaedic Surgeon
Department of Orthopaedic Surgery
Pennsylvania Hospital
Philadelphia, Pennsylvania

Paul A. Lotke, M.D.
Professor of Orthopaedic Surgery
Hospital of the University of Pennsylvania
Philadelphia, Pennsylvania

Martin J. Luber, M.D.
New England Orthopaedic Surgeons Inc.
Springfield, Massachusetts

C. Benjamin Ma, M.D.
Clinical Instructor
Department of Orthopedic Surgery
Center for Sports Medicine
University of Pittsburgh Medical Center
Pittsburgh, Pennsylvania

Mohamed Mahfouz, Ph.D.
Director of Biomedical Imaging Research
Rocky Mountain Musculoskeletal Research
Laboratory
Denver, Colorado

Marc I. Malberg, M.D.
Associate Clinical Professor
Department of Orthopaedics
University of Medicine and Dentistry of New Jersey
Robert Wood Johnson Medical School
University of Medicine and Dentistry of New Jersey
University Hospital
Somerset, New Jersey

Michel Malo, M.D., F.R.C.S.(C.)
Clinical Instructor
Department of Orthopaedic Surgery
University of Montreal, Sacre-Coeur Hospital
Montreal, Quebec, Canada

William J. Maloney, M.D.
Professor of Orthopaedic Surgery
Washington University School of Medicine
St. Louis, Missouri

Henry J. Mankin, M.D.
Edith M. Ashley Distinguished Professor of
Orthopaedic Surgery
Department of Orthopaedic Service
Harvard Medical School
Massachusetts General Hospital
Boston, Massachusetts

Robert G. Marx, M.D., M.Sc., F.R.C.S.(C.)
Assistant Professor of Orthopaedic Surgery
Assistant Professor of Public Health
Weill Medical College of Cornell University
Director of Center for Clinical Outcome Research
Orthopedic Director, The Sports Medicine Institute
for Young Athletes
Assistant Attending Orthopedic Surgeon
Hospital for Special Surgery
New York, New York

Bassam A. Masri, M.D.
Associate Professor of Orthopaedics and Head
Division of Lower Limb Reconstruction
University of British Columbia Faculty of Medicine
Vancouver, British Columbia, Canada

Craig S. Mauro, M.S.
Department of Orthopaedic Surgery
University of Pittsburgh School of Medicine
Pittsburgh, Pennsylvania

M. Gavan McAlinden, B.Sc., Mphil., F.R.C.S.
(Tr. and Orth.)
Consultant in Orthopaedic Surgery
The Ulster Hospital
Belfast, United Kingdom

James P. McAuley, M.D., F.R.C.S.C.
Director of Postgraduate Education
Staff Surgeon
Anderson Orthopaedic Research Institute
Anderson Orthopaedic Clinic
Alexandria, Virginia

John B. Meding, M.D.
Orthopaedic Surgeon
Center for Hip and Knee Surgery
Mooresville, Indiana

Michael H. Metcalf, M.D.
Orthopaedic Specialty Hospital
Salt Lake City, Utah

Jefferey E. Michaelson, M.D.
Clinical Assistant Professor of Orthopaedic Surgery
Director of Orthopaedic Sports Medicine
Wayne State University School of Medicine
Providence Hospital
Detroit, Michigan

Peter J. Millett, M.D., M.Sc.
Clinical Instructor
Department of Orthopaedic Surgery
Harvard Medical School
Brigham and Women's Hospital
Massachusetts General Hospital
Boston, Massachusetts

M. Shannon Moore, M.D., M.P.H.
Orthopaedic Surgeon
Cascade Orthopaedics
Auburn, Washington

Van C. Mow, Ph.D.
Stanley Dicker Professor of Biomedical
  Engineering
Chairman, Department of Biomedical Engineering
Columbia University
New York, New York

Werner Müller, M.D.
Professor of Medicine
Department of Orthopedic Surgery
Kantonsspital Bruderholz
Riehen, Switzerland

Orhun K. Muratoglu, Ph.D.
Alan Gerry Scholar
Assistant Professor
Orthopaedic Surgery
Harvard Medical School
Massachusetts General Hospital
Boston, Massachusetts

David G. Nazarian, M.D.
Clinical Assistant Professor of Orthopaedic
  Surgery
University of Pennsylvania Health System
Philadelphia, Pennsylvania

Mayo A. Noerdlinger, M.D.
Department of Orthopaedics
Portsmouth Regional Hospital
Portsmouth, New Hampshire

Stephen J. O'Brien, M.D.
Department of Sports Medicine
Hospital for Special Surgery
New York, New York

Mary I. O'Connor, M.D.
Associate Professor of Orthopedics
Mayo Medical School
Rochester, Minnesota

John A. Ogden, M.D.
Clinical Professor of Orthopaedics
Department of Orthopaedics
Emory University School of Medicine
Atlanta Medical Center
Atlanta, Georgia

James A. Oliverio, M.D.
Major, United States Army Medical Corps
Chief, Orthopaedic Surgery Service
Ireland Army Community Hospital
Fort Knox, Kentucky

Michael R. O'Rourke, M.D.
Department of Orthopaedics
University of Iowa College of Medicine
Iowa City, Iowa

Mark W. Pagnano, M.D.
Assistant Professor of Orthopedic Surgery
Department of Orthopedics
Mayo Clinic
Rochester, Minnesota

Wayne G. Paprosky, M.D.
Associate Professor of Orthopedic Surgery
Rush Orthopedic Institute
Rush-Presbyterian-St. Luke's Medical Center
Chicago, Illinois

David A. Parker, M.B.B.S., F.R.A.C.S.
Orthopaedic Department
University Hospital
London Health Sciences Centre
London, Ontario, Canada

Christopher L. Peters, M.D.
Associate Professor of Orthopedics
University of Utah School of Medicine
Salt Lake City, Utah

Paul Pollice, M.D.
Adult Reconstructive Surgeon
Orthopaedic Associates of Allentown
Lehigh Valley Hospital and Health Network
Allentown, Pennsylvania

Hollis G. Potter, M.D.
Associate Professor of Radiology
Department of Radiology and Imaging
Hospital for Special Surgery
New York, New York

Ari Pressman, M.D.
Sports Medicine Clinic
Carleton University
Ottawa, Ontario, Canada

Amar S. Ranawat, M.D.
Associate, Ranawat Orthopedic Center
Adjunct Attending
Department of Orthopedic Surgery
Lenox Hill Hospital
New York, New York

Chitranjan S. Ranawat, M.D.
Professor of Orthopaedic Surgery
Weill Medical College of Cornell University
Director, Ranawat Orthopedic Center
Chairman, Department of Orthopedic Surgery
Lenox Hill Hospital
New York, New York

Vijay J. Rasquinha, M.D.
Director of Research
Ranawat Orthopedic Center
Adjunct Attending
Department of Orthopedic Surgery
Lenox Hill Hospital
New York, New York

Anthony M. Reginato, M.D., Ph.D.
Physician
Department of Medicine
Massachusetts General Hospital
Boston, Massachusetts

Lars C. Richardson, M.D.
Instructor
Department of Orthopaedics
Harvard Medical School
Beth Israel Deaconess Medical Center
Boston, Massachusetts

Michael D. Ries, M.D.
Professor of Orthopaedic Surgery
University of California, San Francisco,
*   School of Medicine*
San Francisco, California

Scott A. Rodeo, M.D.
Associate Professor of Orthopedic Surgery
Department of Orthopedic Surgery
Hospital for Special Surgery
New York, New York

David J. Rodricks, M.D.
Chief Resident
Department of Orthopaedic Surgery
University of Medicine and Dentistry of New Jersey
*   Robert Wood Johnson Medical School*
New Brunswick, New Jersey

Joel T. Rohrbough, M.D.
Orthopaedic Surgeon
Summit Center for Orthopaedics and
*   Rehabilitation*
Flagstaff, Arizona

Cecil H. Rorabeck, M.D., F.R.C.S.C.
Professor of Surgery
Division of Orthopaedic Surgery
London Health Sciences Centre
University Hospital
London, Ontario, Canada

Aaron G. Rosenberg, M.D.
Professor of Surgery
Rush Medical College of Rush University
Chicago, Illinois

Andrew E. Rosenberg, M.D.
Associate Professor of Pathology
Harvard Medical School
Massachusetts General Hospital
Boston, Massachusetts

Harry E. Rubash, M.D.
Edith M. Ashley Professor of Orthopaedic Surgery
Harvard Medical School
Chief, Department of Orthopaedic Surgery
Massachusetts General Hospital
Boston, Massachusetts

Thomas A. St. John, M.D.
Orthopaedic Surgeon
Aspen Valley Hospital
Aspen, Colorado

Pamela M. Sanchez, B.S.
Research Assistant
Hospital for Special Surgery
New York, New York

Lisa M. Sasso, B.S.
Research Assistant
Department of Orthopedic Surgery
Rush-Presbyterian-St. Luke's Medical Center
Chicago, Illinois

Thomas P. Schmalzried, M.D.
Associate Director
Joint Replacement Institute
Orthopaedic Hospital
Los Angeles, California

Steven L. Schule, M.D.
Private Practice
Community Memorial Hospital
Ventura, California

Allan Scudamore, M.A., Ph.D.
Research Scientist
Department of Orthopaedic Surgery
King Faisal Specialist Hospital
Riyadh, Saudi Arabia

Thomas P. Sculco, M.D.
Professor of Orthopedic Surgery
Hospital for Special Surgery
New York, New York

Jon K. Sekiya, M.D.
Sports Medicine and Shoulder Fellow
Center for Sports Medicine
University of Pittsburgh Medical Center
Pittsburgh, Pennsylvania

Todd D. Sekundiak, M.D.
St. Boniface Hospital
Winnipeg, Manitoba, Canada

Robert A. Sellards, M.D.
Assistant Professor of Orthopaedic Surgery
Department of Orthopaedics
Louisiana State University School of Medicine in
*   New Orleans*
New Orleans, Louisiana

Peter F. Sharkey, M.D.
Associate Professor
Department of Orthopaedic Surgery
Jefferson Medical College of Thomas
*   Jefferson University*
Philadelphia, Pennsylvania

K. Donald Shelbourne, M.D.
Associate Professor
Department of Orthopaedic Surgery
Indiana University School of Medicine
Indianapolis, Indiana

Mauricio Silva, M.D.
Research Fellow
Joint Replacement Institute
Orthopaedic Hospital—UCLA
Los Angeles, California

Frederick H. Silver, Ph.D.
Chief of Division of Biomaterials
Professor of Pathology and Laboratory Medicine
Department of Pathology and Laboratory Medicine
University of Medicine and Dentistry of New Jersey
*   Robert Wood Johnson Medical School*
Piscataway, New Jersey

Craig D. Silverton, D.O.
Associate Professor of Orthopedics
Department of Orthopedic Surgery
Rush Medical College of Rush University
Chicago, Illinois

Timothy M. Simon, Ph.D.
Orthopaedic Research Institute
Memorial Medical Center
Southern California Center for Sports Medicine
Long Beach, California

Peter T. Simonian, M.D.
Clinical Professor
Department of Orthopaedic Surgery
University of California, San Francisco,
*   School of Medicine*
Fresno, California

William F. Sims, M.D.
Department of Orthopaedic Surgery
University of Washington School of Medicine
Seattle, Washington

Raj K. Sinha, M.D., Ph.D.
Assistant Professor
Department of Orthopaedic Surgery
University of Pittsburgh Medical Center
Pittsburgh, Pennsylvania

Carolyn M. Sofka, M.D.
Assistant Professor of Radiology
Department of Radiology and Imaging
Hospital for Special Surgery
New York, New York

Francis X. Solano, Jr., M.D.
Clinical Professor of Medicine
University of Pittsburgh School of Medicine
Pittsburgh, Pennsylvania

Luis A. Solchaga, Ph.D.
Instructor
Department of Orthopaedics
Case Western Reserve University School of
*   Medicine*
University Hospitals of Cleveland
Cleveland, Ohio

J. Richard Steadman, M.D.
Steadman Hawkins Clinic
Vail, Colorado

James B. Stiehl, M.D.
Clinical Professor of Orthopaedic Surgery
Medical College of Wisconsin
Columbia Hospital
Milwaukee, Wisconsin

Michael G. Sullivan, D.P.T., M.B.A.
Director
Department of Physical and Occupational
*   Therapy*
Massachusetts General Hospital
Boston, Massachusetts

Dale R. Sumner, Ph.D.
Professor and Chair
Department of Anatomy and Cell Biology
Rush Medical College of Rush University
Rush-Presbyterian-St. Luke's Medical Center
Chicago, Illinois

Jonathan W. Surdam, M.D.
Department of Orthopaedics
Lahey Clinic
Burlington, Massachussets

Kyle C. Swanson, M.D.
Orthopaedic Surgeon
Orthopaedic and Fracture Clinic Practice
Mankato, Minnesota

Shinro Takai, M.D., Ph.D.
Assistant Professor of Orthopaedics
Chief of Knee Service
Department of Orthopaedic Surgery
Kyoto Prefectural University of Medicine
Kyoto, Japan

Allan F. Tencer, Ph.D.
Professor
Orthopaedic Science Laboratory
Department of Orthopaedic Surgery
and Sports Medicine
University of Washington School of Medicine
Harborview Medical Center
Seattle, Washington

Kevin M. Terefenko, M.D.
Staff Surgeon
Department of Orthopaedic Surgery
Reading Hospital and Medical Center
West Reading, Pennsylvania

Peter J. Thadani, M.D.
Associate Orthopaedic Surgeon
Kerlan-Jobe Orthopaedic Clinic
Los Angeles, California

Thomas S. Thornhill, M.D.
John B. and Buckminster Brown Professor of
Orthopaedic Surgery
Harvard Medical School
Brigham and Women's Hospital
Boston, Massachusetts

Craig D. Tifford, M.D.
Plancher Orthopaedic and Rehabilitation Associates
Stamford, Connecticut

Scott A. Timmermann, M.D., B.Sc.H.K., B.Ed.,
F.R.C.S.C.
Orthopaedic Surgeon
Department of Surgery
University of Calgary Faculty of Medicine
Calgary, Alberta, Canada

Edwin M. Tingstad, M.D.
Clinical Instructor
Department of Orthopaedics and Sports Medicine
University of Washington School of Medicine
Seattle, Washington

Alison P. Toth, M.D.
Assistant Professor of Orthopaedic Surgery
Department of Surgery
Duke University Medical Center
Durham, North Carolina

Alfred J. Tria, Jr., M.D.
Clinical Professor of Orthopaedic Surgery
Department of Orthopaedic Surgery
University of Medicine and Dentistry of New Jersey
Robert Wood Johnson Medical School
Somerset, New Jersey

Robert T. Trousdale, M.D.
Associate Professor of Orthopedic Surgery
Mayo Graduate School of Medicine
Mayo Clinic
Rochester, Minnesota

Harry Tsigaras, M.D., M.S., F.R.A.C.S.
Adult Reconstruction/Arthroplasty Fellow
Department of Orthopaedic Surgery
London Health Sciences Centre
London, Ontario, Canada

Joshua A. Urban, M.D.
Chief Resident
Department of Orthopaedic Surgery and
Rehabilitation
University of Nebraska Medical Center
Omaha, Nebraska

William F. Urmey, M.D.
Assistant Professor of Clinical Anesthesiology
Weill Medical College of Cornell University
Hospital for Special Surgery
New York, New York

Richard L. Vera, M.D.
Attending/Medical Director
Department of Anesthesiology and Pain Management
Baylor Center for Pain Management
Baylor University Medical Center
Dallas, Texas

Kelly G. Vince, M.D.
Associate Professor
Department of Orthopaedic Surgery—Arthritis
University of Southern California
USC University Hospital
Los Angeles, California

David A. Vittetoe, M.D.
Des Moines Orthopaedic Surgeons
Des Moines, Iowa

Tracy M. Vogrin, M.S.
Medical Student
Department of Orthopaedic Surgery
Center for Sports Medicine
University of Pittsburgh School of Medicine
Pittsburgh, Pennsylvania

Paul D. Warren, M.D.
Orthopaedic Associates of Virginia
Norfolk, Virginia

Russell F. Warren, M.D.
Professor of Orthopaedic Surgery
Department of Orthopaedics
Weill Medical College of Cornell
University
New York, New York

Ray C. Wasielewski, M.S., M.D.
Clinical Associate Professor of Orthopaedic
Surgery
Director of Joint Reconstructive Surgery
Ohio State University College of Medicine and
Public Health
Columbus, Ohio

Steven H. Weeden, M.D.
Texas Hip and Knee Center
Fort Worth, Texas

Craig H. Weinstein, M.D., M.P.H.
Department of Orthopaedic Surgery
Maimonides Medical Center
Brooklyn, New York

Jean F. Welter, M.D., M.Sc., Ph.D.
Assistant Professor of Orthopaedics
Case Western Reserve University School of
Medicine
Cleveland, Ohio

Geoffrey H. Westrich, M.D.
Assistant Professor of Orthopaedic Surgery
Assistant Attending Orthopaedic Surgeon
Weill Medical College of Cornell
University
Hospital for Special Surgery
New York, New York

Leo A. Whiteside, M.D.
Clinical Professor of Orthopaedic Surgery
Department of Orthopaedics
St. Louis University School of Medicine
St. Louis, Missouri

Thomas L. Wickiewicz, M.D.
Professor of Clinical Orthopaedic Surgery
Department of Orthopaedics
Weill Medical College of Cornell
University
Attending Orthopedic Surgeon and Chief
Department of Sports Medicine and Shoulder
Service
Hospital for Special Surgery
New York, New York

Riley J. Williams III, M.D.
Assistant Professor
Department of Orthopaedic Surgery
Weill Medical College of Cornell University
Attending Orthopedic Surgeon
Sports Medicine and Shoulder Service
Hospital for Special Surgery
New York, New York

Russell E. Windsor, M.D.
Professor of Orthopaedic Surgery
Weill Medical School of Cornell University
Co-Chief
The Knee Service
Hospital for Special Surgery
New York, New York

Edward M. Wojtys, M.D.
Professor of Surgery
Department of Orthopedic Surgery
University of Michigan Medical School
Ann Arbor, Michigan

John M. Wright, M.D.
New West Sports Medicine
Good Samaritan Hospital
Kearney, Nebraska

Timothy M. Wright, M.S., Ph.D.
Senior Scientist
Laboratory for Biomedical Mechanics and
Materials
Hospital for Special Surgery
New York, New York

Xu Yang, M.D.
Research Fellow
Orthopedic Research
Hospital for Special Surgery
New York, New York

Nobuyuki Yoshino, M.D., Ph.D.
Director, Department of Orthopaedic Surgery
Kyoto Kujo Hospital
Kyoto, Japan

Bertram Zarins, M.D.
Associate Clinical Professor
Department of Orthopaedic Surgery
Harvard Medical School
Massachusetts General Hospital
Boston, Massachusetts

Shay J. Zayontz, M.B., F.R.A.C.S.
Monash University
Cabrini Hospital
Malvern, Victoria, Australia

Foreword I

Our knowledge of knee functions and methods to repair injured tissues has expanded at an increasing rate. The editors of *The Adult Knee* are to be congratulated for successfully undertaking a daunting project that is comprehensive, well organized, and easily readable. The reader is taken through many of the basic science advances that have aided our treatment of soft tissue injuries, so frequent in sports, and developed a foundation for the operative management of knee pathology. The chapters progress from anatomy to mechanics to our future with cell biology and tissue engineering.

The discussions are well thought out and greatly aid the clinician in dealing with a wide range of problems. The editors selected an outstanding group of authors who were chosen because of their knowledge and understanding of the issues in this field. The chapters lead the reader through difficult problems and improve our care and patient selection. This book is a reference guide for those starting in this field, as well as for specialists with extensive experience. Our patients, in particular, will benefit greatly from this outstanding contribution.

Russell F. Warren, M.D.

Foreword II

The creation of a work of this magnitude is a daunting task. The user-friendly text is divided into 12 well-structured sections covering all aspects of the care and management of the adult knee patient. Of great import, however, is that *The Adult Knee* represents the state-of-the-art of a growing body of knowledge assembled by the leading scientists and surgeons of our day.

I would like to acknowledge:

First, our nonorthopedic colleagues—especially in the fields of basic science, kinematics, and radiology—whose input has, no doubt, greatly improved our understanding of the pathoanatomy of the adult knee.
Second, the editors, who must be congratulated for organizing such an esteemed list of contributors and co-contributors, representing the leading orthopedic knee surgeons of our time, and, perhaps, of times to come.

For its archival value, the reader should pay close attention to the first section on the history of total knee replacement. As for the future, with the recent market-driven interest in unicompartmental and unispacer knee replacement for younger patients, I strongly feel, as George Santayana so eloquently put it, "Those who cannot remember the past are condemned to repeat it."

I have often said, "The eyes only see what the mind knows," and, if you take this comprehensive text to heart, you will see farther and more clearly than most.

The editors and contributors should be proud of their accomplishment in having provided an outstanding compilation and reference for postgraduates and practicing orthopedic surgeons.

Chitranjan S. Ranawat, M.D.

Acknowledgments

My contributions to this book would not be possible without the help of my parents, who promoted intellectual curiosity and the search for truth; my teachers at the Hospital for Special Surgery, including John Insall, Chitranjan Ranawat, Allan Inglis, Thomas Sculco, and Russell Warren, who provided the foundation for my understanding of the adult knee; my friends in The Knee Society, who have pursued similar interests and taught me so much; my students, who have endured the dissemination of my understanding of the knee and who have stimulated many of the questions related to the knee that I have academically pursued over the years; and to my secretary, Lori Yoder, who keeps my professional life in order when I take on such endeavors.

Finally, a sincere acknowledgment to Jim Merritt and his staff at Lippincott Williams & Wilkins who handled every detail in the editing process and, most important, to the authors who have sacrificed their time and energy in the timely preparation of this text.

J.J.C.

The Adult Knee is the twin prodigy of *The Adult Hip*. In the formative stage of *The Adult Hip*, John Callaghan, Aaron Rosenberg, and I envisioned a complementary book—equally detailed, authoritative, and comprehensive—on the adult knee. After many years (and the addition of two outstanding editors), this robust project is finally finished! Many individuals have been instrumental in the development and completion of *The Adult Knee*: my 78-year-old mother, who is a recipient of two CCK total knee arthroplasties for bilateral fixed deformities and who is ambulating without pain, 1.5 in. taller, and in much better spirits; Dr. William H. Harris, my mentor in hip surgery, whose high standards of educational excellence, patient care, and thorough investigational techniques inspired me to pursue my research interests in the knee with the same vigor and enthusiasm as I have in the past with the hip; the late John Insall, whose wisdom and friendship helped to shape my research interest in the patellofemoral joint, the epicondylar axis in total knee arthroplasty, and high flexion after total knee arthroplasty; Edward Hanley, Jr., my friend, colleague, and confidante, who has always been able to help me through complex problems, especially those I have encountered in my new administrative position; my students, residents, and fellows both at the University of Pittsburgh and the Massachusetts General Hospital who have endured my passion for surgical technique, patient care, and pursuit of research studies; Mr. Jim Merritt and his staff at Lippincott Williams & Wilkins who have endured John, Aaron, and me throughout our periods of mania and lethargy; and, finally, but most important, the many authors and coauthors who contributed to this outstanding text.

H.E.R.

To each of the internationally renowned contributors to *The Adult Knee*, whose expertise and dedication made this book possible.

To my mentors, teachers, and colleagues at the University of Washington and the Hospital for Special Surgery.

P.T.S.

To those who have educated me in the past and to those who continue to do so in the present.

T.L.W.

Preface

In the past 30 years, orthopedic surgeons have seen tremendous technical, diagnostic, and philosophic changes that have had a tremendous impact on the practice of orthopedics. Recently, the knee has received more attention than any other single joint and, not surprisingly, has been the subject of numerous publications. However, until now, there has not been a comprehensive, balanced, reference text on the adult knee, an area that clearly is the core of many orthopedic surgeons' practice worldwide. In the planning of this book, we elected not to include fractures or pediatrics—areas that are well covered in other sources—so that we could provide in-depth coverage of *The Adult Knee*. Although comprehensive, we have stressed particularly the technical and practical information that is critical to today's orthopedic surgeon.

The Adult Knee is a complete source for orthopedic surgeons, fellows, and residents, as well as medical students, researchers, or anyone with an interest in knee surgery. The text is presented in two volumes with 12 sections covering all aspects of the adult knee. Volume I presents sections on Historical Perspectives, Basic Science, and Clinical Science, all of which are critical to accurate diagnosis and treatment of knee disorders. Also included in Volume I are sections on Soft Tissue Injury of the Knee, Osteochondral Injury to the Knee, Patella Femoral Disorders, and Alternatives to Arthroplasty for Knee Arthritis. Because of the importance of clear arthroscopic images, Volume I features almost 200 full-color images throughout the chapters. Volume II covers reconstruction of the knee, including sections on Primary Total Knee Arthroplasty, Perioperative Management in Total Knee Replacement, Complications of Total Knee Replacement, and Revision Total Knee Arthroplasty. The book closes with a section on Future Perspectives in this growing area.

A text of this magnitude may be judged best by the authors who have contributed to its creation. We are pleased and honored to have assembled today's leading experts in the field and are indebted to their excellent contributions. In the early stages of planning this book, we also believed it was important to invite a balanced group of writers from all over the world. The list of authors includes distinguished individuals from more than eight countries.

It is immensely satisfying as editors to accomplish the goals we set at the inception of this idea—to create a high-quality, authoritative text on the adult knee. We trust that *The Adult Knee* is an informative and helpful resource serving readers in the years to come.

J.J.C.
A.G.R.
H.E.R.
P.T.S.
T.L.W.

CHAPTER 70

Indications for Total Knee Arthroplasty

Craig J. Della Valle and Aaron G. Rosenberg

Total knee arthroplasty has revolutionized the treatment of patients with end-stage arthritis of the knee. Although early attempts at interpositional arthroplasty and resurfacing procedures routinely met with early failure, the advent of modern total knee surgery offers both surgeons and patients a reliable treatment for arthritis of the knee. When total knee arthroplasty is compared to other medical and surgical interventions for common diseases, the cost of quality-adjusted life-years associated with this procedure is nearly unparalleled (1).

Arthritis of the knee has been shown to be quite prevalent, with radiographic evidence of osteoarthritis in 27% of patients over the age of 70 years (2) and symptomatic osteoarthritis developing among 1% per year among 1,051 surviving subjects of the Framingham study with a mean age of 70 years (3). Furthermore, the natural history of osteoarthritis of the knee has been shown to be poor (4).

Long-term follow-up of total condylar knee arthroplasty has shown survivorship of 77% to 91% at a follow-up of more than 20 years (5,6). With further improvements in operative techniques, instrumentation, and prosthetic design combined with a better understanding of the mechanisms of failure of

total knee arthroplasty, surgical results continue to improve. Given the success of this procedure, surgeons have expanded the surgical indications for it. As with most procedures, appropriate surgical indications are critical to a successful surgical outcome.

Given the aging of the population that is expected to occur over the next several decades, the number of patients requiring treatment of arthritis of the knee will increase greatly, which makes an understanding of the appropriate indications for and limitations of total knee arthroplasty imperative for both orthopedic surgeons and primary care physicians.

INDICATIONS: DEFINING THE TERMS

The terms indications and contraindications, although carrying the ring of specificity, actually represent the end points of a complex decision-making process that must be carried out by the medical practitioner in conjunction with the patient. Any medical decision making requires consideration of the potential risks and benefits of a particular intervention. This type of risk-benefit calculation is relatively uncomplicated for many diagnostic interventions, but there is clearly more at stake in most therapeutic interventions, particularly surgical ones.

Although there is a burgeoning literature devoted to the thought processes and rationale involved in medical decision making, there is no consensus on the specific methods that are most appropriately used to determine when a specific intervention is indicated. Surgical decision making represents a fascinating and complex subset of these processes, commonly undertaken to determine whether or not active intervention and, more specifically, what type of intervention (as well as what timing of the intervention) is in the best interests of the patient. Wide regional variations noted in the rate of performance of multiple surgical techniques (including total joint replacement) demonstrate that "indications" are far from universally agreed on for many surgical procedures. Clearly the consequences of surgical intervention must be carefully evaluated by both the patient and the surgeon, and in more complex cases this may require the full range of the surgeon's analytical skills as well as the ability to communicate effectively with the patient.

Indications can be defined as those situations in which an individual patient will benefit from the intervention in such a way, and with sufficient likelihood, to warrant the specific risks involved in the intervention. Contraindications connote the opposite: the risks involved, or the likelihood of the intervention's failure to achieve the desired results, outweigh the expected benefit of the intervention. Determining whether or not a given procedure is indicated or contraindicated involves the careful evaluation of the patient's complaints, pathology, and overall health status; the weighing of multiple probabilities for various positive and adverse outcomes (many of which are at best based on less than adequate data); and finally arrival at some type of judgment as to whether the final balance of risks and benefits is appropriate for the individual patient under consideration. An important consideration in the performance of any elective surgical procedure is the relative risk of perioperative events that carry with them significant morbidity or mortality. Total knee arthroplasty as initially practiced, and before the risk of thromboembolic disease was well understood, carried with it a mortality risk from pulmonary embolism. Although this incidence has been substantially reduced, as have the initial rates of infection and other serious postsurgical morbidities, the surgeon contemplating elective surgical intervention must essentially compare the potential long-term benefits of pain reduction and improved function with the short-term risks of death and other complications that may potentially occur after surgery.

A simple example of a setting in which a trade-off must be evaluated is consideration of pharmacologic intervention for deep vein thrombosis prophylaxis, in which the benefits of thrombosis and embolism reduction may be accompanied by an increased risk of serious bleeding complications. This type of "apples and oranges" comparison of both short- and long-term risks and potential complications with the expected short- and long-term benefits of a specific intervention is common in reconstructive surgical practice and keeps much of surgical decision making in the realm of heuristic rather than algorithmic problem solving.

Various models of decision making have been evaluated to determine whether they represent a reasonable approximation of the way mature clinicians actually make clinical decisions.

Although none of these models has been found to completely represent the multiple ways in which clinicians think, one of the most widely accepted and useful methods of decision making is based on the theory of expected utility. Its use in decision making is called expected utility analysis. This technique requires the surgeon to list the potential benefits of any intervention and assign to each benefit both a probability for its occurrence and a specific numerical ranking for the expected utility or benefit of such an occurrence. Expected utility theory posits that the decision maker reaches a decision on the potential benefits of a given procedure by summing the products of the expected benefits (utility) and the probabilities of occurrence of those particular outcomes.

Summing these products of the various positive utilities, otherwise known as benefits (pain relief, independence in activities of daily living, return to employment, etc.) and their probabilities, and subtracting from this sum the products of the negative utilities (risks such as death, persistent pain, instability, nerve injury, etc.) and their probabilities leaves an expected utility value, which then may be compared to the utility value generated by other therapeutic choices. Rational decision making would lead the clinician and patient to choose the therapy with the greatest overall utility. This is, in effect, a risk-benefit analysis. An important assumption in this method is that utilities (or outcomes) can be expressed using a common scale. This has not been realistically accomplished for many orthopedic utilities. In business decision making, such utilities are mainly economic factors, and utilities can be compared in common terms such as dollars. Medical decision making, however, in which factors such as pain, various functional parameters, and the ubiquitous "quality of life" must be taken into account, are potentially more complex, and direct conversion to a standard utility rating may be much more difficult. Nonetheless, an approximation of this technique may be quite useful.

For any given procedure, each potential benefit of the procedure can be assigned a utility factor. These can then be listed, with each utility assigned a probability. One can then sum the products of each utility and its probability, which yields a number representing the expected benefit of a particular intervention. The number derived from a similar sum of risk rankings multiplied by their individual probabilities can then be subtracted from the number calculated for the potential benefits of the procedure. Thus, for a given procedure with potential benefits listed as 1, 2, 3, . . . , X, and risks 1, 2, 3, . . . , Y,

$$
\begin{aligned}
\text{Expected utility} = &[(\text{benefit utility 1} \times \text{probability of utility 1}) \\
&+ (\text{benefit utility 2} \times \text{probability of utility 2}) \ldots + (\text{benefit utility X} \times \text{probability of utility X})] \\
&- [(\text{risk utility 1} \times \text{probability of risk 1}) \\
&+ (\text{risk utility 2} \times \text{probability of risk 2}) \ldots + (\text{risk utility Y} \times \text{probability of risk Y})]
\end{aligned}
$$

The resulting value may then be compared to values generated from similar consideration of alternative procedures. Of course, most of the risk and benefit "utilities" are subjective at this time, and there are few hard data on the probabilities of their occurrence in specific unusual or complex settings; hence, the term *subjective utilities analysis* is generally used. Such analysis, however, even on an informal basis, can both assist the surgeon in the complex decision-making process and aid in communicating to the patient all of the potential risks and benefits involved in complex clinical settings with regard to specific interventions. To make such complex decisions, the surgeon not only must accurately assess multiple patient-related factors as noted earlier but must also adequately judge his or her own skill, experience, and resources with regard to any particular procedure.

As mentioned, many of the utilities in question are not associated with well-described or accurate probabilities, nor are clinicians likely to use statistical analytic methods to make specific decisions for individual patients. Nonetheless, these models do yield insight into the complex decision-making process that may occasionally be required in assessing the applicability of total knee arthroplasty in a given patient.

In part, this chapter attempts to review many of those issues facing the orthopedic surgeon and the patient when knee arthroplasty is contemplated. The potential number of factors to be considered in this type of decision is relatively large and makes up a challenging component of the surgical decision-making process. The remainder of this chapter reviews those factors that may be considered appropriate in determining whether knee arthroplasty surgery is or is not indicated.

UNDERLYING ASSUMPTIONS IN TOTAL KNEE ARTHROPLASTY

Although total knee arthroplasty is the operation of choice for severe arthritic knee disease in the vast majority of patients, it is clear that, in several settings, other options may be more appropriate. Decision making regarding total knee arthroplasty is dependent on many factors in addition to the underlying pathology, including the patient's age and activity demands. There are several factors (or assumptions) regarding knee arthroplasty as an interventional choice that must be kept in mind when evaluating an individual for knee replacement surgery.

The first assumption is that the arthroplasty is a time-limited operation. In general, service life can be tied to complications related to fixation longevity, wear, or material failure. Although multiple series demonstrate relatively high component survival with a variety of fixation methods and component designs, even in relatively young and presumably active patients, it is difficult to imagine a young adult with a normal life span outliving a total knee implant. Thus, age becomes an important factor in the decision to proceed with total knee arthroplasty. Assuming no excessive comorbidities, and the presence of symptoms due to knee joint pathology amenable to arthroplasty, older patients are actually better candidates for arthroplasty, in that the operation and implant will most likely outlive the patient. Younger individuals may well require multiple surgeries over their lifetimes, with increased risk and deteriorating function a potential concomitant of multiple surgeries. Ironically, the outstanding clinical result, relative ease of surgery, and normally relatively rapid rehabilitation make arthroplasty an attractive alternative even in patients for whom age and expected longevity would seem to place arthroplasty out of bounds.

It is difficult to say at what patient age a surgeon should strive to find reasonable alternatives to total knee arthroplasty. Yet, the pediatric and young adult patient clearly deserve an attempt at alternative treatment, such as osteotomy or cartilage restoration procedures, if such treatment will relieve symptoms sufficiently to postpone arthroplasty and not make subsequent treatment exceedingly complex.

Another assumption is that nonoperative treatment should be attempted before proceeding with arthroplasty. This may include the use of assistive devices for ambulation, weight loss, systemic or local medications, physiotherapy, bracing, and activity modification. A concerted effort at nonsurgical therapy may be more reasonable in the younger patient than in the elderly, in whom prolonged attempts are time consuming and rarely as effective in relieving symptoms and improving function as total knee arthroplasty. These modalities should be attempted more aggressively in the younger patient than in the elderly. In some settings, the symptoms, physical findings, and radiographic changes are severe enough to warrant consideration of total knee arthroplasty even if the patient has had no prior nonoperative treatment. In most cases, however, particularly in the younger individual, it may be wiser to demonstrate to the patient that conservative or nonsurgical treatment will not relieve symptoms or improve function before recommending more aggressive treatment with more substantial potential risks and complications.

The level of patient activity and symptom severity are other important factors to consider in determining whether arthroplasty is indicated. Although pain is the most common complaint before surgical intervention, in many cases symptoms are activity related. If the patient's symptoms are clearly amenable to activity modification, and if total knee arthroplasty is not an ideal operation due to age, comorbidities, or other factors, the surgeon should opt for nonoperative treatment. An obvious and clear-cut example is a relatively young athletic individual whose knee pain limits only athletic activity. Total knee arthroplasty would not be expected to withstand the rigors of athletic competition, so such activity would be contraindicated after total knee arthroplasty. If the individual has little or no symptoms with activity modification, then activity limitation would be a more reasonable course than proceeding with total knee arthroplasty due to the potential serious long-term consequences of total knee arthroplasty and the relatively small benefit obtained as the patient must abandon competitive athletic competition in either case.

Thus, behavior modification may play a significant role in the treatment of knee disease. In attempting to understand a patient's pain pattern, the clinician must decide whether a patient has realistically modified his or her activity to accommodate the damaged joint. If the patient is unwilling to alter his or her lifestyle to accommodate the degenerative joint, then the likelihood is that this patient will not alter the lifestyle to extend the life of a prosthetic joint. For example, as noted earlier, if the patient is unwilling to give up "cutting" sports or other joint-stressful avocations that cause substantial discomfort, then the patient is probably not having enough pain to warrant surgical intervention in the form of a knee arthroplasty. On the other hand, it seems unreasonable to ask a patient to modify his or her lifestyle to the point of extreme inactivity. Thus, limitation in functional capacity is another important factor in determining the appropriateness of joint arthroplasty. Understanding the patient's requirements for performing activities of daily living is essential in this determination. A patient's ability to perform a job, do household tasks, and maintain personal hygiene can be used as measures of the effect of knee function on the patient's lifestyle. Walking tolerance, defined as the length of time or distance one can walk without rest, can be an important benchmark in assessing the severity of disease and limitation of function. In general, if a patient cannot perform activities of daily living despite nonoperative treatment, knee function has decreased to the point at which intervention is indicated.

Actual decision making in the clinical case of the young patient is usually far from straightforward and often requires consideration of multiple factors before recommendation of total knee arthroplasty. Factors that influence the results and longevity of total knee arthroplasty include weight and expected activity levels. Clearly, the 18-year-old patient with severe multiarticular systemic inflammatory arthritis and persistent contracture impeding any attempts at ambulation would be expected to stress a total knee arthroplasty significantly less than a 30-year-old former professional football player who is 6.5 feet tall, weighs 270 pounds, and suffers from isolated posttraumatic arthritis of the knee.

GOALS OF TOTAL KNEE ARTHROPLASTY

The goals of total knee arthroplasty are to relieve pain and improve function. If these goals are kept in the forefront of a clinician's mind, the task of deciding who will benefit from this procedure is usually not particularly difficult. The appropriateness of this procedure is determined by a clinical decision-making process based on the natural history and severity of the disease, the expected result from intervention, and the risks of complication or failure to achieve the goals of surgery. Patient expectations and compliance are also important variables. Each case must be individualized.

It should be kept in mind that the primary indication for total knee arthroplasty is pain and that different patients have different pain tolerances. What is disabling pain for one patient may be quite tolerable in another. An understanding of this concept is important in deciding the appropriateness of total knee arthroplasty. It is not the clinician's role to argue with the patient's perception of his or her pain pattern. It is the clinician's role, however, to determine if the pain is sufficiently related to the local pathology to warrant intervention. The clinician must adopt an individualized approach in each case and assess the entire patient.

Occasionally, one may encounter a patient who has severe limitation of function, yet has little or no pain referable to the knee joint. Severe flexion contractures can severely affect ambulation and are a good indication for total knee replacement. Similarly, an extremely stiff or ankylosed knee may place excessive stresses on the patient's lower back and ipsilateral hip and ankle, causing severe pain in these remote locations. In addition, there may be settings in which overall function is so limited that knee symptoms are minimized due to generalized activity limitation, or in which the disease process continues to limit function but no longer is associated with severe or even mild pain. Patients who have become wheelchair bound or have severe inflammatory arthropathy may have little pain secondary to their inactivity and nonetheless benefit substantially from total knee arthroplasty. Any intervention in this situation must be carefully considered, and both surgeon and patient must clearly understand the goals of surgical intervention.

A clear understanding of patients' activities of daily living, their functional limitations, as well as their expectations after surgery is mandatory. Generally, only modest gains in function are possible after long-standing contractures. Therefore, the clinician and patient must decide whether the gains anticipated from prosthetic replacement outweigh the risks associated with surgical intervention

Radiographs are extremely helpful in deciding for whom total knee arthroplasty is appropriate. However, the mere existence of moderate to severe degenerative changes radiographically is not an indication for surgery. In this context, the words of the father of modern arthroplasty, Sir John Charnley seem appropriate:

> The x-ray does not influence the surgeon's decision whether or not to operate.

The words above stress the importance of following the goals of total knee arthroplasty in decision making—to decrease pain and increase function. Radiographs are but one small piece of the equation. Most clinicians have seen patients function very well despite severe radiographically apparent changes. Likewise, patients with only moderate changes can be significantly disabled. Therefore, the decision to operate must be a clinical not a radiographic one. The decision to perform surgery immediately because a radiographic picture is sure to deteriorate is also not an appropriate stance. One must be wary of the patient with only mild radiographic changes, reasonable range of motion, and noncharacteristic knee pain. Chances of relieving this type of pain are remote.

In those patients with severe pain and corroborative radiographic changes, this conflict does not exist. Nor does it exist in the opposite situation—in those patients with severe pain and normal radiographs. In such a setting, further evaluative studies of the knee may be indicated, and a search for reasons for pain in this setting may need to be focused elsewhere.

Among the most difficult patients to deal with are those claiming severe pain yet showing only moderate radiographic changes. Only through repeated interview and examination can the clinician understand this patient's pain pattern. The clinician must develop an understanding of what it is like to "walk in this patient's shoes" and strive to understand the patient's lifestyle. In this way, the physician can determine if the patient is putting unrealistic demands on the joint. Such demands may prevent the usual conservative measures from providing tolerable relief.

Failure of nonoperative treatment, on the other hand, is a prime indicator for surgical intervention. Even in those patients with severe disease on initial presentation, a trial of nonoperative treatment has merit. This allows the patient and surgeon a chance to become familiar with each other. It also gives the clinician the chance to understand the patient's lifestyle, pain tolerance, and expectations regarding intervention. It is extremely rare to recommend arthroplasty to a patient on the first encounter.

Behavioral modification can extend the life of a natural knee. Mere avoidance of impact-loading exercise may be all that is necessary to treat a patient successfully. Cane ambulation can significantly offload stress from a degenerative knee. In some societies, however, patients are reluctant to try this, as it appears to be an admission of general infirmity.

Nonsteroidal antiinflammatory medications are widely used to treat arthritis of the knee. The physician is encouraged to trial several different forms of these agents until an effective one is found, as patients may find that one particular agent works best for them. Once an adequate agent is found, liver function, renal function, and hematopoietic function should be monitored routinely to ensure that no adverse effect occurs to the patient as a whole.

Nonoperative treatment is not without its own risks, however, and these should be considered as well. The long-term use of nonsteroidal antiinflammatory agents may have significant morbidity, particularly in older patients. Furthermore, as previously stated, the natural history of arthritis of the knee is poor (4), and an unnecessary delay in surgical intervention is inappropriate and may lead to severe deformity that complicate future total knee arthroplasty. In addition, Lavernia (6a) has demonstrated that patients who delay knee arthroplasty until symptoms become more severe have worse clinical results than those who choose intervention earlier in the course of their disease.

PATIENT SELECTION

In patients older than 60 years, end-stage arthritis of one or more compartments seems to be well treated by total knee arthroplasty. In this age group, activity level has usually diminished and expectations by the patient are reasonable, and thus the clinical results of total knee arthroplasty in this patient group are outstanding. The revision rate in this population is acceptable, and, for the vast majority of patients, the initial operation on their knee will be their last.

In the 40- to 60-year-old age group, however, activity levels remain high and patients' expectations regarding longevity of their implant often exceed the life of the implant itself. Although for many in this age group total knee arthroplasty may be the most appropriate surgical intervention, the timing of this intervention must be chosen carefully. Many of these patients have heard about the clinical successes of their older, more than 60-year-old friends and acquaintances. They frequently demand similar intervention without understanding that in their particular age group early surgical intervention may lead to subsequent revision. Therefore, objective findings must take precedence over subjective complaints in this age group.

> The surgeon should turn a deaf ear to the exaggerated adjectives used to describe pain. . . . Physical signs must take precedence over subjective sensation in this age group. . . . X-ray findings are of great importance in this group.
>
> John Charnley

In those patients younger than 40 years, the stakes regarding surgical intervention go up dramatically. With life expectancy stretching into the seventh and eighth decades in modern society, a prosthetic knee placed in one of these patients cannot be expected to last 40 years. Even in the best circumstances, these patients can count on at least one revision during their lifetime. Behavioral modifications and other conservative modalities must be maximized in this group.

Unfortunately, the success of total knee arthroplasty has colored the patient's perception of nonprosthetic options in treating knee disease. Although knee fusion may be the most appropriate treatment for a manual laborer with a limited education, this option is frequently not accepted by the patient. If an appropriate osteotomy can extend the life of the natural knee, it should be given serious consideration. In this setting, decision making may be at its most complex because the expected life span of the patient is great. It is always necessary for the surgeon who is contemplating total knee arthroplasty in the younger patient to be familiar with the indications for alternative knee salvage procedures so that total knee arthroplasty is not the only option entertained in this patient population. Although familiarity with the specific operative techniques involved in knee salvage is not necessary for all surgeons who treat arthritis of the knee, the surgeon must be able to select out and appropriately refer those younger patients who may benefit substantially from alternative treatments that will reduce pain, improve functional capability, and still allow for total knee arthroplasty at a later date. The reader is thus encouraged to examine the chapters on managing arthritis of the knee by means other than arthroplasty, such as osteotomy and arthrodesis.

It is important to discuss candidly with every young patient the possibility of multiple revisions during his or her lifetime. These patients must understand fully that, to extend the life of their implant, their activity level may need to be lower than that of which they will be capable after the pain relief of total knee arthroplasty.

A final consideration regarding fusion of the knee can be used in determining the wisdom of proceeding with arthroplasty in a young patient. Originally discussed by Charnley with regard to the hip as the "pseudarthroses test," this test at the knee involves determining if a patient with severe knee disease would be no worse off with arthrodesis of the knee than he or she is currently. If that is the case, then prosthetic intervention is probably indicated if the intervention's failure does not prevent one from proceeding with fusion.

TIMING OF SURGICAL INTERVENTION

The timing of surgical intervention is a critical part of the decision making in total knee arthroplasty. There comes a time when a patient has exhausted all nonoperative measures and has met appropriate radiographic and clinical criteria to warrant intervention. As this time approaches, the patient must decide whether symptoms are severe enough to proceed with arthroplasty.

It must be stressed that this is a patient-determined decision and not a radiographically determined one. The clinician's job is to educate patients about their disease, not to make the decision to intervene for them. The decision to have a knee replaced is an informed patient decision after a thorough discussion of treatment alternatives. Even when the alternatives are limited, patients frequently try to have the clinician decide for them.

To help a patient with this decision, once the patient has met appropriate criteria, two questions can be asked: Is your knee keeping you from performing reasonable activities of daily living? Or put another way, Does your knee keep you from doing the things that are important to you on a daily basis? If the answers to these questions are "Yes" and the patient is medically stable and meets objective criteria, then knee replacement is probably in the patient's best interest. Although total knee arthroplasty is a reliable operation for the vast majority of patients, complications do inevitably occur, and the patient must have symptoms severe enough to warrant risking the possibility of a poor outcome.

PATIENT EXPECTATIONS

The surgeon occasionally encounters patients with unrealistic expectations for surgical intervention. These expectations must be tempered by the surgeon's experience and an understanding of the patient's psychological makeup. A patient must understand that knee arthroplasty is not a panacea for multiple musculoskeletal problems. This procedure affects but one joint. Although an improved gait pattern may help an aching back to some degree, it will not have a major impact on other musculoskeletal disorders the patient may have. Indeed, it may be important to explain to the patient that, if multiple joint problems are present, the most severely involved joint may limit their activity to the extent that other arthritic joints currently are not stressed and that, with improvement in the function of the most severely involved joint after arthroplasty, other limiting joints may become more symptomatic.

The patient must also understand that functional limitations may still exist after knee arthroplasty. Normal range of motion may not be restored after years of contracture. Range of motion may be less after surgery than before. These concepts should be discussed preoperatively with the patient.

Finally, it is important to discuss the responsibility patients must assume for their prosthetic knees. Patients must understand that this implant is a walking device designed to relieve pain, and thus patients must be willing to modify their activity to prevent early mechanical failure. Although low-impact activities such as walking, swimming, golf, and doubles tennis are compatible with a long-term successful outcome, higher impact sports or heavy manual labor are not compatible with implant longevity. By assuming responsibility for their actions, patients must realize that abuse of the knee in this regard may result in diminished longevity of the knee and subsequent need for revision surgery. Along these same lines, before embarking on surgical intervention the surgeon must be confident that a given patient is willing and able to comply with the necessary postoperative rehabilitation protocols compatible with a successful outcome.

PATIENT ASSESSMENT

Not unlike in most orthopedic procedures, determining whether total knee arthroplasty is indicated for a given patient consists of obtaining a history consistent with pain and disability, combined with corroborative physical examination and radiographic findings. These three facets of the patient evaluation should all confirm the presence of end-stage arthritis of the knee before the surgeon proceeds with total knee arthroplasty. If any one of these evaluations fails to support this diagnosis, the surgeon should be alerted to the possibility of a mistaken diagnosis or the possibility that the patient's complaints will not be well managed with performance of total knee arthroplasty.

History

The primary indication for total knee arthroplasty is debilitating pain in the knee, as this is the most reliably ameliorated symptom of knee arthritis when total knee arthroplasty is performed. The character and degree of pain is important to document, as is the presence of pain at night or at rest. Presence of these latter two findings should alert the physician to the possibility of joint sepsis or tumor. Once these entities have been excluded (by radiographic and laboratory analysis if deemed appropriate), the presence of night or rest pain often heralds the final stage of knee arthritis that will not respond to nonoperative treatment. Inflammatory arthritis can also be associated with significant discomfort both at rest and at night. If the knee pain is associated with groin or anterior thigh pain, the clinician must be careful to evaluate the hip, as hip pathology may cause pain that is referred to the knee. Pain frequently extends below the knee, but pain down into the foot must be distinguished from radicular pain.

Pain associated with arthritis of the knee is typically related to activity, and the physician should establish the functional disability this has created. Specifically, the physician should determine how the patients' pain has affected their ability to perform their activities of daily living such as shopping, cleaning, and personal hygiene. These facets of the history are important to delineate, as pain is an individual experience that may hamper patients' ability to care for him- or herself and impact their lifestyle in uniquely individual ways. Patients who exhibit both severe pain and functional disability will derive the most benefit from total knee arthroplasty. It is also important to identify those patients with unrealistic expectations from total knee arthroplasty, such as those who only experience pain and disability in the context of intense physical exertion, in whom activity modification, rather than total knee arthroplasty, would be most appropriate.

The patient history should also include an assessment of prior nonoperative and operative treatments. A thorough trial of nonoperative treatment is appropriate for the majority of patients considered for total knee arthroplasty as previously discussed. Nonoperative treatment including activity modification, nonsteroidal antiinflammatory medications, acetaminophen, hyaluronate or corticosteroid injections, the use of an assist device, and bracing should all be considered and discussed with patients as potential forms of nonoperative management of knee arthritis. Failure of these modalities should be considered a good indication for surgery in the presence of corroborative physical examination and radiographic findings.

A prior history of operative treatment is also important to document, as various other operative treatments may influence the operative techniques used and compromise the final outcome if total knee arthroplasty is indicated. If possible, previous operative reports should be reviewed to confirm the surgical findings and treatment rendered.

The patient history should also include an assessment of the patient's general health and any medical problems. Appropriate preoperative medical consultation is imperative to identify medical comorbidities that can be optimized preoperatively or that may argue against elective surgery. A history of disease associated with an immunocompromised state (such as diabetes mellitus, renal failure, or acquired immune deficiency syndrome) is also important to obtain, to more carefully counsel patients on the risks of perioperative or late infection. The history should also seek to identify other medical problems that may be associated with persistent bacteremia such as recurrent urinary tract infections in women, urinary outlet obstruction in men, or dental problems that can be addressed before operative intervention.

Physical Examination

Physical examination should begin with an assessment of gait. An antalgic gait is most commonly encountered; however, the presence of a Trendelenburg gait should alert the physician to a problem with the ipsilateral hip joint, with pain being referred to the knee. A patient's gait is often illustrative of the amount of disability that they are encountering and helps the surgeon to determine if a given patient's arthritis warrants total knee arthroplasty. The alignment of the lower extremity is also noted to assist with preoperative planning of anticipated ligament releases if total knee arthroplasty is in fact indicated.

Inspection of the soft tissue envelope is performed next. The location and age of prior incisions should be noted, as they may impact the surgical approach used in subsequent knee arthroplasty. If there is a question as to the suitability of the soft tissue envelope for surgical intervention, a preoperative consultation with a plastic surgeon is recommended. The presence of cutaneous lesions is also important to note, because they may indicate the cause of arthritis (as in the case of psoriatic arthritis) or may influence the decision to proceed with surgery, as surgery will need to be delayed for patients with active skin lesions until the soft tissue envelope is intact to prevent an unacceptably high rate of infection (7).

A neurovascular examination including the palpation of dorsalis pedis and posterior tibial pulses follows. If they are not palpable, a vascular consultation may be warranted, and the avoidance of a tourniquet intraoperatively should be carefully considered. The neurologic examination may alert the physician to the presence of preoperative neurologic deficits and may also identify a radiculopathy as the cause of the patient's pain.

Examination of the knee itself includes an assessment of range of motion, which is typically decreased. In addition, it is important to recognize that preoperative range of motion is often predictive of postoperative range of motion (8–10). Some patients may seek total knee arthroplasty primarily to increase their range of motion, and the ability to improve their range of motion must be carefully discussed with the patient before surgery. Preoperative flexion contractures are also important to identify so that they can be appropriately addressed at the time of surgery. The knee is next palpated to determine areas of maximal tenderness. The presence of anterior knee pain and peripatellar tenderness is important to note, as some surgeons do not routinely resurface the patellofemoral joint. Ligamentous stability is tested next, as is the ability to correct any valgus or varus deformities if present.

The physical examination should include a thorough assessment of the lower back and hip to ensure that the pain experienced by the patient is not referred from a distant source. In cases in which the cause of the patient's pain is unclear, an intraarticular lidocaine injection can be used to confirm if the pain experienced is arising from the knee joint itself.

Radiographic Analysis

Radiographic confirmation of knee arthritis is important in the evaluation of the patient considered for total knee arthroplasty. Clinical symptoms, however, oftentimes do not correlate directly with the severity of radiographic findings. Specifically, the radiographic presence of severe arthritic changes in the absence of clinical symptoms or disability referable to the knee is clearly not an indication for total knee arthroplasty. Similarly, the absence of radiographic findings should alert the physician to an alternative diagnosis.

Radiographs obtained should include standing anteroposterior, lateral, and patellofemoral views. Standing radiographs are imperative to detect subtle joint space narrowing associated with loss of articular cartilage. A standing view with the knee flexed may further assist in identifying subtle joint space narrowing. It is not uncommon for patients with minimal radiographic changes to undergo an extensive course of nonoperative treatment only for severe cartilaginous destruction to be found at the time of surgery. Thus, radiographs must always be interpreted in the context of clinical symptoms. Magnetic resonance imaging may occasionally be indicated to further evaluate the integrity of the cartilaginous surfaces when plain radiographic findings are unclear. Patellofemoral views are equally important, as total knee arthroplasty is appropriate for older individuals with severe patellofemoral arthritis (11), and, in these cases, anteroposterior and lateral views can underestimate the degree of arthritis present.

ALTERNATIVES TO TOTAL KNEE ARTHROPLASTY

Although total knee arthroplasty is appropriate surgical management for the majority of patients with a severely arthritic knee, the surgeon must be aware of alternate surgical therapies that may be more appropriate for certain patients. Alternative surgical options to total knee arthroplasty include osteotomy, unicompartmental arthroplasty, and arthrodesis. Osteotomy of the knee is reserved for patients who have a focal biomechanical derangement of the knee joint with an adjacent area of intact cartilage available for redirection into the weightbearing portion of the joint. Osteotomy can be performed on either the tibial or femoral side of the joint. A congruous, stable knee with good range of motion is a prerequisite. These procedures are most often used in younger patients with early degenerative arthritis that is limited to either the medial or lateral compartment. Unicompartmental arthroplasty is indicated for patients with unicompartmental tibiofemoral arthritis without significant deformity, concomitant patellofemoral disease, ligamentous instability, or inflammatory arthritis. Arthrodesis of the knee is infrequently indicated except for patients with a clear contraindication to total knee arthroplasty such as active sepsis.

Arthroscopy of the knee may also have a role in the treatment of knee arthritis; however, its indications are controversial. Patients with degenerative arthritis and mechanical symptoms may benefit from operative arthroscopy, but the surgeon should be aware that symptoms may worsen after arthroscopy, which leads to an unhappy patient who may seek further treatment elsewhere. Furthermore, one study has suggested that, in patients with degenerative knee arthritis, arthroscopy had results that were similar to those of a sham operation in which only skin incisions were made (12). Arthroscopic synovectomy may have a role in the treatment of patients with inflammatory arthritis of the knee before severe cartilaginous destruction has occurred; however, the long-term benefits of such intervention are unproven (13).

SPECIFIC PATIENT-RELATED CONSIDERATIONS

Age

When a patient is considered for total knee arthroplasty, it is important to remember that arthroplasty has time-limited results. Although excellent results have been reported for younger, active patients undergoing total knee arthroplasty (14,15), the necessity for revision and possibly multiple revision surgeries must be considered in patients with longer expected life spans, as previously discussed. Younger age should not be considered an absolute contraindication, however, as excellent results have been reported in young patients with inflammatory arthropathies and multiple joint involvement (16). Furthermore, alternative operative interventions are often inappropriate in patients with inflammatory disease.

Good results have also been reported in the very elderly, and likewise advanced age itself should not be considered a contraindication to total knee arthroplasty. Functional improvements, however, may be less than those seen in more youthful patients (17,18). Medical comorbidities may be increased in this patient population, which make the risks of perioperative complications higher.

Weight

Many patients who have arthritis of the knee are obese (19,20), and although weight loss as a treatment for their pain is an attractive option for the surgeon, it is often impossible for the patients to achieve. Obese patients are considered at risk for a higher rate of complications than nonobese controls (21,22). Despite this, it has been reported that these patients can have satisfactory outcomes after total knee arthroplasty (23), and obesity alone should not be considered as a contraindication to total knee arthroplasty. Even morbidly obese patients have been found to have adequate results (24), although functional outcomes are reported to be poorer for this subset of patients. Perioperative complications, particularly wound healing complications, superficial infections, and medial collateral ligament avulsions, are reported more frequently than in nonobese comparative groups. Because of this, care with soft tissue closure and operative technique is imperative in this population. Furthermore, obese patients must be counseled preoperatively on the specific problems of total knee arthroplasty that they may encounter.

Diabetes Mellitus

Patients with diabetes mellitus have been shown to have immune dysfunction secondary to abnormal neutrophil and monocyte activity that makes them predisposed to infection (25). Clinical studies have shown that this patient population has a significantly higher rate of wound complications, deep prosthetic infection, and urinary tract infection after total knee arthroplasty. Deep infection rates ranging from 1.5% to 7.0% in series of patients encompassing from 53 to 109 knees have been reported (26–29). These patients have also been shown to have fewer good and excellent results and lower functional scores than matched controls (27,28).

Given the higher rate of infection found in patients with diabetes mellitus, Chiu et al. (30) studied prospectively the use of antibiotic-impregnated cement in this population. In this study, they found a significantly lower rate of infection with the use of cefuroxime-impregnated cement; no infections occurred in the group of 41 patients in whom antibiotics were used in the cement, compared to five infections in the 37 patients in whom antibiotics were not used in the cement.

Osteonecrosis

Patients with osteonecrosis of the knee may have poor-quality bone that does not adequately support the prosthetic components and leads to a higher rate of failure. It is important to keep in mind, however, that this is a heterogeneous disorder; idiopathic or spontaneous osteonecrosis of the knee occurs in older patients with a more predictable outcome, whereas younger patients with steroid-induced osteonecrosis and diseases such as systemic lupus erythematosus have poorer outcomes. In the latter group of patients, associated diseases such as lupus may make them more susceptible to infection, perioperative medical complications, and a poor functional outcome. Although in general the results of total knee arthroplasty in this population are not as predictable as in patients with osteoarthritis, patients with severe joint involvement may not have other reasonable treatment options.

Mont et al. reported on 31 knees in 21 patients with osteonecrosis of the knee younger than 50 years who had undergone total knee arthroplasty and were taking corticosteroids. These authors found only 55% of patients with good or excellent results and a 37% rate of aseptic loosening requiring revision at a mean of 8 years (31). Similarly, Seldes et al. (32) found a 16% rate of revision among 31 knees with three cases of aseptic loosening and two deep infections among patients with steroid-induced osteonecrosis after 5 years of follow-up. In a later study by Mont et al. (33), 48 knees treated with total knee arthroplasty for atraumatic osteonecrosis of the knee had a similarly disappointing rate of 71% clinically successful results at 9 years. Bergman and Rand (34), however, reported somewhat better results among 38 knees at a mean of 4 years, with 85% survival of the prosthesis at a shorter follow-up period of 5 years.

Hemophilic Arthropathy

In severely affected patients with hemophilia, severe joint destruction and stiffness may occur. These patients may also have concomitant transfusion-related human immunodeficiency virus infection. Specific problems encountered include poor bone quality and severe soft tissue fibrosis, which leads to a high rate of complications. Hematologic consultation before and after surgery is essential to assist in the maintenance of factor levels at 100% in the perioperative period. The presence of inhibitors (antibodies directed against the deficient factors) is a contraindication to total knee arthroplasty.

Figgie et al. (34a) reported on 19 knees with an average follow-up of 9.5 years and found a 32% rate of fair and poor results. Thomason et al. (35) reported even poorer results among 23 knees treated with total knee arthroplasty in 15 patients with hemophilic arthropathy of the knee. At a mean of 7.5 years postoperatively, 19 knees were rated as fair or poor with four infections (all of these patients tested positive for human immunodeficiency virus infection). Both groups also documented high rates of radiographic evidence of prosthetic loosening. Despite the problems encountered in this patient population, patient satisfaction is high with significant improvements in quality of life documented after total knee arthroplasty (36).

Ipsilateral Hip Fusion

Patients with a fusion of the hip may experience pain and arthrosis of the lumbar spine, ipsilateral knee, or contralateral hip. In general, it is advisable to perform a conversion arthroplasty of the hip before total knee arthroplasty, as patients may have significant pain relief in their knee after fusion takedown (37–40). In addition, total knee arthroplasty with an ipsilateral hip fusion is technically challenging. Patients may have a frontal plane knee deformity if the ipsilateral hip is fused in excessive abduction or adduction, and ligamentous instability is common (37).

Romness and Morrey (41) reported on 16 knees in patients with an ipsilateral hip fusion; 12 patients had undergone total knee arthroplasty after conversion arthroplasty of the hip and 4 before such intervention. At a mean of 5.5 years, 15 of 16 patients had no or minimal pain, and there had been no revisions. Garvin et al. (42) reported on nine knees that had undergone total knee arthroplasty with an ipsilateral hip fusion. Although eight of the nine knees had good or excellent results at 7 years, all patients had at least one complication: Seven knees required manipulation under anesthesia for poor range of motion, two experienced peroneal nerve palsies (both in patients with valgus deformity preoperatively), and one deep infection occurred.

Paget's Disease

Paget's disease of bone is a disorder of abnormal bone remodeling with increased osteoclastic resorption followed by a secondary increase in reactive bone formation (43,44). It is found in 3% to 4% of the population over 50 years of age, although it is usually asymptomatic and often found incidentally on radiographs obtained for other reasons. The increased metabolic state leads to highly vascular bone that is weaker than normal (43).

Radiographic features include coarsened trabeculae with a blastic appearance with remodeling that leads to bony enlargement and deformity. The femur and tibia are frequently involved, and the disease process can cause severe deformity, pain, and degenerative joint disease of the hip and knee. At times, it may be difficult to differentiate pain secondary to the disease process itself from pain in an adjacent joint secondary to arthritis. In these cases, an intraarticular injection of lidocaine into the knee can assist in differentiating the origin of pain.

A sudden increase in pain may herald a pathologic fracture or the transformation of a pagetic lesion into sarcoma, which should be ruled out. In these cases, radiographs may show cortical destruction and advanced imaging studies reveal an associated soft tissue mass.

Medical treatment before surgical intervention is recommended as it may decrease pain and thus obviate the need for surgery. In addition, if surgical intervention is indicated, medical management may decrease blood loss associated with operating on highly vascular pagetic bone.

Clinical experience with total knee arthroplasty in patients with Paget's disease is limited to several small series of patients (45–47). These studies report difficulty in obtaining appropriate alignment secondary to deformity, and extramedullary alignment systems are often required. Clinical and radiographic results have been good, however, with little difference seen between these patients and matched osteoarthritic control patients.

Posttraumatic Arthritis

Patients with posttraumatic arthritis of the knee may have previously undergone surgical intervention or have had severe soft tissue injuries that may complicate total knee arthroplasty. The location of previous incisions should be carefully noted, as should the overall condition of the overlying soft tissue envelope. These patients may also have severe deformities, bone loss, or associated ligamentous deficiencies that need to be addressed at the time of surgery. Furthermore, the removal of internal fixation devices may both complicate the operative approach and mandate the use of stemmed components to span areas of potential weakness. If prior operative intervention has been carried out, the presence of an infection must also be considered.

Roffi and Merritt (48) reported on 13 knees, of which 8 were considered to show successful results with a short-term follow-up averaging 27 months. Saleh et al. (49) reported on 15 total knee arthroplasties performed after open reduction and internal fixation of a tibial plateau fracture. Perioperative complications included four knees with poor wound healing (which led to a deep infection in three cases), two patellar ligament ruptures, and three knees that required a manipulation under anesthesia for stiffness. At a mean of 6 years postoperatively, 12 of the 15 patients had good or excellent results. Given the high rate of infection observed, the authors recommended preoperative joint aspiration and the use of antibiotic-loaded cement.

Neurologic Dysfunction

Neurologic diseases can affect the results of total knee arthroplasty. In a series of patients with Parkinson's disease, although overall results were found to be acceptable, functional scores were poor in those in whom Parkinson's disease progressed (50,51). Poliomyelitis may similarly affect the results of total knee arthroplasty, particularly if significant knee instability or quadriceps weakness is present. Although there is little literature available on this topic, Patterson and Insall reported on nine patients with polio who had undergone total knee arthroplasty (52). Three of these nine patients required a revision for instability at an average follow-up of 6.8 years, and thus these authors recommended the use of more constrained implants. The presence of chronic neurologic diseases has also been associated with a higher rate of morbidity after total knee arthroplasty (53).

Workers' Compensation

Patients receiving workers' compensation have been shown to have significantly poorer outcomes than matched subjects not receiving workers' compensation after total knee arthroplasty (15,54,55). Interestingly, whereas objective postoperative indicators such as range of motion and radiographic findings are similar to those in matched patients, subjective findings, particularly measures of pain, and overall outcomes are far worse. Although receipt of workers' compensation is not a contraindication to total knee arthroplasty, the surgeon should spend a substantial amount of time getting to know such patients preoperatively to build a strong relationship with them and to attempt to understand their motivations in seeking surgical intervention.

CONTRAINDICATIONS TO TOTAL KNEE ARTHROPLASTY

There are few absolute contraindications to total knee arthroplasty. Relative contraindications include morbid obesity, neurologic dysfunction, and remote local infection. Although in each of these conditions there may be a higher failure rate, substantial reduction in pain and improvement in function may overshadow the potential risks in these populations.

Another confounding factor is specific anatomic abnormalities of soft tissue or bone that would place the patient at substantial increased risk from the surgical procedure itself. For example, an elderly patient having an ancient femoral neck fracture malunion with substantial shortening and rotational deformity with concomitant severe atherosclerotic femoral vessels may be at substantially increased risk of femoral artery thrombosis due to the lengthening and rotational release required to perform the surgery. Again, the risks of surgery must be balanced against the patient's symptoms.

Active Sepsis

Active sepsis of the knee joint or systemic sepsis that could lead to bacterial seeding of the knee joint is the most rigid contraindication to total knee arthroplasty, as the implantation of a metallic prosthesis in this setting will surely lead to deep infection and failure. Patients with a remote history of sepsis of the knee who subsequently undergo total knee arthroplasty also have a high rate of recurrent infection, with Jerry et al. (56) reporting an infection rate of 7.7% (5 of 65 knees).

In cases in which active or persistent infection is suspected, a thorough preoperative investigation including laboratory testing (white blood cell count, erythrocyte sedimentation rate and C-reactive protein level) and knee joint aspiration (with cell count and culture) are mandatory. In cases in which the presence of active infection is undetermined, the patient can undergo a two-stage exchange protocol, with resection of all bony surfaces, insertion of an antibiotic spacer, and an extended course of intravenous antibiotics. The surgeon must realize, however, that osteomyelitis of bone may be more recalcitrant to treatment than a periprosthetic infection, and the patient should be willing to accept a high risk of failure and the possibility of both knee arthrodesis and amputation if this course of treatment is selected. In patients with persistent knee joint sepsis and pain, arthrodesis is the preferred surgical option.

Incompetent Extensor Mechanism

Incompetence of the extensor mechanism is a contraindication to total knee arthroplasty. Extensor mechanism dysfunction leads to persistent knee instability. The surgeon faced with such a patient may try to perform allograft extensor mechanism reconstruction at the time of primary knee arthroplasty; however, the results of this type of reconstruction following extensor mechanism disruption after total knee arthroplasty have been mixed (57), and Leopold et al. (58) reported a high rate of persistent extensor lag.

Neuropathic Arthropathy

Neuropathic or Charcot arthropathy is a chronic, progressive degenerative process that develops secondary to a disturbance in the normal sensory innervation of joints (59). Neuropathic arthropathy is most commonly associated with diabetes mellitus, syphilis, and syringomyelia but may be seen in patients with leprosy, spinal dysraphism, amyloidosis, Charcot-Marie-Tooth disease, multiple sclerosis, and congenital insensitivity to pain. Patients typically present with a warm, swollen, erythematous joint, and although the condition is classically viewed as painless, many patients present with significant pain as well as instability. Radiographs typically show severe joint destruction with periarticular bone formation, osteophytes, fractures, and osseous debris (59). If neuropathic arthropathy is suspected, a neurologic consultation is mandatory to identify the underlying neurologic disorder. In these cases, it may be difficult to differentiate neuropathic arthropathy from infection, and joint aspiration and culture should be considered if the diagnosis is unclear.

Total knee arthroplasty is controversial in this patient population as there is minimal clinical experience reported in the literature. For the majority of patients, initial treatment should include protective bracing. If this fails, arthrodesis of the knee has been reported to be successful (60–62). Soudry et al. (63) reported on nine neuropathic knees in seven patients treated with total knee arthroplasty and found that the results were excellent in eight knees at an average of 3 years after surgery. Yoshino et al. (64) reported on three neuropathic knees that were treated with total knee arthroplasty and found that two had a successful result. Both reports stressed the importance of correcting bone loss (with bone grafts or metal wedges), reestablishing alignment, and achieving ligamentous balance.

Knee Arthrodesis

Conversion of a knee that has undergone previous operative arthrodesis or spontaneous ankylosis to a total knee arthroplasty is controversial. Most surgeons believe that these conditions are a contraindication to total knee arthroplasty because of the severe muscular and ligamentous atrophy that follows knee arthrodesis, which makes postoperative instability of great concern. As many knee fusions (both surgical and spontaneous) follow joint infections, the rate of recurrent infection is high, as are wound-healing complications, and postoperative range of motion is often poor. The overall complication rate has been reported to range from 53% to 57% in series encompassing from 17 to 37 knees (65–68). Although patients are often happy with the improved mobility of the knee, given the high rate of complications associated with the conversion of a knee fusion to a total knee arthroplasty, most surgeons do not recommend this procedure.

Severe Medical Comorbidities

As previously discussed, a thorough preoperative general medical evaluation is mandatory before total knee arthroplasty. Certain patients may have severe medical comorbidities that make any type of elective surgery unsafe. The risks of perioperative mortality after surgical intervention must be carefully weighed against the expected functional improvement and pain relief that can be expected with any type of surgical intervention. In these patients, the risks of surgical intervention may outweigh the benefits of total knee arthroplasty if the risk of perioperative morbidity and mortality are excessive.

Severe Peripheral Vascular Disease

Severe peripheral vascular disease can result in wound complications (secondary to poor perfusion to the area of the incision) or more catastrophic limb ischemia that may necessitate amputation or cause death after total knee arthroplasty. In one report of vascular injuries after total knee arthroplasty, 6 of 14 patients (43%) required an amputation and one patient died of sepsis (69). These injuries are most commonly secondary to compression of an atherosclerotic plaque with acute thrombosis by a tourniquet, although injury can occur secondary to manipulation alone or via stretching of the vessel secondary to correction of a flexion contracture. Calligaro et al. reviewed 4,097 total knee arthroplasties and found seven cases of acute ischemia (0.17%) secondary to occlusion in patients with underlying chronic occlusive atherosclerotic disease (70). The most common risk factors cited are a history of arterial insufficiency (intermittent claudication, pain at rest, or prior arterial ulcers), prior vascular surgery, absent or asymmetric distal pulses, and presence of vascular calcifications on plain radiographs (71). If vascular insufficiency is suspected, the ankle-brachial index should be determined, and if it is less than 0.9, a vascular surgery consultation should be obtained (72). If the ankle-brachial index is less than 0.5, vascular bypass may be necessary preoperatively (70).

Unrealistic Patient Expectations

As discussed previously, patients must have realistic expectations for total knee arthroplasty. Surgeons contemplating total knee arthroplasty must ensure that their patients have a realistic picture of the potential benefits and complications that may occur after total knee arthroplasty. Furthermore, patients must be willing to comply with postoperative activity restrictions that are consistent with longevity of the prosthesis and must be willing to participate actively in an intensive postoperative physical therapy program. Patients with an uncontrolled lifestyle such as active intravenous drug users are also poor candidates for total knee arthroplasty. If the surgeon is unsure if the patient fits these criteria, options include asking the patient to seek a second opinion from another surgeon or offering alternative treatments.

CONCLUSION

Surgical decision making can vary from simple to complex. In making the decision to replace the knee joint, it is the job of the surgeon to assess all of the relevant patient-related factors involved in the surgical decision while communicating effectively to the patient alternative treatment options, the risks of operative intervention, and the expected results of surgery. Such communication must be tempered by an understanding of the patient's psychological makeup and intellectual capabilities. This informing of the patient may occasionally be both a time-consuming and difficult undertaking. Specifically, in cases in which the surgeon does not have good data regarding the outcomes and risks in specific conditions or in cases of specific anatomic variations, it may be difficult to assess the real benefits or risks of surgery. Nonetheless, time spent in this exercise will reward the surgeon with patients who fully understand the goals of surgery, are better able to cooperate with their own recovery, and have a greater understanding of expected outcomes. In our experience, this tends to make for a happier patient population and a more satisfying surgical practice—perhaps the ultimate goals of the knee arthroplasty surgeon.

REFERENCES

1. Lavernia CJ, Guzman JF, Gachupin-Garcia A. Cost effectiveness and quality of life in knee arthroplasty. *Clin Orthop* 1997;345:134.
2. Felson DT, Zhang Y, Hannan MT, et al. The incidence and natural history of knee osteoarthritis in the elderly. The Framingham Osteoarthritis Study. *Arthritis Rheum* 1995;38(10):1500.
3. Felson DT, Naimark A, Anderson J, et al. The prevalence of knee osteoarthritis in the elderly. The Framingham Osteoarthritis Study. *Arthritis Rheum* 1987;30(8):914.
4. Dieppe PA, Cushnaghan J, Shepstone L. The Bristol "OA500" study: progression of osteoarthritis (OA) over 3 years and the relationship between clinical and radiographic changes at the knee joint. *Osteoarthritis Cartilage* 1997;5(2):87.
5. Pavone V, Boettner F, Fickert S, et al. Total condylar knee arthroplasty: a long-term followup. *Clin Orthop* 2001;388:18.
6. Rodriguez JA, Bhende H, Ranawat CS. Total condylar knee replacement: a 20-year followup study. *Clin Orthop* 2001;388:10.
6a. Lavernia CJ, Sierra R, Hernandez R. The timing of arthroplasty: Optimize the outcome. Presented at: Annual Meeting of the American Academy of Orthopaedic Surgeons; 2002; Dallas.
7. Stern SH, Insall JN, Windsor RE, et al. Total knee arthroplasty in patients with psoriasis. *Clin Orthop* 1989;248:108.
8. Anouchi YS, McShane M, Kelly F Jr, et al. Range of motion in total knee replacement. *Clin Orthop* 1996;331:87.
9. Kawamura H, Bourne RB. Factors affecting range of flexion after total knee replacement. *J Orthop Sci* 2001;6(3):248.
10. Lizaur A, Marco L, Cebrian R. Preoperative factors influencing the range of movement after total knee arthroplasty for severe osteoarthritis. *J Bone Joint Surg Br* 1997;79(4):626.
11. Laskin RS, van Steijn M. Total knee replacement for patients with patellofemoral arthritis. *Clin Orthop* 1999;367:89.
12. Moseley JB Jr, Wray NP, Kuykendall D, et al. Arthroscopic treatment of osteoarthritis of the knee: a prospective, randomized, placebo-controlled trial. Results of a pilot study. *Am J Sports Med* 1996;24(1):28.
13. Klug S, Wittmann G, Weseloh G. Arthroscopic synovectomy of the knee joint in early cases of rheumatoid arthritis: follow-up results of a multicenter study. *Arthroscopy* 2000;16(3):262.
14. Diduch DR, Insall JN, Scott WN, et al. Total knee replacement in young, active patients. Long-term follow-up and functional outcome. *J Bone Joint Surg Am* 1997;79(4):575.
15. Lonner JH, Hershman S, Mont M, et al. Total knee arthroplasty in patients 40 years of age and younger with osteoarthritis. *Clin Orthop* 2000;380:85.
16. Cage DJ, Granberry WM, Tullos HS. Long-term results of total arthroplasty in adolescents with debilitating polyarthropathy. *Clin Orthop* 1992;283:156.
17. Belmar CJ, Barth P, Lonner JH, et al. Total knee arthroplasty in patients 90 years of age and older. *J Arthroplasty* 1999;14(8):911.

18. Jones CA, Voaklander DC, Johnston DW, et al. The effect of age on pain, function, and quality of life after total hip and knee arthroplasty. *Arch Intern Med* 2001;161(3):454.

19. Bray GA. Complications of obesity. *Ann Intern Med* 1985;103[6 (Pt 2)]:1052.

20. Leach RE, Baumgard S, Broom J. Obesity: its relationship to osteoarthritis of the knee. *Clin Orthop* 1973;93:271.

21. Ahlberg A, Lunden A. Secondary operations after knee joint replacement. *Clin Orthop* 1981;156:170.

22. Stern SH, Insall JN. Total knee arthroplasty in obese patients. *J Bone Joint Surg Am* 1990;72(9):1400.

23. Mont MA, Mathur SK, Krackow KA, et al. Cementless total knee arthroplasty in obese patients. A comparison with a matched control group. *J Arthroplasty* 1996;11(2):153.

24. Winiarsky R, Barth P, Lotke P. Total knee arthroplasty in morbidly obese patients. *J Bone Joint Surg Am* 1998;80(12):1770.

25. Calvet HM, Yoshikawa TT. Infections in diabetes. *Infect Dis Clin North Am* 2001;15(2):407.

26. England SP, Stern SH, Insall JN, et al. Total knee arthroplasty in diabetes mellitus. *Clin Orthop* 1990;260:130.

27. Papagelopoulos PJ, Idusuyi OB, Wallrichs SL, et al. Long term outcome and survivorship analysis of primary total knee arthroplasty in patients with diabetes mellitus. *Clin Orthop* 1996;330:124.

28. Serna F, Mont MA, Krackow KA, et al. Total knee arthroplasty in diabetic patients. Comparison to a matched control group. *J Arthroplasty* 1994;9(4):375.

29. Yang K, Yeo SJ, Lee BP, et al. Total knee arthroplasty in diabetic patients: a study of 109 consecutive cases. *J Arthroplasty* 2001;16(1):102.

30. Chiu FY, Lin CF, Chen CM, et al. Cefuroxime-impregnated cement at primary total knee arthroplasty in diabetes mellitus. A prospective, randomised study. *J Bone Joint Surg Br* 2001;83(5):691.

31. Mont MA, Myers TH, Krackow KA, et al. Total knee arthroplasty for corticosteroid associated avascular necrosis of the knee. *Clin Orthop* 1997;338:124.

32. Seldes RM, Tan V, Duffy G, et al. Total knee arthroplasty for steroid-induced osteonecrosis. *J Arthroplasty* 1999;14(5):533.

33. Mont MA, Baumgarten KM, Rifai A, et al. Atraumatic osteonecrosis of the knee. *J Bone Joint Surg Am* 2000;82(9):1279.

34. Bergman NR, Rand JA. Total knee arthroplasty in osteonecrosis. *Clin Orthop* 1991;273:77.

34a. Figgie MP, Goldberg VM, Figgie HE, et al. Total knee arthroplasty for the treatment of chronic hemophilic arthropathy. *Clin Orthop* 1989;(248):98–107.

35. Thomason HC 3rd, Wilson FC, Lachiewicz PF, et al. Knee arthroplasty in hemophilic arthropathy. *Clin Orthop* 1999;360:169.

36. Schick M, Stucki G, Rodriguez M, et al. Haemophilic arthropathy: assessment of quality of life after total knee arthroplasty. *Clin Rheumatol* 1999;18(6):468.

37. Amstutz HC, Sakai DN. Total joint replacement for ankylosed hips. *J Bone Joint Surg Am* 1975;57:619.

38. Hamadouche M, Kerboull L, Meunier A, et al. Total hip arthroplasty for the treatment of ankylosed hips: a five to twenty-one-year follow-up study. *J Bone Joint Surg Am* 2001;83(7):992.

39. Hardinge K, Murphy JC, Frenyo S. Conversion of hip fusion to Charnley low-friction arthroplasty. *Clin Orthop* 1986;211:173.

40. Kilgus DJ, Amstutz HC, Wolgin MA, et al. Joint replacement for ankylosed hips. *J Bone Joint Surg Am* 1990;72(1):45.

41. Romness DW, Morrey BF. Total knee arthroplasty in patients with prior ipsilateral hip fusion. *J Arthroplasty* 1992;7(1):63.

42. Garvin KL, Pellicci PM, Windsor RE, et al. Contralateral total hip arthroplasty or ipsilateral total knee arthroplasty in patients who have a long-standing fusion of the hip. *J Bone Joint Surg Am* 1989;71(9):1355.

43. Kaplan FS, Singer FR. Paget's disease of bone: pathophysiology, diagnosis, and management. *J Am Acad Orthop Surg* 1995;3(6):336.

44. Merkow RL, Lane JM. Paget's disease of bone. *Orthop Clin North Am* 1990;21(1):171.

45. Broberg MA, Cass JR. Total knee arthroplasty in Paget's disease of the knee. *J Arthroplasty* 1986;1(2):139.

46. Gabel GT, Rand JA, Sim FH. Total knee arthroplasty for osteoarthrosis in patients who have Paget disease of bone at the knee. *J Bone Joint Surg Am* 1991;73(5):739.

47. Schai PA, Scott RD, Younger AS. Total knee arthroplasty in Paget's disease: technical problems and results. *Orthopedics* 1999;22(1):21.

48. Roffi RP, Merritt PO. Total knee replacement after fractures about the knee. *Orthop Rev* 1990;19(7):614.

49. Saleh KJ, Sherman P, Katkin P, et al. Total knee arthroplasty after open reduction and internal fixation of fractures of the tibial plateau: a minimum five-year follow-up study. *J Bone Joint Surg Am* 2001;83(8):1144.

50. Duffy GP, Trousdale RT. Total knee arthroplasty in patients with Parkinson's disease. *J Arthroplasty* 1996;11(8):899.

51. Vince KG, Insall JN, Bannerman CE. Total knee arthroplasty in the patient with Parkinson's disease. *J Bone Joint Surg Br* 1989;71(1):51.

52. Patterson BM, Insall JN. Surgical management of gonarthrosis in patients with poliomyelitis. *J Arthroplasty* 1992;7[Suppl]:419.

53. Perka C, Arnold U, Buttgereit F. Influencing factors on perioperative morbidity in knee arthroplasty. *Clin Orthop* 2000;378:183.

54. Brinker MR, Savory CG, Weeden SH, et al. The results of total knee arthroplasty in workers' compensation patients. *Bull Hosp Joint Dis* 1998;57(2):80.

55. Mont MA, Mayerson JA, Krackow KA, et al. Total knee arthroplasty in patients receiving workers' compensation. *J Bone Joint Surg Am* 1998;80(9):1285.

56. Jerry GJ Jr, Rand JA, Ilstrup D. Old sepsis prior to total knee arthroplasty. *Clin Orthop* 1988;236:135.

57. Emerson RH Jr, Head WC, Malinin TI. Extensor mechanism reconstruction with an allograft after total knee arthroplasty. *Clin Orthop* 1994;303:79.

58. Leopold SS, Greidanus N, Paprosky WG, et al. High rate of failure of allograft reconstruction of the extensor mechanism after total knee arthroplasty. *J Bone Joint Surg Am* 1999;81(11):1574.

59. Alpert SW, Koval KJ, Zuckerman JD. Neuropathic arthropathy: review of current knowledge. *J Am Acad Orthop Surg* 1996;4(2):100.

60. Drennan DB, Fahey JJ, Maylahn DJ. Important factors in achieving arthrodesis of the Charcot knee. *J Bone Joint Surg Am* 1971;53(6):1180.

61. Fahmy NR, Barnes KL, Noble J. A technique for difficult arthrodesis of the knee. *J Bone Joint Surg Br* 1984;66(3):367.

62. Incavo SJ, Lilly JW, Bartlett CS, et al. Arthrodesis of the knee: experience with intramedullary nailing. *J Arthroplasty* 2000;15(7):871.

63. Soudry M, Binazzi R, Johanson NA, et al. Total knee arthroplasty in Charcot and Charcot-like joints. *Clin Orthop* 1986;208:199.

64. Yoshino S, Fujimori J, Kajino A, et al. Total knee arthroplasty in Charcot's joint. *J Arthroplasty* 1993;8(3):335

65. Cameron HU, Hu C. Results of total knee arthroplasty following takedown of formal knee fusion. *J Arthroplasty* 1996;11(6):732.

66. Kim YH, Cho SH, Kim JS. Total knee arthroplasty in bony ankylosis in gross flexion. *J Bone Joint Surg Br* 1999;81(2):296.

67. Kim YH, Kim JS, Cho SH. Total knee arthroplasty after spontaneous osseous ankylosis and takedown of formal knee fusion. *J Arthroplasty* 2000;15(4):453.

68. Naranja RJ Jr, Lotke PA, Pagnano MW, et al. Total knee arthroplasty in a previously ankylosed or arthrodesed knee. *Clin Orthop* 1996;331:234.

69. Kumar SN, Chapman JA, Rawlins I. Vascular injuries in total knee arthroplasty. A review of the problem with special reference to the possible effects of the tourniquet. *J Arthroplasty* 1998;13(2):211.

70. Calligaro KD, DeLaurentis DA, Booth RE, et al. Acute arterial thrombosis associated with total knee arthroplasty. *J Vasc Surg* 1994;20(6):927.

71. Smith DE, McGraw RW, Taylor DC, et al. Arterial complications and total knee arthroplasty. *J Am Acad Orthop Surg* 2001;9(4):253.

72. DeLaurentis DA, Levitsky KA, Booth RE, et al. Arterial and ischemic aspects of total knee arthroplasty. *Am J Surg* 1992;164(3):237.

CHAPTER 71

Implant Options in Primary Total Knee Replacement

John J. Callaghan and Michael R. O'Rourke

Many options are available to the orthopedic surgeon today in terms of implant selection for primary total knee arthroplasty. For the routine case, most surgeons select a specific implant that in their hands has worked well. There are select situations, however, in which surgeons must have various options at their disposal. This chapter outlines the various total knee arthroplasty options available to the orthopedic surgeon today.

FEMORAL COMPONENT OPTIONS

For the femoral component of a total knee replacement, the surgeon should be familiar with several options that are available in terms of fixation, sagittal contour of the implant, metallurgy, constraint, stem availability, stem variations, and potential for metal augmentation. Initially, all the femoral components in the total knee arthroplasty construct were cemented. In the early and mid-1980s, cementless fixation on the femoral side of the total knee construct also became available (1–5). Although there was much initial enthusiasm for cementless fixation in the total knee arthroplasty construct and although there are still champions of this approach, including Whiteside (5), the majority of implants today are placed with cemented fixation. Cementless fixation of the femoral component has fared better than cementless fixation of the tibial component, however, and many surgeons still use the option of a cementless femoral component with a cemented tibial component, as the predictability of ingrowth on the femoral side has been excellent in many series (2,6). Among cemented femoral implants, most components provide indentation pockets on the undersurface of the implant so that cement can interdigitate with the implant (Fig. 1). Most of these contact surfaces are also relatively rough rather than polished. In cementless femoral fixation implants, both beaded and fiber mesh surfaces are available (Fig. 2) (1,5). A number of autopsy retrieval studies have shown excellent bony ingrowth fixation into both of these surfaces (1,5,6). Hydroxyapatite-coated surfaces have not been commonly used in cementless fixation of either the femoral component or the tibial component; however, some manufacturers provide this option.

The sagittal contour of the femoral component varies among various implants. In general, the term for the sagittal contour is the J curve. This terminology has developed because the patellar flange is usually longer than the posterior condylar flange of the implant, which gives the appearance of a J. Femoral components can have a changing radius from anterior to posterior or a constant radius (Fig. 3). It is still unclear whether one of these alternatives is more beneficial. Those surgeons that champion the constant-radius approach believe that the patellofemoral mechanics are improved. Implants with longer J curves may also provide more friendly patellofemoral joint mechanics and less soft tissue impingement, although no study has definitely demonstrated this theoretical advantage.

The femoral component of the total knee arthroplasty construct was initially chrome cobalt in most cases. In the early 1980s, titanium surfaces became available. In most cases, the titanium surface was ion-bombarded to harden that surface. Although femoral scratching has been noted on the retrieval of some components, in general both the titanium and chrome cobalt surfaces have provided a durable bearing surface. More recently, ceramic and zirconium oxide femoral bearing surfaces have been developed to potentially decrease any femoral component scratching (Fig. 4). Their material properties are harder than those of the chrome cobalt and titanium surfaces used today. Although not approved

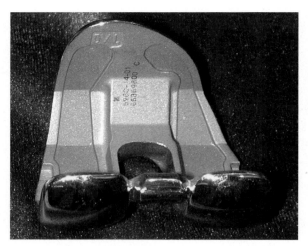

FIG. 1. Typical femoral component used for cemented application with pocket indentations for cement capture.

for use in this country, ceramic femoral components have been developed and used in Japan and other countries.

In terms of the potential to direct the kinematic motions of the knee to promote or constrain motions in various directions, the surgeon has the option to use posterior cruciate–retaining devices, posterior cruciate–sacrificing devices, posterior cruciate–substituting devices, and the more constraining Total Condylar III (Zimmer, Warsaw, IN) types of devices (7–21). All posterior cruciate–retaining devices spare intercondylar notch bone. In addition, all are anatomic in that there are both right and left components. The original posterior cruciate–sacrificing devices as well as the posterior cruciate–substituting devices were symmetrical medially and laterally; hence, right and left devices were not needed. Presently, however, even with posterior cruciate–sacrificing and posterior cruciate–substituting devices, many companies have anatomic patellofemoral grooves, so that right and left components are

required. Especially in the revision setting, it is important for the orthopedic surgeon to recognize these differences in planning the operation. Among posterior cruciate–substituting devices, some are open boxed, which some designers believe is beneficial because less intercondylar notch bone is sacrificed, and some are closed boxed (Fig. 3). There are a number of constraining components available today (11,22). The original device in this category was the Total Condylar III (11). The surgeon should be aware of the amount of constraint provided by the femoral implant and tibial spine of the implant he or she is using.

On the femoral side of the total knee arthroplasty construct, pegs have been used for added femoral fixation in most posterior cruciate–retaining designs. The femoral box provides added fixation for the posterior cruciate–substituting designs; however, at least one posterior cruciate–substituting design also has peg augmentation along with the fixation provided by the femoral box (Fig. 5). In most systems today, cemented or cementless stems can be added to the femoral component, and although these are not commonly used in the primary total knee arthroplasty construct, there are certain situations in which they may be employed (Fig. 6). These include cases in which there are large areas of osteonecrosis of the femoral condyles; cases in which the anterior femoral cortex has been notched intraoperatively, especially in patients with osteopenia; and cases in which femoral osteotomies have been incorporated into the total knee construct, that is, when extraarticular deformity is present and in both very active and very osteopenic patients (23). The benefit of cemented stems is that they provide the most secure fixation; cementless stems provide less secure fixation but are more easily retrievable in the case of revision or infection. The main purpose of these stems is to prevent bending moments around the implant-bone interface.

Metal modular femoral augments, both distal and posterior, are available in most total knee arthroplasty systems (Fig. 7). In cases of previous trauma or markedly deficient femoral condyles, these augments can be beneficial in the primary replacement setting.

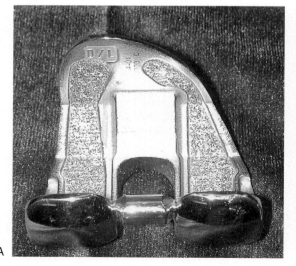

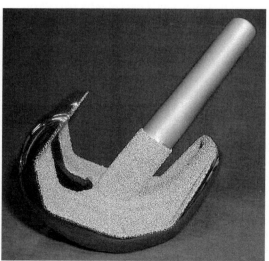

FIG. 2. Typical femoral components used for cementless application with fiber metal **(A)** or porous bead **(B)** ingrowth surfaces.

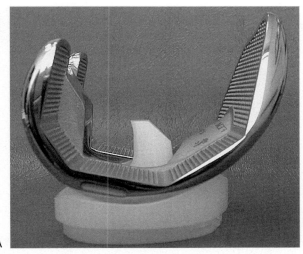
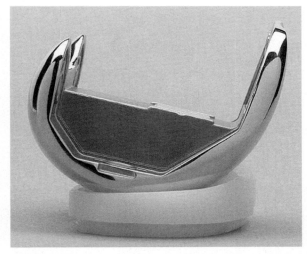

FIG. 3. Sagittal view of femoral components with single radius of curvature **(A)** and changing radius **(B)**. The same components demonstrate an open box **(A)** and closed box **(B)** posterior cruciate–substituting mechanism.

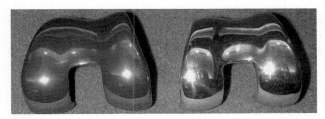

FIG. 4. Femoral components with zirconium oxide **(left)** and chrome cobalt **(right)** material.

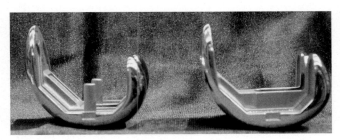

FIG. 5. Typical posterior cruciate–retaining femoral component with peg fixation **(left)** and posterior cruciate–substituting femoral component with central box fixation **(right)**.

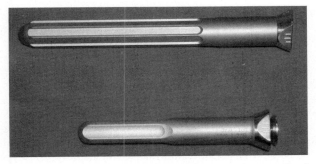

FIG. 6. Typical fluted femoral stem **(top)** for cementless fixation and smoother tapered stem **(bottom)** for cemented fixation.

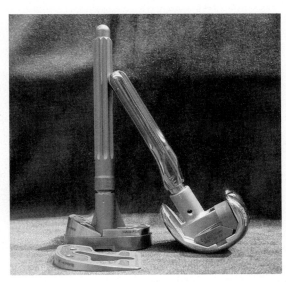

FIG. 7. Offset modular femoral stem with modular distal femoral augments and modular tibial wedge and block augments.

TIBIAL COMPONENT OPTIONS

For the tibial component, there are various fixation options, metallurgy options, polyethylene constraint, tibial tray option, stem options, and augment options. Both cemented and cementless tibial component fixation options are available in most total knee systems. Although the majority of tibial components are cemented, cementless fixation is still championed by several renowned knee replacement surgeons (5,6,24). For cemented fixation, the options include the use of keels or center post versus resurfacing of the tibial surface only (Figs. 8 and 9). Freeman initially championed simple resurfacing of the tibial surface, and this approach was later supported from Montreal (6) (Fig. 8). The original Miller-Galante prosthesis with this form of fixation has provided durable results in the hands of

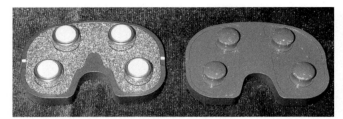

FIG. 8. Tibial resurfacing components for cementless **(left)** and cemented **(right)** fixation.

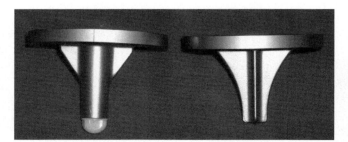

FIG. 9. Modular **(left)** and keel **(right)** tibial stems.

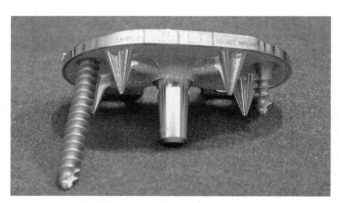

FIG. 10. Tibial tray for cementless fixation with post, spikes, and screw augmentation.

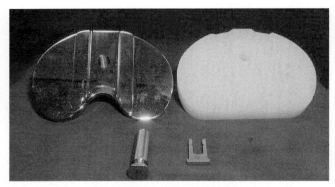

FIG. 11. Polished tibial tray.

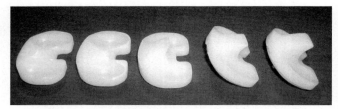

FIG. 12. Modular tibial inserts with increasing conformity and constraint from left to right, starting with a flat posterior cruciate–retaining liner and ending at the right with a constraining Total Condylar III–type inset.

selected surgeons (6). Most components today rely on keel or post fixation to counteract bending moments around the tray. Keels can be cemented or left without cement with only resurfacing of the cut tibial surface (25). For cementless tibial fixation, options also include resurfacing types or keel-type stem supports (Figs. 8 through 10). In most cementless designs, screws or spikes are also added to better secure the implant to the cut tibial surface, as autopsy retrievals have in general shown limited ingrowth into the tibial surfaces, especially compared to the ingrowth documented on the femoral side of the construct (5). With regard to the metallurgy of the tibial component, both titanium and chrome cobalt surfaces have been used. Many tibial trays have been made of titanium, especially those with the modular design, as it is simpler to machine the capturing mechanism into the softer titanium surfaces. With the recognition of backside wear noted with modular tibial trays (26–29), there is enthusiasm for returning to harder chrome cobalt metallurgy,

with polishing of the top of the tibial trays so as to limit the potential for abrasive wear between the tray and polyethylene liner insert when micromotion occurs (Fig. 11).

In terms of the constraint provided by the tibial surface articulating with the femoral component, a number of options are available (Fig. 12). With the original posterior cruciate–retaining designs, most articulating polyethylene surfaces were relatively flat to avoid constraint in the kinematics between the femoral component and tibial component so that the posterior cruciate ligament could function optimally. With time, however, consideration of the trade-off between the avoidance of constraint and the potential for adding more surface area of contact between polyethylene and femoral component led to the development of more conforming curved insets (9,10). Posterior cruciate–sacrificing devices have always had relatively large amounts of conformity between the femoral component and the polyethylene surface, and posterior cruciate–sacrificing components have become increasingly available (ultracongruent liners) (30). For posterior cruciate–substituting devices, the surgeon should recognize that every tibial post is different and is positioned differently in the anterior/posterior plane. In addition, all tibial posts provide different amounts of rotational constraint. Some concerns over femoral box tibial post impingement and wear have been recognized (17,27). All designs may not be equally susceptible to this problem; however, the optimal design for preventing this difficulty is still under investigation. Finally, more constraining Total Condylar III–type posts are available that provide anterior-posterior and medial-lateral stability. These are not commonly used in the primary knee replacement construct; however, in cases of large valgus deformity, medial col-

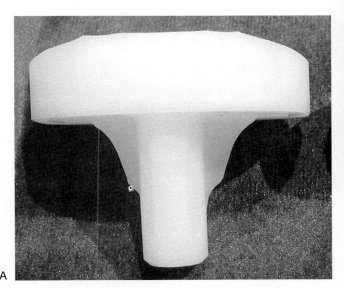

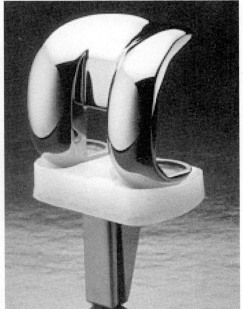

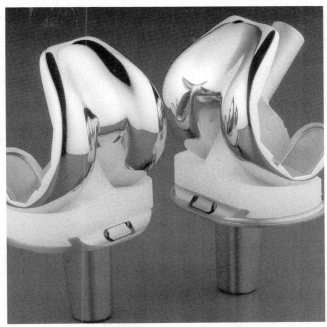

FIG. 13. Typical evolution of tibial component options from all polyethylene component **(A)**, to monoblock metal component **(B)**, to modular metal-backed component **(C)**.

lateral ligament rupture, and relative instability in older patients, these constructs can be useful in primary total knee replacement (11,22). For the tibial tray, all-polyethylene components, modular metal-backed components, and mono-blocked metal-back components in which the polyethylene has been applied to the metal tray by the manufacturer are available (Fig. 13). Proponents of the all-polyethylene trays are concerned with the problems related to backside wear of modular components (31,32). However, the modular components provide maximum versatility. The monoblocked tibial trays offer the benefit of protecting the tibial bone cement interface provided by a metal-backed tray without the clinical problems associated with backside wear. Tibial stems and

posts are available for both cemented and cementless fixation. In addition, in the primary situation, especially when there has been a prior tibial osteotomy, tibial offset stems may provide fixation while avoiding penetration of the tibial stem into the tibial-fibular interosseous membrane (Fig. 14). Also, although not commonly needed in the primary situation, wedges and block metal augments should be available for the surgeon in cases of severe intraarticular or extraarticular deformities created by trauma or congenital or developmental defects. The potential benefit of blocks over wedges is that they provide less shear stresses between the implant and bone; however, the potential downside is that more bone must be resected to accommodate these blocks.

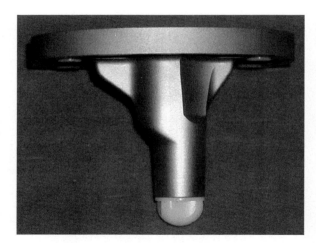

FIG. 14. Modular offset tibial stem.

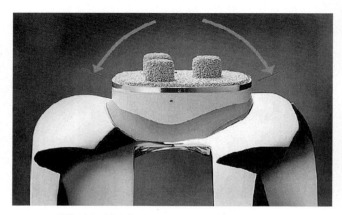

FIG. 15. Mobile bearing patellar component.

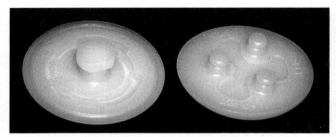

FIG. 16. Central (left) versus peripheral (right) peg options on patellar components.

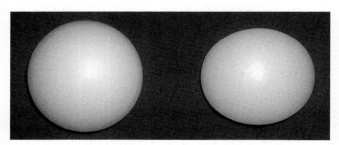

FIG. 17. Round (left) and oval (right) patellar component options.

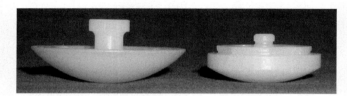

FIG. 18. Resurfacing (left) and inset (right) patellar component options.

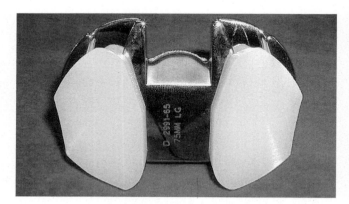

FIG. 19. Meniscal bearing mobile bearing knee replacement.

PATELLAR COMPONENT OPTIONS

In determining the patella component to be used in the total knee arthroplasty construct, if it is to be used at all, the considerations are the type of fixation, use of multiple pegs versus center posts, use of anatomic versus spherical components, use of all-polyethylene versus metal-backed components, and the use of a fixed versus mobile bearing component if metal backing is used. Although cementless patellar fixation has been reported to provide durable results in selected series, numerous series have shown more problems related to fracture of the metal pegs, delamination of the polyethylene from the metal backing, and wear when either cementless or cemented metal-backed components are used (33–35). Because of these reported problems, most patellar components are cemented today. One exception to this cited in the literature is cases in which a mobile bearing cementless patellar component was used (36) (Fig. 15).

With regard to design features of the component, fixation can be provided by multiple pegs or a central post (Fig. 16). Both designs have provided durable results long term (36). Those who favor multiple-peg fixation do so because mechanical studies have shown the best bone of the patella to be in the central portion. Both anatomic and oval or spherical components have

been used (Fig. 17). Both have provided durable results in many series (36). Inset patellar components are also available (Fig. 18). The metal backing of cemented patella components has fallen into disfavor in recent years because of the poor durability of these components compared to cemented components of similar design (33).

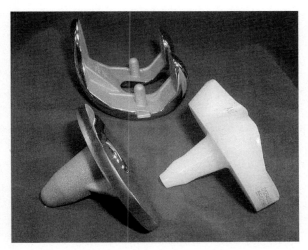

FIG. 20. Rotating platform mobile bearing knee replacement.

MOBILE BEARING KNEE TECHNOLOGY

Mobile bearing knee technology has been available for close to a quarter of a century and, in several series, has demonstrated durable long-term results with favorable wear characteristics for the implant. More recently, however, enthusiasm for these devices has arisen because of the concern for backside wear of modular tibial trays, the fact that total knee replacements are being performed in younger and younger patients, and the hope for improving knee kinematics (37,38). These components can provide meniscal-type bearing or rotating platform–type bearing surfaces (Figs. 19 and 20). Many of the newer designs have bumpers to limit motion in various directions as well as to promote motion in other directions. Some have a changing sagittal-plane radius, whereas some provide a uniform sagittal-plane radius. The surgeon should recognize the design features of the mobile-bearing implant he or she is selecting, as every manufacturer has different design criteria.

Even in the primary situation, use of a hinged or hinged type of component is occasionally indicated (39–42). Especially in osteopenic intercondylar and supracondylar fractures in the elderly, these devices can provide a quick solution for returning the patient to optimal function (40). Both fixed- and mobile-bearing designs are available (Fig. 21).

CONCLUSION

With regard to femoral, tibial, and patellar implant options, the orthopedic surgeon today has multiple choices. Although the surgeon may select one design for the routine case, he or she should be aware of the multiple options available for dealing with any particular clinical situation that presents.

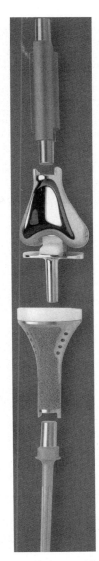

FIG. 21. Modular rotating hinge total knee replacement components.

REFERENCES

1. Berger RA, Lyon JH, Jacobs JJ, et al. Problems with cementless total knee arthroplasty at 11 years followup. *Clin Orthop* 2001;392:196.
2. Campbell MD, Duffy GP, Trousdale RT. Femoral component failure in hybrid total knee arthroplasty. *Clin Orthop* 1998;356:58.
3. Duffy GP, Berry DJ, Rand JA. Cement versus cementless fixation in total knee arthroplasty. *Clin Orthop* 1998;356:66.
4. McCaskie AW, Deehan DJ, Green TP, et al. Randomised, prospective study comparing cemented and cementless total knee replacement: results of press-fit condylar total knee replacement at five years. *J Bone Joint Surg Br* 1998;80:971.
5. Whiteside LA. Cementless total knee replacement: 9- to 11-year results and 10-year survivorship analysis. *Clin Orthop* 1994;309:185.
6. Silverton C, Rosenberg AO, Barden RM, et al. The prosthesis-bone interface adjacent to tibial components inserted without cement: clinical and radiographic follow-up at nine to twelve years. *J Bone Joint Surg Am* 1996;78:340.
7. Benjamin J, Szivek J, Dersam G, et al. Linear and volumetric wear of tibial inserts in posterior cruciate-retaining knee arthroplasties. *Clin Orthop* 2001;392:131.
8. Colizza WA, Insall JN, Scuderi GR. The posterior stabilized total knee prosthesis. Assessment of polyethylene damage and osteolysis after a ten-year-minimum follow-up. *J Bone Joint Surg Am* 1995;77:1713.
9. D'Lima DD, Chen PC, Colwell CW. Polyethylene contact stresses, articular congruity, and knee alignment. *Clin Orthop* 2001;392:232.
10. D'Lima DD, Hermida JC, Chen PC, et al. Polyethylene wear and variations in knee kinematics. *Clin Orthop* 2001;392:124.
11. Easley ME, Insall JN, Scuderi GR, et al. Primary constrained

condylar knee arthroplasty for the arthritic valgus knee. *Clin Orthop* 2000;380:58.

12. Font-Rodriguez DE, Scuderi GR, Insall JN. Survivorship of cemented total knee arthroplasty. *Clin Orthop* 1997;345:79.

13. Hirsch HS, Lotke PA, Morrison LD. The posterior cruciate ligament in total knee surgery: save, sacrifice, or substitute? *Clin Orthop* 1994;309:64.

14. Lombardi AV, Mallory TH, Fada RA, et al. An algorithm for the posterior cruciate ligament in total knee arthroplasty. *Clin Orthop* 2001;392:75.

15. Lonner JH, Hershman S, Mont M, et al. Total knee arthroplasty in patients 40 years of age and younger with osteonecrosis. *Clin Orthop* 2000;380:85.

16. Malkani AL, Rand JA, Bryan RS, et al. Total knee arthroplasty with the kinematic condylar prosthesis: a ten-year follow-up study. *J Bone Joint Surg Am* 1995;77:423.

17. Mikulak SA, Mahoney OM, Dela Rosa MA, et al. Loosening and osteolysis with the press-fit condylar posterior-cruciate-substituting total knee replacement. *J Bone Joint Surg Am* 2001;83:398.

18. Pagnano MW, Cushner FD, Scott WN. Role of the posterior cruciate ligament in total knee arthroplasty. *J Am Acad Orthop Surg* 1998;6:176.

19. Rand JA, Ilstrup DM. Survivorship analysis of total knee arthroplasty: cumulative rates of survival of 9200 total knee arthroplasties. *J Bone Joint Surg Am* 1991;73:397.

20. Scuderi GR, Insall JN, Windsor RE, et al. Survivorship of cemented knee replacements. *J Bone Joint Surg Br* 1989;71:798.

21. Thadani PJ, Vince KG, Ortaaslan SG, et al. The Insall award. Ten- to 12-year followup of the Insall-Burnstein I total knee prosthesis. *Clin Orthop* 2000;380:17.

22. Scuderi GR. Revision total knee arthroplasty: how much constraint is enough? *Clin Orthop* 2001;392:300.

23. Rodrigo JJ, Hazelwood SJ, Farver TB, et al. Total knee replacement with interlocking stems: a preliminary report. *Clin Orthop* 2001;392:139.

24. Engh GA, Bobyn JD, Petersen TL. Radiographic and histologic study of porous coated tibial component fixation in cementless total knee arthroplasty. *Orthopedics* 1988;5:725.

25. Bert JM, McShane M. Is it necessary to cement the tibial stem in cemented total knee arthroplasty? *Clin Orthop* 1998;356:73.

26. Parks NL, Engh GA, Topoleski T, et al. The Coventry Award: modular tibial insert micromotion: a concern with contemporary knee implants. *Clin Orthop* 1998;356:10.

27. Puloski SKT, McCalden RW, MacDonald SJ, et al. Tibial post wear in posterior stabilized total knee arthroplasty: an unrecognized source of polyethylene debris. *J Bone Joint Surg Am* 2001;83:390.

28. Wasielewski RC, Galante JO, Leighty RM, et al. Wear patterns on retrieved polyethylene tibial inserts and their relationship to technical considerations during total knee arthroplasty. *Clin Orthop* 1994;299:31.

29. Wasielewski RC, Parks N, Williams I, et al. Tibial insert undersurface as a contributing source of polyethylene wear debris. *Clin Orthop* 1997;345:53.

30. Laskin RS, Maruyama Y, Villaneuva M, et al. Deep-dish congruent tibial component use in total knee arthroplasty: a randomized prospective study. *Clin Orthop* 2000;380:36.

31. Gioe TJ, Bowman KR. A randomized comparison of all-polyethylene and metal-backed tibial components. *Clin Orthop* 2000;380:108.

32. Rodriguez JA, Baez N, Rasquinha V, et al. Metal-backed and all-polyethylene tibial components in total knee replacement. *Clin Orthop* 2001;392:174.

33. Bayley JC, Scott RD, Ewald FC, et al. Failure of the metal-backed patellar component after total knee replacement. *J Bone Joint Surg Am* 1988;70:668.

34. Kraay MJ, Darr OJ, Salata MJ, et al. Outcome of metal-backed cementless patellar components: the effect of implant design. *Clin Orthop* 2001;392:239.

35. Rosenberg AG, Andriacchi TP, Barden R, et al. Patellar component failure in cementless total knee arthroplasty. *Clin Orthop* 1988;236:106.

36. Larson CM, McDowell CM, Lachiewicz PF. One-peg versus three-peg patella component fixation in total knee arthroplasty. *Clin Orthop* 2001;392:94.

37. Callaghan JJ. Mobile-bearing knee replacement: clinical results: a review of the literature. *Clin Orthop* 2001;392:221.

38. D'Lima DD, Trice M, Urquhart AG, et al. Comparison between the kinematics of fixed and rotating bearing knee prostheses. *Clin Orthop* 2000;380:151.

39. Barrack RL. Evolution of the rotating hinge for complex total knee arthroplasty. *Clin Orthop* 2001;392:292.

40. Bell KM, Johnstone AJ, Court-Brown CM, et al. Primary knee arthroplasty for distal femoral fractures in elderly patients. *J Bone Joint Surg Br* 1992;74:400.

41. Jones RE, Barrack RL, Skedros J. Modular, mobile-bearing hinge total knee arthroplasty. *Clin Orthop* 2001;392:306.

42. Springer BD, Hanseen AD, Sim FH, et al. The kinematic rotating hinge prosthesis for complex knee arthroplasty. *Clin Orthop* 2001;392:283.

CHAPTER 72

Implant Fixation—Cement

Edward Michael Keating and John B. Meding

Cement remains the "gold standard" for implant fixation in total knee replacement (TKR). Long-term data support the use of cement as the fixation method of choice. Twelve- to 15-year follow-up studies of cemented TKR using multiple prosthetic designs are common and have shown good to excellent results, with more than 85% survivorship at 12 years and beyond. These designs include the total condylar (1–8), posterior cruciate condylar (9–12), kinematic (13–15), Insall-Burstein posterior stabilized (Zimmer, Warsaw, IN) (16–18), low-contact stress (19,20), and the Anatomic Graduated Components (Biomet, Warsaw, IN) (21,22). Although much less common, several studies have shown similar results with cementless fixation using the Ortholoc and the Press-Fit Condylar designs (23,24). Based on the overwhelming success of cemented TKR, surgeons must carefully consider whether or not a reason exists *not* to use cement in almost any age or diagnostic group.

The advantages of cemented fixation in TKR include the allowance of immediate weightbearing. This advantage may be even more important in patients with polyarticular arthritis where upper extremity disease may preclude the protracted use of crutches or a walker. Some authors have even shown increased failure rates when uncemented fixation is used with certain prosthetic designs. In a prospective study from the Mayo Clinic, Duffy et al. reported 10-year survival rates of 72% and 94% in uncemented and cemented knees, respectively (25). Ezzet et al. (26) also reported higher rates of osteolysis in uncemented knees compared with knees with cemented fixation of all three components. Finally, because of the higher polyethylene wear rates associated with uncemented metal-backed patellar components placing the femoral component at risk as well (27), most TKR designs include an all-polyethylene cemented button.

Obtaining rigid initial fixation at the prosthesis–cement–bone interface is one of the most important factors in preventing mechanical loosening and achieving satisfactory long-term results in TKR (28). Even if this initial fixation is obtained, cemented implant migration may occur as a result of failure at any level between the implant and bone, including the bone cement. However, because both the compressive and tensile strength of polymethylmethacrylate is greater than bone, failure, when it does occur, is most likely to occur from bone fatigue than from cement fatigue (29). As such, many prosthetic designs use metal backing of the tibial components to minimize

the increased stress to cancellous bone that is known to occur during loading after TKR (29). Interestingly, little variation in cemented tibial component migration has been noted between stem designs of the tray (30). While metal trays may reduce bone stresses, failure at this level may still occur during extreme loading conditions such as occurs in cases of instability, component malposition, and malalignment. Thus, cement technique is only one of several surgeon-dependent variables that will affect the success or failure of cemented component fixation.

Cement technique in TKR may vary but usually involves the use of high-pressure and/or high-volume lavage. This technique not only removes fat and blood debris, both associated with venous clot formation in cemented TKR (31), but also increases the penetration of cement into cancellous bone (32,33). Inadequate preparation of the bony surfaces has been associated with a higher incidence of radiolucent lines about the bone–cement interface (33,34). Furthermore, such improper preparation has resulted in significantly lower implant survival up to 10 years postoperatively (33). The use of high-volume and high-pressure pulsed lavage to thoroughly clean the cancellous bone and remove fat and marrow elements has almost completely eliminated these radiolucent lines (Fig. 1).

Because the quality of the interlock between the bone–cement and the cement–prosthesis interface affects the mechanical strength, some surgeons prefer cement pressurization rather than finger packing to increase the penetration of cement into bone (35). Although such penetration may improve the tensile and shear strength at the bone–cement interface, cement pressurization, as opposed to simple finger packing, has not necessarily been associated with improved implant survival (33). Similarly, nearly all cemented knee components use a roughened or porous surface to enhance the mechanical strength between the prosthesis and cement. In contradistinction, implant stability was enhanced with certain prosthetic designs with the addition of cement surrounding the tibial stem or keel (36).

The author's preferred technique includes a thorough high-pressure and high-volume pulsatile lavage of the osseous surfaces, suction drying, and pressurization of a low-viscosity polymethylmethacrylate cement. Suction drying of all the bony surfaces, however, generally allows adequate pressurization of normal viscosity cement (Fig. 2). All three components are generally cemented after one vacuum mix, beginning with the tibial

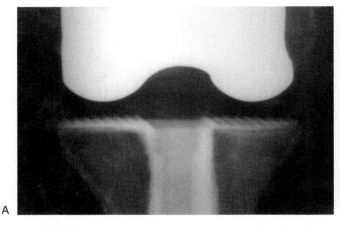

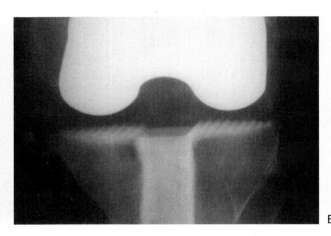

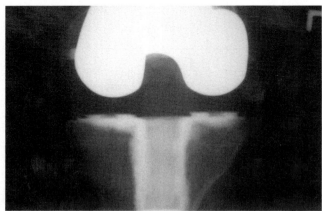

FIG. 1. Radiographs of bone-cement interface after three different cementing techniques. **A:** Depicts finger packing of cement after no preparation of the bony surfaces. Note the interface radiolucencies in the medial and lateral tibial zones on the 2-month postoperative radiograph. After jet lavage and suction drying, radiolucencies are not present, but cement penetration into the bone is minimal with finger packing **(B)**. Further penetration of cement into bone is evident when pressurization of cement is added after proper bone preparation **(C)**.

prosthesis if a posterior cruciate retaining prosthesis is used. If a posterior cruciate sacrificing prosthesis is used, the femoral component is cemented first. All cement excrescences are removed and the knee is thoroughly irrigated with the same high-pressure, high-volume jet lavage to avoid third-body wear. Helmers et al. (37) reported that the amount of particulate debris removed after irrigation continues up to 6 L of pressurized irrigant. However, the vast majority of the material was removed during the 4 L of irrigation. As such, irrigation with more than three to four liters of fluid is probably not necessary.

Many brands of cement are commercially available. Variations may therefore exist in the elastic modulus, fatigue strength, and tensile and compressive strengths of the different preparations. Further variability may be added with attempts at porosity reduction including vacuum mixing and centrifugation. Yet, to our knowledge, only Boneloc bone cement has been

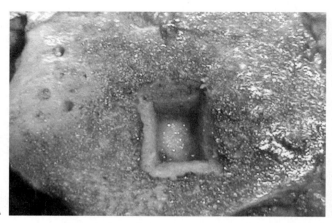

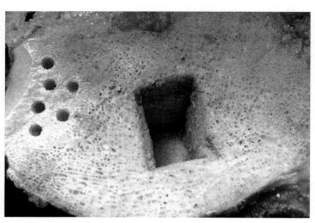

FIG. 2. Intraoperative examples of inadequate and proper bone preparation. **A:** Shows blood and debris on the bony surfaces that can clearly limit cement penetration. After jet lavage and suction drying, the bony surfaces are ready for cementation **(B)**.

reported in the literature to be associated with inferior clinical results in cemented TKR (38).

Several long-term series (more than 10-year follow-up) have been reported, with *survivorship* defined as loosening or revision of any component (excluding infection). Some of these reports have also included the incidence of radiolucent lines. In general, radiolucencies are considered important only if they are global—that is, in all zones about a prosthesis—or if they are more than 1 to 2 mm and/or progressive. These reviews testify to the success of cemented TKR.

A 20-year follow-up study of 220 total condylar replacements noted 85% survival at 21 years, with a 42% and 49% incidence of radiolucent lines about the tibial and femoral components, respectively (39). Another report of 120 total condylar replacements with an average follow-up of 14 years noted 91% survivorship at 23 years (40).

In a minimum 10-year follow-up study comparing 101 Insall-Burstein I and 117 Insall-Burstein II prostheses, 96% and 98% survival, respectively, was reported. The incidence of radiolucent lines was 11% in the Insall-Burstein I and 29% in the Insall-Burstein II. No radiolucent lines were reported around the femoral components (41).

The Mayo Clinic reviewed 168 kinematic condylar prostheses with an average follow-up of 15 years and reported 85% survival (42). A 20-year survival of 98% was reported in 64 rotating platform Low Contact Stress total knees, with an average follow-up of 12 years. No radiolucent lines were reported about any knees (43). Survivorship of 4,583 Anatomic Graduated Component replacements at 15 years was 99%. Follow-up averaged 11 years (44).

Ten-year survival rates of 172 Miller-Galante I and 109 Miller-Galante II knee systems were 84% and 100%, respectively. Radiolucencies were seen approximately 14% and 13% of the tibial components, respectively; 10% and 11% of the femoral components, respectively; and 7% and 1.4% of patellar components, respectively (45).

Finally, a 10-year review of 100 Genesis total knees reported a 97% survival. Radiolucent lines were seen in approximately 14% of tibial components (46).

In summary, cemented TKR has achieved a high rate of success. It is generally accepted that cemented fixation be used for older, less active patients and uncemented fixation be reserved for younger patients. Yet, long-term data suggest that cemented TKR, which involves meticulous bone preparation at surgery, may be indicated for all age groups.

REFERENCES

1. Font-Rodriguez DE, Scuderi GR, Insall JN. Survivorship of cemented total knee arthroplasty. *Clin Orthop* 1997;345:79–85.
2. Gill GS, Joshi AB, Mills DM. Total condylar knee arthroplasty. 16 to 21 year results. *Clin Orthop* 1999;367:210–215.
3. Goldberg VM, Figgie MP, Figgie HE, et al. Use of a total condylar knee prosthesis for treatment of osteoarthritis and rheumatoid arthritis. Long term results. *J Bone Joint Surg* 1988;70:802–811.
4. Ranawat CS, Flynn WF, Deshmukh RG. Impact of modern technique on long-term results of total condylar knee arthroplasty. *Clin Orthop* 1995;309:131–135.
5. Ranawat CS, Flynn WF, Saddler S, et al. Long-term results of total condylar knee arthroplasty. A 15-year survivorship study. *Clin Orthop* 1993;286:94–102.
6. Ranawat CS, Boacjie-Aadjei O. Survivorship analysis and results of total condylar knee arthroplasty. Eight- to 11-year follow-up period. *Clin Orthop* 1988;226:6–13.
7. Scuderi GR, Insall JN, Windsor RE, Morgan MC. Survivorship of cemented knee replacements. *J Bone Joint Surg Br* 1989;71:798–803.
8. Vince KG, Insall JN, Kelly MA. The total condylar prosthesis. 10- to 12-year results of a cemented knee replacement. *J Bone Joint Surg Br* 1989;71:793–797.
9. Dennis DA, Clayton ML, O'Donnell S, et al. Posterior cruciate condylar total knee arthroplasty. Average 11-year follow-up evaluation. *Clin Orthop* 1992;281:168–176.
10. Rand JA. Comparison of metal-backed and all-polyethylene tibial components in cruciate condylar total knee arthroplasty. *J Arthroplasty* 1993;8:307–313.
11. Ritter MA, Campbell E, Faris PM, et al. Long-term survival analysis of the posterior cruciate condylar total knee arthroplasty. A 10-year evaluation. *J Arthroplasty* 1989;4:293–296.
12. Ritter MA, Herbst SA, Keating EM, et al. Long-term survival analysis of a posterior cruciate-retaining total condylar total knee arthroplasty. *Clin Orthop* 1994;309:36–145.
13. Ewald FC, Wright RJ, Poss R, et al. Kinematic total knee arthroplasty. A 10- to 14-year prospective follow-up review. *J Arthroplasty* 1999;14:473–480.
14. Malkani AL, Rand JA, Bryan RS, et al. Total knee arthroplasty with the kinematic condylar prosthesis. A ten-year follow-up study. *J Bone Joint Surg Am* 1995;77:423–431.
15. Weir J, Moran CG, Pinder IM. Kinematic condylar total knee arthroplasty. 14-year survivorship analysis of 208 consecutive cases. *J Bone Joint Surg Br* 1996;78:907–911.
16. Colizza WA, Insall JN, Scuderi GR. The posterior stabilized total knee prosthesis. Assessment of polyethylene damage and osteolysis after a ten-year minimum follow-up. *J Bone Joint Surg Am* 1995;77:1713–1720.
17. Scott WN, Rubenstein M, Scuderi G. Results after total knee replacement with a posterior cruciate-substituting prosthesis. *J Bone Joint Surg Am* 1988;70:1163–1173.
18. Stern SH, Insall JN. Posterior stabilized prosthesis. Results after follow-up of nine to twelve years. *J Bone Joint Surg Am* 1992;74:980–986.
19. Callaghan JJ, Squire MW, Goetz DD, et al. Cemented rotating-platform total knee replacement. A nine to twelve-year study. *J Bone Joint Surg Am* 2000;82:705–711.
20. Sorrells RB. Primary knee arthroplasty: long-term outcomes. The rotating platform mobile bearing TKA. *Orthopaedics* 1996;19:793–796.
21. Emerson RH, Higgins LL, Head WC. The AGC total knee prosthesis at average 11 years. *J Arthroplasty* 2000;15:418–421.
22. Ritter MA, Worland R, Saliski J, et al. Flat-on-flat, nonconstrained, compression molded polyethylene total knee replacement. *Clin Orthop* 1995;321:79–85.
23. Whiteside LA. Cementless total knee replacement. Nine- to 11-year results and 10-year survivorship analysis. *Clin Orthop* 1994;309:185–192.
24. Schai PA, Thornhill TS, Scott RD. Total knee arthroplasty with the PFC system. Results at a minimum of ten years and survivorship analysis. *J Bone Joint Surg Br* 1998;80:850–858.
25. Duffy GP, Berry DJ, Rand JA. Cement versus cementless fixation in total knee arthroplasty. *Clin Orthop* 1998;356:66–72.
26. Ezzet KA, Garcia R, Barrack RL. Effect of component fixation method on osteolysis in total knee arthroplasty. *Clin Orthop* 1995;321:86–91.
27. Rosenberg AG, Andriacchi TP, Barden R, et al. Patellar component failure in cementless total knee arthroplasty. *Clin Orthop* 1988;236:106–114.
28. Ryd L, Lindstrand A, Rosenquist R, et al. Tibial component fixation in knee arthroplasty. *Clin Orthop* 1986;213:144–149.
29. Burstein AH, Wright TM. Biomechanics. In: Insall JN, et al., eds. *Surgery of the knee*, 2nd ed. New York: Churchill Livingstone, 1993:61.
30. Stern SH, Wills, RD, Gilbert JL. The effect of tibial stem design on component micromotion in knee arthroplasty. *Clin Orthop* 1997;345:44–52.

31. Berman AT, Parmet JL, Harding SP, et al. Emboli observed with use of transesophageal echocardiography immediately after tourniquet release during total knee arthroplasty with cement. *J Bone Joint Surg Am* 1998;80:389–396.

32. Maistrelli GL, Antonelli L, Fornasier V, et al. Cement penetration with pulsed lavage versus syringe irrigation in total knee arthroplasty. *Clin Orthop* 1995;312:261–265.

33. Ritter MA, Herbst SA, Keating EM, et al. Radiolucency at the bone-cement interface in total knee replacement. *J Bone Joint Surg Am* 1994;76:60–65.

34. Insall JN, Hood RW, Flawn LB, et al. The total condylar knee prosthesis in gonarthrosis. A five to nine-year follow-up of the first one hundred consecutive replacements. *J Bone Joint Surg Am* 1983;65:619–628.

35. Krause WR, Krug W, Eng B, et al. Strength of the cement-bone interface. *Clin Orthop* 1982;163:290–299.

36. Bert JM, McShane M. Is it necessary to cement the tibial stem in cemented total knee arthroplasty? *Clin Orthop* 1998;356:73–78.

37. Helmers S, Sharkey PF, McGuigan FX. Efficacy of irrigation for removal of particulate debris after cemented total knee arthroplasty. *J Arthroplasty* 1999;14:549–552.

38. Nilsson KG, Dalen T. Inferior performance of Boneloc bone cement in total knee arthroplasty. A prospective randomized study comparing Boneloc with Palacos using radiostereometry (RSA) in 19 patients. *Acta Orthop Scand* 1998;69:479–483.

39. Rodriguez JA, Bhende H, Ranawat CS. Total condylar knee replacement. A 20-year followup study. *Clin Orthop* 2001;388:10–17.

40. Pavone V, Boettner F, Fickert S, et al. Total condylar knee arthroplasty. A long-term followup. *Clin Orthop* 2001;388:18–25.

41. Bassard MF, Insall JN, Scuderi GR, et al. Does modularity affect clinical success? A comparison with a minimum 10-year followup. *Clin Orthop* 2001;388:26–32.

42. Sextro GS, Berry DJ, Rand JA. Total knee arthroplasty using cruciate-retaining kinematic condylar prosthesis. *Clin Orthop* 2001;388:33–40.

43. Buechel FF Sr, Buechel FF Jr, Pappas MJ, et al. Twenty-year evaluation of meniscal bearing and rotating platform knee replacements. *Clin Orthop* 2001;388:41–50.

44. Ritter MA, Berend ME, Meding JB, et al. Long-term followup of anatomic graduated components posterior cruciate-retaining total knee replacement. *Clin Orthop* 2001;388:51–57.

45. Berger RA, Rosenberg AG, Barden RM, et al. Long-term followup of the Miller-Galante total knee replacement. *Clin Orthop* 2001;388:58–67.

46. Laskin, RS. The Genesis total knee prosthesis. A 10-year followup study. *Clin Orthop* 2001;388:95–102.

CHAPTER 73

Cementless Fixation in Primary Total Knee Arthroplasty

Aaron A. Hofmann and John David Evanich

The decision to use cemented or cementless implant fixation has been debated since the advent of modern total knee arthroplasty. Although many of the early prostheses were implanted without cement (1–3), cemented fixation soon became the mainstay of total knee replacement. During the 1980s, a resurgence of interest in cementless fixation was spurred in part by the dissatisfaction with cemented fixation (4). Cement failure by fragmentation and debonding resulted in loosening of the prosthesis. These failures combined with the trend of total knee arthroplasty in younger, more active patients led to the exploration for a more durable, secure, and biologically viable form of implant fixation (5).

The advantages of modern cementless fixation over cemented fixation include a more durable method of fixation (6), a relatively bone-sparing technique (Fig. 1) (6,7), and the avoidance of cement complications such as cement disease (8). Aside from relieving pain and restoring function, cementless fixation in total knee arthroplasty attempts to offer a permanent fixation solution to those patients with disabling degenerative knee disease. Through a biologic microinterlock with dynamic remodeling capabilities between patient's bone and the prosthetic porous surface, cementless fixation aims to offer a total knee replacement that can last a lifetime.

BONE INGROWTH

Lasting mechanical stability in cementless total knee implants requires bone ingrowth into the porous surface. Successful bone ingrowth is known to be dependent on several factors. Many studies have demonstrated the importance of pore size (9–15), porous surface composition (9,16–26), intimate bone-implant apposition (27–34), and relative lack of motion at the bone-implant interface (35–47).

Pore Size

Optimal pore size favorable to bone ingrowth has been investigated (9,10). Bobyn et al. (9) examined the growth of osseous tissue into cobalt alloy rods coated with cobalt alloy powder of four different particle sizes. This coating method produced surfaces with pore sizes of 20 to 800 μm and fully interconnecting voids. After implanting these rods into the lateral cortex of beagle femurs, the rate of bone ingrowth and maximum fixation strengths attained were measured. Implants with pore sizes of less than 50 μm had incomplete ingrowth of calcified tissue and inferior mechanical strength at all time periods. Those with pore sizes

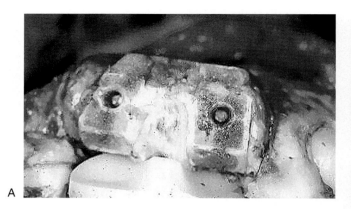

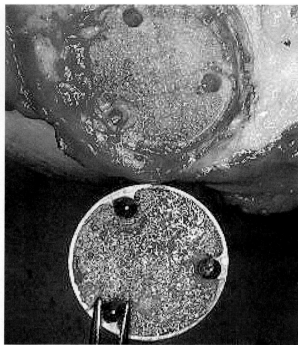

FIG. 1. Excellent preservation of bone stock noted at time of revision of well-fixed femoral **(A)** and patellar **(B)** components.

of 50 to 400 μm had complete bone ingrowth at 8 weeks. Bone and fibrous tissue was apparent at 8 and 12 weeks in those implants with pore sizes of more than 400 μm. Implants with pore sizes of 50 to 400 μm developed a greater maximal strength of fixation more quickly than those with pore sizes of more than 400 μm. It was theorized that because the pore size was smaller, bone more quickly filled the pore spaces, and in turn, the implant reached maximum fixation more rapidly. Thus, a 50- to 400-μm pore size was considered optimal for biologic fixation of porous-surfaced implants. Hulbert et al. (12) demonstrated that a pore size of 100 μm allowed for bone ingrowth, but a pore size of 150 μm was required for osteon formation. Through his analysis of the vascular requirements of bone relative to pore size, Skinner (14) theorized that an effective porous structure in humans would require interconnecting pores of 300 to 1,000 μm. In humans, implant retrieval studies have shown that pore sizes of 400 to 600 μm allow for consistent bone ingrowth (28,48–52).

Porous Surface Composition

Titanium and cobalt chromium alloys are the most common materials used in modern porous surface preparations. Animal studies have demonstrated bone ingrowth into both of these alloy materials (9,16,17). Investigators have cautioned against extrapolating animal bone ingrowth data into human applications because of possible species differences (10,27,53). Hofmann (19) studied the difference between titanium and cobalt chromium alloy implants in human subjects. Identically structured cylinders were implanted in the load-bearing surface of distal femoral condyles of humans with osteoarthritis. The amount of bone ingrowth and the mineral apposition rate (a measurement of new mineralized bone laid down per unit of time) were quantified after explantation. A significant difference

in bone ingrowth existed, with the titanium implants experiencing ingrowth almost double the amount measured in the cobalt chromium porous coatings. The mineral apposition rates were similar between the two alloys, but the direction of cancellous bone remodeling differed. The cancellous bone advanced toward the titanium but away from the cobalt chromium. These differences suggest that titanium alloy is more biocompatible than cobalt chromium as a porous surface material.

Ceramics, particularly hydroxyapatite, have been investigated as a possible augment to porous-coating fixation in total knee arthroplasty (18,20–25). Calcium phosphate (hydroxyapatite) is thought to act as an osteoconductive scaffolding, promoting the growth of bone into the porous surface. This ingrowth, in turn, enhances the initial stability of the prosthesis (26). Hofmann et al. (20) compared human cancellous bone remodeling with titanium- and hydroxyapatite-coated implants. The use of hydroxyapatite increased bone ingrowth by 8%, but a significantly lower bone mineral content at the implant interface was measured. Gaps of 50 to 500 μm filled with fibrous tissue were observed on both the titanium- and hydroxyapatite-coated implants, suggesting that hydroxyapatite-coated devices still require precise surgical placement and intimate bone–implant contact. The use of hydroxyapatite to enhance the fixation of knee prostheses has been evaluated only with limited follow-up of 2 to 5 years (21–25). Comparisons of porous-coated implants to those augmented with hydroxyapatite showed a slight increase in subsidence (using radiostereometric analysis) of the nonaugmented implants, but no significant clinical differences were measured at 2 years (21,24,25). When comparing hydroxyapatite-coated implants with cemented implants, hydroxyapatite-coated implants had increased initial migration that stabilized at 3 months; no difference in overall micromotion existed at 24 months (23).

The use of ceramic coating is not without risks. Nilsson et al. (22) reported on an early failure, with complete debonding of the hydroxyapatite from the entire medial tibial plateau undersurface at 8 weeks. The marginal and equivocal improvements gained by the use of hydroxyapatite, coupled with its increased cost, have limited the widespread use of this technology in cementless total knee arthroplasty.

Intimate Bone–Implant Apposition

Intimate bone–implant apposition is required for bone ingrowth to occur (27,29). Bloebaum et al. (27) noted that bone ingrowth did not occur when bone was over 50 μm from the porous coating. A cadaver study evaluating flatness of the tibial condyles after bone resection found that the clinically flat tibial plateau had a maximum roughness of 1.4 mm (34). This measurement was the distance between the uppermost and lowermost points on the resected tibial plateau. Bloebaum et al. (54) found that 76% of the surface area of the proximal tibia consisted of bone marrow space. Hofmann et al. (30,32,55) and Bloebaum et al. (28) have shown that by placing morselized autograft bone chips at the bone-implant interface, one can decrease the cancellous bone porosity and smooth out the roughness of the resected proximal tibial plateau, thereby immediately increasing the contact between the host bone and porous coating. This increased initial contact has been shown to directly correlate with increased bone ingrowth (32). Surgical technique is very important in attaining this close contact and cannot be overlooked (27,33,56). The use of precision cutting instruments and a high degree of technical accomplishment are required for successful cementless knee implantation.

Lack of Motion at Bone-Implant Interface

A microinterlock between the bone and a porous-coated implant is required for bone ingrowth to occur. Initial implant movement relative to bone may prevent bone ingrowth and promote fibrous tissue ingrowth instead (36,37,41). Evaluating porous-coated staple pullout strength in mongrel dogs, Cameron et al. (36) concluded that ingrowth can occur with micromovement but not macromovement. Freeman and Tennant (37) hypothesized that initial micromotion equal to the pore size (typically 250 to 600 μm) of the porous-coated implant would prevent ingrowth of any tissue into the pores, in particular, bone ingrowth. Pilliar et al. (41) determined that bone ingrowth can, in the presence of some movement (up to 28 μm) and excess movement (150 μm or more), result in the attachment of connective tissue. Modern cementless knee systems incorporate various forms of adjunctive fixation to help increase initial stability. Multiple studies have confirmed an improvement in initial implant stability with the use of press-fit stems/pegs and screw fixation (35,38–40,42,43–47).

COMPONENT DESIGN CONSIDERATIONS

Cementless designs for knee replacement incorporate the current understanding of the basic science principles involving bone ingrowth. The designs by anatomic location of the individual knee components reflect many of the concepts previously discussed.

Femoral Component

The porous-coated femoral component has been used successfully in both hybrid and cementless total knee arthroplasty (6,55,57). Reliable fixation to bone and good clinical results have been demonstrated in both applications. Problems with femoral component fixation are rare because of the femoral chamfer cuts and the inherent three-dimensional structure of the distal femur, which together allow for a stable press-fit.

Porous-coated pegs have been shown to cause adverse changes and the loss of bone mineral density in the distal femur (58). A significant increase in the bone adjacent to the porous-coated fixation pegs resulted in stress shielding of the bone anteriorly at as early as 1 year. This relative osteopenic area has correlated with areas of significant bone loss at the time of revision. Porous-coated pegs also increased the possibility of a distal femoral periprosthetic fracture secondary to an osteopenic stress riser. Fixation pegs can be helpful in maintaining rotational alignment, but the clinical experience and literature demonstrate they should be smooth and not porous coated (6,58).

With regard to the patellofemoral articulation, avoidance of a box-shaped femoral component and use of a femoral component with a deep trochlear inset and generous radius profile have been shown to prevent excess loads on the patellar component while allowing good range of motion (Fig. 2) (6,59,60).

Tibial Component

As in cemented total knee arthroplasty, the tibial component has been the biggest challenge in obtaining lasting, secure fixation. Some initial designs were flat with short pegs. These designs demonstrated difficulty in obtaining and maintaining fixation, often resulting in subsidence or lift-off (61–64). Biomechanical studies have shown that when loading tibial components fixed only with short pegs, the loaded side subsides and the opposite side lifts off (44). The addition of stems and screws to the initial designs helped stabilize the component and eliminated excess micromotion (Fig. 2) (35,38–40,43–47,65). Metal backing of polyethylene tibial components also increased their rigidity and decreased the maximal cancellous compressive stresses of the proximal tibia (66). All of these improvements aimed at increasing rigidity and improving stability decreased micromotion between the bone and the implant and, in turn, allowed for bone ingrowth (28,48).

The use of adjunctive tibial screw fixation has been associated with osteolysis in some clinical studies (6,67–69). The screw hole and screw are thought to provide a conduit for polyethylene wear debris to the undersurface of the tibia. The reported incidence of screw track osteolysis varies from 0% to 31% in large reported clinical series (6,68,69). Lewis et al. (68) reviewed radiographs of 217 cementless knees of various designs and found a 31% incidence of screw osteolysis. They hypothesized that the design of the components, particularly the polyethylene attachment mechanism, was responsible for the difference in the frequency of osteolysis among the various designs. Hofmann et al. (6) reported no cases of screw track osteolysis in 176 cementless Natural

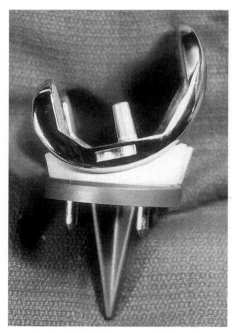

FIG. 2. Example of generous radius curvature of femoral component and cruciate stem augmentation of tibial component (Natural Knee).

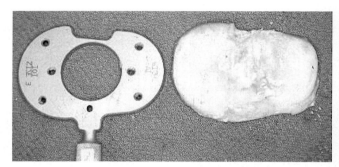

FIG. 3. Asymmetric proximal tibial drill guide and resected proximal tibial wafer.

Knees at a minimum follow-up of 10 years. They attributed the lack of screw-associated osteolysis to a secure tibial insert locking mechanism, intimate screw hole and head fit, and screw hole sealing from the plastic creep of the undersurface of the polyethylene inserts noted in postmortem retrievals (48).

Whiteside (70) studied the effect of porous-coating configuration on tibial osteolysis after total knee arthroplasty. He observed that smooth metal tracks between the patch porous coating on the undersurface of the tibial component appeared to allow the migration of polyethylene debris from the joint area to the area surrounding the stem and screws. Approximately 20% of his reported knee arthroplasties performed with this design displayed evidence of osteolysis and bone loss at 2 to 4 years postoperatively. Subsequent arthroplasties performed with a newly designed tibial component that was fully porous-coated revealed no evidence of osteolysis at 4 to 8 years postimplantation. Engh et al. (71) also found that smooth metal surfaces provided minimal resistance to osteolysis but reported that porous-coated metal interfaces with bone were more resistant to osteolysis. Therefore, the clinical data support that the undersurface of the tibial component should be fully porous-coated.

The proximal tibia displays asymmetric anatomy, with the medial plateau larger than the lateral plateau. Anatomic regional analysis of the proximal tibia has shown significantly higher bone quantities in the posterior medial and medial regions as compared with the anterior and anterolateral regions (54). Carter and Hayes (72) have shown that the load-carrying capacity of cancellous bone is not improved by the presence of bone marrow. Thus, maximum contact between the cortical and cancellous bone of the proximal tibia and the tibial component is desired. An asymmetric tibial component, with a larger medial side, is advantageous in improving surface area contact between the tibial component and resected tibial surface; the asymmetric design improves coverage while attempting to avoid soft tissue impingement secondary to lateral component overhang (Fig. 3). The increased coverage allows a more uniform load transmission to the cancellous bone of the proximal tibia (66) and provides more surface area available for bone ingrowth, thereby improving fixation and clinical results (6,48,55).

Patellar Component

Early metal-backed patellar component designs met with varying degrees of failure and success (60,73–80). Wear or fracture of the polyethylene, dissociation of the polyethylene from the base plate, and dissociation of the base plate from the fixation pegs were the most common modes of failure. These failures led to metal-on-metal articulation, proliferative synovitis, and pain. The complications were attributed both to femoral and patellar component design along with surgical technique.

A box-shaped femoral component with a shallow trochlear groove produced excessive forces at the patellofemoral joint (59). In contrast, a generously curved femoral component with a deep trochlear groove decreased patellofemoral load, captured the patellar component, and allowed for a greater range of motion (6,55).

Deleterious patellar design factors included thin polyethylene, a metal endoskeleton for the polyethylene, and porous-coated peg fixation. Significant forces are placed on the patella, particularly in weightbearing flexion (e.g., ascending stairs). Greenwald et al. (81) showed that the contact stresses on the patella during activities of daily living exceed the yield point of polyethylene; thus, some deformation of the plastic always occurs. Therefore it is important to attempt to minimize the forces at the patellofemoral joint and maximize the patellar polyethylene thickness. Many metal-backed patellae were implanted using an onset technique, in which the metal backing of the patellar component was implanted flush with the cut surface of the patella. This technique required the polyethylene to be thin to maintain the overall patellar bone–implant construct thickness. By insetting the metal backing of the patellar component, thicker polyethylene could be used, which minimized wear and fracture complications (75,76). The use of a metal endoskeleton also decreased the thickness of the polyethylene, particularly at the periphery, resulting in the same complications associated with thin polyethylene (77,80). Porous-coated pegs resulted in the same stress shielding complications discussed in Femoral Design. Rosenberg et al. (60) noted bone ingrowth into the porous-coated pegs with variable ingrowth into the plate portion of the patellar component. He observed that peg fixation without plate fixation resulted in high eccentric shear forces at the peg-plate junction, with resultant failure at this junction.

Excellent clinical results have been reported using a fully porous-coated metal-backed patella implanted using an inset technique that countersinks the metal backing and allows for the use of thicker polyethylene (6,75,76). Hofmann et al. (6) reported a 95.1% survival at 10 years of 176 smooth-pegged, metal-backed patellae implanted inset and centered over the anatomic sagittal ridge. Laskin and Bucknell (76) had no revisions of 451 inset metal-backed patellae at an average follow-up of 4 years.

PATIENT SELECTION

Age

Younger patients (younger than 60 years) are often considered excellent candidates for cementless total knee arthroplasty, whereas older patients with compromised bone strength are generally thought to be better served by cemented fixation (82). The literature shows that cementless arthroplasty is appropriate for both younger and older patients (83–85). Hungerford et al. (84) evaluated 52 porous-coated anatomic knee prostheses implanted in 43 patients younger than age 50 years. At an average follow-up of 51 months, the average Hospital for Special Surgery knee score increased from 41 to 90 postoperatively, which compared favorably with reported cemented results. Hofmann (83) evaluated cementless arthroplasty of the knee in patients older than age 65 years. Ninety-seven patients, averaging 71 years of age, were followed for 31 months. Average Hospital for Special Surgery knee scores improved 44 points to 99 at 2 years; knee flexion increased from 109 degrees preoperatively to 123 degrees 2 years postoperatively. Based on these early results, he concluded that cementless total knee arthroplasty can be successful in patients older than 65 years of age and need not be reserved for younger patients. In evaluating the pain relief response of his second-generation cementless knee, Whiteside (85) observed that age made no difference in ultimate pain relief obtained after cementless knee implantation.

Weight

A significant percentage of total knee candidates are obese (86). Weight has not been shown to be an adverse risk factor to cementless total knee arthroplasty (6,87). Mont et al. (87) evaluated 45 obese patients who underwent cementless knee arthroplasty. This group was compared with a matched control group with respect to age, gender, diagnosis, and preoperative deformity. All obese patients weighed more than 94 kg and had a body mass index of greater than 40, with a score of 30 indicating obesity. At a 7-year average follow-up period, no significant differences in the combined percentage of good and excellent clinical results were noted between the two groups.

Bone Quality

Significantly osteoporotic bone has been shown to be a relative contraindication to cementless total knee arthroplasty. Biomechanical studies in synthetic models and cadaver bone have demonstrated that poor bone quality decreases implant stability (40,88). In a biomechanical load study in cadaver tibias, Miura et al. (40) showed that an increase in bone strength significantly reduced the degree of lift-off and micromotion of securely fixed tibial components. Hofmann (83) recommended cementing all components in those patients whose bone appeared soft and was indentable by thumb pressure over the central portion of the resected proximal tibia.

Inflammatory Arthritis

Patients with inflammatory arthritis are often excluded from cementless total knee arthroplasty because of concerns of compromised bone, implant fixation, and bone ingrowth (89). Several studies evaluating patients with rheumatoid arthritis with cementless total knee arthroplasty have shown good to excellent results with short- and intermediate-term follow-up (89–92). Boublik et al. (91) found that knee arthroplasty with cementless components gave results comparable with reported cemented series in patients with juvenile rheumatoid arthritis patients. Fourteen patients, at an average age of 26 years, improved their Knee Society knee scores from 18 to 92 at almost 4 years postoperatively. In Armstrong and Whiteside's (90) study, older rheumatoid patients improved their knee scores from 32 to 88 over a 1- to 7-year follow-up period. At their most recent follow-up, 98% of these older patients reported to be pain-free or had only mild discomfort with weightbearing. Comparing cementless with cemented fixation in knee arthroplasty in rheumatoid patients, Ebert et al. (92) found good to excellent clinical results for 91% in the cementless group versus 81% in the cemented group at an average follow-up of 65 months. The more sedentary activity of the typical rheumatoid patient may place less demand on any knee prosthesis and thereby result in better clinical results.

SURGICAL TECHNIQUE

Cementless total knee arthroplasty requires significant attention to operative detail to obtain successful clinical results. Specific techniques have contributed to long-term component survivorship in the University of Utah experience (6,56). These include the use of precision-cutting instrumentation (56), irrigation of all saw cuts (56,93), proximal tibia resection along the posterior slope (54,94,95), the use of autograft bone chips (27,28,31,32), and exacting patellar preparation (6,56,75).

Precision-cutting instrumentation is essential for cementless total knee arthroplasty. As previously discussed, intimate bone–implant apposition is required for bone ingrowth. Small cancellous surface irregularities that can be tolerated when using acrylic cement, which acts as a grouting agent, are not well tolerated in cementless fixation. In cementless total knee arthroplasty, complete contact of the implant to the bone is required for both initial stability and subsequent biologic ingrowth (27,29). The use of precision instrumentation with exacting tolerances, the use of new cutting blades for each case, and application of attentive operative technique help make successful cementless arthroplasty possible.

Thermal necrosis of bone occurs at 55°C (93). As cementless knee arthroplasty requires viable bone to attach to an implant's porous coating, specific protection against thermal necrosis must be used routinely. Irrigation during bone resection main-

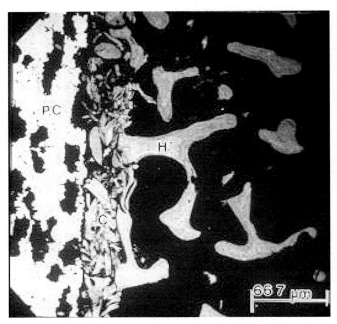

FIG. 4. Postmortem retrieval of tibial component from patient who died of a postoperative myocardial infarction showing autograft bone chips (C) filling the gap between the porous coating (PC) and the host bone (H).

tains the bone temperature at 38°C. Without irrigation, any type of drilling or sawing maneuver may increase the temperature of bone to as high as 170°C (93).

Proximal tibia resection in line with the patient's natural posterior slope improves initial tibial component stability and protects against anterior subsidence (54,94,95). Trabecular bone orientation of the proximal tibia is nearly perpendicular to the anatomic surface (94). Thus, proximal tibial bone resected in line with the natural posterior slope allows the bone to be loaded in compression, perpendicular to the cancellous trabeculae. Conversely, proximal tibial bone resected perpendicular to the long axis of the tibia loads these same trabeculae with a bending moment. From basic mechanics theory, as the trabeculae are angled further from vertical, the mode of failure changes from

buckling to bending, and the load carrying capability decreases (94). Results of mechanical testing have indicated that proximal tibial bone resected parallel to the surface exhibited a 40% greater load-carrying capacity and 70% greater stiffness than bone resected perpendicular to the tibial long axis (94,95).

Autograft bone chips spread on the cancellous surfaces of the tibia, femur, and patella during implantation increase initial bone-implant contact and improve ultimate fixation (27,28,31, 32). The bone chips form a low-viscosity "biologic bone cement" when obtained from the undersurface of the cut cancellous bone surface of the resected tibia wafer when using gentle pressure and a patellar reamer (56). The slurry of bone acts like a grouting agent, filling in inherent gaps within the cancellous bone and smoothing out small irregularities in the cut bone surface (Fig. 4). Aside from decreasing the porosity of the cut bone surfaces and improving initial bone-implant contact, the application of bone chips also increases the speed and amount of bone ingrowth by significantly increasing the mineral apposition rate and host bone available for ingrowth (27,28,31,32). The viability of the autograft bone chips has been established by tetracycline-labeling studies in humans (32).

Patellar-measured resection with component medialization and countersinking has produced excellent clinical results for certain cementless metal-backed patellae (6,75). The measured resection technique dictates that only the thickness of bone that is removed can be replaced. This prevents exceeding the original thickness, which may limit postoperative flexion or subject the component to excessive loads. In an effort to improve patellar tracking, the patellar component should be centered over the sagittal ridge, which is anatomically medial to the center of the patella (Fig. 5) (56). By countersinking (or insetting) the metal backing of the patellar component, thicker patellar polyethylene can be used, which minimizes polyethylene wear and fracture complications (75,76).

MANAGEMENT OF BONE DEFECTS

In primary knee arthroplasty, bone deficiencies are often eliminated with standard bone cuts. Occasionally, bone defects remain after routine preparation of the distal femur and proximal tibia. Limited bone defects can be managed with either autogenous bone graft or metal spacers.

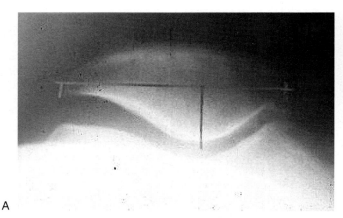
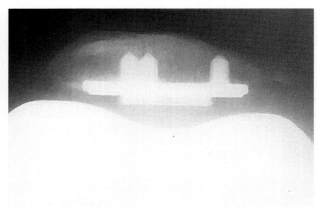

A   B

FIG. 5. Medial location of the sagittal ridge in the native patella **(A)** reproduced by medialization of the resurfaced patella **(B)**.

Contained defects comprising less than 15% to 20% of the surface area of the proximal tibia and distal femur are packed with autogenous bone slurry obtained from the undersurface of the resected tibia wafer (56). As these bone chips are viable (32), bony incorporation into the defect and ingrowth into the porous prosthesis are characteristic.

Uncontained defects are more often seen in the severe varus or valgus knee. In these cases, the deformity is often the direct result of significant bone loss. Small (less than 3 mm), uncontained defects of the tibial plateau may be undercut and replaced with a thicker polyethylene insert. In cases of larger (more than 3 mm) uncontained bone deficiencies of either the medial or lateral tibial plateau, metal spacers may be used for augmentation. Precision-cutting instrumentation is required to ensure intimate bone–prosthesis contact. Uncontained defects of the distal femur often require cemented or revision components, and bone grafting or metal augmentation of the distal femur in cementless knee arthroplasty is not recommended.

COMPLICATIONS

Reported complications of cementless total knee arthroplasty have included metal-backed patellar failure, osteolysis, bone stress shielding, and component fracture. Metal-backed patellar failure, bone stress shielding, and screw-associated osteolysis have been previously discussed in Patellar Component, Femoral Component, and Tibial Component, respectively. Discussions of osteolysis, other than screw-associated, and component fracture are presented here.

Complications secondary to osteolysis have plagued both cemented and cementless methods of fixation. Wear debris osteolysis is an important factor in aseptic implant loosening (96). Articulating surfaces and contact interfaces are potential sources of wear debris regardless of fixation method (97). Knee pain, effusion, and new asymmetric coronal instability are hallmarks of polyethylene wear (98). Risk factors for increased polyethylene wear of tibial inserts include thin (less than 6 mm) insert constructs, heat-pressed manufacturing, increased crystallinity, poor locking mechanisms with resultant backside wear, and use with excessively unconstrained and incongruent knee designs (69,98–103). Peters et al. (69) reported on the high incidence of osteolysis with the Synatomic and Arizona (DePuy, Warsaw, IN) knee designs. The use of thin polyethylene tibial inserts and the abutment of the femoral component on the proud tibial insert spine were implicated as the main contributors to the polyethylene wear debris and ultimate failure of the prostheses. A high incidence of osteolysis with use of the porous-coated anatomic knee also has been well documented (98,99,101,103–105). Bloebaum et al. (99) reported on the early delamination and surface failure of heat-pressed tibial inserts. The use of these heat-pressed tibial inserts and the nature of the unconstrained and incongruent design of the porous-coated anatomic knee were cited as principal reasons for osteolysis in this knee design.

Component fracture in cementless and cemented total knee arthroplasty is exceedingly rare. Using cementless fixation, 37 cases of fractured femoral components have been reported (106–109). Thirty-six fractures have involved the Ortholoc II (Dow Corning Wright, Arlington, TN) femoral component (106,108,109). All fractures occurred at a junction of the beveled surfaces along the distal aspect of the component. More fractures occurred in smaller components and in those components with a double layer (vs. single layer) of sintered beads (109). All components demonstrated evidence of fatigue failure. It was theorized that the combination of the thinness of the metal at the beveled junctions, the decrease in thickness necessary to accommodate the porous coating, the notch effect of the beaded surface, and the weakened base metal secondary to bead sintering were collectively responsible for the component fracture sensitivity (109). Huang et al. (107) reported on regional osteonecrosis as a reason for femoral component fracture in the New Jersey low contact stress knee. Osteonecrosis of the medial femoral condyle caused a loss of medial osseous support for the femoral component. This loss of support coupled with the significant bone ingrowth of the central and lateral flanges resulted in the formation of a medial lever arm, with subsequent fracture of medial flange.

IMPLANT RETRIEVAL STUDIES

Knowledge of basic research analysis terminology proves to be helpful in evaluating and comparing implant retrieval studies. The bone around the implant is often divided into three regions: inside the porous coating (i.e., bone ingrowth) (Fig. 6), in contact with the porous coating (i.e., appositional bone), and within the metaphysis (i.e., host bone) (49). The appositional bone index measures the amount of bone in apparent contact with the porous coating (48). The volume fraction of bone measures the amount of bone per unit area in a specified location.

Implant retrieval studies can be divided into those evaluating malfunctioning components obtained at revision surgery and those analyzing well-functioning prostheses obtained postmortem. Cook et al. (110) reported on 62 total knee components of various designs retrieved primarily at revision surgery at an average of 12 months postimplantation. Revision indications included infection, implant malposition, and unexplained pain. Quantification analysis using a point-counting technique showed no more than 10% of porous coating ingrown with bone in all components; one-third of the components exhibited only fibrous connective tissue ingrowth with no evidence of bone ingrowth. No significant differences in the patterns of tissue

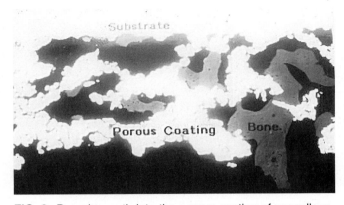

FIG. 6. Bone ingrowth into the porous coating of cancellous-structured titanium (CSTi, Sulzer Orthopedics, Austin, TX).

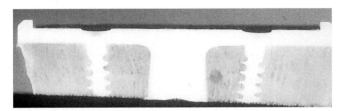

FIG. 7. Contact radiograph showing intimate contact and appositional bone of a postmortem retrieved tibial component with screws. Note the lack of osteolysis about the screw threads.

ingrowth were noted in comparing components based on anatomic location and different designs.

Sumner et al. (111) evaluated 13 Miller-Galante I tibial components revised primarily for unexplained pain and found 9.5% average bone ingrowth. Preferential ingrowth was observed along the porous-coated fixation pegs. The depth and orientation of the resection plane were found to influence the pattern of bone ingrowth. Deeper posterior resections and resections parallel to the tibia surface correlated with increased bone ingrowth. Increased implant stability secondary to the surface parallel orientation of the resection plane likely resulted in increased bone ingrowth.

When evaluating well-functioning prostheses obtained at autopsy, more encouraging results have been reported (48,49,111–113). Vigorita et al. (113) reported on five clinically successful porous-coated anatomic knee implants evaluated histomorphometrically and histologically for bone ingrowth. Average bone ingrowth varied by component, with patellae at 29%, tibias 6%, and femora 8%. Appositional bone at the patellar interface averaged 53%, tibial 36%, and femoral 32%. Bloebaum and colleague's (48) postmortem analysis of eight consecutively retrieved porous-coated Natural Knee tibial components also revealed 6% average bone ingrowth, with an average of 73% appositional bone present (Fig. 7). The 6% bone ingrowth into the porous coating must be considered in light of the fact that the volume fraction of host bone in the tibial metaphysis averages only 10% (48). Thus, 60% (six of ten) of the host bone

available for ingrowth was within the porous coating. Higher percentages of bone ingrowth (8% to 22%) were separately reported by Bloebaum et al. (28) when analyzing 10 asymmetric tibial components removed for various reasons at 1 week to 48 months postimplantation. It was noted that there was a steady increase in bone ingrowth over time, with the ingrown volume fraction of bone stabilizing between 13 and 48 months. The effectiveness of using autograft bone chips to promote fixation was also confirmed. These bone chips, applied to the bone-implant interface during implantation, were integrated and connected to the host bone at 3 to 6 months. Eleven porous-coated metal-backed patellar components evaluated postmortem by Bloebaum et al. (49) demonstrated secure fixation, with an average of 86% appositional bone and 13% bone ingrowth. Higher bone indexes were thought to be partially due to the creation and mechanical impaction of autograft bone chips through patellar reaming. Based on these studies of well-functioning implants, it can be concluded that small (6% to 22%) volume fractions of bone ingrowth into an implant's porous coating, coupled with significant appositional bone support, can yield successful clinical results.

CLINICAL RESULTS

Several studies have evaluated the effectiveness of cementless knee arthroplasty. Many studies, generally with follow-up of less than 5 years, were published to describe the early clinical experience with specific designs (55,114–127). Intermediate and long-term results provide more information regarding the durability and clinical success of any prosthetic design. Table 1 lists the implant survivorship for those prostheses with average clinical follow-up of more than 5 years (6,7,128–137). Cementless total knee replacement has shown to be successful over the long-term when using specific designs to attain biologic fixation (Fig. 8) (6,7). These long-term results are comparable to reported long-term cemented fixation clinical results (138). The ability to achieve these excellent survivorship results in younger, heavier, and often more active patients suggests that cementless biologic fixation could be the answer to a knee replacement that lasts a lifetime (6).

TABLE 1. *Implant survivorship for prostheses with average clinical follow-up of more than 5 years*

Device	Study	Number	Average follow-up (yr) (range)	Survivorship (%) (revision as an end point)	Postoperative range of motion (degrees)	Comments
Intermediate-term results						
Freeman-Samuelson	Samuelson and Nelson (137)	221	7 (5–9)	87.1 at 9 yr	113	All-polyethylene tibial component used Medial subsidence of tibial component characterized failures Abrasion noted on undersurface of tibial components in revision cases Survivorship decreases to 82% when including radiographic subsidence
Freeman-Samuelson	Regner et al. (136)	144	6.8	79 at 10 yr	101	10-yr survival rates decrease to 66% when including clinical failures; decrease to 33% with clinical and radiographic failures Progressive varus tilting of tibial component was early sign of failure Cementless fixation with only macrointerlocking pegs not recommended
Miller-Galante I	Fanning et al. (132)	42	6.4 (5.4–7.0)	Femoral 95 Tibial 93 Patellar 55	—	Large patellar component failure rate Black carbon, fiber-reinforced polyethylene used 39% tibial component lucencies Primary prosthesis no longer available
Performance	Bassett (128)	549	5.2 (3.0–7.9)	Femoral 99 Tibial 99	120	Cemented all-polyethylene patellar component used No screw-associated osteolysis noted
PCA	Dodd et al. (130)	18	5.7	Femoral 100 Tibial 100 Patellar 94	106	Staged, paired knees in cement versus cementless study One-third of patients preferred cementless knee; one-third preferred cemented; one-third found no difference Functional and clinical results equal
PCA	Moran et al. (135)	108	5 (3–8)	84 at 5 yr 78 at 6 yr	103	No patellar resurfacing Collapse of anteromedial plateau most common failure Authors do not recommend use of this design
PCA	Kim and Oh (133)	56	7	Femoral 100 Tibial 100 Patellar 89 Overall 89	112	Additional 30% patellae with evidence of loosening 89% tibial components with evidence of osteolysis 75% polyethylene inserts with evidence of wear Authors do not support continued use of this design
PFC	McKaskie et al. (139)	58	5	98 at 5 yr	102	No patellar resurfacing One revision for infection No clinical differences when compared to cemented cohort
Tricon-M	Cameron and Jung (129)	252	5 (3–8)	86 at 5 yr	—	Polyethylene wear was most common reason for revision Failures associated with metal-backed patellae and thin (<6 mm) tibial inserts Prior high tibial osteotomy had higher incidence of revision
Long-term results						
Natural	Hofmann et al. (6)	176	12 (10–14)	Femoral 99.1 Tibial 99.6 Patellar 95.1 Overall 93.4	120	No screw-associated osteolysis noted Advocates use of autograft bone chips to enhance fixation Overall survivorship includes revisions secondary to infection and late posterior cruciate ligament failure
PFC	Duffy et al. (131)	55	10	Femoral 87.6 Tibial 87.6 Patellar 64.8	100	Large patellar component failure Indications limited to young age, good bone stock, and stable initial implant fixation Survivorship of femoral and tibial components decreases to 72.7% when including radiographic failure
Whiteside Ortholoc	Whiteside (7)	163	10 (9–11)	94.1 at 10 yr	115	60/265 knees (23%) lost to follow-up Excellent remaining bone stock noted at revision surgery

PCA, porous-coated anatomic knee; PFC, PFC Sigma.

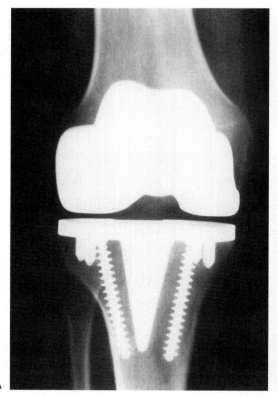 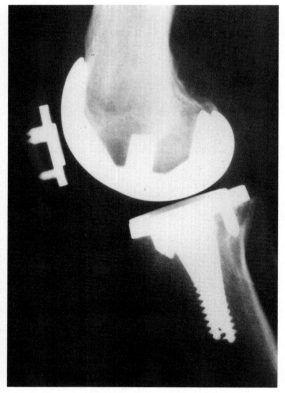

A

B

FIG. 8. Anteroposterior **(A)** and lateral knee **(B)** radiographs of an active 71-year-old patient 10 years status postimplantation of a cementless Natural Knee.

REFERENCES

1. Jones GB. Arthroplasty of the knee by the Walldius prosthesis. *J Bone Joint Surg Br* 1968;50:505–510.
2. Ring PA. Uncemented surface replacement of the knee joint. *Clin Orthop* 1980;148:106–111.
3. Walldius B. Arthroplasty of the knee using an endoprosthesis. *Acta Orthop Scand* 1957;24:8–16.
4. Miller J. Fixation in total knee arthroplasty. In: Insall JN, ed. *Surgery of the knee*. New York: Churchill Livingstone 1984:717–728.
5. Landon GC, Galante JO, Casini J. Essay on total knee arthroplasty. *Clin Orthop* 1985;192:69–74.
6. Hofmann AA, Evanich JD, Ferguson R, et al. Ten- to 14-year clinical follow-up of the cementless Natural Knee system. *Clin Orthop* 2001;388:85–94.
7. Whiteside LA. Cementless total knee replacement: nine to eleven year results and ten year survivorship analysis. *Clin Orthop* 1994;309:185–192.
8. Jones LC, Hungerford DS. Cement disease. *Clin Orthop* 1987;225:192–206.
9. Bobyn JD, Pilliar RM, Cameron HU, et al. The optimum pore size for the fixation of porous-surfaced metal implants by the ingrowth of bone. *Clin Orthop* 1980;150:263–270.
10. Bobyn JD, Pilliar RM, Cameron HU, et al. Osteogenic phenomena across endosteal bone-implant spaces with porous surfaced intramedullary implants. *Acta Orthop Scand* 1981;52:145–153.
11. Galante J, Rostoker W, Lueck R, et al. Sintered fiber metal composites as a basis for attachment of implants to bone. *J Bone Joint Surg Am* 1971;53:101–114.
12. Hulbert SF, Klawitter JJ, Talbert CD, et al. *Research in dental and medical materials*. New York: Plenum Press 1969.
13. Landon GC, Galante JO, Maley MM. Noncemented total knee arthroplasty. *Clin Orthop* 1986;205:49–57.
14. Skinner H. Analysis of the oxygen supply to porous implants in bone. *Med Inform* 1979;4:143.
15. Welsh RP, Pilliar RM, Macnab I. Surgical implants: the role of surface porosity in fixation to bone and acrylic. *J Bone Joint Surg Am* 1971;53:963–975.
16. Bachus KN, Hofmann AA, Dauterman LA. Canine and human cancellous bony ingrowth into cobalt chrome and titanium porous coated implants—a backscattered electron microscopic analysis. *Trans Orthopaed Res Soc* 1988;13:308.
17. Bobyn JD, Cameron HU, Abdulla D, et al. Biologic fixation and bone modeling with an unconstrained canine total knee prosthesis. *Clin Orthop* 1982;166:301–312.
18. Carlsson L, Regner L, Johansson C, et al. Bone response to hydroxyapatite-coated and commercially pure titanium implants in the human arthritic knee. *J Orthop Res* 1994;12:274–285.
19. Hofmann AA. Response of human cancellous bone to identically structured commercially pure titanium and cobalt chromium alloy porous-coated cylinders. *Clin Mater* 1993;14:101–115.
20. Hofmann AA, Bachus KN, Bloebaum RD. Comparative study of human cancellous bone remodeling to titanium and hydroxyapatite-coated implants. *J Arthroplasty* 1993;8:157–166.
21. Nelissen RGHH, Valstar ER, Rozing PM. The effect of hydroxyapatite on the micromotion of total knee prostheses. A prospective, randomized, double-blind study. *J Bone Joint Surg Am* 1998;80:1665–1672.
22. Nilsson KG, Cajander S, Karrholm J. Early failure of hydroxyapatite-coating in total knee arthroplasty. A case report. *Acta Orthop Scand* 1994;65:212–214.
23. Nilsson KG, Karrholm J, Carlsson L, et al. Hydroxyapatite coating versus cemented fixation of the tibial component in total knee arthroplasty: prospective randomized comparison of hydroxyapatite-coated and cemented tibial components with 5-year follow-up using radiostereometry. *J Arthroplasty* 1999;14:9–20.
24. Onsten I, Nordqvist A, Carlsson AS, et al. Hydroxyapatite augmentation of the porous coating improves fixation of tibial components. A randomised RSA study in 116 patients. *J Bone Joint Surg Br* 1998;80:417–425.
25. Regner L, Carlsson L, Karrholm J, et al. Ceramic coating improves

tibial component fixation in total knee arthroplasty. *J Arthroplasty* 1998;13:882–889.

26. Søballe K, Hansen ES, Brockstedt-Rasmussen H, et al. Hydroxyapatite coating enhances fixation of porous coated implants. *Acta Orthop Scand* 1990;61:299–306.

27. Bloebaum RD, Bachus KN, Momberger NG, et al. Mineral apposition rates of human cancellous bone at the interface of porous coated implants. *J Biomed Mater Res* 1994;28:537–544.

28. Bloebaum RD, Rubman MH, Hofmann AA. Bone ingrowth into porous-coated tibial components implanted with autograft bone chips: analysis of ten consecutively retrieved implants. *J Arthroplasty* 1992;7:483–493.

29. Carlsson L, Rostlund T, Albrektsson B, et al. Implant fixation improved by close fit. Cylindrical implant-bone interface studied in rabbits. *Acta Orthop Scand* 1988;59:272–275.

30. Hofmann AA. The cementless alternative to TKA. *Orthopedics* 1996;19:789–791.

31. Hofmann AA, Bloebaum RD, Bachus KN. Progression of human bone ingrowth into porous-coated implants. *Acta Orthop Scand* 1997;68:161–166.

32. Hofmann AA, Bloebaum RD, Rubman MH, et al. Microscopic analysis of autograft bone applied at the interface of porous-coated devices in human cancellous bone. *Int Orthop* 1992;16:349–358.

33. Hungerford DS. The technique of cementless total knee replacement. *Techniques Orthop* 1991;6:1–7.

34. Toksvig-Larsen S, Ryd L. Surface flatness after bone cutting: a cadaver study of tibial condyles. *Acta Orthop Scand* 1991;62:15–18.

35. Cameron HU. Noncemented tibial components: does a stem help? *Contemp Orthop* 1992;24:326–330.

36. Cameron HU, Pilliar RM, Macnab I. The effect of movement on the bonding of porous metal to bone. *J Biomed Mater Res* 1973;7:301–311.

37. Freeman MAR, Tennant R. The scientific basis of cement vs. cementless fixation. *Clin Orthop* 1992;276:19–25.

38. Kaiser AD, Whiteside LA. The effect of screws and pegs on the initial fixation stability of an uncemented unicondylar knee replacement. *Clin Orthop* 1990;259:169–187.

39. Kraemer WJ, Harrington IJ, Hearn TC. Micromotion secondary to axial, torsional, and shear loads in two models of cementless tibial components. *J Arthroplasty* 1995;10:227–235.

40. Miura H, Whiteside LA, Easley JC, et al. Effects of screws and a sleeve on initial fixation in uncemented total knee tibial components. *Clin Orthop* 1990;259:160–168.

41. Pilliar RM, Lee JM, Maniatopoulos C. Observations on the effect of movement on bone ingrowth into porous-surfaced implants. *Clin Orthop* 1986;208:108–113.

42. Shimagaki H, Bechtold JE, Sherman RE, et al. Stability of initial fixation of the tibial component in cementless total knee arthroplasty. *J Orthop Res* 1990;8:64–71.

43. Sumner DR, Turner TM, Dawson D, et al. Effect of pegs and screws on bone ingrowth in cementless total knee arthroplasty. *Clin Orthop* 1994;309:150–155.

44. Volz RG, Nisbet JK, Lee RW, et al. The mechanical stability of various noncemented tibial components. *Clin Orthop* 1988;226:38–42.

45. Whiteside LA. Four screws for fixation of the tibial component in cementless total knee arthroplasty. *Clin Orthop* 1994;299:72–76.

46. Wyatt RWB, Alpert JP, Daniels AU, et al. The effect of screw fixation on initial rigidity of tibial knee components. *J Appl Biomater* 1991;2:109–113.

47. Yoshii I, Whiteside L, Milliano M, et al. The effect of central stem and stem length on micromovement of the tibial tray. *J Arthroplasty* 1992;7:433–438.

48. Bloebaum RD, Bachus KN, Jensen JW, et al. Postmortem analysis of consecutively retrieved asymmetric porous-coated tibial components. *J Arthroplasty* 1997;12:920–929.

49. Bloebaum RD, Bachus KN, Jensen JW, et al. Porous-coated metal-backed patellar components in total knee replacement. *J Bone Joint Surg Am* 1998;80:518–528.

50. Bloebaum RD, Bachus KN, Rubman MH, et al. Postmortem comparative analysis of titanium and hydroxyapatite porous coated femoral implants retrieved from the same patient. *J Arthroplasty* 1993;8:203–211.

51. Engh CA, Hooten JP Jr., Zettl-Schaffer KF, et al. Evaluation of bone ingrowth in proximally and extensively porous-coated anatomic medullary locking prostheses retrieved at autopsy. *J Bone Joint Surg Am* 1995;77:903–910.

52. Pidhorz LE, Urban RM, Jacobs JJ, et al. A quantitative study of bone and soft tissues in cementless porous-coated acetabular components retrieved at autopsy. *J Arthroplasty* 1993;8:213–225.

53. Kuo TY, Skedros JG, Bloebaum RD. Comparison of human, primate, and canine femora: implications for biomaterials testing in total hip replacement. *J Biomed Mater Res* 1998;40:475–489.

54. Bloebaum RD, Bachus KN, Mitchell W, et al. Analysis of the bone surface area in resected tibia. Implications in tibial component subsidence and fixation. *Clin Orthop* 1994;309:2–10.

55. Hofmann AA, Murdock LE, Wyatt RWB, Alpert JP. Total knee arthroplasty: two- to four-year experience using an asymmetric tibial tray and a deep trochlear-grooved femoral component. *Clin Orthop* 1991;269:78–88.

56. Hofmann AA. Total knee replacement using the Natural-Knee system. *Techniques Orthop* 1987;1:1–17.

57. Kobs J, Lachiewicz P. Hybrid total knee arthroplasty: two- to five-year results using the Miller-Galante prosthesis. *Clin Orthop* 1993;286:78–87.

58. Petersen MM, Olsen C, Lauritzen JB, et al. Changes in bone mineral density of the distal femur following uncemented total knee arthroplasty. *J Arthroplasty* 1995;10:7–11.

59. Firestone TP, Teeny SM, Krackow KA, et al. The clinical and roentgenographic results of cementless porous-coated patellar fixation. *Clin Orthop* 1991;273:184–189.

60. Rosenberg AG, Andriacchi TP, Barden R, et al. Patellar component failure in cementless total knee arthroplasty. *Clin Orthop* 1988;236:106–114.

61. Branson PJ, Steege J, Wixson RL, et al. Rigidity of initial fixation with uncemented tibial knee implants. *J Arthroplasty* 1989;4:21–26.

62. Nilsson KG, Karrholm J, Ekelund L, et al. Evaluation of micromotion in cemented vs. uncemented knee arthroplasty in osteoarthrosis and rheumatoid arthritis: randomized study using roentgen stereophotogrammetric analysis. *J Arthroplasty* 1991;6:265–278.

63. Ryd L. Micromotion in knee arthroplasty: a roentgen stereophotogrammetric analysis of tibial component fixation. *Acta Orthop Scand* 1986;57:3–71.

64. Ryd L, Lindstrand A, Stenstrom A, et al. Porous coated anatomic tricompartmental tibial components: the relationship between prosthetic position and micromotion. *Clin Orthop* 1990;251:189–197.

65. Volz RG, Kantor SG, Howe C, et al. Factors affecting tibial component stability: a comparative study. In: Rand JA, Lawrence DD, eds. *Total arthroplasty of the knee: proceedings of the Knee Society 1985–1986.* Rockville, MD: Aspen Publishers, 1987:109–120.

66. Murase K, Crowninshield RD, Pedersen DR, et al. An analysis of tibial component design in total knee arthroplasty. *J Biomech* 1983;16:13–22.

67. Engh GA, Parks NL, Ammeen DJ. Tibial osteolysis in cementless total knee arthroplasty. A review of 25 cases treated with and without tibial component revision. *Clin Orthop* 1994;309:33–43.

68. Lewis PL, Rorabeck CH, Bourne RB. Screw osteolysis after cementless total knee replacement. *Clin Orthop* 1995;321:173–177.

69. Peters PC, Engh GA, Dwyer KA, et al. Osteolysis after total knee arthroplasty without cement. *J Bone Joint Surg Am* 1992;74:864–876.

70. Whiteside LA. Effect of porous-coating configuration on tibial osteolysis after total knee arthroplasty. *Clin Orthop* 1995;321:92–97.

71. Engh G, Dwyer K, Hanes C. Polyethylene wear of metal-backed tibial components in total and unicompartmental knee prostheses. *J Bone Joint Surg Br* 1992;74:9–17.

72. Carter DB, Hayes WD. The compressive behavior of bone as a two-phase porous structure. *J Bone Joint Surg Am* 1977;59:954–962.

73. Bayley JC, Scott RD. Further observations on metal-backed patellar component failure. *Clin Orthop* 1988;236:82–87.

74. Bayley JC, Scott RD, Ewald FC, et al. Failure of the metal-backed patellar component after total knee replacement. *J Bone Joint Surg Am* 1988;70:668–674.

75. Evanich CJ, Tkach T, von Glinski S, et al. 6- to 10-year experience using countersunk metal-backed patellas. *J Arthroplasty* 1997;12:149–154.

76. Laskin R, Bucknell A. The use of metal-backed patellar prostheses in total knee arthroplasty. *Clin Orthop* 1990;260:52–55.

77. Lombardi AV, Engh GA, Volz RG, et al. Fracture/dissociation of the polyethylene in metal-backed patellar components in total knee arthroplasty. *J Bone Joint Surg Am* 1988;70:675–679.

78. Mont MA, Becher OJ, Lee CW, et al. Patellofemoral complications after total knee arthroplasty: a comparison of Modular Porous-Coated Anatomic with Duracon prostheses. *Am J Orthop* 1999;24:241–247.

79. Rader CP, Lohr J, Wittmann R, et al. Results of total arthroplasty with a metal-backed patellar component: a 6-year follow-up study. *J Arthroplasty* 1996;11:923–930.

80. Stulberg SD, Stulberg BN, Hamati Y, et al. Failure mechanisms of metal-backed patellar components. *Clin Orthop* 1988;236:88–105.

81. Greenwald A, Cepulo A, Black J, et al. Mechanical characteristics of the patello-femoral replacement. *Orthop Trans* 1983;8:41.

82. Krakow KA. Uncemented total knee arthroplasty: a two to eight years survey and analysis of multi-center, multi-system results. *Am J Knee Surgery* 1988;1:42.

83. Hofmann AA. Cementless total knee arthroplasty in patients over 65 years old. *Clin Orthop* 1991;271:28–34.

84. Hungerford DS, Krackow KA, Kenna RV. Cementless total knee replacement in patients 50 years old and under. *Orthop Clin North Am* 1989;20:131–145.

85. Whiteside LA. The effect of patient age, gender, and tibial component fixation on pain relief after cementless total knee arthroplasty. *Clin Orthop* 1991;271:21–27.

86. Leach RE, Baumgard S, Broom J. Obesity: its relationship to osteoarthritis of the knee. *Clin Orthop* 1973;93:271–273.

87. Mont MA, Mathur SK, Krackow KA, et al. Cementless total knee arthroplasty in obese patients: a comparison with a matched control group. *J Arthroplasty* 1996;11:153–156.

88. Lee R, Volz R, Sheridan D. The role of fixation and bone quality on the mechanical stability of tibial knee components. *Clin Orthop* 1991;273:177–183.

89. Stuchin SA, Ruoff M, Matarese W. Cementless total knee arthroplasty in patients with inflammatory arthritis and compromised bone. *Clin Orthop* 1991;273:42–51.

90. Armstrong RA, Whiteside LA. Results of cementless total knee arthroplasty in an older rheumatoid arthritis population. *J Arthroplasty* 1991;6:357–362.

91. Boublik M, Tsahakis PJ, Scott RD. Cementless total knee arthroplasty in juvenile onset rheumatoid arthritis. *Clin Orthop* 1995;286:88–93.

92. Ebert FR, Krackow KA, Lennox DW, et al. Minimum 4-year follow-up of the PCA total knee arthroplasty in rheumatoid patients. *J Arthroplasty* 1992;7:101–108.

93. Krause WR, Bradbury DW, Kelly JE, et al. Temperature elevations in orthopaedic cutting operations. *J Biomech* 1982;15:267–275.

94. Bachus KN, Harman MK, Bloebaum RD. Stereoscopic analysis of trabecular bone orientation in proximal human tibias. *Cells Mater* 1992;2:13–20.

95. Hofmann AA, Bachus KN, Wyatt RWB. Effect of the tibial cut on subsidence following total knee arthroplasty. *Clin Orthop* 1991;269:63–69.

96. Amstutz HC, Campbell P, Kossovsky N, et al. Mechanism and clinical significance of wear debris-induced osteolysis. *Clin Orthop* 1992;276:7–18.

97. Robinson EJ, Mulliken BD, Bourne RB, et al. Catastrophic osteolysis in total knee replacement: a report of 17 cases. *Clin Orthop* 1995;321:98–105.

98. Jones SMG, Pinder IM, Moran CG, et al. Polyethylene wear in uncemented knee replacements. *J Bone Joint Surg Br* 1992;74:18–22.

99. Bloebaum RD, Nelson K, Dorr LD, et al. Investigation of early surface delamination observed in retrieved heat-pressed tibial inserts. *Clin Orthop* 1991;269:120–127.

100. Collier JP, Mayor MB, McNamara JL, et al. Analysis of the failure of 122 polyethylene inserts from uncemented tibial components. *Clin Orthop* 1991;283:232–242.

101. Kim Y-H, Oh J-H, Oh S-H. Osteolysis around cementless porous-coated anatomic knee prostheses. *J Bone Joint Surg Br* 1995;77:236–241.

102. Plante-Bordeneuve P, Freeman MAR. Tibial high-density polyethylene wear in conforming tibiofemoral prostheses. *J Bone Joint Surg Br* 1993;75:630–636.

103. Tsao A, Mintz L, McRae C, et al. Failure of the porous-coated anatomic prosthesis in total knee arthroplasty due to severe polyethylene wear. *J Bone Joint Surg Am* 1993;75:19–26.

104. Berry DJ, Wold LE, Rand JA. Extensive osteolysis around an aseptic, stable, uncemented total knee replacement. *Clin Orthop* 1993;293:204–207.

105. Engh G. Failure of the polyethylene surface of a total knee replacement within four years. A case report. *J Bone Joint Surg Am* 1988;70:1093–1096.

106. Cook SD, Thomas KA. Fatigue failure of noncemented porous-coated implants. A retrieval study. *J Bone Joint Surg Br* 1991;73:20–24.

107. Huang C-H, Yang C-Y, Cheng C-K. Fracture of the femoral component associated with polyethylene wear and osteolysis after total knee arthroplasty. *J Arthroplasty* 1999;14:375–379.

108. Wada M, Imura S, Bo A, et al. Stress fracture of the femoral component in total knee replacement: a report of 3 cases. *Int Orthop* 1997;21:54.

109. Whiteside LA, Fosco DR, Brooks JG. Fracture of the femoral component in cementless total knee arthroplasty. *Clin Orthop* 1993;286:71–77.

110. Cook SD, Thomas KA, Haddad RJ Jr. Histologic analysis of retrieved human porous-coated total joint components. *Clin Orthop* 1988;234:90–101.

111. Sumner DR, Kienapfel H, Jacobs JJ, et al. Bone ingrowth and wear debris in well-fixed cementless porous-coated tibial components removed from patients. *J Arthroplasty* 1995;10:157–167.

112. Bloebaum RD, Rhodes DM, Rubman MH, et al. Bilateral tibial components of different cementless designs and materials: microradiographic, backscattered imaging, and histologic analysis. *Clin Orthop* 1991;268:179–187.

113. Vigorita VJ, Minkowitz B, Dichiara JF, et al. A histomorphometric and histologic analysis of the implant interface in five successful, autopsy-retrieved, noncemented porous-coated knee arthroplasties. *Clin Orthop* 1993;293:211–218.

114. Blaha JD, Insler HP, Freeman MAR, et al. The fixation of a proximal tibial polyethylene prosthesis without cement. *J Bone Joint Surg Br* 1982;64:326–335.

115. Cameron HU, Jung YB. Noncemented stem tibial component in total knee replacement: the 2- to 6-year results. *Can J Surg* 1993;36:555–559.

116. Engh GA, Bobyn JD, Petersen TL. Radiographic and histologic study of porous coated tibial component fixation in cementless total knee arthroplasty. *Orthopedics* 1988;11:725–731.

117. Freeman MAR, Bradley GW, Blaha JD, et al. Cementless fixation of the tibial component for the ICLH knee. *J R Soc Med* 1982;75:418–424.

118. Freeman MAR, Samuelson KM, Levack B, et al. Knee arthroplasty at the London Hospital: 1975–1984. *Clin Orthop* 1986;205:12–20.

119. Hungerford DS, Kenna RV. Preliminary experience with a total knee prosthesis with porous coating used without cement. *Clin Orthop* 1983;176:96–107.

120. Hungerford DS, Krakow KA. Total joint arthroplasty of the knee. *Clin Orthop* 1985;192:23–33.

121. Joseph J, Kaufman EE. Preliminary results of Miller-Galante uncemented total knee arthroplasty. *Orthopedics* 1990;13:511–516.

122. Laskin RS. Tricon-M uncemented total knee arthroplasty: a review of 96 knees followed for longer than 2 years. *J Arthroplasty* 1988;3:27–38.

123. Nafei A, Nielsen S, Kristensen O, et al. The press-fit Kinemax knee arthroplasty: high failure rate of non-cemented implants. *J Bone Joint Surg Br* 1992;74:243–246.

124. Nilsson KG, Karrholm J, Linder L. Femoral component migration in total knee arthroplasty: randomized study comparing cemented and uncemented fixation of the Miller-Galante I design. *J Orthop Res* 1995;13:347–356.

125. Rackemann S, Mintzer CM, Walker PS, et al. Uncemented press-fit total knee arthroplasty. *J Arthroplasty* 1990;5:307–314.

126. Stuchin SA, Kuschner SH, Ergas E. Results of total knee replacement using an uncemented tibial component. *Bull Hosp Jt Dis Orthop Inst* 1985;45:133–142.

127. Yamamoto S, Nakata S, Kondoh Y. A follow-up study of an uncemented knee replacement: the results of 312 knees using the Kodama-Yamamoto prosthesis. *J Bone Joint Surg Br* 1989;71:505–508.
128. Bassett RW. Results of 1,000 performance knees: cementless versus cemented fixation. *J Arthroplasty* 1998;13:409–413.
129. Cameron HU, Jung YB. Noncemented, porous ingrowth knee prosthesis: the 3- to 8-year results. *Can J Surg* 1993;36:560–564.
130. Dodd CAF, Hungerford DS, Krackow KA. Total knee arthroplasty fixation: comparison of the early results of paired cemented versus uncemented porous coated anatomic knee prostheses. *Clin Orthop* 1990;260:66–70.
131. Duffy GP, Berry DJ, Rand JA. Cement versus cementless fixation in total knee arthroplasty. *Clin Orthop* 1998;356:66–72.
132. Fanning JW, Joseph J, Kaufman EE. Follow up on uncemented total knee arthroplasty. *Orthopedics* 1996;19:933–999.
133. Kim Y, Oh J. Evaluation of the anatomic patellar prosthesis in uncemented porous-coated total knee arthroplasty: seven-year results. *Am J Orthop* 1995;24:412–419.
134. McCaskie AW, Deehan DJ, Green TP, et al. Randomised, prospective study comparing cemented and cementless total knee replacement. *J Bone Joint Surg Br* 1998;80:971–975.
135. Moran CG, Pinder IM, Lees TA, et al. Survivorship analysis of the uncemented porous-coated anatomic knee replacement. *J Bone Joint Surg Am* 1991;73:848–857.
136. Regner L, Carlsson L, Karrholm J, et al. Clinical and radiologic survivorship of cementless tibial components fixed with finned polyethylene pegs. *J Arthroplasty* 1997;12:751–758.
137. Samuelson K, Nelson L. An all-polyethylene cementless tibial component: a five-to nine-year follow-up study. *Clin Orthop* 1990;260:93–97.
138. Ranawat CS, Flynn WF Jr., Saddler S, et al. Long-term results of the total condylar knee arthroplasty. A 15-year survivorship study. *Clin Orthop* 1993;286:94–102.
139. McKaskie AW, Deechen DJ, Green TP, et al. Randomised, prospective study comparing cemented and cementless total knee replacement. *J Bone Joint Surg Br* 1998;80:971–975.

CHAPTER 74

Principles of Instrumentation and Component Alignment

Paul Pollice, Paul A. Lotke, and Jess H. Lonner

Current instrumentation for total knee replacement facilitates the ability of the surgeon to make reproducible and accurate bone cuts that consistently restore the mechanical axis of the limb. Additionally, instruments may have the versatility to make adjustments that can accommodate for bone deficiency, ligament imbalances, and anatomic variations. This chapter focuses on the role and application of instruments in total knee replacement.

NORMAL ANATOMY

There is great variation in limb alignment. Individual differences in height, weight, and bone morphology affect the static knee alignment, and these differences are further affected by eccentric and asymmetric degenerative changes that are typically associated with the arthritic knee.

The mechanical axis of a knee normally aligned in the coronal plane is defined as a line drawn from the center of the femoral head passing through the center of the knee and ending in the center of the ankle joint. The *anatomic axis* refers to the intersection of a line down the axis of the femoral and tibial shafts (Fig. 1). On average, the anatomic axis of the knee is 5 to 7 degrees of valgus. This angle represents a combination of the valgus alignment for the femoral condyles (a mean of 7 degrees) and the varus tilt of the tibial plateau (a mean of 3 degrees) (1).

The axis of rotation of the femur (flexion) also had wide deviation, as the amount of the posterior condyles that falls below the transepicondylar axis can vary greatly. This is important if we make a transverse cut in the tibia and want to establish a rectangular space in flexion during total knee arthroplasty.

The flexion axis of rotation is complex but generally believed to transect the medial and lateral epicondyles at the origins of the collateral ligaments. It is transverse to the long axis of the tibia. At 90 degrees of flexion, the medial condyle extends approximately 3 degrees (1 to 6 degrees) below (more posterior) the lateral condyles (Fig. 2).

BIOMECHANICS

In a limb with anatomic alignment of 7 degrees of valgus, during normal gait, 60% to 70% of weightbearing forces in stance phase pass through the medial compartment of the knee. Small changes in alignment can lead to substantial changes in load distribution in each of the compartments, which ultimately may predispose to arthritis (2–5). This may explain why there is often asymmetric chondral degeneration noted with progressive varus or valgus deformity in osteoarthritis.

Restoration of limb and component alignment during total knee arthroplasty normalizes the distribution of forces across the implant and enhances implant survival and performance. Lotke and Ecker (6) first established the overall importance of limb alignment and subsequent balance of soft tissues to optimize the results of total condylar knee replacement. Hsu et al. (7) demonstrated that a 5-degree axial malalignment can change in load distribution up to 40%. These studies were corroborated by Ritter et al. (8), who showed that early failures occurred with tibial varus of more than 5 degrees.

ALIGNMENT, OSTEOTOMIES, AND COMPONENT PLACEMENT

The potential for errors of component implantation is great when we consider that the femoral and tibial components each

1085

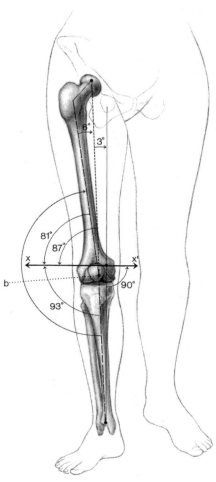

FIG. 1. The reference axes for correct alignment are the anatomic axis along the shaft of the bone, and the mechanical axis, from the femoral head to the center of the ankle.

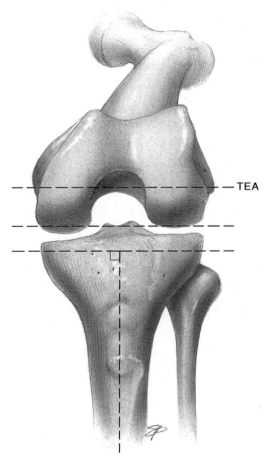

FIG. 2. In flexion, the posterior medial condyle falls approximately 3 degrees (3 mm) further below the transepicondylar axis (TEA) than the lateral posterior condyle. The medial tibial plateau is approximately 3 degrees (3 mm) more distal than the lateral tibial plateau. If you make a transverse tibial osteotomy, to maintain a balanced rectangular flexion space, you will resect more bone from the medial posterior condyle.

have 6 degrees of freedom in which they can be implanted: varus-valgus tilt, flexion-extension, proximal-distal position, internal-external rotation, anterior-posterior translation, and medial-lateral translation. The overall limb alignment and patella each have 3 degrees of freedom. Combining all of the possibilities of implanting the components in relationship to each other, there exist more than 11,000 ways to get component alignment wrong. Fortunately, proper placement and alignment of components can be thought of as a range of satisfactory positions; however, implantation errors can be minimized by adhering to proven principles of total knee arthroplasty.

Alignment Goals

Restoring the mechanical limb alignment to neutral is a primary goal of total knee arthroplasty. It is commonly believed that tibiofemoral alignment should be restored to 6 ± 1 to 2 degrees of valgus. This may vary depending on conditions such as obesity, premorbid alignment, and medial collateral ligament integrity. Although the average knee has a 3-degree varus tilt in the tibia, a transverse osteotomy of the proximal tibia is most commonly preferred. This is believed to be more reproducible and is associated with the highest chance of success and prosthetic survivorship. Therefore, the femur should be cut in 4 to 7 degrees of valgus.

Two techniques are used to integrate the tibial and femoral cuts: the measured resection technique and the tensioned gap technique.

The measured resection technique restores knee anatomy by replacing what is removed or eroded by arthritis. For example, if 10 mm is removed from the proximal tibia, 10 mm of tibial tray and polyethylene should be used to restore the anatomy. Posterior and distal femoral condylar resections should be equal to the thickness of the condyles of the implant component (Fig. 3).

The tension technique keys off the initial transverse tibial resection and attempts to make equal and rectangular gaps in flexion and extension (Fig. 4). It is critical with the tensioning technique that all osteophytes are removed and ligaments balanced before bone cuts, allowing the surgeon to properly gauge

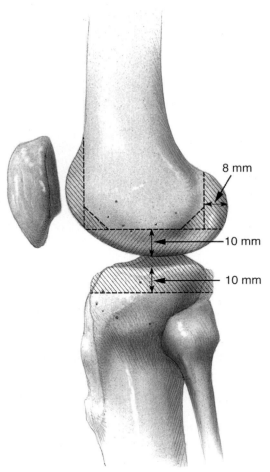

FIG. 3. The measured resection technique removes as much bone and/or cartilage as to be replaced by the thickness of the arthroplasty components. This method attempts to restore the anatomic joint line level.

the size of the flexion–extension gaps. The technique mandates an accurate tibial resection; otherwise, reciprocal errors in the femur will occur.

Alignment Osteotomies

Three osteotomies are required to correctly align and balance the total knee: the proximal tibia, the distal femur, and the anterior and posterior femur condylar resection—rotation (Fig. 5).

Tibial Osteotomy

Instruments are used to make a cut perpendicular to the long axis of the tibial shaft in the coronal plane. Extramedullary and intramedullary (IM) instruments can be equally effective for the tibial osteotomy (Fig. 6) (9). The extramedullary guide is placed parallel to the tibial crest in the coronal plane, with ability to adjust for a posterior slope. Extramedullary systems bypass any potential deformity of the tibial shaft, which can bias alignment. They also reduce the risk of fat embolism syndrome and allow

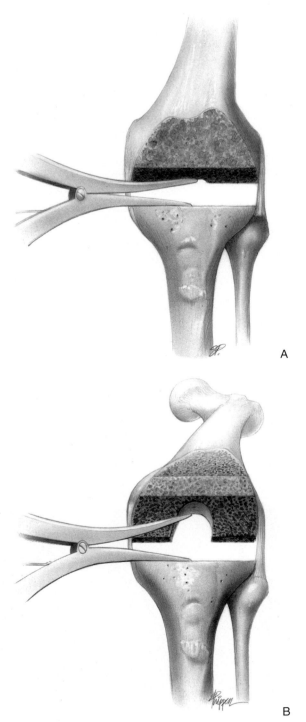

FIG. 4. The tension technique makes a transverse tibial osteotomy first **(A)**, and the femoral osteotomy is determined with tension to make equal rectangular spaces in flexion and extension **(B)**.

for easy adjustment of alignment in all planes. Although this technique can be highly effective and accurate, Cates et al. (10) reviewed alignment of the proximal tibial cut with the use of extramedullary guides and found a disturbing percentage of

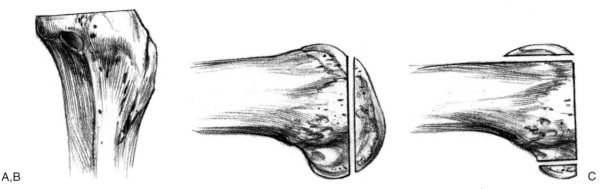

A,B

C

FIG. 5. Three osteotomy cuts determine the alignment of the knee: the proximal tibia **(A)**, distal femur **(B)**, and anterior and posterior cuts of the distal femur **(C)**.

alignment errors. In morbidly obese patients, in whom external landmarks are obscure, these guides have greater potential for error.

IM guides can also create reproducible osteotomies (11,12). This technique is applicable for most knees, except when there is significant tibial deformity or obstruction of the tibial canal by previous fracture or hardware. IM instrumentation is placed through a drill hole in the tibial plateau. The pilot hole is often started at the junction of the insertion of the anterior cruciate ligament and the anterior horn of the lateral meniscus. Proximally, the drill hole should be wide enough so the guide is not biased at this level and marrow pressures can be released during rod insertion. It has been shown that a 12.7-mm drill hole can reduce the risk of intraoperative oxygen desaturation when using an 8-mm alignment rod designed to allow venting of the canal (13).

It has also been shown that fluted and hollow rods significantly reduce IM pressures within the canal (14), offering an explanation in the mechanism of reduced fat embolization.

Both IM and extramedullary guides have telescoping elements that are used to place a cutting block at the desired resection level (Fig. 7). The varus and valgus alignment is adjusted to parallel the mechanical axis of the tibia, and the posterior slope is "dialed in" by the cutting block to approximate the native posterior slope. The block is pinned at an appropriate resection level and osteotomy performed. A measuring guide (stylus) can be used to accurately determine the amount of bone to be resected, generally seeking to remove 10 mm of bone and cartilage from the less arthritic hemiplateau. Adjustments in placement of the stylus may be necessary in the presence of subchondral loss and abnormal contouring of the plateau. In the measured resection

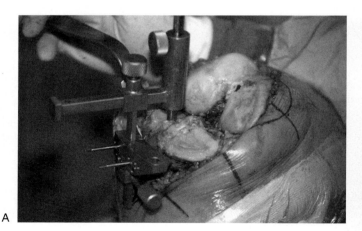

A

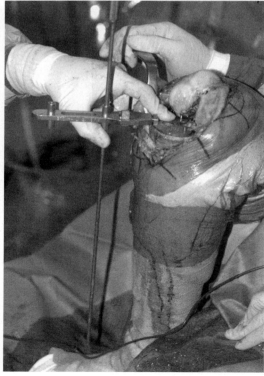

B

FIG. 6. Intramedullary **(A)** or extramedullary **(B)** guides may be used to make a transverse osteotomy of the tibia.

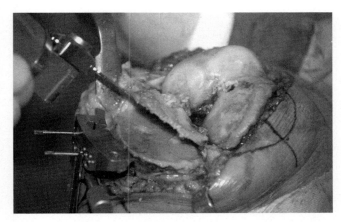

FIG. 7. A tibial cutting block is fixed in place and used to guide the transverse tibial osteotomy.

technique, the amount of resection should be approximate to the preferred thickness of the tibial component.

In the tensioning technique, a transverse tibial osteotomy is also made; however, the depth of resection is not always determined, and some surgeons using this technique prefer to resect a minimal amount of bone, arguing that the more conservative the resection, the better the osseous support. Distal femoral and posterior femoral condylar resection may be excessive if inadequate tibial resection is performed to use a polyethylene insert of ample thickness. In this scenario, the joint line is elevated, and the gap kinematics may be compromised. With newer implant designs and wider size ranges, the tension technique no longer requires elevation of the joint line, and successful alignment and kinematics can be routinely anticipated.

Femoral Osteotomy

There are two important femoral osteotomies. The distal osteotomy sets axial alignment, and the anterior-posterior osteotomies determine rotational alignment.

Distal Femur

With the distal femoral osteotomy, most surgeons will try to align the distal osteotomy in 4 to 7 degrees of valgus. IM and extramedullary guides are available for the distal femoral resection. However, most surgeons find that the IM devices are reproducible, easy, and applicable in the vast majority of cases (Fig. 8) (3,10,15–20). Cates et al. (10) reviewed 200 consecutive total knee arthroplasties in which IM femoral guides were used in 125 cases, and extramedullary femoral guides in 75 cases. The distal femoral resection angle was outside the accepted range (4 to 10 degrees of femoral valgus) in 28% of the extramedullary group and in only 14% of the IM group. Joint line orientation was also outside the normal range twice as frequently in the extramedullary alignment group. The authors suggested that IM guides improve the accuracy of distal femoral osteotomy. Teter et al. (15) reviewed 201 total knee arthroplasties in which IM femoral guides were used. Distal femoral alignment was considered inaccurate in only 8% of the x-rays. Risk factors for inaccurate alignment included capacious femoral canals and distal

femoral bowing. Regardless of the technique, IM or extramedullary, attention to detail and confirmatory assessments are critical in minimizing alignment errors.

If opting to use an IM system, a drill hole is made in the femoral notch anterior to the origin of the posterior cruciate ligament, with the knee flexed. Standard full-length femoral radiographs can show the optimal placement of the drill hole to access the femoral canal. This position is usually slightly medial to the center of the apex of the intercondylar notch. Insertion of the IM guide too far medially leads to a relative varus cut; too far laterally leads to a valgus cut. The canal is overdrilled at the entry so as to not bias the IM guide, allowing the rod to engage diaphyseal bone. This also allows for the release of medullary contents and minimizes pressure within the canal (13). Fluted rods placed in the canal have been shown to decrease IM pressures and possibly reduce the incidence of fat emboli syndrome (13,14). Most jigs allow for adjustment of the valgus angle of the distal cut from 4 to 7 degrees.

Femoral Osteotomy by the Tensioning Technique

When using the tensioning technique, the femoral resection is keyed off of the tibial osteotomy. Adequate distal and posterior femoral resection needs to be performed to accommodate the implants. Once the flexion space is created under tension by resecting enough posterior femoral condyle (see below), the distal femoral osteotomy is completed under equal tension to produce an equal extension gap. Femoral external rotation (posterior condyle cut) and femoral valgus (distal femoral cut) are determined during tensioning so that rectangular gaps are created. Before making the bone cuts, the surgeon should remove osteophytes and ensure that the soft tissue envelope is balanced. For example, in the varus-aligned knee with a tight medial sleeve, the distal femur may be cut in excessive valgus if the only goal were to create a rectangular extension gap. It is also important to ensure that the tibial cut is accurate before femoral resection because errors will otherwise be compounded.

Anterior and Posterior Femur Condylar Resection—Rotation

In the measured resection technique, the distal femoral resection removes the amount of bone replaced by the prosthesis. Once a satisfactory distal femoral cut is created in 4 to 7 degrees of valgus, the size of the distal femur is determined by either anterior or posterior referencing.

Anterior referencing creates a measured resection with the anterior surface of the femur as a guide (Fig. 9). If cut at the level of the anterior cortex, it reduces the risk of overstuffing the patellofemoral joint and notching the anterior femur. When the sizing is perfect no compromise is made, and the posterior femoral resection is determined. A disadvantage of anterior referencing is encountered when the condylar anatomy falls "between" sizes. In this situation the smaller size implant is selected; avoid overstuffing the flexion gap, as this may increase the relative flexion gap. This option should not be used in cruciate-retaining knees because this effectively elongates the posterior cruciate ligament.

Posterior referencing has the advantage of optimizing the posterior condylar cut to maintain tension of a retained posterior

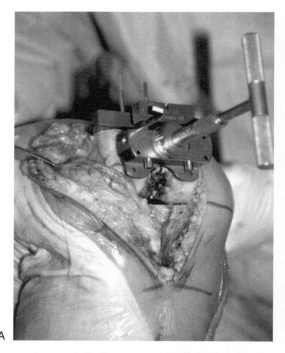

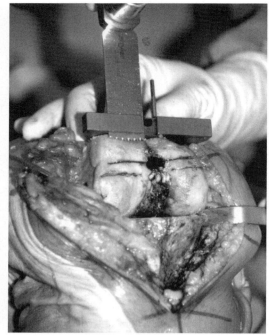

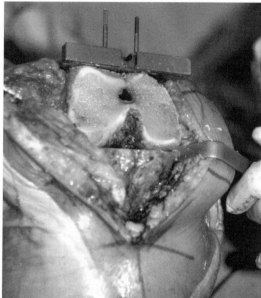

FIG. 8. An intramedullary guide is set at 4 to 6 degrees of valgus and placed into the femur **(A)**. The rod is removed, and the osteotomy is taken in the distal femur **(B)**. The contour of the cut surface should approximate a "figure of eight" **(C)**.

cruciate ligament. Between-size knees are problematic, as the use of oversized components will overstuff the patellofemoral joint and an undersized cutting block may cause notching of the femur (Fig. 10). Again, compromises must be made to balance a possible mismatch in size.

With posterior cruciate ligament–substituting designs, the surgeon should be aware that the release of the posterior cruciate ligament will result in an increase in the flexion space by 2 to 3 mm. This will need to be compensated by a comparable amount of additional resection of the distal femur. In addition, femoral resections should avoid creating flexion in the femoral component, which can cause impingement of the femoral component at the tibial post.

Determining Rotation of the Femoral Component

External rotation of the femoral component is the key to creating a rectangular flexion gap and facilitating patella tracking (21,22). Several methods are used to determine femoral component rotation. Each is effective but has some inherent errors (Fig. 11).

1. The transepicondylar axis—a line drawn between the medial and lateral epicondyles (23). Some surgeons find this anatomy difficult to identify (Fig. 2).
2. The anterior-posterior line of Whiteside (24,25)—a line from the deepest portion of the trochlea, to the center of the

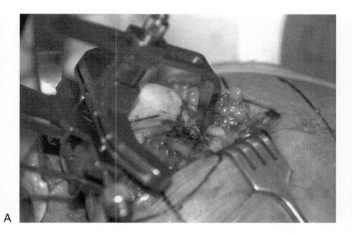

A

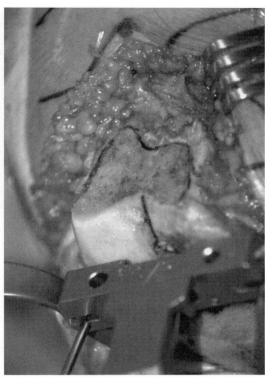

B

FIG. 9. A: Anterior references systems place a guide on the anterior femoral cortex. This generally prevents anterior notching of the femur but can lead to overcorrection or undercorrection of the posterior femoral condyle. **B:** When the appropriate anterior osteotomy has been completed, the contours of the osteotomy should have a "bimodal" shape and enough area to receive the anterior flange of the femoral component.

intercondylar notch. A line drawn perpendicular to this is considered to be an effective degree of femoral component external rotation (Fig. 11). This technique relies on consistent trochlear anatomy, which can be destroyed by patellofemoral arthritis (26).

3. Posterior condylar axis—a line drawn between the posterior surface of the medial and lateral condyles with a prefixed use of a 3-degree external rotation guide (27) (Fig. 2). With cartilage wear and bone defects of the posterior femoral condyles, this technique can be unreliable (28).

4. Tensioned gap technique—this places a spreader to tension the flexion gap. Osteotomies are made to establish a rectan-

gular gap in flexion with the tibial shaft axis (29). This technique may be difficult when there is a substantial preexisting ligamentous imbalance. Errors in tibial resection can compromise femoral component rotation (Fig. 4).

These various techniques have had several advocates and detractors in the literature.

Olcott and Scott (30) prospectively analyzed 100 total knee arthroplasties and compared how these intraoperative femoral landmarks performed. Using the tensioning rectangular flexion space as the control, the transepicondylar axis most consistently created a balanced flexion gap when they compared the antero-

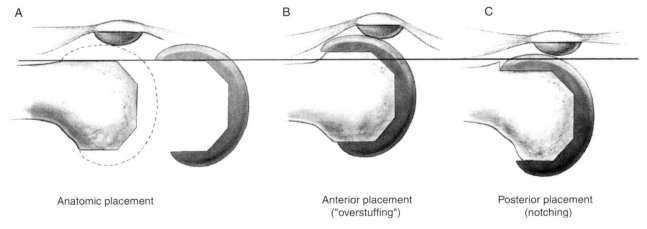

A   B   C

Anatomic placement   Anterior placement   Posterior placement
                            ("overstuffing")   (notching)

FIG. 10. A perfectly fit femur will have contours that conform to normal anatomy **(A)**. If the component is placed too far anteriorly, it will lead to flexion laxity and overstuffing of the patellofemoral joint **(B)**. If it is placed too far posteriorly, it will notch the femur and narrow the flexion gap, preventing good flexion **(C)**.

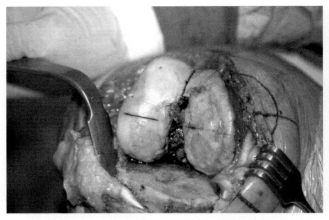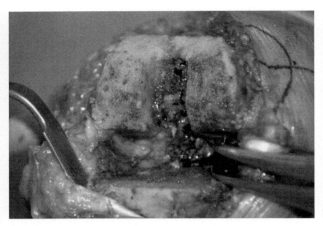

FIG. 11. A knee with a transepicondylar axis and white slides drawn on the distal femur **(A)**. After the posterior condylar osteotomy, the flexion gap should be rectangular under tension of a laminar spreader **(B)**.

posterior "line of Whiteside" and 3 degrees of external rotation of the posterior condyles. Three degrees of external rotation performed least favorably, especially in preoperative valgus-aligned knees. Akagi et al. (31) reported similar inaccuracies with the use of posterior condylar axis. They performed computed tomography scans on 111 knees with symptomatic arthritis and evaluated the transepicondylar axes (clinical and surgical), the posterior condylar axis, and the anteroposterior axis. These values were then compared with the tibiofemoral and femoral valgus angles of the individual patients studied. The authors found that when tibiofemoral valgus exceeded 9 degrees, the posterior femoral axis became increasingly unreliable. In 25% of the cases, the surgical transepicondylar axis could not be reconstructed due to medial epicondylar sulcus being unrecognized. In knees with greater valgus alignment, the authors believe the anteroposterior axis is more reliable. The authors advocate computed tomography scans in severe valgus cases to help define femoral component rotation. Katz et al. (32) showed that the tension technique was the most reliable and that estimating the transepicondylar axis had the greatest variation.

Because of the vagaries and errors of any one technique, most surgeons will use several of these techniques in combination during each case to estimate femoral component rotation. We have found that for routine total knees, without too much deformity, we have relied more on the tension technique at 90 degrees of flexion to confirm a rectangular flexion gap.

Another check for proper rotation is the "footprint" created by the anterior osteotomy. It should look like a low and high bimodal curve (Fig. 9B). If a reasonable contour is obtained, it can be a crude estimate of appropriate rotation.

Patellofemoral tracking is directly influenced by rotation of the femoral component (21,33). External rotation of the femoral component brings the trochlea in closer proximity to the center of the patella. In addition, internal rotation leads to underresection of the medial femoral condyle and a tight medial flexion gap. If this malrotation is not identified, unnecessary release of the medial structures may be performed. Problems with maltracking of the patella or a tight medial sleeve may be indications of a femoral component internal rotation. Excessive external rotation does not adversely affect patellofemoral tracking. However, it does create a trapezoidal flexion space and a flexion imbalance. Therefore, an appropriate rotational alignment is essential for creating the perfect total knee.

CONCLUSION

Alignment in total knee replacement has evolved over the last decade and better instrumentation has enabled the surgeon to perform total knee replacements with increasing consistency and reliability. The techniques outlined are the parameters we used to aid in the proper alignment and placement of femoral and tibial implants. Understanding the goals and principles of restoring limb alignment is essential in creating a well-balanced total knee replacement and will ultimately contribute to the success of the implant; contemporary instruments can aid in achieving these goals.

REFERENCES

1. Johnson F, Leitl S, Waugh W. The distribution of load across the knee. *J Bone Joint Surg Br* 1992;62:346.
2. Harrington IJ. A bioengineering analysis of force actions at the knee in normal and pathologic gait. *Biomed Eng* 1976;11:167.
3. Harrington IJ. Static and dynamic loading patterns in knee joints with deformities. *J Bone Joint Surg Am* 1983;65:247–259.
4. Hsu RWW, Himeno S, Coventry MB. Normal axial alignment of the lower extremity and load-bearing distribution at the knee. *Clin Orthop* 1990;255:215–217.
5. Morrison JB. Bioengineering analysis of force actions transmitted by the knee joint. *Biomed Eng* 1968;3:164.
6. Lotke PA, Ecker ML. Influence of positioning of prosthesis in total knee replacement. *J Bone Joint Surg Am* 1977;59:77.
7. Hsu HP, Garg A, Walker PS, et al. Effect on knee component alignment on tibial load distribution with clinical correlation. *Clin Orthop* 1989;248:135.
8. Ritter MA, Faris PM, Keating EM, et al. Postoperative alignment of total knee replacement. Its effect on survival. *Clin Orthop* 1994;299:153–156.
9. Dennis DA, Channer M, Susman MH, et al. Intramedullary versus extramedullary tibial alignment systems in total knee arthroplasty. *J Arthroplasty* 1993;8:43.
10. Cates HE, Ritter MA, Keating EM, et al. Intramedullary versus extramedullary alignment systems in total knee replacement. *Clin Orthop* 1993;286:32–39.
11. Laskin RS, Turtel A. the use of an intramedullary tibial alignment guide in total knee replacement. *Am J Knee Surg* 1989;2:123.

12. Simmons ED Jr, Sullivan JA, Rackemann S, et al. The accuracy of tibial intramedullary alignment devices in total knee arthroplasty. *J Arthroplasty* 1991;6:45.

13. Fahmy NR, Chandler HP, Danylchuk K, et al. Blood-gas and circulatory changes during total knee replacement. Role of the intramedullary alignment rod. *J Bone Joint Surg Am* 1990;72:19–26.

14. Gleitz M, Hopf T, Hess T. [Experimental studies on the role of intramedullary alignment rods in the etiology of fat embolisms in knee endoprosthesis.] *Z Orthop Ihre Grenzgeb* 1996;134:254–259.

15. Teter KE, Bregman D, Colwell CW Jr. The efficacy of intramedullary alignment in total knee replacement. *Clin Orthop* 1995;321:117–121.

16. Engh GA, Peterson TL. Comparative experience with intramedullary and extramedullary alignment in total knee arthroplasty. *J Arthroplasty* 1990;5:1.

17. Manning M, Elloy M, Johnson R. The accuracy of intramedullary alignment in total knee replacement. *J Bone Joint Surg Br* 1988;70:852.

18. Ritter MA, Campbell ED. A model for easy location of the center of the femoral head during total knee arthroplasty. *J Arthroplasty* 1988;3(Suppl):S59.

19. Siegel JL, Shall LM. Femoral instrumentation using the anterosuperior iliac spine as a landmark in total knee arthroplasty. *J Arthroplasty* 1991;6:317.

20. Tillett ED, Engh GA, Petersen T. A comparative study of extramedullary and intramedullary alignment systems in total knee arthroplasty. *Clin Orthop* 1988;230:176.

21. Anouchi YS, Whiteside LA, Kaiser AD. The effects of axial rotational alignment of the femoral component on instability and patellar tracking in total knee arthroplasty demonstrated on autopsy specimens. *Clin Orthop* 1993;287:170.

22. Rhoads DD, Noble PC, Reuben JD, et al. The effect of femoral component position on patellar tracking after total knee arthroplasty. *Clin Orthop* 1990;260:43.

23. Stiehl JB, Abbott BD. Morphology of the transepicondylar axis and its application in primary and revision total knee arthroplasty. *J Arthroplasty* 1995;10:785–789.

24. Arima J, Whiteside LA, McCarthy DS, et al. Femoral rotational alignment, based on the anteroposterior axis in total knee arthroplasty in a valgus knee: a technical note. *J Bone Joint Surg Am* 1995;77:1331–1334.

25. Whiteside LA, Arima J. The anteroposterior axis for femoral rotational alignment in valgus total knee arthroplasty. *Clin Orthop* 1995;321:168.

26. Poilvache PL, Insall JN, Scuderi GR, et al. Rotational landmarks and sizing of the distal femur in total knee arthroplasty. *Clin Orthop* 1996;331:35–46.

27. Berger RA, Rubash HE, Seel MJ, et al. Determining the rotational alignment of the femoral component in total knee arthroplasty using the epicondylar axis. *Clin Orthop* 1993;286:40–47.

28. Griffin FM, Insall NJ, Scuderi GR. The posterior condylar angle in osteoarthritis knees. *J Arthroplasty* 1988;13:812.

29. Stiehl JB, Cherveny PM. Femoral rotational alignment using the tibial shaft axis in total knee arthroplasty. *Clin Orthop* 1996;331:47.

30. Olcott CW, Scott RD. A comparison of 4 intraoperative methods to determine femoral component rotation during total knee arthroplasty. *J Arthroplasty* 2000;15:22–26.

31. Akagi M, Yamashita E, Nakagawa T, et al. Relationship between frontal knee alignment and reference axes in the distal femur. *Clin Orthop* 2001;388:147–156.

32. Katz, MA, Beck TD, Silber JS, et al. Determining femoral rotational alignment in total knee arthroplasty: reliability of techniques. *J Arthroplasty* 2001;16:301.

33. Berger RA, Crossett LS, Jacobs JJ, et al. Malrotation causing patellofemoral complications after total knee arthroplasty. *Clin Orthop* 1998;356:144.

CHAPTER 75

Surgical Exposure for Primary Total Knee Arthroplasty

David A. Parker, Harry Tsigaras, and Cecil H. Rorabeck

Choice of surgical approach for a primary total knee arthroplasty (TKA) is an important decision for the arthroplasty surgeon. The surgical approach should be one that a surgeon finds readily reproducible and provides adequate exposure to perform the procedure without compromise. It should also have the flexibility to allow for intraoperative modifications, should these be necessary in more difficult cases. In this chapter, we describe the various approaches for primary TKA, describe the theoretical advantages and disadvantages of each, and compare one with another with the aim of providing recommendations for the most appropriate approach to use.

SKIN INCISIONS

Preservation of skin viability is essential for any arthroplasty to succeed, particularly over the anterior aspect of the knee, where soft tissue coverage is thin. It is important for the surgeon to be familiar with the local anatomy in this area. The vascularity of the skin of the anterior aspect of the knee is medially based, mostly from the saphenous and descending geniculate arteries, and therefore the lateral flap is generally more hypoxic (1–3). Vessels perforate the deep fascia and form an anastomosis superficial to the deep fascia (Fig. 1). As there is minimal communication between vessels in the superficial layer, dissection should be deep to the fascial layer to preserve this anastomosis and the blood supply to the skin (1).

Choice of skin incision is based on ease of subsequent exposure, extensibility, cosmesis, and potential for uncomplicated healing. The medial parapatellar incision has been shown to be better ori-

ented relative to Langer's lines (4) and subjected to less tension with knee flexion when compared with an anterior midline incision (5). This theoretical advantage has not been borne out in clinical studies. In a comparative study by Johnson (3), decreased oxygenation was found in the lateral flap of anterior midline, medial parapatellar, and curved medial approaches. Oxygenation was lowest in the curved medial approach, with subsequent wound problems, but no significant difference was found between anterior midline and medial parapatellar incisions. Although both of these incisions can be used, the anterior midline skin incision is the classic extensile approach and is the authors' preference if there are no previous incisions to take into account. The incision is centered over the patella and extends proximally and distally approximately 10 cm, ending distally 1 cm medial to the tibial tubercle. Proximal and distal extension of this incision allows development of large flaps if necessary, exposing anterior, medial, and lateral supporting structures. The incision is also readily used again should revision surgery be necessary.

Previous incisions need to be carefully considered. Generally speaking, if previous incisions are present, it is preferable to incorporate longitudinal components if possible and incise at right angles to previous horizontal incisions. Intersecting incisions are at increased risk of necrosis at their junctions; hence, acute angles of intersection should be avoided. If more than one previous longitudinal incision is present, it is preferable to use the more lateral of these to preserve the vascularity of the skin flaps, assuming the incision is not too lateral to make the procedure technically possible. Scars that are adherent to underlying bone or tendon should be excised, and if any soft tissue defi-

1095

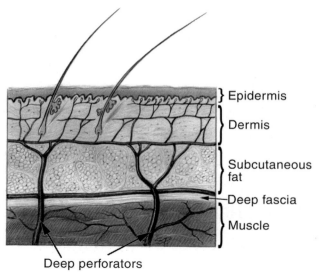

A

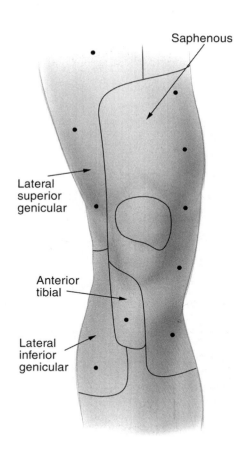

B

FIG. 1. A: Microvascular anatomy of the skin of the thigh. The vessels just superficial to the deep fascia form an anastomosis. The skin blood supply arises from this anastomosis, with little communication in the subcutaneous tissues. The deep perforators supply the anastomosis above the deep fascia. **B:** Areas supplied by the deep vessels (*solid circles* indicate approximate position of deep perforators). Most of the blood supply comes from the medial side; therefore, using a medial incision will increase the chance of skin-edge necrosis. (From Younger AS, Duncan CP, Masri BA. Surgical exposures in revision total knee arthroplasty. *J Am Acad Orthop Surg* 1998;6:56, Figs. 1A and B, with permission.)

ciency is predicted, preoperative consultation with a plastic surgeon is advisable. The most common scenario is old incisions for open meniscectomy, and it is usually possible to incorporate these into a curved parapatellar incision if they are not too distant from the immediate parapatellar region. Incisions that are further away from the midline, especially if old, can usually be ignored in favor of a straight midline approach.

Once the skin incision is made, dissection should be carried directly down completely through the fat layer to the underlying extensor mechanism. Medial and lateral mobilization of these flaps should be sufficient to allow exposure for the ensuing arthrotomy but no further, to avoid further tissue devascularization and dead space creation. Mobilization of the medial flap needs to be sufficient to allow exposure of the planned arthrotomy, whereas that of the lateral flap only needs to be sufficient to allow room for patellar resurfacing instruments. In obese patients, this lateral flap can also be mobilized to create a pocket for the everted patella. This incision routinely sacrifices the infrapatellar branch of the saphenous nerve, and although this is not usually a cause of any significant morbidity, it is important to warn patients, of the resulting area of lateral numbness they should expect postoperatively (6). Careful consideration of skin incisions and avoidance of excessive subcutaneous dissection are critical in minimizing complications relating to the TKA wound.

MEDIAL PARAPATELLAR APPROACH

Also known as the *median parapatellar* or *paramedian approach*, the medial parapatellar approach was initially

described by Von Langenbeck in 1879 and more recently popularized by Insall (7). It has become a popular approach among arthroplasty surgeons and offers an easily reproducible technique that provides excellent exposure of the knee. The classic version of this approach splits the quadriceps tendon in its medial one-third, releasing part of both the rectus femoris tendon and vastus medialis fibers from the patella (Fig. 2). Subsequent modification of this involves a more medial quadriceps incision, leaving the majority of the quadriceps tendon intact and releasing the vastus medialis from the patella. In Insall's modification, the extensor mechanism dissection is carried in a straight line over the anterior surface of the patella and along the medial border of the patellar tendon (7). The quadriceps expansion is peeled from the anterior surface of the patella by sharp dissection until the medial border of the patella is seen. The synovium is then divided and the fat pad split in the midline. The patella is then everted laterally.

This is the preferred approach of the authors and has been modified slightly from Insall's description. An anterior midline incision is used starting a hand's breadth proximal to the patella and extending distally to the medial and inferior aspect of the tibial tubercle (Fig. 3). The knee is flexed for the skin incision and then brought into extension for the remainder of the arthrotomy. Dissection is carried down through the fat and superficial fascial and medial and lateral flaps developed as described above. The quadriceps tendon is transversely marked with a marking pen just proximal to the patella as a guide for later closure (Fig. 4). The arthrotomy is then performed from proximal to distal curving around the medial edge of the patella. A cuff of tendon approximately 5 mm in width is left on the lateral aspect

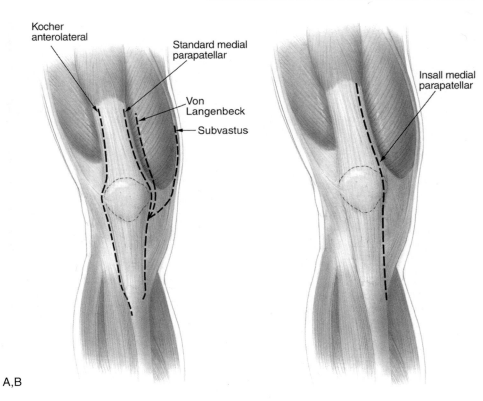

A,B

FIG. 2. A, B: Capsular incisions used for revision total knee arthroplasty. All can be reached from any skin incision by subfascial dissection, but this should be kept to a minimum to prevent skin necrosis. (From Younger AS, Duncan CP, Masri BA. Surgical exposures in revision total knee arthroplasty. *J Am Acad Orthop Surg* 1998;6:59, Fig. 3, with permission.)

of the vastus medialis muscle and on the medial aspect of the patella for later closure. The incision is carried distally through the medial retinaculum approximately 5 mm medial to the patellar tendon, also to assist in closure later. The infrapatellar fat pad is excised as necessary and a medial release is initially carried

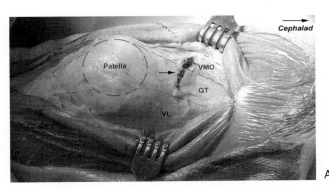

A

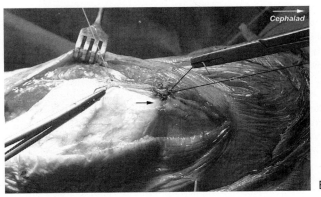

B

FIG. 4. A: An approximation mark (*dark arrow*) is made over the quadriceps tendon (QT) and vastus medialis obliquus (VMO). This is made before the arthrotomy and guides closure of the capsular layer at the end of the procedure **(B)**. VL, vastus lateralis. [From photo library—Department of Orthopaedics (Adult Reconstruction), London Health Sciences Centre, London, Ontario, Canada, with permission.]

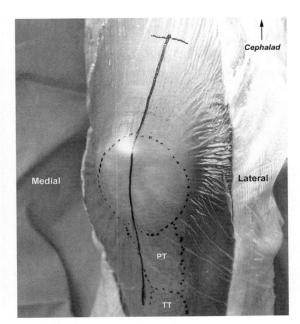

FIG. 3. Author's preferred skin incision. The skin and fat are incised with the knee in a flexed position. PT, patella tendon; TT, tibial tuberosity. [From photo library—Department of Orthopaedics (Adult Reconstruction), London Health Sciences Centre, London, Ontario, Canada, with permission.]

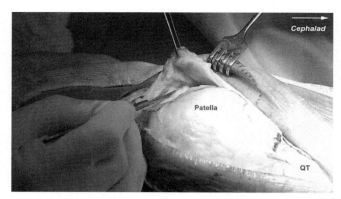

FIG. 5. The medial release from the proximal tibia is performed with sharp subperiosteal dissection. Its limit depends on the severity of the varus deformity—mild to moderate deformities require a release to at least the midcoronal plane; more severe deformities require the release to extend to the posteromedial corner. QT, quadriceps tendon. [From photo library—Department of Orthopaedics (Adult Reconstruction), London Health Sciences Centre, London, Ontario, Canada, with permission.]

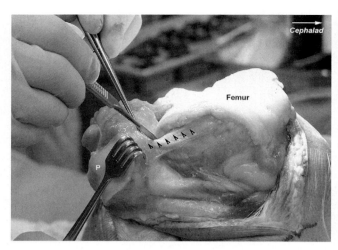

FIG. 6. Release of the lateral patellofemoral ligament (*dark arrowheads*) assists patella eversion. P, patella. [From photo library—Department of Orthopaedics (Adult Reconstruction), London Health Sciences Centre, London, Ontario, Canada, with permission.]

out to the midcoronal plane (Fig. 5). In a large varus deformity, the release needs to be continued around to include the entire posteromedial corner. This allows for correction of this deformity as well as allows external rotation of the tibia to assist in patella eversion. If a valgus deformity is present, the release is limited only to that part of the deep collateral ligament attached above the level of the proposed bony resection and is rarely continued posterior to the midcoronal plane.

Infrapatellar tissue is released from the tibia down to the tendon attachment and across to the anterior aspect of the lateral plateau. The patella is then everted and the knee flexed, with the surgeon taking care to watch for avulsion of the patellar tendon from the tibial tubercle. If there is undue tension on the patellar tendon making eversion difficult and putting the patellar tendon at risk, other techniques can be used, as discussed later. Placing a pin in the tuberosity can help in providing some protection against tendon avulsion. The synovium and fat pad overlying the supracondylar aspect of the femur are incised and reflected medially and laterally to clearly define the bony anatomy here, particularly if an anterior referencing system is to be used. With the patella everted and a retractor applying tension laterally to the patella, the lateral patellofemoral ligament is released, further decreasing tension on the everted extensor mechanism (Fig. 6). The initial exposure is now completed.

After completion of the arthroplasty, patellar tracking is assessed and a lateral release performed from outside in if necessary, although this is rare in the author's experience. Closure is completed over a drain, using interrupted no. 1 absorbable suture in the extensor mechanism adjacent to the patella and the same suture proximal and distal to this in a continuous fashion. Masri et al. (8) have shown in a randomized prospective trial that whether closure is performed in either flexion or extension has no effect on outcome, and it is the authors' practice to close with the knee in extension. This closure is tested by flexing the knee beyond 90 degrees, after which the fat and superficial fascial layer is closed as one layer with a continuous 2-0 absorbable suture and skin with metal staples. The benefits of this approach are its relative technical simplicity, the excellent exposure it provides, and its extensile nature that allows for further extension should stan-

dard technique provide inadequate exposure. The potential disadvantages of this approach are that it does detach the vastus medialis muscle from the remainder of the extensor mechanism as well as interrupt the medial vascularity of the patella (9,10), although no corresponding clinical morbidity has been consistently demonstrated as a result of these theoretical disadvantages.

MIDVASTUS APPROACH

The midvastus approach has been described and popularized by Engh and Parks (11). It differs from the medial parapatellar and subvastus approaches by opening an interval in the midsub-

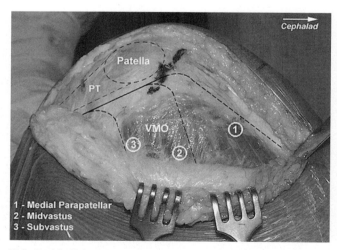

FIG. 7. Medial perspective of a flexed knee after dissection of the superficial tissues. The three common "medial" approaches are outlined. PT, patella tendon; VMO, vastus medialis obliquus. [From photo library—Department of Orthopaedics (Adult Reconstruction), London Health Sciences Centre, London, Ontario, Canada, with permission.]

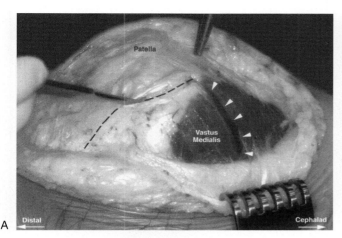
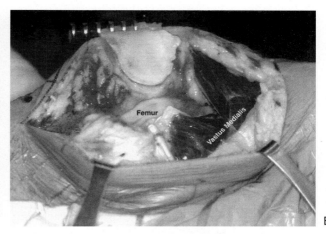

FIG. 8. A: Right knee in 90 degrees flexion, with the midvastus approach shown as a dashed line. The muscular segment of the incision (*white arrowheads*) is parallel to the muscle fibers of the vastus medialis and ends at the superomedial pole of the patella. **B:** The patella is easily everted once the retinacular segment of the incision is made. (From Engh GA, Parks NL. Surgical technique of the midvastus arthrotomy. *Clin Orthop* 1998;351:271, Figs. 2B and C, with permission.)

stance of the vastus medialis muscle starting at the superomedial border of the patella (Fig. 7). The stated advantages of this approach are that it avoids incision of the quadriceps tendon and vastus medialis muscle, thereby maintaining an intact extensor mechanism above the patella. Proponents of the approach also claim that the exposure achieved is excellent and that there is less compromise of the patellar vascularity compared with the medial parapatellar arthrotomy.

A standard anterior midline incision is made with the knee in flexion and dissection continued down directly through fat and superficial fascia. The fascia is reflected to expose the medial aspect of the patella and vastus medialis at its insertion into the quadriceps tendon. The prepatellar bursa is reflected medially from the anterior surface of the patella, and the dissection distally is limited to skin and fat only. The superomedial corner of the patella is identified with the knee in flexion and the vastus medialis split by blunt finger dissection parallel to its fibers through the full thickness of the muscle, beginning 4 cm from and extending to the superomedial border of the patella. The amount of muscle split can be titrated once the patella is everted (Fig. 8).

The joint capsule is entered proximal to the patella and deep to the split vastus medialis. The capsular folds of the suprapatellar pouch need to be released to allow full eversion of the patella. The retinaculum and capsule along the medial side of the patella are then incised, leaving a cuff on the patella for later repair. This is carried distally approximately 1 cm medial of the patellar tendon insertion into the tibial tubercle, down to the distal limit of the tubercle. A subperiosteal medial release is performed to the mid-coronal plane. Capsule and synovium behind the patellar tendon are reflected to the medial border of the tubercle and tissue is released from the proximal tibia across to the retropatellar bursa. The patella is then everted, the lateral patellofemoral ligament is released, a portion of the fat pad is excised, and the joint capsule above the patellar tendon insertion is reflected until the lateral plateau is clearly exposed. Closure is performed in 60 degrees of flexion, commencing with a suture at the intersection of the capsular and muscle splitting components of the incision. No suturing of the muscle split is necessary.

The authors claim that innervation of the muscle is not compromised and that the approach does not extend far enough medially to encounter the femoral artery or saphenous nerve (Fig. 9). The geniculate arteries and branches are also rarely

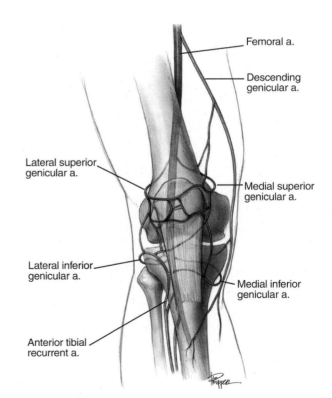

FIG. 9. Blood supply to the patella. Medial retinacular incisions will disrupt the three medial blood vessels, contributing to the anastomosis around the patella. If a lateral retinacular release is added, one or both of the lateral vessels will be disrupted. (From Engh GA, Parks NL. Surgical technique of the midvastus arthrotomy. *Clin Orthop* 1998;351:273, Fig. 3, with permission.)

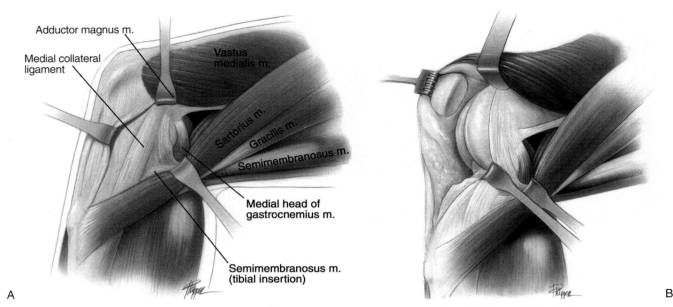

FIG. 10. A, B: The subvastus approach. (From Scuderi G. Chapter 7. In: Insall N, Scott WN, eds. *Surgery of the knee*, 3rd ed, vol 1. Philadelphia: WB Saunders, 2000:195, Fig. 7.5, with permission.)

encountered. Cooper et al. (12) studied this approach using a cadaver model, finding that the average distance between the start of the muscle split at the patella and the popliteal vessels was 8.8 cm, with a range from 6.5 to 12.3 cm. They concluded the maximal safe distance from the patellar margin for sharp dissection was 4.5 cm, but that further blunt muscle splitting was safe beyond this. Examination of the innervation of the muscle showed extensive branching of the femoral nerve within the muscle. The authors concluded that denervation of the distal segment of the muscle would occur only if the fibers were split to the point of attachment to the vastoadductor membrane, as the nerve is directly deep to this membrane. However, in a prospective randomized study, Parentis et al. (13) found electromyographic evidence of nerve injury in 9 of 21 patients after midvastus arthrotomy but no denervation after medial parapatellar arthrotomy. No corresponding clinical difference was found and the authors concluded longer-term studies would be necessary before the significance of this is determined.

Engh and Parks (11) listed some recommendations for the use of this approach. Obesity, hypertrophic arthritis, flexion of less than 80 degrees, and previous high tibial osteotomy are all listed as relative contraindications, and the authors suggested that the standard medial parapatellar arthrotomy may provide superior exposure. If a quadriceps snip is predicted to be necessary, this approach is not advised. They stated that revision surgery can be done through this approach, ideally in patients with flexion of more than 90 degrees who have had a previous midvastus approach.

SUBVASTUS (SOUTHERN) APPROACH

The subvastus approach first was described in the German literature in 1929 but has received relatively little attention in the subsequent literature. It has been described and popularized more recently by Hofmann et al. (14), who consider it a more anatomic approach than the standard medial parapatellar approach, with a number of subsequent advantages, as outlined below. A direct anterior midline incision is made with the knee flexed to 90 degrees, and dissection is carried down directly through the fat layer to identify the superficial fascia. This fascia is incised proximally in line with the skin incision and at the level of the patella slightly medial to avoid damage to the prepatellar plexus of vessels. Blunt finger dissection is used to separate this fascial layer from the perimuscular fascia of the vastus medialis down to its insertion site. The inferior edge of the vastus is identified and the muscle is lifted off the periosteum and intermuscular septum with blunt finger dissection for a distance of approximately 10 cm proximal to the adductor tubercle.

The muscle belly is placed under tension, allowing identification of the 2- to 3-cm-wide tendinous insertion of the vastus medialis to the medial capsule, which is transversely incised at the midpatellar level. Care is taken not to incise the synovium. The remainder of the vastus medialis remains attached to the patella and quadriceps tendon. The extensor mechanism is retracted anterolaterally and a curvilinear medial arthrotomy is made from the suprapatellar pouch to the tibial tubercle (Fig. 10). The fat pad is incised along its medial edge and sharp soft tissue release is performed from the proximal tibia. The patella is everted and dislocated laterally with the knee in full extension. The knee is then slowly flexed while the vastus medialis muscle belly is bluntly dissected off the intermuscular septum more proximally. This avoids overstretching of the vastus and excessive tension on the patellar tendon insertion.

Once the arthroplasty is completed, patellar tracking can be observed through the inferomedial window. If a lateral release is required it is performed from outside in with the knee in full flexion, with the surgeon releasing only that part of the capsule that is tight to palpation or visualization. The capsular closure is initiated with a suture at the apex of the L-shaped incision and completed with interrupted closure of the capsule and fascial layer.

The advantages of this approach lie in the more anatomic nature of the arthrotomy. The main theoretical advantages of this approach over the medial parapatellar approach are that the extensor mechanism is left intact and the medial vascularity of the patella is undamaged, which is particularly relevant if a lateral release is required. The proponents of the approach admit some limitations and suggest that relative contraindications to its use include revision arthroplasties or any previous arthrotomy about the knee, previous high tibial osteotomy, and patients weighing more than 200 lb. In these knees and in any other knee in which eversion of the patella is believed to be potentially difficult, the nonextensile subvastus approach may be a difficult technique with which to obtain satisfactory exposure. In addition, although a good exposure of the medial compartment can usually be achieved, it can be difficult to gain similarly good access to the lateral side, particularly in a knee with significant deformity or stiffness. Nonetheless, this approach is promoted as a more natural and logical choice than the medial parapatellar approach for the above-mentioned reasons and as a simple technique that can be easily mastered without adding to operating time (14,15).

MEDIAL TRIVECTOR–RETAINING APPROACH

The medial trivector–retaining approach was described by Bramlett, with potential advantages over the medial parapatellar and subvastus approaches (16). The principle of the technique lies in the concept that the quadriceps muscle has medial, lateral, and superior vectors. By taking the extensor mechanism incision through the vastus medialis, the muscle is not completely detached from the quadriceps tendon, thereby preserving a significant portion of the medial vector. Proponents of the technique believe that it combines the extensile nature of the medial parapatellar approach and the preservation of the vastus medialis insertion of the subvastus approach. The approach is done through a standard anterior midline skin incision, with dissection carried down directly through fat and superficial fascia to expose the underlying extensor mechanism. The extensor mechanism incision is commenced approximately 6 cm proximal to the patella and extended distally through the vastus medialis muscle approximately 10 to 15 mm medial to the attachment to the quadriceps tendon. This is then continued distally 1 cm medial to the patella down to the tibia medial to the tibial tubercle, and the patella is then everted. The exposure and closure are done in flexion.

Proponents of this approach claim that it allows good exposure similar to the medial parapatellar approach but with the advantage of retaining a significant portion of the medial vector of the extensor mechanism, with subsequent improved quadriceps function postoperatively. Fisher et al. (17) compared this approach with the medial parapatellar approach in ten patients undergoing bilateral TKA, finding that the trivector approach resulted in independent straight leg raising 2 days earlier than the medial parapatellar but no other significant differences between the groups. The small number of patients in the study makes it impossible to draw definite conclusions and no other studies are currently available. This approach has some potential disadvantages. It can compromise the medial vascularity of the patella similar to the medial parapatellar approach, and the effect of dividing the muscle fibers of the vastus medialis has not

been well studied, particularly in terms of potential for hematoma formation, healing capacity of the muscle fibers, and possible denervation. Further study is therefore necessary before the theoretical advantages of this approach can translate to a general recommendation for its usage.

LATERAL APPROACH

The lateral approach for TKA was first described by Keblish (18), who developed the technique after first using a more limited approach for lateral unicompartmental arthroplasty. He considered the medial arthrotomy to be inappropriate for knees with significant valgus deformity for several reasons, including the indirect access to tight lateral structures, exacerbation of external tibial rotation, the invariable need for lateral release that isolates the patella from its major blood supply, and increased frequency of postoperative patellar problems. He also believed there was an increased risk for skin problems and tentative rehabilitation due to extensive and at times unsatisfactory medial soft tissue closure.

A long anterior midline skin incision is made following the Q angle and ending 1 to 2 cm lateral to the tibial tubercle. The dissection is carried directly through fat and superficial fascia to expose the extensor mechanism. The arthrotomy begins proximally along the lateral border of the quadriceps tendon, extending distally 1 to 2 cm lateral to the patella and through the medial edge of Gerdy's tubercle, ending in the anterior compartment fascia approximately 2 cm lateral to the tibial tubercle (Fig. 11A). It is important to avoid going through the fat pad to preserve the lateral blood supply with mobilization of the fat pad, which is essential for soft tissue gap closure. The availability of soft tissue to close the anticipated gap should be analyzed and dissection from lateral to medial done in such a way as to maximize soft tissue preservation. The mobilization involves sharp dissection under the patellar tendon across to the medial aspect of the intermeniscal ligament, which is incised down to bone. The dissection is then continued back laterally to include a rim of lateral meniscus and this composite graft of fat pad, intermeniscal ligament, and lateral meniscal rim is mobilized on the lateral vascular pedicle. This flap is protected throughout the rest of the procedure and subsequently used to close the lateral defect at the end of the procedure.

If the knee is not correctable to a neutral alignment, Keblish recommends releasing the iliotibial band approximately 10 cm proximal to the joint line as part of the exposure. If the deformity is more than 40 degrees, the release is done by elevating Gerdy's tubercle with a sleeve of fascia. The lateral 50% of the tibial tubercle is elevated with a wide osteotome to create a sleeve of tendon, tubercle, and anterior compartment fascia that assists in medial eversion of the patella. This is done in flexion while applying a varus moment to the knee. Any blocking adhesions or large patellar osteophytes are removed if necessary to assist with eversion. Lateral osteophytes are removed. Visualization of the posterolateral corner is usually excellent at this stage, and if necessary, an osteoperiosteal release can be done at this stage from the femoral side. To assist with visualization of the medial side a curved retractor is placed behind the posteromedial plateau and the assistant rotates the tibia back to a neutral position.

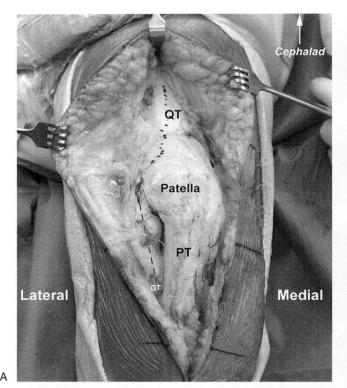

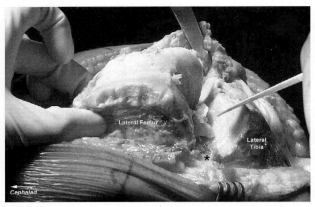

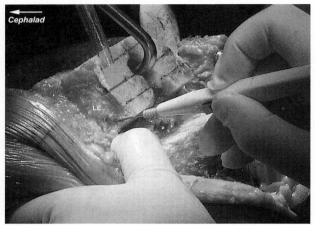

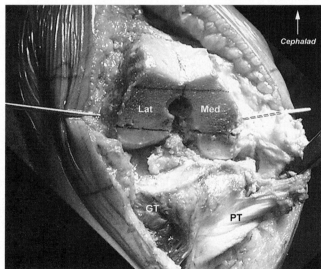

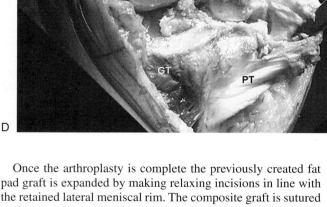

FIG. 11. A: The authors' anterolateral approach. The incision along the lateral border of the quadriceps tendon (QT) is indicated. The distal limb of the incision is centered over Gerdy's tubercle (GT), approximately 1 cm lateral to the margin of the patella tendon (PT). B: In a fixed valgus knee, a lateral subperiosteal sleeve (incorporating the iliotibial band insertion) is lifted from the proximal tibia to the level of the fibular head (*asterisk*). C: A subperiosteal release of the structures from the lateral epicondyle (LE)—the popliteus tendon and the lateral collateral ligament—is performed with the knee in flexion. D: Final view afforded by an anterolateral approach to a fixed, valgus knee. [From photo library—Department of Orthopaedics (Adult Reconstruction), London Health Sciences Centre, London, Ontario, Canada, with permission.]

Once the arthroplasty is complete the previously created fat pad graft is expanded by making relaxing incisions in line with the retained lateral meniscal rim. The composite graft is sutured to the capsule proximally and the lateral aspect of the quadriceps and patellar tendons. Vastus lateralis closure is then completed and the lateral defect is now closed. The distal patellar tendon sleeve is left unsutured. Closure is then completed over a drain.

Several modifications of this approach have been described (19–22). Buechel (19) uses a similar exposure but describes a sequential release for deformity correction. Mild deformities usually only require release of the iliotibial band from Gerdy's tubercle (Fig. 11B). Moderate fixed valgus of 10 to 20 degrees

requires this plus release of collateral ligament and popliteus tendon as a proximally based flap on the femoral side, releasing the amount of tissue necessary to correct the deformity (Fig. 11C). This release is done in flexion of 90 degrees. For severe deformities, the knee is held once again at 90 degrees, the entire periosteum is elevated from the fibular head, and the fibular head is then resected. If the tibia is subsequently translating forward and unable to be displaced beneath the femur at 90 degrees, the posterior cruciate ligament should be released. Fiddian et al. (20) modified the approach by extending the quadriceps tendon incision proximally 2 to 3 cm beneath the fat and skin to completely release the contracted vastus lateralis from the patella and quadriceps tendon. To close the arthrotomy, the knee is held at 75 degrees and the vastus lateralis and lateral quadriceps tendon sutured to the medial tendon under gentle tension, effectively repositioning the vastus lateralis proximally. They make no attempt to close the residual defect distally and claim that the modification avoids the need for elevation of the tibial tubercle and improves patellofemoral tracking and contact pressures. Hendel and Weisbort (21) also described a technique to avoid the tubercle elevation with the use of a medial quadriceps snip, whereas Burki et al. (22) combined the lateral approach with a tubercle osteotomy, with both groups claiming excellent exposure of the joint.

The lateral approach is certainly a logical option for arthroplasty in the valgus knee. The advantages are that it provides a more direct access to the area of bony pathology and soft tissue contractures that require releasing, possibly allowing a more conservative and appropriate release to correct deformity. It naturally corrects the external rotation deformity of the tibia, which is invariably associated with valgus knees, and the often-required lateral release is incorporated into the exposure, minimizing the damage to the vascularity of the patella. The stability of the medial structures is also uncompromised by the approach and patellofemoral problems are thought to be reduced. The disadvantages of the procedure are relatively poor visualization of the medial side, difficulty everting the patella, more difficult orientation with the anatomy reversed compared with the more familiar medial approach, and a large lateral defect invariably ensues. This is probably the technique of choice for knees with significant valgus deformity associated with patellar subluxation, but the surgeon certainly needs to be familiar with this more technically demanding approach to reap all of its theoretical benefits (Fig. 11D).

DIFFICULT EXPOSURE: SPECIALIZED TECHNIQUES

Exposure of certain TKAs can be particularly difficult, requiring supplementary techniques to the previously described approaches. It is important to attempt to identify those patients with potentially difficult exposures during the preoperative planning. This allows planning the approach to maximize exposure while decreasing the chance of complications such as patellar tendon avulsion, which can have disastrous consequences. Patients with severe valgus or varus deformities and those with flexion contractures or flexion of less than 90 degrees will often provide a particular challenge to achieve adequate exposure. Radiographic evidence of patella baja or significant deformity is also a warning sign of a potentially difficult exposure. The following techniques have all been described to supplement standard exposure techniques in such cases of difficult exposure.

Medial Epicondylar Osteotomy

The medial epicondylar osteotomy has been popularized by Engh (23) as a method of correcting soft tissue contractures associated with varus deformity and flexion deformity in difficult primary and revision arthroplasties. Specifically, the technique is said to be a useful procedure in difficult exposures such as capsular fibrosis, conversion of a knee arthrodesis, allograft distal femur reconstruction, and revision of a posterior dislocation of a cruciate-retaining arthroplasty. The procedure is performed

through a medial arthrotomy and the capsule is incised and reflected from the medial tibial metaphysis to the midcoronal plane. The epicondylar osteotomy is performed with the knee in 90 degrees of flexion or at maximum flexion if 90 degrees is not possible. Osteophytes are removed to allow clear visualization of the epicondyle and the adductor tubercle and insertion of the adductor magnus tendon are identified by palpating the proximal end of the medial femoral condyle. The synovium is incised with cautery to demarcate the osteotomy. The osteotomy is begun just proximal to the rim of excised osteophytes. The osteotome is oriented parallel to the long axis of the femur and is advanced to release a segment of bone 1 cm thick and 4 cm in diameter, with the attachments of medial collateral ligament and adductor magnus tendon. The segment of bone is hinged open when the fragment is displaced posterior to the condyle. This allows easy access to the posterior compartment from the medial side if further release is necessary. Posteromedial capsule is released if necessary to fully correct a varus deformity (Fig. 12).

Knee stability in extension is maintained through the proximal-to-distal continuity of the attached soft tissue sleeve, akin to the attached sleeve of a trochanteric slide in total hip arthroplasty, and stability in flexion is established when the epicondyle is reattached. This is done with the knee in 90 degrees of flexion, bringing the epicondyle into position as far anterior on the condyle as permitted by the medial collateral ligament attachment. A cortical bridge is maintained between the anterior femoral resection and the epicondylar osteotomy, which serves as an anchor for sutures passed through the condyle. Two or three No. 2 sutures are placed through the epicondyle and under the cortical bridge and secured, and stability is tested. Postoperative rehabilitation is not restricted unless the fragment cannot be satisfactorily reattached, in which case a brace is used for 6 weeks to limit flexion. Heterotopic bone and fibrous union are reported, but the authors report no clinical problems resulting form either of these scenarios.

Engh states that advantages of this technique include the avoidance of extensive stripping or sectioning of ligaments, enhanced exposure of the posterior capsule for additional releases that may be necessary, and good restoration of stability with repair of the osteotomy. He warns against creation of a fragment that is too thin and may subsequently fragment and also advises that large deformities may require additional division of the posteromedial capsule. If the fragment is difficult to reduce, the cautery should be used to divide tissues attached to the posterior rim of the fragment to allow a more anterior approximation on the condyle. With correction of severe varus deformities, the attachment may become more distal, in which case the position of the fragment is accepted and any joint line overhang is trimmed with a rongeur. The authors deny experiencing any clinical problems with this technique, which they describe as a valuable tool for gaining exposure, correcting deformity, and restoring knee stability without damage to ligamentous structures. It is, however, difficult to provide general recommendations for the use of this approach until these positive results are further substantiated by clinical studies from other centers.

Tibial Tubercle Osteotomy

Osteotomy of the tibial tubercle is a useful technique that allows distal extension of the approach in difficult exposures. This tech-

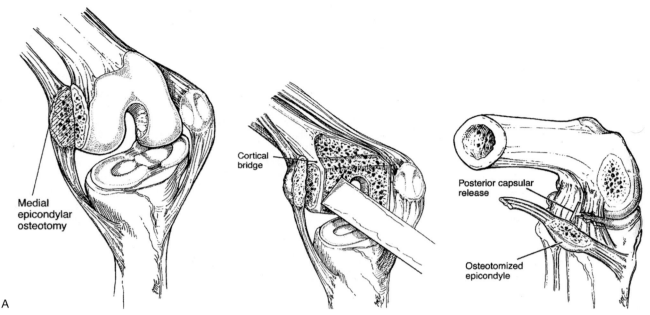

A

B,C

FIG. 12. A: The osteotomized epicondyle with intact adductor magnus tendon and collateral ligaments is displaced posterior to the medial femoral condyle. Exposure is enhanced by external rotation and varus angulation of the knee in a flexed position. **B:** A cortical bridge is established between the anterior femoral bone resection and the osteotomized medial femoral epicondyle. Sutures are passed beneath this bridge of cortical bone to anchor the repair of the epicondyle. **C:** The posteromedial capsule, including fibers of the posterior oblique ligament, is released with cautery to fully correct varus deformity and flexion contracture of the knee. (From Engh GA. Medial epicondylar osteotomy: a technique used with primary and revision total knee arthroplasty to improve surgical exposure and correct varus deformity. *Instr Course Lect* 1999;48:153–156, Figs. 1 to 3, with permission.)

nique was first described for TKA by Dolin (24) and has subsequently been modified and popularized by Whiteside (25) and used by many other authors (26,27). Earlier reports (28) of this technique reported a high incidence of complications, including nonunion, tendon rupture, and infection, resulting in a poor reputation for the procedure, which is therefore often discouraged by many authors in favor of other techniques such as quadriceps turndown. More recent reports (25–27,29) with improved techniques have, however, shown the technique to be a useful adjunct that, if done properly, has a relatively low complication rate. Specific advantages include the ability to reposition the tubercle, for example more proximally in cases of patellar baja and more medially in cases of patellar subluxation. The osteotomy also allows access for removal of tibial component stems in revision scenarios.

Several variations of tibial tubercle osteotomy have been described, mostly for treatment of patellofemoral instability or pain. The technique used by the authors for TKA exposure is similar to that described by Whiteside (25) (Fig. 13). The most important aspects of the technique are to take a fragment of adequate thickness and length, to leave a lateral soft tissue hinge intact, and to achieve stable fixation. It is also important to bypass the defect with a stemmed tibial component to avoid a postoperative fracture. In performing the osteotomy, the edges of the patellar tendon are clearly defined and the proposed osteotomy is marked out, taking the full thickness of the tubercle proximally with all of the patellar tendon insertion and extending distally approximately 8 cm, beveling the fragment toward the anterior cortex distally. This is in contrast to Whiteside, who performs a transverse cut distally, which

leaves a significantly greater stress riser at this level than the beveled cut. The osteotomy can be done with a saw or osteotomes but should leave the lateral soft tissues and distal periosteal sleeve intact, hinging the fragment laterally to evert the patella. Fixation can be done either with screws or wires, with the authors' preference for wires. If screws are used, two are usually placed with offset entry points on the tubercle to avoid splitting the fragment, and diverging away from the tibial component stem. If wires are used, three Luque wires are usually used, with the first through the fragment and the distal two around the fragment. The wires are angled distally from lateral to medial to tension the fragment distally. All should be placed through the thick posteromedial cortex to achieve solid fixation when tightened (Figs. 13C and D).

Postoperative rehabilitation is not restricted with this approach and is the same as for routine primary arthroplasty patients. Additional specific advantages over other techniques such as quadriceps turndown include the ability to reposition the tubercle if necessary, bone-to-bone healing, and maintenance of quadriceps power. Good results have been reported with this technique (25–27), and in the authors' experience this is a technique that, although rarely required in primary arthroplasty, provides a useful extensile exposure distally for cases in which exposure is difficult.

Quadriceps (Rectus) Snip

The quadriceps or rectus snip has been popularized by Garvin et al. (30) and provides an effective adjunct to exposure of the

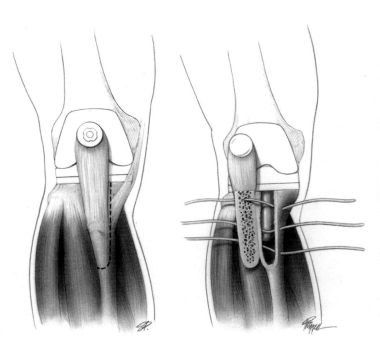

A,B

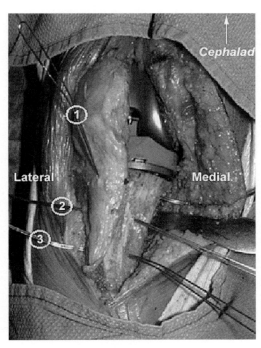

C

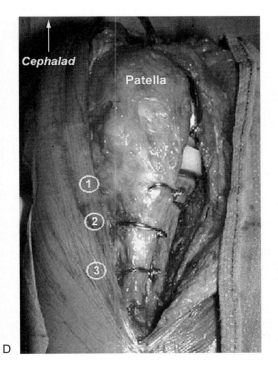

D

FIG. 13. A: The bone cut for the tibial tubercle osteotomy is outlined. The osteotomy should be 5 to 7 cm in length and should be at least 1 cm thick to prevent fracture of the fragment. The osteotomy is performed with the use of a saw from medial to lateral and can be completed with osteotomes. The osteotomy is hinged on the lateral soft tissues, which are left intact to maintain blood supply. **B:** The tibial shaft can be accessed for cement removal, which reduces tension on the extensor mechanism by displacing the tibial tubercle laterally. Note that the three wires have been inserted before implantation of the revision, stemmed tibial component. **C:** The osteotomy is closed by passing three wires (through drill holes) and is then stabilized by compression of the cortical bone. Wire No. 1 is actually passed through the osteotomized fragment to avoid fragment "escape." The lower wires (2 and 3) are placed through lateral drill holes that are placed more proximally than the medial drill holes; this draws the osteotomy distally with compression. **D:** Stability of fixation is assessed by observing the wires while putting the knee through an arc of flexion-extension. [**A** and **B** from Younger AS, Duncan CP, Masri BA. Surgical exposures in revision total knee arthroplasty. *J Am Acad Orthop Surg* 1998;6:63; **C** and **D** from photo library—Department of Orthopaedics (Adult Reconstruction), London Health Sciences Centre, London, Ontario, Canada, with permission.]

stiff knee that has been shown to have little if any added morbidity when compared with a standard medial parapatellar approach (Fig. 14). If the knee is very stiff, it is important to keep in mind that the snip will give only a certain amount of additional exposure, and if significant difficulty is anticipated, other techniques need to be considered and incorporated into the planning. A standard medial parapatellar arthrotomy is performed, and if there is significant difficulty everting the patella, placing the patellar tendon at risk, a rectus snip is performed. This involves extending the proximal limit of the quadriceps

incision proximally and laterally at approximately 45 degrees to transect the rectus femoris tendon near its musculotendinous junction. This allows the patella to be mobilized distally and laterally. If eversion of the patella remains difficult, it is important to ensure that all hypertrophic scar tissue has been excised, and if necessary, a lateral retinacular release can be added. If exposure is still inadequate, the quadriceps incision can then be carried inferiorly and laterally to achieve a quadriceps turndown, although this is rarely necessary. The rectus snip is a technically simple procedure to perform that predictably improves expo-

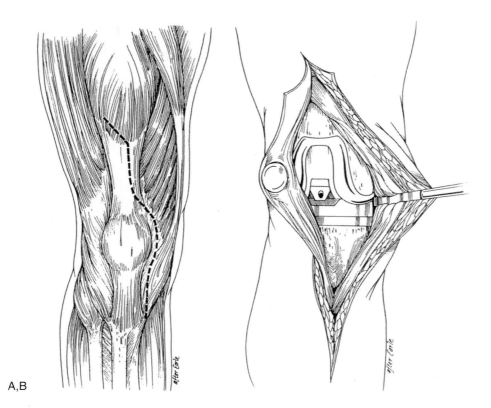

A,B

FIG. 14. The quadriceps snip. A standard medial parapatellar incision is used **(A)**, with further exposure of the knee being obtained by dividing the quadriceps muscle proximally, with extension of the incision laterally **(B)**. A greater degree of exposure will be obtained with a more distal and transverse cut. (From Younger AS, Duncan CP, Masri BA. Surgical exposures in revision total knee arthroplasty. *J Am Acad Orthop Surg* 1998;6:61, Figs. 5A and B, with permission.)

sure. In contrast to the quadriceps turndown, it spares the superior lateral genicular artery, there is no need for any alteration in the postoperative rehabilitation, and there is no significant effect on the recovery of quadriceps function postoperatively (31).

Quadriceps Turndown and V-Y Quadricepsplasty

The quadriceps turndown procedure was initially described by Coonse and Adams (32) and has subsequently been modified by other authors (33). The initial description was of a distally based inverted V with the apex at the proximal central limit of the quadriceps tendon. Subsequent modifications have been designed (30) to allow for conversion of initial standard approaches intraoperatively if necessary. The exposure allows distal and lateral displacement of the extensor mechanism for wide exposure and release of distal tension on the patellar tendon in stiff or ankylosed knees. The approach also allows for lengthening of the extensor mechanism as a V-Y plasty in cases of stiff knees with limited flexion. The procedure is not without problems, however, particularly the virtually complete devascularization of the patella with increased risk of avascular necrosis and the almost invariable presence of an extensor lag postoperatively.

The procedure can be performed as a spectrum of increasing quadriceps incisions depending on the exposure obtained with each step. Initial exposure is done through a medial parapatellar arthrotomy as described previously, and if after the standard exposure excessive tension is on the patellar tendon, an ancillary procedure is required. If the surgeon believes that this may not be achieved with a rectus snip, the initial step must allow for possible conversion to a quadriceps turndown. Having taken the quadriceps incision to the proximal extent of the tendon an

oblique cut is made laterally across the quadriceps tendon, angling 45 degrees distally, in contrast to the snip, which is angled proximally. This may be sufficient and if so leaves the vastus lateralis intact and allows for direct suture of the tendon after the procedure. Although rarely necessary, if exposure remains inadequate, this can be continued distally across the vastus lateralis tendon and upper portion of the iliotibial tract, completing the patellar turndown to give excellent exposure (Fig. 15). Easy access to the lateral gutter is obtained, allowing for release of dense adhesions and mobilization of the extensor mechanism (31). This has the advantage of stopping proximal to the inferior lateral geniculate artery, although this is only theoretical, as this artery is usually sacrificed later in the procedure when the lateral meniscus is excised. Scott and Siliski (33) modified the turndown to avoid division of the superior lateral geniculate artery. In this case, the distal extent of the incision is taken across the vastus lateralis insertion, stopping proximal to the superior lateral geniculate artery and not including a lateral release. They described this approach as a modified V-Y quadricepsplasty. Once again, the advantages of preservation of the artery are unproven, as Ritter and Campbell (34) found no increase in patellofemoral complications with sacrifice of this artery, although in the authors' experience the quadriceps turndown has been associated with a high rate of patellar avascular necrosis.

Repair of the turndown should be completed with heavy nonabsorbable sutures at the appropriate degree of tension. This is difficult to judge but as a general guide should be done as close as possible to an anatomic repair while allowing flexion close to 90 degrees. As extensor lag is a common complication of this approach, it is critical to avoid any overlengthening of the tendon. In cases such as ankylosis in which there is chronic short-

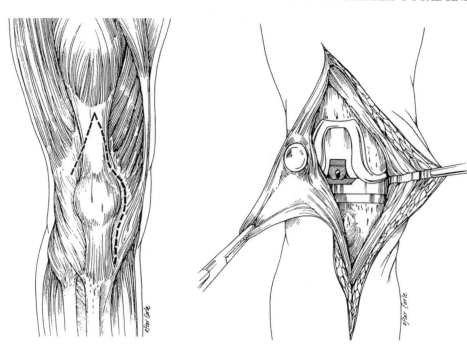

A,B

FIG. 15. The incision **(A)** and the exposure obtained **(B)** with the patella turndown. The quadriceps tendon should be repaired with the use of a non-absorbable suture and should be protected postoperatively. (From Younger AS, Duncan CP, Masri BA. Surgical exposures in revision total knee arthroplasty. *J Am Acad Orthop Surg* 1998;6:62, Figs. 6A and B, with permission.)

ening of the extensor mechanism, the tendon can be lengthened by conversion to a Y but once again avoiding any overlengthening. The lateral retinaculum is often left open as a lateral release. The point at which the repair comes under tension should be noted and the postoperative rehabilitation limited to this range for approximately 6 weeks to allow some tendon healing. Active extension should also probably be avoided for a similar timeframe. Another drawback of this approach is in using it more than once, such as in infection, where multiple procedures may be necessary. Although the turndown is technically a relatively straightforward approach that provides excellent exposure, its use is not without significant potential morbidity and should therefore be restricted to cases in which no other method will provide adequate exposure without additional morbidity.

COMPARATIVE STUDIES

Several clinical studies have been performed to compare different approaches, including four recent studies published within the same year comparing the medial parapatellar and midvastus arthrotomies. White et al. (35) looked at 109 patients who had a medial parapatellar approach in one knee and a midvastus approach in the other. Significant differences were found in number of lateral retinacular releases, pain at 8 days and 6 weeks, and straight leg raising at 8 days, all favoring the midvastus approach. No increased difficulty was encountered using the midvastus approach for severe deformity. At 6 months, both patient groups were identical to clinical assessment, suggesting the advantages of the midvastus approach lie in the immediate postoperative recovery. These results were duplicated by Dalury and Jiranek (36). In contrast, Keating et al. (37) found no significant difference between the two approaches in a randomized prospective trial, including the parameters found to be different in the two previously mentioned studies. They did find the midvastus approach to be more difficult in obese patients and had a

higher rate of complications, although not a significant difference. Parentis et al. (13), in another randomized prospective study, found a greater number of lateral releases and higher blood loss in the parapatellar group but no other significant difference postoperatively. They did, however, perform electromyography postoperatively in all patients, finding 43% of electromyograms to be abnormal in the midvastus approach. No corresponding clinical deficit was detected and the significance of this denervation remains uncertain. Comparison of these two approaches has certainly been investigated thoroughly with properly designed studies. It is not possible on the basis of these studies to identify a clearly superior technique that should be recommended, and each can obviously be used with success. The main disadvantage of the midvastus approach when compared with the parapatellar is its nonextensile nature proximally, which could be a significant disadvantage in knees that are difficult to expose.

In other comparative studies, Matsueda and Gustilo (38) compared the subvastus with the parapatellar approach, finding improved patellar tracking and decreased need for lateral release in the subvastus group but no other significant difference. The retrospective nature of this study, particularly involving an earlier time frame for the parapatellar group, means that these results may have also been affected by factors such as improved surgical technique over the 9-year period. In a comparative study of approaches in revision surgery, Barrack et al. (39) compared patients undergoing the standard medial parapatellar approach with patients requiring a rectus snip and patients requiring either a quadriceps turndown or tibial tubercle osteotomy. No difference was found between the rectus snip group and the standard approach for all parameters. The osteotomy and turndown groups had equivalent postoperative scores that were significantly lower than the other groups. The osteotomy group had less extensor lag than the turndown group but had greater difficulty squatting and kneeling. The turndown group had a greater improvement in arc of motion than the osteotomy

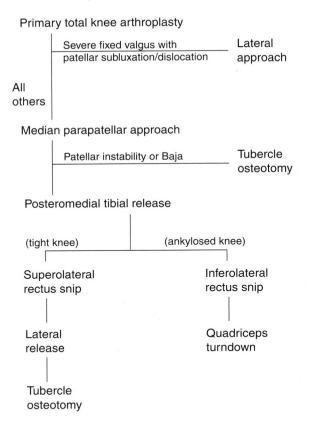

FIG. 16. Algorithm for choice of approach. Progression to each next step in the pathway should be made on the basis of inadequate exposure.

group and a higher degree of patient satisfaction. This study had a number of design flaws, including a tendency for osteotomy to be used in the more difficult cases, making the findings less of a scientific basis for strong recommendations.

The overall summary of these comparative studies seems to be that no basis has been found for strongly recommending one technique over another. Those techniques that preserve some or all of the vastus medialis attachment such as the midvastus and subvastus may have advantages in improving patellofemoral tracking, at least intraoperatively, as well as enhancing the early recovery of function. However, they also have the disadvantages of being nonextensile and potentially difficult in certain patients. The rectus snip seems to add no increased morbidity to a standard approach, whereas tibial tubercle osteotomy and quadriceps turndown have specific well-recognized disadvantages, making them procedures to use only after careful consideration and when absolutely necessary.

CONCLUSION

Approach to the primary TKA should be a straightforward exercise in most cases. Careful preoperative planning will identify those cases that are likely to be more difficult and require modifications of the standard approach. Thorough attention to detail with each step from skin incision to closure should ensure excellent exposure that does not compromise implantation and

is not associated with any unnecessary morbidity. The previous discussion is a comprehensive account of all of the commonly used techniques available. It is the arthroplasty surgeon's responsibility to be familiar with each of these to appreciate which is the most appropriate in each scenario. For the vast majority of cases, the authors' preference is to use the medial parapatellar approach. The algorithm in Figure 16 outlines a general pathway for choice of the appropriate approach and ancillary procedures. With appropriate choice of technique, it should be possible to achieve an excellent exposure for all TKAs using these guidelines.

REFERENCES

1. Haertsch PA. The blood supply to the skin of the leg: a post-mortem investigation. *Br J Plast Surg* 1981;34:470–477.
2. Younger ASE, Duncan CP, Masri BA. Surgical exposures in revision total knee arthroplasty. *J Am Acad Orthop Surg* 1998;6:55–64.
3. Johnson DP. Midline or parapatellar incision for knee arthroplasty. *J Bone Joint Surg Br* 1988;70:656–658.
4. Langer K. On the anatomy and physiology of the skin. *Br J Plast Surg* 1978;31:3–8.
5. Johnson DP, Houghton TA, Radford P. Anterior midline or medial parapatellar incision for arthroplasty of the knee. *J Bone Joint Surg Br* 1986;68:812–814.
6. Chambers GH. The prepatellar nerve. *Clin Orthop* 1972;82:157–159.
7. Insall J. A midline approach to the knee. *J Bone Joint Surg Am* 1971;53:1584–1586.
8. Masri BA, Laskin RS, Windsor RE, et al. Knee closure in total knee replacement: a randomized prospective trial. *Clin Orthop* 1996;331:81–86.
9. Bonutti PM, Miller BG, Cremens MJ. Intraosseous patellar blood supply after medial parapatellar arthrotomy. *Clin Orthop* 1998;352:202–214.
10. Kayler D, Lyttle D. Surgical interruption of patellar blood supply by total knee arthroplasty. *Clin Orthop* 1988;229:221–227.
11. Engh GA, Parks NL. Surgical technique of the midvastus arthrotomy. *Clin Orthop* 1998;351:270–274.
12. Cooper RE Jr., Trinidad G, Buck WR. Midvastus approach in total knee arthroplasty: a description and a cadaveric study determining the distance of the popliteal artery from the patellar margin of the incision. *J Arthroplasty* 1999;14:505–508.
13. Parentis MA, Rumi MN, Deol GS, et al. A comparison of the vastus splitting and median parapatellar approaches in total knee arthroplasty. *Clin Orthop* 1999;367:107–116.
14. Hofmann AA, Plaster RL, Murdock LE. Subvastus (southern) approach for primary total knee arthroplasty. *Clin Orthop* 1991;269:70–77.
15. Faure BT, Benjamin JB, Lindsey B, et al. Comparison of the subvastus and paramedian surgical approaches in bilateral knee arthroplasty. *J Arthroplasty* 1993;8:511–516.
16. Stern SH. Surgical exposure in total knee arthroplasty. In: Fu FH, Harner CD, Vince KG, eds. *Knee surgery*, vol. 2. Baltimore: Williams & Wilkins, 1994:1289–1302.
17. Fisher DA, Trimble SM, Breedlove K. The medial trivector approach in total knee arthroplasty. *Orthopedics* 1998;21:53–56.
18. Keblish P. The lateral approach to the valgus knee. Surgical technique and analysis of 53 cases with over two-year follow-up evaluation. *Clin Orthop* 1991;271:52–62.
19. Buechel FF. A sequential three-step lateral release for correcting fixed valgus knee deformities during total knee arthroplasty. *Clin Orthop* 1990;260:170–175.
20. Fiddian NJ, Blakeway C, Kumar A. Replacement arthroplasty of the valgus knee. A modified lateral capsular approach with repositioning of vastus lateralis. *J Bone Joint Surg Br* 1998;80:859–861.
21. Hendel D, Weisbort M. Modified lateral approach for knee arthroplasty in a fixed valgus knee—the medial quadriceps snip. *Acta Orthop Scand* 2000;71:204–205.
22. Burki H, von Knoch M, Heiss C, et al. Lateral approach with osteotomy of the tibial tubercle in primary total knee arthroplasty. *Clin Orthop* 1999;362:156–161.
23. Engh GA. Medial epicondylar osteotomy: a technique used with pri-

mary and revision total knee arthroplasty to improve surgical exposure and correct varus deformity. *Instr Course Lect* 1999;48:153–156.

24. Dolin MG. Osteotomy of the tibial tubercle in total knee replacement. *J Bone Joint Surg Am* 1983;65:704–706.

25. Whiteside LA. Exposure in difficult total knee arthroplasty using tibial tubercle osteotomy. *Clin Orthop* 1995;321:32–35.

26. Masini MA, Stulberg SD. A new surgical technique for tibial tubercle transfer in total knee arthroplasty. *J Arthroplasty* 1992;7:81–86.

27. Ries MD, Richman JA. Extended tibial tubercle osteotomy in total knee arthroplasty. *J Arthroplasty* 1996;11:964–967.

28. Grace JN, Rand JA. Patellar instability after total knee arthroplasty. *Clin Orthop* 1988;237:184–189.

29. Whiteside LA. Distal realignment of the patellar tendon to correct abnormal patellar tracking. *Clin Orthop* 1997;344:284–289.

30. Garvin KL, Scuderi G, Insall JN. Evolution of the quadriceps snip. *Clin Orthop* 1995;321:131–137.

31. Barrack RI. Specialized surgical exposure for revision total knee: quadriceps snip and patellar turndown. *Instr Course Lect* 1999;48:149–152.

32. Coonse K, Adams JD. A new operative approach to the knee joint. *Surg Gynecol Obstet* 1943;77:344–347.

33. Scott RD, Siliski JM. The use of a modified V-Y quadricepsplasty during total knee replacement to gain exposure and improve flexion in the ankylosed knee. *Orthopedics* 1985;8:45–48.

34. Ritter MA, Campbell ED. Postoperative patellar complications with or without lateral release during total knee arthroplasty. *Clin Orthop* 1987;219:163–168.

35. White RE Jr., Allman JK, Trauger JA, et al. Clinical comparison of the midvastus and medial parapatellar surgical approaches. *Clin Orthop* 1999;367:117–122.

36. Dalury DF, Jiranek WA. A comparison of the midvastus and paramedian approaches for total knee arthroplasty. *J Arthroplasty* 1999;14:33–37.

37. Keating EM, Faris PM, Meding JB, et al. Comparison of the midvastus muscle-splitting approach with the median parapatellar approach in total knee arthroplasty. *J Arthroplasty* 1999;14:29–32.

38. Matsueda M, Gustilo RB. Subvastus and medial parapatellar approaches in total knee arthroplasty. *Clin Orthop* 2000;371:161–168.

39. Barrack RL, Smith P, Munn B, et al. The Ranawat Award. Comparison of surgical approaches in total knee arthroplasty. *Clin Orthop* 1998;356:16–21.

CHAPTER 76

Unicompartmental Knee Arthroplasty

Amir A. Jamali, David J. Rodricks, Marc I. Malberg, Alfred J. Tria, Jr.,
Harry E. Rubash, and Andrew A. Freiberg

Surgical options for arthritis of one compartment of the tibiofemoral joint have been limited. These include arthroscopic chondral débridement, allograft or autograft surface replacement, high tibial osteotomy (HTO), unicompartmental arthroplasty,* and total knee arthroplasty (TKA) (Fig. 1). In this chapter, the developmental history, theoretical advantages, indications, clinical follow-up, and surgical technique of unicompartmental knee arthroplasty (UKA) are discussed.

The first unicompartmental arthroplasties were inserted in the early 1950s. McKeever used a flat metallic insert that included a keel for press-fit fixation on the tibial plateau (1). MacIntosh experimented with several different materials and ultimately removed the keel, relying on the soft tissues to hold his prosthesis in place (2). The base of the tibial tray had a roughened surface to improve contact with the cut tibial plateau. The major source of failure in these implants was loss of articular cartilage

on the femoral side. Gunston published the first paper on the cemented polycentric knee in 1971 (3). With this prosthesis, the medial and lateral compartments were resurfaced independently. Marmor, based on the experience with the tibial plateau prostheses, addressed the femoral side with a metal component and thus inserted the first cemented unicompartmental knee replacement in the United States (4). The all-polyethylene† tibial component was modeled on the tibial plateau prostheses. In 1978, Goodfellow and O'Connor designed the first meniscal bearing prosthesis, with a spheric femoral component, a flat metallic tibial component, and a fully congruent polyethylene liner to allow rotation and translation of the liner between the femur and tibia (5–7). During the early years of development, many of these prostheses were used on both the medial and lateral side of the same knee (3,4,8,9). These bicompartmental modular arthroplasties proved to be more technically difficult

---

*In this chapter, the term *unicompartmental knee arthroplasty* is used synonymously with *unicondylar knee arthroplasty* and *unicompartmental arthroplasty*.

---

†The term *polyethylene* used in this chapter refers to the polymer ultrahigh molecular weight polyethylene.

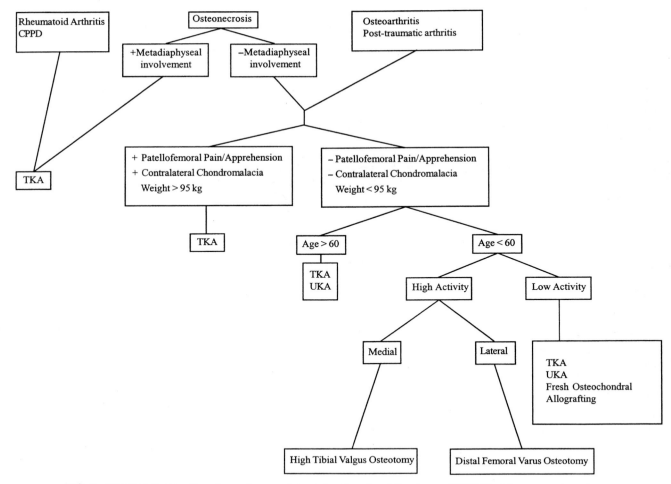

FIG. 1. Treatment algorithm for unicompartmental arthrosis of the knee. CPPD, calcium pyrophosphate dihydrate deposition; TKA, total knee arthroplasty; UKA, unicompartmental knee arthroplasty.

and less reliable than standard TKA and fell out of favor by the early 1980s.

UKA was conceived as a less invasive approach to treatment of isolated arthrosis of one compartment of the knee (4). The early advocates believed that UKA provided an intermediate operation that, if needed, could later be revised to a TKA. Short- and medium-term follow-up results from Insall et al., at the Hospital for Special Surgery (HSS), demonstrated poor results, particularly with medial compartment arthroplasty (10,11). However, this series was characterized by an incidence of patellectomy of more than 50%, which some authors have since considered a relative contraindication to UKA (12). The varus knees in this series were corrected from an average of 8 degrees varus to 4 degrees valgus. Recent experience with UKA has found that overcorrection can lead to accelerated degeneration in the contralateral compartment (12–14). Laskin reinforced these findings in 37 patients at short-term follow-up (13). He described recurrent pain, contralateral degeneration, and settling of the tibial component. Thirty-five percent of patients in the series had activity-related knee pain. In 35% of patients, there was a more than 2 mm of subsidence of the tibial component, indicating that the tibial components may have been undersized or that excessive bone was resected before implanta-

tion. These medial compartment arthroplasties generally performed poorly, with a 24% reoperation rate. One-half of these reoperations were due to contralateral degeneration, associated with overcorrection. Since the time of these original reports, more encouraging results have been reported, with survival rates at 10 years in the 85% to 98% range (Table 1) (15–21).

INDICATIONS

Classically, the indications for UKA have been degenerative arthritis in one compartment of the knee in a low-demand, elderly, thin patient (older than 60 years) (see Table 2 for contraindications). Competence of both the cruciates and collateral ligaments has been considered critical to knee kinematics in these patients. Underlying osteoarthritis (22–25), rheumatoid arthritis (RA) (26,27), and osteonecrosis (28,29) have all been successfully treated with UKA.

In 1989, Kozinn and Scott (30) summarized the currently accepted patient selection criteria for UKA. Their indications included patients older than age 60 years and weighing less than 180 lb (82 kg), with a low level of activity and minimal rest pain. Range of motion should be a minimum arc of at least 90

TABLE 1. *Long-term results of unicompartmental knee arthroplasty*

Study	Year	Implant	Patient series	Patient age at operation (yr)	Follow-up period (yr)	Number of knees initially in series	Number of knees available at follow-up	Survival based on revision rate or survivorship analysis	95% confidence interval	Diagnosis (percent of total)	Laterality (percent medial/lateral)	Comments
Marmor (46)	1988	Marmor	One surgeon	65 (31–85)	11 (10–13)	87	60	69% (10 yr)	N/A	Osteoarthritis 90% Posttraumatic 10%	88/12	HSS score (49): 63% good/excellent Pain relief in 87%
Scott et al. (21)	1991	Brigham	One center	71 (41–85)	10 (8–12)	100	64	85% (10 yr)	67–69%	Osteoarthritis 94% Osteonecrosis 4% Rheumatoid 2%	88/12	87% of knees with no significant pain at follow-up
Capra and Fehring (17)	1992	Marmor, Compartmental II	Three surgeons	63 (30–81)	8.3 (8–12)	52	39	94% (10 yr)	N/A	Osteoarthritis 86.5% Posttraumatic 11.5% Rheumatoid 2%	77/13	HSS score (49): 80% good/excellent
Heck et al. (18)	1993	Zimmer, Compartmental I; Zimmer, Compartmental II; Marmor	Three surgeons, three centers	68.2 (22–92)	6 (N/A–15)	294	250	91.4 ± 2.8% (10 yr)	N/A	Osteoarthritis 85% Osteonecrosis 9% Posttraumatic 4% Unknown 2%	87/13	Average weight for patient requiring revision: 90.4 kg Average weight for successful outcome: 67 kg HSS score (49): 86% good/excellent (one center) Knee Society score (72): 99% good/excellent (two centers)
Weale and Newman (70)	1994	St. Georg Sledge	One center	71	12.8 (12–17)	52	42	10% (10 yr)	N/A	Osteoarthritis 100%	N/A	80% with mild or no pain at follow-up
Cartier et al. (15)	1996	Marmor	One surgeon	65 (28–82)	12 (10–18)	207	60	93% (10 yr)	80.7–100%	Osteoarthritis 66% Posttraumatic 22% Osteonecrosis 14%	88/12	Knee Society score (72): Knee score: 95% good/excellent Function score: 77% good/excellent—due to pain developing elsewhere
Ansari et al. (16)	1997	St. Georg Sledge	Four surgeons	70 (46–93)	4 (1–17)	461	437	88% (10 yr)	81–93%	Osteoarthritis 100%	100% medial	Bristol Knee score (76): 92% good/excellent

Continued.

TABLE 1. *Continued.*

Study	Year	Implant	Patient series	Patient age at operation (yr)	Follow-up period (yr)	Number of knees initially in series	Number of knees available at follow-up	Survival based on revision rate or survivorship analysis	95% confidence interval	Diagnosis (percent of total)	Laterality (percent medial/lateral)	Comments
Tabor and Tabor (87)	1998	Marmor	Two surgeons	61 (41–80)	9.7 (5–20)	73	58	84% (10 yr)	N/A	Osteoarthritis 100%	91/9	Knee Society score (72): Average knee score: 91 (range of 48–100) Average functional score: 77 (5–100)
Murray et al. (20)	1998	Oxford	One surgeon	70.7 (34.6–90.6)	7.6 (N/A–13.8)	144	109	97% (10 yr)	91–100%	Osteoarthritis 100%	100% medial	—
Squire et al. (45)	1998	Marmor	One surgeon	70.9 (51–94)	18 (15–22)	140	48	84 ± 9% (22 yr)	N/A	Osteoarthritis 97% Posttraumatic 1.4% Rheumatoid 0.7% Osteonecrosis 0.7%	89/11	Knee Society score (72): Knee score: Preoperative–31 (15–50); follow-up–85 (49–100) Functional score: preoperative–42 (5–70); postoperative–71 (0–100) HSS: preoperative–57 (43–77); postoperative–82 (65–97)
Berger et al. (44)	1999	Zimmer Miller-Galante	One center	68 (51–84)	7.5 (6–10)	62	61	98% (10 yr)	96–100%	Osteoarthritis 85% Osteonecrosis 15%	95/5	HSS score (49): preoperative–55 (30–79); follow-up–92 (60–100) 98% good/excellent results

HSS, Hospital for Special Surgery; N/A, not available.

TABLE 2. *General unicompartmental knee arthroplasty contraindications*

Age <60 yr
Weight >95 kg
High activity level
Patellofemoral pain, apprehension
Contralateral tibiofemoral joint:
   Joint space narrowing
   Osteophytes
Inflammatory arthritis
   Calcium pyrophosphate dihydrate deposition
   Rheumatoid arthritis
Symptomatic anterior cruciate ligament insufficiency
Posterior cruciate ligament insufficiency
Collateral ligament insufficiency
Varus deformity greater than 10 degrees
Valgus deformity greater than 15 degrees
Flexion contracture greater than 10 degrees

degrees, with a flexion contracture of no greater than 5 degrees, and a passively correctable angular deformity no greater than 10 degrees varus or 15 degrees valgus. These authors considered inflammatory diseases, such as RA and chondrocalcinosis, as contraindications to this procedure because of the risk of contralateral degeneration and ongoing synovitis. They recommended UKA for both isolated medial and lateral disease.

The indications for UKA have continued to evolve since its introduction in the early 1970s. Several studies have used lax inclusion criteria, including severe unicompartmental arthrosis (31–33) and insufficiency of the anterior cruciate ligament (ACL) (32). These studies have had lower patient satisfaction and higher revision rates than those of tricompartmental arthroplasty. Patients exhibiting inflammatory signs characterized by effusion, significant rest pain, and/or synovitis are best treated with standard TKA (34).

Increased patient weight has been implicated as a risk factor for failure after UKA. Heck et al. emphasized the direct relationship between patient weight and need for revision after UKA (18). Using an arbitrary cutoff of 81 kg, this association was noted to be statistically significant. In this series of 294 knees, the average weight of patients requiring revision was 90.4 kg, compared with 67 kg in nonrevised cases. Stockelman and Pohl found increased functional pain in patients heavier than 90 kg (35). In general, we recommend avoidance of UKA in patients weighing more than 95 kg.

Involvement of other compartments of the knee with chondromalacia or degenerative arthritis is an intuitive contraindication to UKA. This was studied by Corpe and Engh, who reported 89% excellent results at 32-month follow-up, despite the presence of Outerbridge (37) grade III and IV changes in the unreplaced femorotibial compartment. These authors assessed the various knee compartments intraoperatively and accepted up to 10% eburnated bone in the contralateral compartment (37).

Most authors do not consider patellofemoral chondromalacia a contraindication to UKA (16,20,30). However, in our experience, patients who have complaints of predominantly anterior knee pain at rest, who have anterior pain with squatting and stair climbing, or who have a positive patellar apprehension test may be better treated with tricompartmental knee arthroplasty.

CRUCIATE LIGAMENTS AND ANTEROMEDIAL ARTHRITIS

In 1991, White et al. studied the tibial articular surfaces removed during surgery from 46 knees that had been treated with UKA (38). All knees had an intact ACL. In every case, the origin of the articular cartilage lesion was in the anterior portion of the tibial plateau and the posterior articular cartilage was preserved (Fig. 2). The varus deformity visible on standing disappeared on anteroposterior (AP) radiographs taken with the knee in flexion, presumably as a result of maintenance of the posteromedial tibial articular cartilage and rollback of the femur on this region of the tibia. One important finding in these patients is that all the varus deformities were correctable with manual stress. This indicates normal length of the medial collateral ligament (MCL). With flexion, these authors proposed that the femoral rollback stretches the MCL out to its proper length. The term *anteromedial arthritis* was coined as a pathologic entity that arises in the setting of an intact ACL. With the absence of the ACL, these authors proposed that fixed deformity would follow along with eventual degenerative changes in the posteromedial aspect of the knee as well as the lateral compartment. Thus, UKA would be an ideal treatment in cases of isolated anteromedial arthritis. Radiographic assessment of 200 knees with AP varus stress films and lateral radiographs was performed by Keyes et al. (39). These authors were able to predict integrity of the ACL with 95% accuracy and rupture of the ACL with 100% accuracy on preoperative films. This provided the surgeons with important information about intraoperative findings and facilitated preoperative planning of the operation. Magnetic resonance imaging has been used preoperatively by Sharpe et al. in cases of anteromedial arthritis of the knee to assess the integrity of the ACL (40). These authors found that 33% of patients with

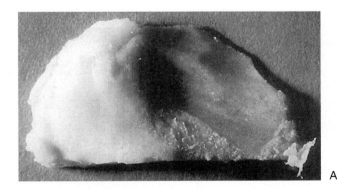

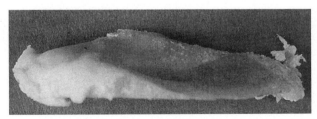

FIG. 2. A: Anteromedial arthritis of the knee (top view). **B:** Anteromedial arthritis of the knee (side view). (From White SH, Ludkowski PF, Goodfellow JW. Anteromedial osteoarthritis of the knee. *J Bone Joint Surg Br* 1991;73:582–586, with permission.)

this specific pattern of arthritis had degenerative changes by magnetic resonance imaging. This was in contrast to intraoperative evidence of degeneration in 13% of knees. They concluded that magnetic resonance imaging overestimates clinically relevant ACL insufficiency and should not be used for preoperative selection of TKA over UKA.

The pattern of wear after UKA with an intact ACL was studied by McCallum and Scott in 14 cases (41). These authors found a wear pattern on the anterior portion of the polyethylene liner in every implant studied. Preoperative radiographs confirmed anterior arthritis of the tibial plateau. They hypothesized that the same loads that cause anteromedial arthritis were responsible for this pattern of polyethylene wear.

Because of the decreased constraints of most UKA systems, ligamentous stability is vital for long-term function. The ACL is believed to be critical to the long-term success of mobile bearing UKA. The importance of a functional ACL for fixed bearing UKA is controversial.

Anterior subluxation of the tibia can lead to early arthritic changes in the contralateral compartment (34,37,42). Soft tissue tension plays an important role in maintaining the polyethylene liner in position in mobile (meniscal) bearing implants. One theoretical advantage of the Oxford prosthesis is the lack of constraint, which may allow the cruciate and collateral ligaments to function in a kinematically more normal fashion (8). Increased laxity may predispose the knee to accelerated polyethylene wear and early failure as a result of increased shear stress across the bone–implant interfaces. The posterior cruciate ligament (PCL) plays a similar role in maintaining soft tissue tension and normal joint kinematics. There is universal agreement that knees with clinical and intraoperative PCL deficiency and knee arthritis should be treated with posterior-stabilized TKA.

The role of the ACL and PCL in knee joint proprioception after UKA, compared with posterior-stabilized and PCL-retaining TKA, was studied by Simmons et al. (43). Passive motion thresholds were used to measure joint proprioception. These authors found that proprioception declines early in the course of knee arthritis. This correlated with histologic loss of mechanoreceptors in mild knee arthritis. This study demonstrated no difference in joint proprioception in UKA with cruciate ligament preservation compared with either type of TKA.

LATERAL VERSUS MEDIAL DISEASE

UKA has been successfully performed in both medial and lateral gonarthrosis. Early reports by Insall (10,11) and Laskin (13) suggested improved results with lateral UKA compared with procedures on the medial side. The medial side is involved in the majority of unicompartmental knee arthritis. For example, in Christensen's series of 575 knees, 521 medial, 51 lateral, and three bilateral unicompartmental arthroplasties were performed (32). Lateral procedures make up approximately 5% to 15% of all UKAs in a number of series (15,18,19,21,44–46).

Marmor reported on 14 lateral UKAs at average follow-up of 89 months. Eleven patients had excellent results (47). These results were corroborated by Ohdera et al., with 16 of 18 knees treated by lateral unicompartmental arthroplasty with satisfactory function based on the HSS knee score at minimum 5-year follow-up (48,49). In some recent reports, lateral unicompartmental arthroplasty has been associated with suboptimal out-comes compared with medial UKA. Ansari et al. reported only 62% survival in lateral procedures at 10 years (50). The leading causes for revision were progression of arthritis in other compartments and prosthetic loosening. The Oxford UKA, performed on the lateral side, had a 21% revision rate at 5 years in a series of 53 patients, as reported by Gunther et al. (51). This is in strong contrast to results on the medial side, with 98% survival at 10 years (20). The majority of the revisions on the lateral side were due to dislocation of the meniscal bearing of the Oxford implant. This was in contrast to a series of 121 medial procedures performed by the same group, with only one case of bearing dislocation. The authors believed this difference is due to variability in the elastic properties of the MCL compared with the relatively lax lateral collateral ligament in positions of knee flexion (52). To alleviate the problem, the authors developed new instrumentation to achieve more precise balance, started performing a lateral parapatellar arthrotomy to improve exposure, released the popliteus to keep it from bowstringing around the back of the meniscal bearing, and increased the height of the posterior lip of the bearing (51).

In spite of the variety of published results, we believe that lateral compartment arthroplasty does have a role in select patients. Such patients should have a correctable valgus deformity that is no more than 15 degrees, preservation of medial and patellofemoral joint space, age older than 60 years, low activity level, and flexion deformity of less than 10 degrees.

OSTEONECROSIS

Osteonecrosis of the knee is a common cause of knee pain in the elderly population. This disease is commonly divided into spontaneous osteonecrosis of the knee primarily involving the medial femoral condyle, steroid-induced or atraumatic osteonecrosis, and posttraumatic osteonecrosis (53,54). Spontaneous osteonecrosis of the knee is predominantly unilateral, associated with age older than 55 years, and confined to the epiphysis and subchondral region. Tibial lesions in older patients can often be confused with degenerative meniscal tears. The atraumatic or secondary form can involve the tibia or femur (55). This entity can be associated with systemic lupus erythematosus, sickle cell disease, alcoholism, and corticosteroid use (55). Patients with secondary osteonecrosis are usually younger than 55 years old; often have involvement of the other knee or other joints; and can have involvement of the epiphysis, metaphysis, or diaphysis. Mont et al., in a review of 248 knees in 136 patients with atraumatic osteonecrosis, found that the least favorable prognosis was associated with large lesions and lesions involving the epiphysis (55). A high index of suspicion is required to make the diagnosis, which can then be confirmed with imaging studies. Initial treatment is nonoperative, consisting of antiinflammatory medications and protected weightbearing. In more advanced cases, with large lesions, operative treatment is advised. Surgical management has included arthroscopic débridement with drilling, osteotomy, allografting, and prosthetic replacement (54,56). UKA has been used with success in the treatment of spontaneous or idiopathic osteonecrosis of the knee. Marmor (29) reported on 34 knees with medial femoral condyle osteonecrosis treated with UKA. Thirty-two knees were diagnosed with spontaneous osteonecrosis and two knees with steroid induced osteonecrosis. At a mean follow-up of 5.5 years, 89% reported good or excellent results based on the HSS score (49). Of the four clinical failures in this series, two were due to osteonecrosis of the contralateral femoral condyle and two were due to subsidence into compromised bone stock. Imaging studies to assess the extent and location of involvement of osteonecrosis are critical in surgical planning. Based on the risk of disease progression with secondary osteonecrosis, we believe that UKA is indicated only for spontaneous osteonecrosis of the knee, localized to the subchondral region. Treatment with TKA is recommended if there is any involvement of the epiphyseal or metaphyseal bone. Depending on the extent of involvement, use of stemmed TKA implants is occasionally required (54).

RHEUMATOID ARTHRITIS

Patients with RA have been included in multiple series treated with UKA (26,27,45,57). In spite of this, RA makes up a small minority of patients within most series. Due to the global synovitis, ligamentous laxity, and risk of progression, RA is a relative contraindication to UKA.

The treatment of RA of the knee was a primary impetus in the development of early UKA implants (4,9,57–59). Initially, unicompartmental hemiarthroplasty was used by Potter et al. and MacIntosh in treating RA of the knee (57–60). MacIntosh advocated the use of the hemiarthroplasty in cases in which disease was confined to one compartment, with the stipulation that contralateral surgery may be needed later (58).

Kay and Martins (61) presented results with the MacIntosh hemiprosthesis in 44 knees with RA at 27-month average follow-up. Eighty-five percent of the patients were relieved of pain. Fifteen knees had only one compartment replaced. Two of these patients had severe pain at latest follow-up. Swanson et al. reported on 26 knees at 5-year average follow-up treated with hemiarthroplasty for RA (60). They treated 22 of 26 knees with RA with bicompartmental implants. One patient with RA required revision to TKA at 6 months due to rapid progression in the contralateral side. Based on these two studies, RA treated with hemiarthroplasty demonstrated best results when both compartments were treated (60,61).

Knutson et al. published data from the Swedish National Knee Registry on UKA in RA (19). Using actuarial methods, they studied UKA for osteoarthritis in 2,345 patients and for RA in 222 patients. The revision rate within the first 6 years was 6% for a diagnosis of osteoarthritis and 17.5% for a diagnosis or RA. Robertsson et al. demonstrated a five-times-higher 10-year cumulative revision rate after UKA compared with TKA in data on 4,381 patients with RA from the Swedish National Knee Registry (25% vs. 5%) (62). Regarding deep infection, Bengtson et al., in another study from the Swedish National Knee Registry, found that the 10-year cumulative risk of infection after TKA for RA is 4.6% (2,866 knees) compared with 2.4% (291 knees) for UKA (63). Based on the predictable results after TKA and in spite of the higher infection rate with TKA, we believe that treatment of RA with UKA is not indicated. Complications of RA treated with UKA include increased failure rate, ongoing pain due to synovitis (30), and degeneration in the untreated compartments of the knee.

ALTERNATIVES TO UNICOMPARTMENTAL KNEE ARTHROPLASTY

Advantages of UKA over TKA include minimal bone loss (64), preservation of ligamentous structures (64), shorter operative time (65), and increased range of motion (65,66). Other procedures such as HTO address only the alignment and not the articular surface. UKA preserves the visibly normal portion of the knee, which may play a role in improved proprioception, decreased frictional coefficient relative to metal on polyethylene, and more normal joint kinematics.

Unicompartmental Knee Arthroplasty versus High Tibial Osteotomy

HTO has traditionally been indicated in young, active patients with unicompartmental arthritis of the medial compartment. In comparison with UKA, results with HTO have been inferior. Five-year follow-up studies of HTO reveal 65% to 90% good or excellent results (67,68). However, these results drop by 10 years to approximately 30% to 60% good or excellent outcomes (68,69). Several studies have shown statistically better long-term outcome after unicompartmental arthroplasty compared with HTO in similar patient populations. A direct comparison of HTO with UKA was performed in Bristol, United Kingdom, and reported by Broughton et al. (24) at 5 to 10 years and by Weale and Newman (70) at 12 to 17 years. They compared a group of 49 knees with UKA (average age at latest follow-up of 80) with a group of 42 knees treated with HTO (average age at latest follow-up of 74). Preoperative characteristics were similar between the groups. At 12- to 17-year follow-up, pain was absent or mild in 80% of the UKA group and in only 43% of the HTO group. The HTO patients had a higher reoperation rate than the UKA group (35% vs. 12%) (Fig. 3). There was a higher complication rate in the HTO group, with more wound problems, neurovascular complications, and higher rate of deep venous thrombosis (24). A prospective, randomized study was undertaken by Stukenborg-Colsman et al. on 60 patients treated either with HTO or UKA (71). The average age of the patients was 67 years old. At 7- to 10-year follow-up, these authors could show no significant difference in Knee Society scores (72) or survivorship. One weakness of this study was that the patients were not matched based on the severity of their preoperative arthritis. The majority of complications were in the HTO group and included deep venous thrombosis, superficial wound infection, delayed union, loosening of hardware, and fracture. These results are further supported when complication rates of different series of UKA are compared with those of HTO (21,32,68).

In patients with varus deformity of greater than 10 degrees, Marmor recommends UKA over HTO because of the risk of mediolateral instability due to bone loss (46).

The results of HTO revised to UKA have been studied by Rees et al. in a series of 18 patients (5.4-year mean follow-up). This group was compared to 613 primary UKAs (5.8-year mean follow-up) (73). Of the primary UKA subjects, 3.1% had been revised compared with 27.8% of the HTO revision UKA group. These authors recommend that UKA should not be used in cases of failed HTO.

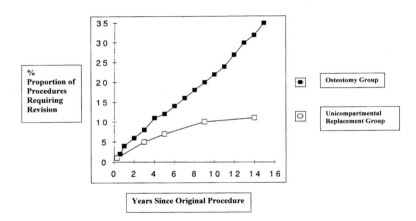

FIG. 3. Cumulative failure rate of unicompartmental knee arthroplasty compared with high tibial osteotomy. (From Weale AE, Newman JH. Unicompartmental arthroplasty and high tibial osteotomy for osteoarthrosis of the knee. A comparative study with a 12- to 17-year follow-up period. *Clin Orthop* 1994;302:134–137, with permission.)

Unicompartmental versus Tricompartmental Knee Arthroplasty

UKA has been compared with TKA in a number of reports. Cameron and Jung compared 20 patients with UKA and contralateral TKA at average follow-up of 3 years, reporting no difference in patient preference in spite of increased range of motion in the UKA patients (74). Length of hospitalization was slightly less in the UKA group, with more rapid recovery. Both early and late complications were higher in the UKA group. Cobb et al. reported on 42 patients at intermediate follow-up, asking them to rate whether they preferred UKA or the contralateral TKA. Fifty percent preferred the UKA, 21% preferred the TKA, and 29% could not tell the difference (75). Laurencin et al. attempted to control for timing of surgery by prospectively studying 26 patients who underwent UKA and contralateral TKA during the same hospitalization (66). Patients were divided into resurfaced and unresurfaced patella groups. For the overall group, at 81-month average follow-up, twice as many patients preferred the UKA to the TKA. However, 44% could not tell any difference. In a randomized, controlled study, Newman et al. compared clinical and radiographic results of UKA and TKA in patients with isolated unicompartmental arthritis (76). Knee scores improved significantly in both groups using the Bristol knee score. This instrument evaluates pain, function, range of motion, deformity, and stability. These authors recorded improved knee scores in both groups. However, no significant difference was noted between the UKA scores and the TKA scores. There were significantly more patients with an excellent rating in the UKA group (75.6% vs. 56.5%). Range of motion was higher in the UKA, with approximately 70% reaching 120 degrees of flexion (compared with 17% of TKA group) at 5 years postoperatively. On average, patients in the UKA left the hospital 3 days sooner than the TKA group. Weale et al. cited the unreliability of knee scoring systems and differences between physician and patient definition of success (78), leading them to a study of UKA compared with TKA based on questionnaires filled out by patients in the early postoperative period (6 months to 4 years). They found no significant difference in pain or functional outcome. Patients who had been treated with UKA could descend stairs more easily ($p = .07$). The average age of patients was lower in the UKA group (62.4 vs. 71.3 years), potentially confounding the results of this study. For example, the older TKA patients may have had lower muscle power, diminishing the ability to walk down stairs, whereas the younger UKA patients may be more active, leading to more joint pain.

In addition to functional comparisons between UKA and TKA, the incidence of patella baja (infera) after each operation has been studied (78). Patella baja has been correlated with restriction of motion and pain. In a randomized, prospective series of 84 patients, no increased risk of patella baja was found after UKA, compared with a 34% risk after TKA. This implies that revision operations, specifically exposure and patellar eversion, may be technically easier after UKA compared with TKA.

UKA provides a subjectively more natural knee joint, with improved or equivalent patient satisfaction, improved function, decreased hospital stay, and decreased implant cost.

MINIMALLY INVASIVE SURGERY

The term *minimally invasive surgery* has been used to describe operations with smaller skin incisions and less dissection. The results of laparoscopic versus open hernia repair have been compared in large prospective, randomized studies (79,80). Earlier return to work and better function have been reported with the less invasive procedures. Repicci and Eberle showed that it was possible to resurface one compartment of the knee using a 3-in. incision extending from the proximal medial tip of the patella to a point 1 in. below the tibial articular surface (81). A 1-in. proximal transverse capsular incision was also made extending from the medial edge of the patella as well as a 1.5-in. incision of the medial capsule from the tibial plateau. Using this technique, 80% of their patients had the procedure done as an outpatient procedure. These authors advocated preoperative arthroscopic examination to evaluate for involvement of other compartments. Using this technique, the estimated average cost of UKA was $7,000 compared with $16,000 for UKA with a standard knee incision and arthrotomy with patellar eversion (81). Price et al. prospectively compared the technique of UKA through a short medial incision without patellar dislocation with UKA through a standard open incision with patellar dislocation and with TKA through a standard incision (82). Recovery in the minimally invasive group was twice as rapid as in the open UKA group and three times as rapid as in the TKA group. Evaluation of postoperative radiographs did not demonstrate compromise of implant position with the minimally invasive procedure.

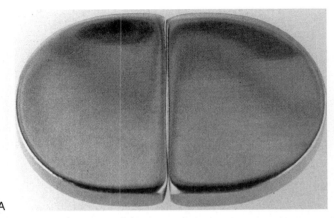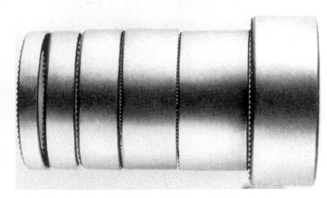

A   B

FIG. 4. A: MacIntosh tibial hemiarthroplasty implant (top view). **B:** MacIntosh tibial hemiarthroplasty implant (side view). (From MacIntosh DL, Hunter GA. The use of the hemiarthroplasty prosthesis for advanced osteoarthritis and rheumatoid arthritis of the knee. *J Bone Joint Surg Br* 1972;54:244–255, with permission.)

Cost analysis of UKA compared with TKA was performed by Robertsson et al. (83). They compared matched patients from the Swedish Knee Registry; for UKA, the hospital stay was shorter, the mean hospital stay cost $700 less, and the cost of the implants was approximately 60% of the cost of TKA.

SELECTED IMPLANTS

Unicompartmental Hemiarthroplasty

MacIntosh has described the history of tibial hemiarthroplasty starting in 1954, at Toronto General Hospital. A patient with a severe yet correctable valgus deformity was admitted. The lateral ligaments became taut with varus stress, restoring stability. In the operating room, "an acrylic prosthesis for replacement of the whole upper end of the tibia" was cut in half and placed in the joint to correct the deformity (58). The patient lived a pain-free life for the next 12 years. Acrylic was later abandoned due to poor results in hip arthroplasty. Teflon had been tried, with poor success due to high wear and foreign body reaction. Titanium was also tried but failed due to metallosis. Ultimately, the Vitallium MacIntosh prosthesis was introduced in 1964 (Fig. 4). The top of the prosthesis had a smooth concave contoured surface. The undersurface was flat, with multiple serrations. Early results on these hemiarthroplasty series were encouraging. At minimum 6-month follow-up, MacIntosh reported good results in 70% of patients (2). Contraindications to the operation were lateral subluxation, patellofemoral disease, deep infection, a fixed deformity, previous fusion, advanced disease, and poor patient compliance (58). Potter et al. reported good to excellent results in 17 of 19 patients at average 3-year follow-up in patients with unicompartmental and bicompartmental osteoarthritis and RA (57).

McKeever developed a metal resurfacing of the arthritic tibial plateau in the late 1950s (1). The McKeever was also composed of Vitallium, was available in thicknesses of 2 to 6 mm, and was inserted without cement (Fig. 5). The implant had a T-

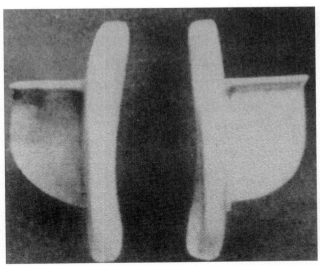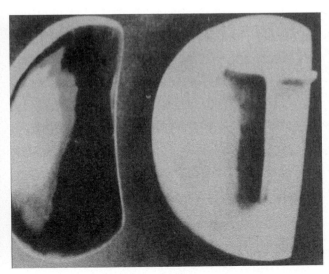

FIG. 5. McKeever tibial hemiarthroplasty. (From McKeever D. Tibial plateau prosthesis. *Clin Orthop* 1960;18:86–95, with permission.)

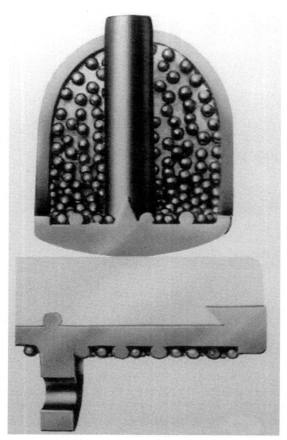

FIG. 6. Cross-sectional representation of Endo-Model Sled (latest generation St. Georg sledge) prosthesis demonstrating spheric attachments on cobalt-chromium undersurface and flat, convex, femoral component articulating with flat polyethylene liner. (Courtesy of Waldemar Link, Hamburg, Germany.)

shaped fin for stability. Slots were cut in the bone with a reciprocating saw, through the subchondral bone, to allow ease of insertion of the prosthesis. The transverse portion of the fin was measured and cut approximately 0.5 in. from the anterior tibial plateau (1). Emerson et al. reviewed 61 patients with isolated unicompartmental osteoarthritis treated with the McKeever implant (84). At average 5-year follow-up, 72% had a good to excellent clinical result based on a clinical rating scale developed by Potter et al. (57). They observed that poor results were associated with arthritis within the ipsilateral unresurfaced compartment. Scott et al. treated 44 knees with a McKeever hemiarthroplasty (85). At average 8-year (range of 5- to 13-year) follow-up, 70% had good or excellent results based on the Potter rating system.

Swanson, having used the above implants and finding them to be occasionally unstable, designed a cobalt-chromium alloy implant with a 15-mm vertical fin. He believed that the single fin was easier to insert than the McKeever T-shaped fin and more stable than the MacIntosh implant. The designer reported on a series of ten unicompartmental cases and 20 bicompartmental cases at 5-year (2- to 14-year) follow-up. At latest follow-up, 87.5% of the knees were not painful with activity (60). The role of the hemiarthroplasty of the knee is primarily in young, active

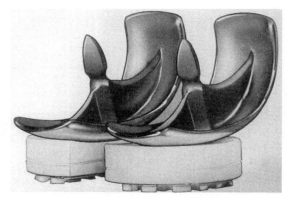

FIG. 7. Marmor modular knee. (From Marmor L. The modular knee. *Clin Orthop* 1973;94: 242–248, with permission.)

patients who are not candidates for osteotomy or who have failed a previous osteotomy. The operation requires a lengthy period of rehabilitation, with the use of crutches for up to 3 months. Its advantage lies in the minimal bone resection, which may make revision to a TKA relatively straightforward. Scott et al. delineated the main advantages of this hemiarthroplasty over HTO (85). These include removal of torn meniscal fragments and bony impingement at time of surgery, release of intraarticular adhesions to improve both flexion and extension, and decreased need for postoperative immobilization, leading to a hypothetically decreased risk of venous thrombosis. Additionally, the risk of delayed union or nonunion is avoided with the hemiarthroplasty.

St. Georg Sledge

The St. Georg modular prosthesis (Waldemar Link, Hamburg, Germany) has been in clinical use since 1969 (9,86). It consists of a biconcave metal femoral component and a flat, cemented, all-polyethylene tibial component. The curved-on-flat design does lead to increased pressure on the polyethylene liner due to the small contact area (Fig. 6). In spite of this, the prosthesis has enjoyed very good long-term results. According to Newman et al., wear has not been a problem because "a suitably congruous indentation forms in the tibia resulting in slow wear" (76). The design philosophy of this implant was to allow full freedom of motion of the femoral component on the tibia to minimize constraint. The lack of constraint allows the femur to follow a path across the tibia that is determined by soft tissue tension. Theoretically, this decreases the torque across the prosthesis. Excellent long-term data have been presented with this implant. Weale et al. (14) reported on 42 knees treated with this implant at 12- to 17-year follow-up. Five revisions were performed in this series (70). Ansari et al. reported 92% good or excellent results at average 4-year (range of 1- to 17-year) follow-up using this prosthesis for medial gonarthrosis (16). Adequate pain relief was achieved in 90% of patients.

Marmor

The Marmor modular UKA (Smith & Nephew, Memphis, TN) was first performed in the early 1970s (4). The original

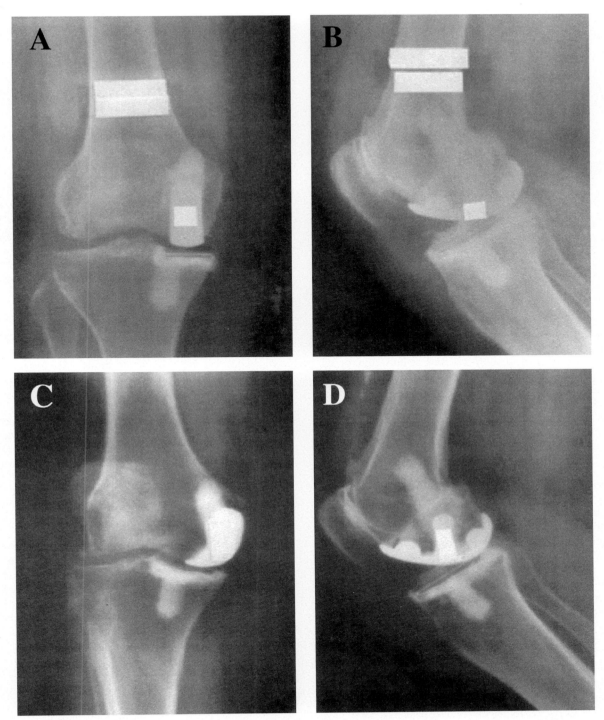

FIG. 8. Marmor unicompartmental knee arthroplasty. **A:** Postoperative anteroposterior radiograph. **B:** Postoperative lateral radiograph. **C:** Anteroposterior radiograph obtained at 16-year follow-up. **D:** Lateral radiograph obtained at 16-year follow-up of the knee of a woman who was 75 years of age at the time of surgery. (From Squire MW, et al. Unicompartmental knee replacement. A minimum 15 year followup study. *Clin Orthop* 1999;367:61–72, with permission.)

prosthesis was composed of a stainless steel femoral component and an all-polyethylene tibia (Fig. 7). This implant was initially designed for bicondylar knee replacement, resurfacing both femoral condyles and tibial plateaus independently. Unicompartmental replacement was an alternative indication. The advantage of the implant according to the designer was the preservation of cortical bone, the option of variable thickness of the implant on each side, and increased freedom of rotation. Marmor reported minimum 10-year data on 60 knees with 70% survivorship and 63% good/excellent results (46). Squire et al.

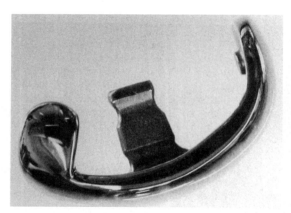

FIG. 9. Brigham unicompartmental arthroplasty femoral component with intercondylar portion of the prosthesis turned up as an anterior and medial tab to provide additional rotatory fixation. (From Scott RD, Santore RF. Unicondylar unicompartmental replacement for osteoarthritis of the knee. *J Bone Joint Surg Am* 1981;63:536–544, with permission.)

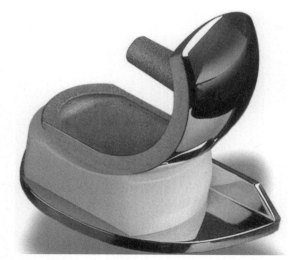

FIG. 10. Oxford unicompartmental knee prosthesis. (Courtesy of Biomet, Warsaw, IN.)

reported the University of Iowa experience with the Marmor implant at minimum 15-year follow-up on 140 knees (45). They used relatively lax inclusion criteria such as no weight or age limitations and the presence of large angular deformities, contralateral osteophytes, and tibial subluxation. In spite of this, for the overall series, 14 (10%) were revised (Fig. 8). Indications for revision included tibial loosening, disease progression, and pain. Other series with this prosthesis have demonstrated 10-year survivorship of 84% (87) and 93% (15).

Brigham

The Brigham (Johnson & Johnson, New Brunswick, NJ) unicompartmental prosthesis was introduced in 1974, at the Robert Breck Brigham Hospital. The femoral component was notable for the intercondylar portion of the prosthesis, which was turned up as an anterior and medial tab to provide additional rotatory fixation (Fig. 9). The femoral component was modified in 1981 with a broader design. The tibial component was initially all polyethylene and conforming to the femoral component. In 1977, the polyethylene concavity in AP plane was eliminated to allow the femoral component to slide anteroposteriorly with knee flexion. In 1981, a metal-backed tibial design was introduced. Scott and Santore reported average 3.5-year follow-up data (range of 2 to 6 years) on the first 100 consecutive patients (22). Ninety-two percent of patients had good to excellent results. Scott et al. published the 8- to 12-year follow-up on these patients (21). Eighty-seven percent of the 64 available knees demonstrated no pain. At 10 years, this implant had 85% survivorship. All-polyethylene components were used in every case of this series. In the 1980s, attempts to improve fixation of the tibial component led to the use of metal-backed components. The next generation Brigham prosthesis was marketed with a titanium-backed tibial component. Metal-backed tibial components forced the surgeon to use a thinner polyethylene liner to maintain a minimal bony resection from the tibia. Early catastrophic wear was described by Palmer et al. in 1998, with seven cases in a cohort of 32 patients (88). The average time to revision in this series was 52 months (23–80). Intraoperatively, severe soft tissue staining and metallosis were noted in the synovium with a pronounced granulomatous response. In several cases, both the polyethylene liner and the metal tibial component were completely worn through. The mean polyethylene thickness in these patients was 6.3 mm (range of 6 to 8 mm). The authors concluded that several factors were responsible for the high early failure rate. These included thin polyethylene liners, malalignment, manufacturing defects with subsurface cracks, sterilization defects due to gamma irradiation in air, and inadequate polyethylene fixation to the tibial baseplate. Newer designs have emphasized thicker polyethylene, improved polyethylene quality, and alternative sterilization modalities.

Oxford

The Oxford mobile bearing prosthesis (Biomet, Warsaw, IN) was introduced by Goodfellow and O'Connor in 1978 (6). It was theorized that the design would simulate the normal meniscus of the knee with a mobile, congruous design (Fig. 10). The femoral condyle is spheric to allow for congruity in all positions of flexion. The tibial tray is a flat, metallic component. Both components are cemented. The polyethylene liner is fully congruent with the femoral component and has a flat undersurface, which rests on the flat tibial component. It is maintained in a reduced position by the shapes of the femoral and tibial components and by soft tissue tension. This prosthesis depends on precise equality of the flexion and extension gaps. The instrumentation has been revised twice since the initial design. In 1985, instrumentation was introduced to prepare the femoral cut surface in a spheric fashion. The tibial surface and posterior femur are initially cut. This determines the "flexion gap," the space required by the prosthesis in flexion. Subsequently, the distal femur is incrementally milled until the "extension gap," the space taken up by the prosthesis in extension, matches the flexion gap. This permits equivalent ligamentous tension in flexion and extension. This constant tension is critical to normal knee mechanics and the maintenance of the polyethylene liner between the metal components (Fig. 11). The congruent nature of the Oxford knee provides approximately 6 cm^2 of contact at both surfaces (8,89,90). This high degree of congruity between the femoral component and the polyethylene liner

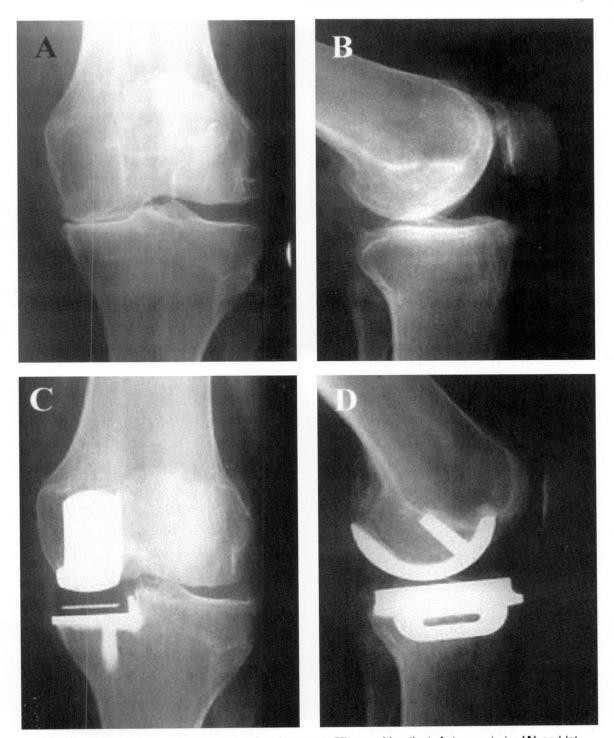

FIG. 11. Oxford medial unicompartmental replacement: 77-year-old patient. Anteroposterior **(A)** and lateral **(B)** views of stage III osteoarthritis with anteromedial erosion of the tibial plateau on the lateral projection. Anteroposterior **(C)** and lateral **(D)** views showing satisfactory postoperative alignment of unicompartmental components. (From Weale AE, et al. Perceptions of outcomes after unicompartmental and total knee replacements. *Clin Orthop* 2001;382:143–153, with permission.)

has led to very low wear rates, an average of 0.01 to 0.03 mm per year (89,90). A primary disadvantage of this implant is the technical difficulty of the surgery. The bearings can dislocate and more tibial bone must be resected compared with other designs that use all-polyethylene components.

Porous-Coated Anatomic Knee

The constrained Porous-Coated Anatomic (PCA) knee (Howmedica, Allendale, NJ) was introduced in the 1980s. The tibial surface had a convex surface leading to a small contact area

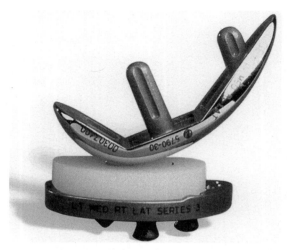

FIG. 12. Miller-Galante unicompartmental knee prosthesis. (Courtesy of Zimmer, Warsaw, IN.)

between the femur and tibia. Ivarsson showed that the tensile strain was higher in the anteromedial region (91). This led the femoral component to ride up the central slope of the tibial component, promoting wear in this region.

The polyethylene of the PCA knee was treated with a heat treatment to decrease friction and to increase wear resistance. This led to a more fragile material. This is a proposed source of flaking of the polyethylene with increased stress (25). An additional factor was the decreased thickness of the PCA knee polyethylene liner due to the metal-backed tibial component. In some cases, the polyethylene was as thin as 4.5 mm (23,25).

Riebel et al. retrospectively reported on 100 patients treated with the PCA implant. At an average of 26 months, 20 patients had failed treatment (92). Fourteen patients demonstrated radiographic femoral component loosening that was confirmed at operation. These authors then performed comparitive biomechanical testing between the PCA and Oxford femoral components. These two designs differ in that the PCA bone–implant interface consists of an angled surface with straight limbs, whereas the Oxford has a biconcave design in both the coronal and sagittal planes. These components were implanted on cadaver limbs with a press-fit technique. Cyclical loading was performed to simulate gait up to 5,000 cycles. The position of the implant relative to the bone was measured using photographs. The PCA femoral component resulted in motion in as few as ten cycles. The average change in angular position of the PCA was 1.9 degrees relative to the Oxford's 0.5 degrees. Average translations of the implant were also higher for the PCA compared with the Oxford (1.1 mm vs. 0.3 mm). Contact with the posterior aspect of the femoral implant caused the anterior portion of the implant to separate from its bony base. Increased motion of the femoral component was attributed to the large flat surfaces, which the authors believed made this design less resistant to shear stresses at the bone–implant interface. Based on these results, UKA femoral components with biconcave designs have improved stability and fixation greater than devices with angled bone–implant surfaces.

Bergenudd reported on 90 knees treated with the PCA prosthesis at 3- to 9-year follow-up (25). Based on the HSS knee score (49), 61% of patients had a good or excellent result, whereas 39%

had a fair or poor result, including 27 (30%) with indications for revision. The majority of these were for femoral component and tibial component aseptic loosening. Poor clinical results with this prosthesis were confirmed in several other studies (93,94).

Miller-Galante

The Miller-Galante (Zimmer, Warsaw, IN) unicompartmental knee system is a modular system with a cobalt-chromium alloy femoral component (Fig. 12). Tibial options include a metal-backed titanium tray or an all-polyethylene component. The tibial articular surface is relatively flat to allow for unconstrained motion of the femoral component. Multiple sizes are available for each component to allow precise matching to the patient's anatomy. Intermediate results at 6 to 10 years have been reported on 62 knees in 51 patients by Berger et al. using strict inclusion criteria (44). They attempted to include patients with a range of motion of at least 90 degrees; maximum varus and valgus deformity of 10 degrees and 15 degrees, respectively; normal contralateral and patellofemoral radiographs; minimal rest pain; sedentary lifestyle; absence of obesity; and age older than 60 years. Of 50 available patients, one patient underwent revision. All other patients had good to excellent results (98%). Kaplan-Meier 10-year survival was 98%. The average HSS knee score (49) increased from 55 (range of 30 to 79) to 92 (range of 60 to 100). These authors highlighted the importance of strict selection criteria, unconstrained geometry, and thicker polyethylene liners.

Repicci

The Repicci UKA prosthesis (Biomet), currently marketed as the Repicci II, consists of a cobalt-chromium femoral component and an all-polyethylene tibial component (Fig. 13). The design principle of the femoral component is to rest on the subchondral bone and to require minimal bony resection. Unlike other systems with a formal distal femoral resection, the Repicci depends on rounding of the distal condyle with minimal bony resection using a handheld motorized burr without a cutting

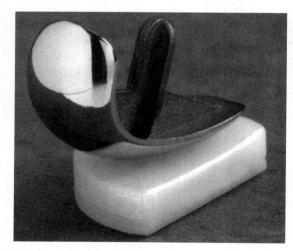

FIG. 13. Repicci unicompartmental knee prosthesis. (Courtesy of Biomet, Warsaw, IN.)

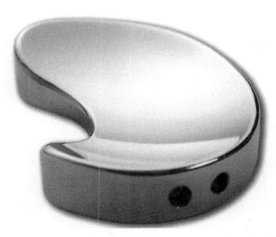

FIG. 14. UniSpacer interpositional knee prosthesis. (Courtesy of Sulzer, Austin, TX.)

block. Although other femoral components, such as the Oxford, Miller-Galante, and St. Georg sledge, have centrally located posts on the inner femoral component, the Repicci uses a central keel and post configuration. The tibial articular surface conforms to the shape of the femoral component in an attempt to reduce contact stresses. Both components are implanted with cement. In 2002, Romanowski and Repicci presented data on 136 consecutive medial UKAs (95). All were performed through small incisions. Sixty percent of patients had excellent results, 26% had good results, and 14% had fair or poor results. Using the Ahlback classification of knee osteoarthritis (96), 25% of the patients with severe disease (Ahlback stage 4) required revision, compared with 4% of the less severely involved group (Ahlback stages 2 and 3). At 8-year follow-up, there was 93% survivorship for the entire series of patients.

Interpositional Implants

Recently, an interpositional implant has been developed for use in younger patients with unicompartmental arthritis. The device, marketed as UniSpacer (Sulzer, Austin, TX), has been approved for use by the U.S. Food and Drug Administration based on substantial similarities to previous hemiarthroplasty implants such as the MacIntosh and McKeever. The implant is composed of a cobalt-chromium alloy (Fig. 14). It comes in several sizes and thicknesses. The surgical technique involves arthroscopic débridement and meniscectomy. The size of the implant in the AP plane is measured in the AP direction with an arthroscopically visualized measuring device. After arthroscopy a small incision is made and the implant is inserted, without any bony resection or cement fixation. According to the manufacturer, early results have been encouraging. Follow-up studies are currently under way.

REVISION OF UNICOMPARTMENTAL KNEE ARTHROPLASTY

Early reports on the revision of UKA to TKA were not encouraging. Padgett et al. (97) described a "major osseous defect" in 76% of cases. They challenged the theoretically conservative nature of the UKA compared with standard TKA. In the 1990s, a fundamental change occurred in the revision of UKA. With minimal bone cuts on the tibial surface, improved instrumentation, and surgical technique, most recent series have had low rates of large osseous defects. Levine et al. required no structural allografts in a series of 31 knees undergoing revision to TKA (26). McAuley et al. were able to revise 32 knees without structural allografting (98). In their series, the predominant mode of failure had shifted to polyethylene wear. Nine patients had failed due to loosening.

Involvement of the contralateral tibiofemoral compartment or patellofemoral joint has been reported as a cause of failure. Barrett and Scott reported 31% of failures due to progression to the opposite compartment and 7% failed due to patellofemoral symptoms (27). Technical error played a role in 55% of cases in their series of 29 knees (27). In the majority of these, there was overcorrection or undercorrection of the deformity, presumably leading to abnormal loading. These authors commented on malposition of the femoral component, placing it too close to the central axis of the femur in the coronal plane. They hypothesized that this led to lateral subluxation of the tibia with implant articulation, with subsequent central tibial spine impingement on the lateral femoral condyle. Another pitfall of femoral component application is placement of the component in an excessively anterior position. Anteriorization of the femoral component has been associated with decreased stair-climbing ability (99).

The choice of salvage procedures remains controversial. We prefer to revise failed unicompartmental arthroplasty with a standard tricompartmental arthroplasty. Lewold et al. noted that after only 5 years, UKAs revised with a new UKA have a three times higher rate of rerevision than those revised with TKA (100).

POLYETHYLENE WEAR IN UNICOMPARTMENTAL KNEE ARTHROPLASTY

The issue of polyethylene wear has been addressed in several retrieval studies. The critical factors responsible for accelerated wear are the contact area between the femoral component and the polyethylene, the *in vivo* alignment of the components, and the composition and thickness of the polyethylene. Bartel et al. have shown that subsurface stresses increase greatly with decreasing polyethylene thickness (101,102). Additionally, in certain designs, such as the PCA, heat processing of the polyethylene led to poor wear resistance (103).

Congruence, the degree of match between the convex femoral component and the tibial component, has been implicated as having a role in polyethylene wear. Incongruent designs, such as the St. Georg sledge, in which the femoral component contacts a flat polyethylene liner, have markedly increased contact pressures (104). In these designs, the minimal bony resection has led many surgeons to use relatively thin polyethylene. This, combined with preservation of the cruciate ligaments, leads the femoral component to slide and roll on the polyethylene surface. The stage is potentially set for increased polyethylene wear. The Oxford prosthesis has benefited from a large contact area as a result of the conforming polyethylene liner, which is analogous to the normal meniscus. In a retrieval study of 16 Oxford UKA specimens at 0.8 to 12.8 years after implantation, Psychoyios et

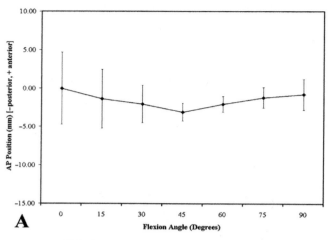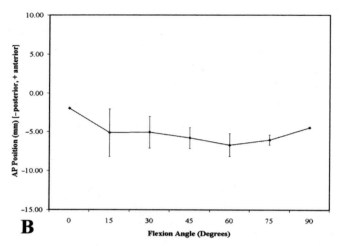

FIG. 15. A: Average anteroposterior (AP) contact position in the sagittal plane in subjects with a medial unicompartmental knee replacement. **B:** Average AP contact position in the sagittal plane in subjects with a lateral unicompartmental knee replacement. [From Dennis BD, et al. In vivo three-dimensional determination of kinematics for subjects with a normal knee or a unicompartmental or total knee replacement. *J Bone Joint Surg Am* 2002;83(Suppl 2):104–105, with permission.]

al. measured the actual polyethylene thickness using a dial gauge (90). To correct for any inaccuracies of measurement, these were compared with measurements of components with known thicknesses. Using this technique, they reported the rate of wear of this implant at 0.01 to 0.03 mm per year.

The material properties of the polyethylene play an important role in the rate of wear. Fusion defects in the polyethylene have been implicated as a site of subsurface crack initiation and increased wear (90,103). Heat pressing of the polyethylene in the PCA has led to early and sometimes catastrophic delamination of the component (93,103,105). Impingement of the femoral component on the polyethylene liner leads to abnormal stresses and accelerated wear (90,105). The ultimate key to control of wear in UKA appears to involve proper alignment of the femoral and tibial components and use of thick polyethylene liners, with minimization of fusion defects. The use of highly cross-linked polyethylene may allow for safe use of thinner implants and decreased bone resection and is currently under clinical and laboratory investigation.

KINEMATICS

Three-dimensional analysis of the kinematics of UKA was performed by Dennis et al. in 20 knees (17 medial and three lateral) (111). These authors used fluoroscopic imaging and a superimposed three-dimensional overlay to assess the translation and axial rotation of the femoral and tibial components of UKA relative to one another at 15-degree intervals from full extension to 90 degrees flexion. The sagittal midpoint of the tibial component was assigned as the reference point. Contact positions anterior to this were denoted as positive and those posterior denoted as negative. At full extension, the average medial UKA had a contact point of 0.0 mm (range of 10.7 to –6.8 mm) (Fig. 15). The lateral UKA average contact position was –1.95 mm (range of 0.0 to –3.9 mm). With flexion, the medial UKA contact position moved posteriorly to –3.1 mm (range of 4.9 to –12.7 mm) at 45 degrees and then gradually trended to the neutral position with flexion of 90 degrees. The lateral UKA demonstrated increased posterior translation, with a maximum of –6.7 mm (range of –1.0 to –11.2 mm) at 60 degrees of flexion.

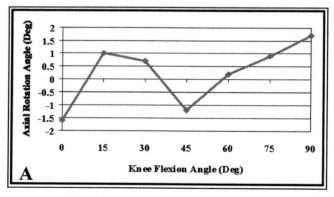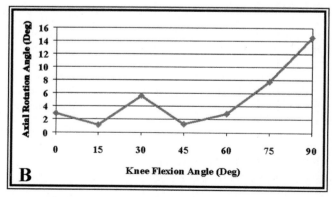

FIG. 16. A: Average axial rotation pattern in subjects with a medial unicompartmental knee replacement. **B:** Average axial rotation pattern in subjects with a lateral unicompartmental knee replacement.

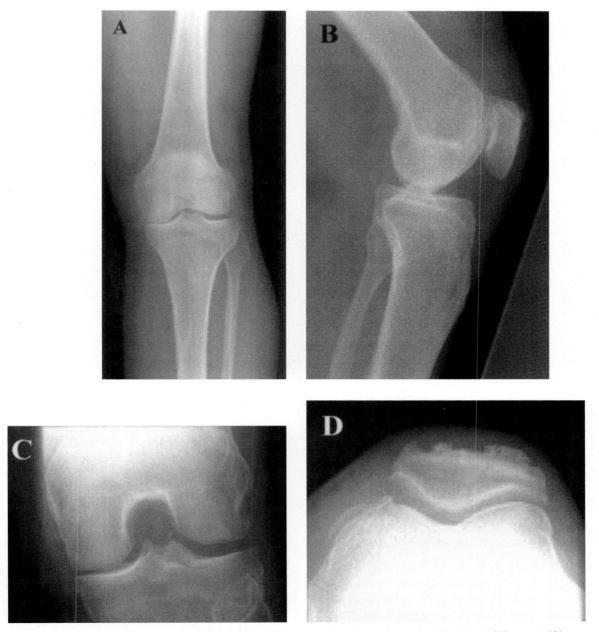

FIG. 17. Preoperative planning radiographs, including standing anteroposterior **(A)**, lateral **(B)**, notch **(C)**, and sunrise **(D)** views.

Lateral UKA demonstrated 11.2 degrees of axial rotation compared with 3.3 degrees for the medial UKA during a flexion arc from full extension to 90 degrees of flexion (Fig. 16). It is notable that these data were characterized by a large degree of variability between patients. Twelve of the 20 patients had a posterior contact point in full extension. These authors believed that this represented inadequate function of the ACL because the ligament was unable to provide an anteriorly directed force on the femur to bring it forward on the tibia in full extension. They hypothesized that this functional deficit may be partially responsible for premature polyethylene wear after UKA.

IMPLANT FIXATION

Most early unicompartmental arthroplasties were performed with the use of polymethylmethacrylate cement. The PCA implant was available in a cementless configuration (23). The use of noncemented unicompartmental arthroplasty has been associated with increased femoral and tibial loosening and osteolysis (93,94,103,105). This factor is confounded by suboptimal mechanical properties of the polyethylene, as discussed previously. Cementation techniques have been compared by Miskovsky et al. (106). These authors compared fixation of the

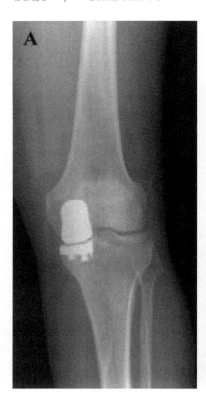

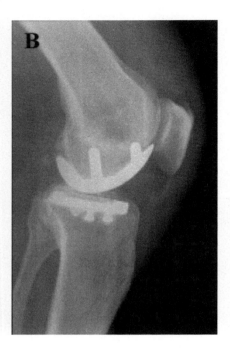

FIG. 18. A, B: Postoperative radiographs of the patient from Figure 17 after Miller-Galante unicompartmental knee arthroplasty, demonstrating full coverage of the medial femoral condyle with the prosthesis, matching of the anatomic tibial slope with the tibial component, and avoidance of overcorrection of varus deformity on the anteroposterior view: anteroposterior radiograph **(A)**, lateral radiograph **(B)**.

tibial plate with three preparations: minimal cut with exposure of cancellous bone, additional perforations of the bone with a drill with use of pulse lavage, and removal of the cartilage only. Significantly improved fixation was achieved with the second group using multiple perforations and pulse lavage to improve cement interdigitation and removal of loose fragments. Currently, we recommend use of polymethylmethacrylate cement in both the femoral and tibial component of all unicompartmental knee arthroplasties. In addition, multiple surface perforations are performed if the bone surfaces are sclerotic.

In vitro biomechanical studies have noted improved performance of metal-backed tibial components in TKA (107,108). The role of metal-backing of the tibial component in UKA was evaluated by Hyldahl et al. in a clinical series using the Miller-Galante prosthesis and radiostereometric analysis (109). In a prospective study, all-polyethylene components were compared with metal-backed implants of the same design. Patients were assessed clinically using the HSS score (49), with no difference noted between groups. Radiographically, joint alignment and implant position were evaluated, in addition to radiostereometric analysis being performed for evidence of implant migration. No significant differences were noted between the all-polyethylene and metal-backed series at 2-year follow-up. Based on this study, the authors recommend use of the all-polyethylene component due to decreased cost and the ability to use a thicker polyethylene liner. The main disadvantages of the all-polyethylene components are lack of modularity and the ability to adjust implant thickness after cementation.

PREOPERATIVE PLANNING

We obtain multiple radiographs as part of preoperative planning for UKA (Fig. 17, with postoperative radiographs of the same knee shown in Fig. 18). A standard weightbearing AP pro-

vides information about the loss of articular cartilage in full extension. The lateral radiograph can be used to assess the normal tibial slope and the location of tibial cartilage loss as described by White et al. (38). It can be helpful in predicting the need for TKA versus UKA based on the tibial wear pattern as described by Keyes et al. (39). The long-cassette AP view provides important information about the location of the mechanical axis as well as any specific deformities localized to the femur or tibia. Skyline knee radiographs are used in assessing the degree of involvement of the patellofemoral joint. Notch radiographs are obtained to assess the degree of articular cartilage loss on the posterior femoral condyles, which may not be seen in standing radiographs. The mechanical axis of the femur is drawn from the center of the femoral head to the center of the intercondylar notch, the point of entry of the intramedullary femoral guide. The anatomic axis is a line passing down the center of the femoral shaft. The difference between the mechanical and anatomic axes of the femur determines the valgus distal femoral cut. The key difference in planning for the UKA is that this angle does not determine the overall limb alignment but rather the alignment of the implants relative to the femur and tibia. The distal femoral angle, or distal femoral valgus angle, is defined as the angle between the anatomic axis of the femur and a line connecting the distal femoral condyles. This angle is usually 5 to 7 degrees of valgus.

SURGICAL TECHNIQUE

When performing a medial compartment arthroplasty, we prefer to use an 8-cm medial incision, approximately 1 cm medial to the patellar tendon. We routinely use perioperative antibiotics and a pneumatic tourniquet. The knee is flexed to 90 degrees. The incision starts at the superior pole of the patella and extends distally to the tibial tubercle (Fig. 19A). After the skin

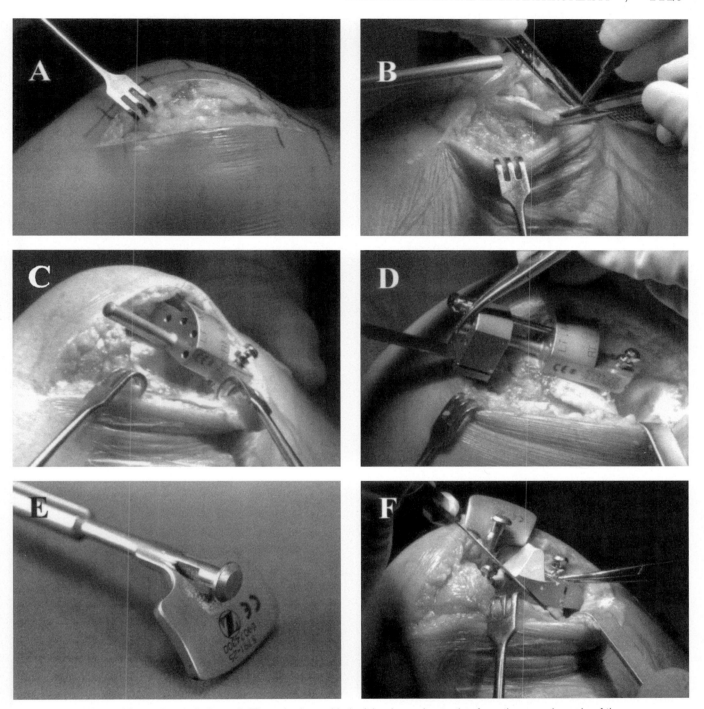

FIG. 19. Operative technique. **A:** Three-in.-long skin incision is made starting from the superior pole of the patella and extending distally to the tibial tubercle, 1 cm medial to the medial pole of the patella. **B:** A medial arthrotomy is made in line with the skin incision. **C:** A distal femoral intramedullary cutting guide is passed into the femur. **D:** A cutting block is passed over the anterior post of the cutting guide, allowing rotation and fine adjustment of the angle of the femoral cut. **E:** After opening the femoral intramedullary canal, an intramedullary patellar retractor is used to expose the joint. **F:** The femoral sizing guide is attached and the chamfer cuts are performed, along with drilling of the lug holes for the femoral component.

incision, a medial arthrotomy is made in line with the skin incision (Fig. 19B). Care is taken to avoid injury to the ACL, the MCL, and the anterior horn of the lateral meniscus during the exposure. A thorough débridement of the medial compartment is required, including the remnants of the meniscus, any mar-

ginal and intercondylar notch osteophytes, loose bodies, and synovium. The articular cartilage of the distal femoral condyle and tibial plateau is then visually inspected. The patellofemoral and lateral compartments are inspected for chondromalacia. Exposure depends on retraction of the patella laterally. The

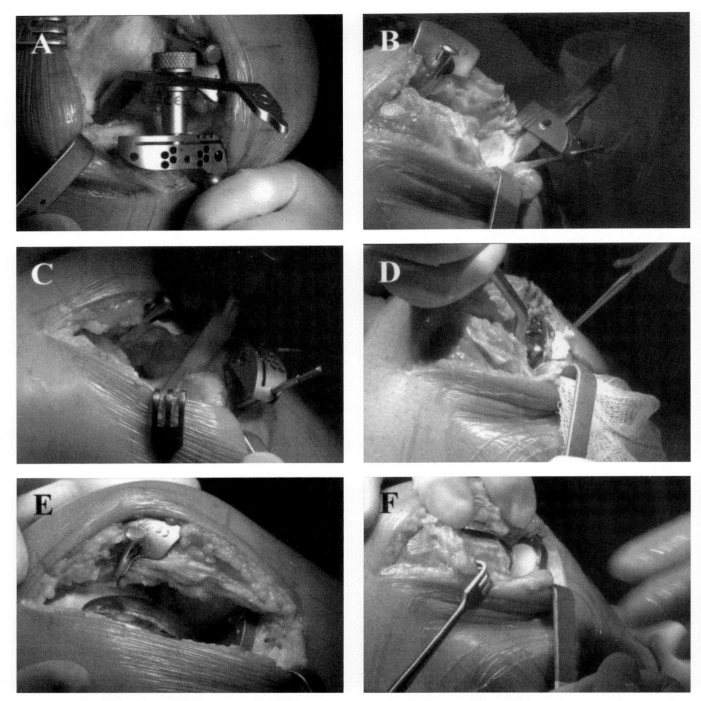

FIG. 20. Operative technique continued. **A:** The external tibial alignment guide is applied, taking approximately 2 mm of bone from the involved medial tibial plateau. **B:** The transverse tibial cut is performed with a reciprocating saw. **C:** The sagittal cut of the tibia is performed, just medial to the anterior cruciate ligament insertion. **D:** After trials have been completed, the final implants are cemented into place and the excess cement is removed. **E:** With use of a metal backed tibia, the thickness of the polyethylene can be adjusted after implant cementation to optimize stability. **F:** The final polyethylene liner is impacted in position.

patella is subluxated with a rake retractor. The femoral cuts are performed using an intramedullary alignment system. Extramedullary systems are available as well. The starting hole for the intramedullary guide is just anterior to intercondylar notch and the PCL attachment. The canal is opened with an 8-mm drill.

The canal is irrigated and suctioned to minimize risk of embolism of marrow contents. The intramedullary rod of the distal femoral cutting guide is passed into the femur (Fig. 19C). The guide can be rotated in the axial plane. It is then pinned in position parallel to the tibial surface and perpendicular to the shaft of the tibia, with the knee in 90 degrees of flexion. Next, a distal femoral cutting block is mounted on the anterior portion of the intramedullary resection guide (Fig. 19D). This guide determines the angle of the distal femoral cut compared with the anatomic axis. The correct angle is determined on preoperative planning. The distal femoral cut is made perpendicular to the mechanical axis of the femur, taking approximately 6 mm of bone from this region. This standard femoral cut is made if the distal femoral valgus angle is less than 6 degrees. If it is greater than or equal to 6 degrees, a 2 mm more proximal cut is made, taking 8 mm off the distal femoral condyle. In lateral-side unicompartmental arthroplasties, we perform a standard 6-mm cut on all patients. Next the distal femoral cutting block is removed.

The intramedullary patellar retractor is then passed into the canal (Fig. 19E). This instrument retracts the patella and exposes the cut surface of the distal femur. At this point, the distal femur is sized with one of seven sizing and finishing guides. If there is inadequate room to seat the sizing guides, this step can be performed after the tibial cut is completed. The goal of the femoral sizing is to allow 1 to 2 mm of bone around the perimeter of the femoral component. The sizing guides have a foot, which rests on the posterior condyle. This prevents placement of the femoral component in an excessively anterior position. The appropriate sizing guide is pinned in position and the chamfer cut, and posterior cuts are performed with a reciprocating saw (Fig. 19F). The lug holes for the implant are drilled through the guide. At this point, the sizing and finishing guide is removed and attention is diverted to the tibia. We use the extramedullary tibial cutting guide (Fig. 20A). Proximally, the center of the guide is placed at the junction of the middle and medial third of the tibial tubercle. The rod is placed parallel with the tibial crest and in line with the second metatarsal distally. It should pass directly anterior to the center of the tibiotalar joint. We base our tibial slope cut on the patient's preoperative tibial slope as seen on the preoperative lateral radiograph. The axial tibial cut is made with a reciprocating saw. We prefer to take a 2-mm cut from the lowest point on the involved medial tibial plateau (Fig. 20B). The sagittal cut is made next with the reciprocating saw (Fig. 20C). This cut should be made as lateral as possible, adjacent to the tibial spine but taking care to protect the ACL. The tibial component is sized with one of five tibial sizers. Every attempt should be made to rest the tibial component on cortical bone around its perimeter. Each sizer has a fin, which can be impacted into the cancellous tibial bone to stabilize the component. It is further stabilized with pins. The tibial component has two large peg holes that are drilled. At this point a provisional femoral component is impacted into position, followed by a trial polyethylene liner. The selection of the trial liner is critical, as it determines the tension in the collateral ligaments as well as the correction of any deformity. We use a liner that allows 2 mm of medial joint opening with stress yet does not overcorrect the alignment. The knee is checked thoroughly at this point. The checklist includes clinical limb alignment in extension and component alignment in extension. Laxity to varus and valgus stress is checked in full extension, 10 degrees of flexion, 45 degrees of flexion, and 90 degrees of flexion. Maximum flexion should be at least 120 degrees. Anterior and posterior tibial translation is noted. In cases of excessive varus or valgus alignment or laxity, the thickness of the tibial provisional component can be varied. If flexion is inadequate, the

tibia can be recut with slightly increased slope. Many systems allow the option of an all-polyethylene or metal-backed titanium component. The advantage of the all-polyethylene component lies in thicker polyethylene, avoidance of "backside" wear (the wear between the modular polyethylene liner and the tibial tray), and avoidance of a locking mechanism, which can occasionally malfunction. According to clinical and radiostereometric studies, no disadvantage in fixation has been noted with the use of the all-polyethylene component (109). The advantages of the metal-backed tibial tray are the ability to adjust the alignment or laxity of the extremity after cementation of the implants, the ability to change the liner at time of revision, and increased ease of cementation of the implants. On the medial side, a dry sponge is passed into the posterior joint and secured in position with a Z retractor. All cut surfaces are thoroughly irrigated with pulse lavage irrigation to remove loose debris and blood. Polymethylmethacrylate cement is used in a doughy state (Fig. 20D). We typically allow the cement to become somewhat firm or doughy before final application to control its location and decrease the risk of escape of the cement into the posterior joint. A small amount of doughy cement is applied to the tibial surface and hand pressurized. Another portion of cement is applied to the tibial component, mainly near the anterior edge. The tibial component is then applied. The sponge in the posterior joint is removed, usually bringing with it any loose cement. The femoral component is applied next (Fig. 20E). Final checks are performed with various thicknesses of the provisional polyethylene liner. Caution is required throughout the operation to avoid overcorrecting any deformity, with its risks of increased progression of arthritis on the contralateral side. The final polyethylene liner is opened and impacted into the tibial tray (Fig. 20F). The wound is irrigated and closed in layers over a small closed-suction drain. We use a running or interrupted No. 1 monofilament, absorbable suture in the anterior capsule. The subcutaneous layer is closed with a running No. 00 monofilament, absorbable suture. The skin is usually closed with skin staples. After closure, approximately 15 to 20 mL of 0.25% bupivacaine (Marcaine) is injected into the joint and the region of the incision.

REHABILITATION

Repicci and Eberle, using a short incision, without patellar eversion, described an accelerated rehabilitation program for UKA (81). Their program involves early ambulation with a knee immobilizer and walker starting on the day of surgery. On postoperative day 2 or 3, the patient is started on passive knee flexion as tolerated. On postoperative day 4, knee exercises are initiated. The goal is to achieve 90 degrees of knee flexion by 1 week postoperatively. Starting in the second week, patients can discontinue their walking aids and begin to resume normal activity. The patient can resume all normal activities by 6 weeks postoperatively. In our experience, patients are mobile by 24 hours after surgery. We start continuous passive motion and gentle active and passive range of motion exercises on the day of surgery. Patients receive one to two sessions per day with physical therapists and ambulate several times per day. The use of a knee immobilizer is optional. Patients are usually discharged to home by 48 hours. Deep venous thrombosis prophylaxis has not been specifically studied in patients with UKA. However, there is a small but definite risk of deep venous thrombosis and pulmonary embolism. We routinely use low-molecular-weight heparin followed by a short course of aspirin.

CONCLUSION

UKA has a history that parallels TKA. It has enjoyed variable popularity over the last three decades. Over this course of time, we have learned a great deal about the proper indications, optimal designs, and the best surgical technique to achieve a successful outcome (Table 1). Some opponents of UKA have argued that TKA provides a more reliable treatment alternative, even in younger patients. This will remain a controversial issue. The goal of UKA should be to provide pain relief and long-term implant survival comparable to TKA while providing improved knee range of motion and patient satisfaction. Several new studies have demonstrated this (20,44). From a theoretical point of view, in the setting of intact cruciate and collateral ligaments and a specific lesion such as anteromedial arthritis (38) of the tibia, this resurfacing may provide an indefinite surgical solution. The current indications for UKA are unicompartmental osteoarthritis or post-traumatic arthritis in an older patient with low activity level; minimal flexion deformity; minimal, correctable varus or valgus deformity; and intact cruciate and collateral ligaments. Newer implants use improved instrumentation for more precise cuts and better exposure. Currently, optimal fixation of implants to bone is achieved with polymethylmethacrylate cement. Future directions in UKA include increased wear resistance of polyethylene, more precise instrumentation based on a better understanding of knee kinematics, and improved fixation, possibly including a revival of uncemented implants. If our knowledge of this procedure and its pitfalls is incorporated into surgical decision making, this operation can provide long-term results comparable to TKA, with the additional benefit of decreased cost (83), shorter hospital stay (82), more rapid recovery (74,76,82), improved range of motion (66,74), decreased transfusion requirement (81,110), and higher patient satisfaction (66).

REFERENCES

1. McKeever D. Tibial plateau prosthesis. *Clin Orthop* 1960;18:86–95.
2. MacIntosh D. Hemiarthroplasty of the knee using a space occupying prosthesis for painful varus and valgus deformities. In Proceedings of the Joint Meeting of the Orthopaedic Associations of the English-Speaking World. *J Bone Joint Surg Am* 1958; 40A:1431.
3. Gunston FH. Polycentric knee arthroplasty. Prosthetic simulation of normal knee movement. *J Bone Joint Surg Br* 1971;53:272–277.
4. Marmor L. The modular knee. *Clin Orthop* 1973;94:242–248.
5. Goodfellow JW, O'Connor J. Clinical results of the Oxford knee. Surface arthroplasty of the tibiofemoral joint with a meniscal bearing prosthesis. *Clin Orthop* 1986;205:21–42.
6. Goodfellow J, O'Connor J. The mechanics of the knee and prosthesis design. *J Bone Joint Surg Br* 1978;60:358–369.
7. Goodfellow JW, et al. Unicompartmental Oxford meniscal knee arthroplasty. *J Arthroplasty* 1987;2:1–9.
8. Callaghan JJ, et al. Mobile-bearing knee replacement: concepts and results. *Instr Course Lect* 2001;50:431–449.
9. Engelbrecht E, et al. Statistics of total knee replacement: partial and total knee replacement, design St. Georg: a review of a 4-year observation. *Clin Orthop* 1976;120:54–64.
10. Insall J, Walker P. Unicondylar knee replacement. *Clin Orthop* 1976;120:83–85.
11. Insall J, Aglietti P. A five to seven-year follow-up of unicondylar arthroplasty. *J Bone Joint Surg Am* 1980;62:1329–1337.
12. Laskin RS. Unicompartmental knee replacement: some unanswered questions. *Clin Orthop* 2001;392:267–271.
13. Laskin RS. Unicompartmental tibiofemoral resurfacing arthroplasty. *J Bone Joint Surg Am* 1978;60:182–185.
14. Weale AE, et al. Radiological changes five years after unicompartmental knee replacement. *J Bone Joint Surg Br* 2000;82:996–1000.
15. Cartier P, Sanouiller JL, Grelsamer RP. Unicompartmental knee arthroplasty surgery. 10-year minimum follow-up period. *J Arthroplasty* 1996;11:782–788.
16. Ansari S, Newman JH, Ackroyd CE. St. Georg sledge for medial compartment knee replacement. 461 arthroplasties followed for 4 (1–17) years. *Acta Orthop Scand* 1997;68:430–434.
17. Capra SW Jr., Fehring TK. Unicondylar arthroplasty. A survivorship analysis. *J Arthroplasty* 1992;7:247–251.
18. Heck DA, et al. Unicompartmental knee arthroplasty. A multicenter investigation with long-term follow-up evaluation. *Clin Orthop* 1993;286:154–159.
19. Knutson K, Lindstrand A, Lidgren L. Survival of knee arthroplasties. A nation-wide multicentre investigation of 8000 cases. *J Bone Joint Surg Br* 1986;68:795–803.
20. Murray DW, Goodfellow JW, O'Connor JJ. The Oxford medial unicompartmental arthroplasty: a ten-year survival study. *J Bone Joint Surg Br* 1998;80:983–989.
21. Scott RD, et al. Unicompartmental knee arthroplasty. Eight- to 12-year follow-up evaluation with survivorship analysis. *Clin Orthop* 1991;271:96–100.
22. Scott RD, Santore RF. Unicondylar unicompartmental replacement for osteoarthritis of the knee. *J Bone Joint Surg Am* 1981;63:536–544.
23. Magnussen PA, Bartlett RJ. Cementless PCA unicompartmental joint arthroplasty for osteoarthritis of the knee. A prospective study of 51 cases. *J Arthroplasty* 1990;5:151–158.
24. Broughton NS, Newman JH, Baily RA. Unicompartmental replacement and high tibial osteotomy for osteoarthritis of the knee. A comparative study after 5–10 years' follow-up. *J Bone Joint Surg Br* 1986;68:447–452.
25. Bergenudd H. Porous-coated anatomic unicompartmental knee arthroplasty in osteoarthritis. A 3- to 9-year follow-up study. *J Arthroplasty* 1995;10(Suppl):S8–S13.
26. Levine WN, et al. Conversion of failed modern unicompartmental arthroplasty to total knee arthroplasty. *J Arthroplasty* 1996;11:797–801.
27. Barrett WP, Scott RD. Revision of failed unicondylar unicompartmental knee arthroplasty. *J Bone Joint Surg Am* 1987;69:1328–1335.
28. Atsui K, et al. Ceramic unicompartmental knee arthroplasty for spontaneous osteonecrosis of the knee joint. *Bull Hosp Joint Dis* 1997;56:233–236.
29. Marmor L. Unicompartmental arthroplasty for osteonecrosis of the knee joint. *Clin Orthop* 1993;294:247–253.
30. Kozinn SC, Scott R. Unicondylar knee arthroplasty. *J Bone Joint Surg Am* 1989;71:145–150.
31. Barck AL. 10-year evaluation of compartmental knee arthroplasty. *J Arthroplasty* 1989;4(Suppl):S49–S54.
32. Christensen NO. Unicompartmental prosthesis for gonarthrosis. A nine-year series of 575 knees from a Swedish hospital. *Clin Orthop* 1991;273:165–169.
33. Larsson SE, Larsson S, Lundkvist S. Unicompartmental knee arthroplasty. A prospective consecutive series followed for six to 11 years. *Clin Orthop* 1988;232:174–181.
34. Barnes CL, Scott RD. Unicompartmental knee arthroplasty. *Instr Course Lect* 1993;42:309–314.
35. Stockelman RE, Pohl KP. The long-term efficacy of unicompartmental arthroplasty of the knee. *Clin Orthop* 1991;271:88–95.
36. Reference deleted in text.
37. Corpe RS, Engh GA. A quantitative assessment of degenerative changes acceptable in the unoperated compartments of knees undergoing unicompartmental replacement. *Orthopedics* 1990;13:319–323.
38. White SH, Ludkowski PF, Goodfellow JW. Anteromedial osteoarthritis of the knee. *J Bone Joint Surg Br* 1991;73:582–586.

39. Keyes GW, et al. The radiographic classification of medial gonarthrosis. Correlation with operation methods in 200 knees. *Acta Orthop Scand* 1992;63:497–501.

40. Sharpe I, Tyrrell PN, White SH. Magnetic resonance imaging assessment for unicompartmental knee replacement: a limited role. *Knee* 2001;8:213–218.

41. McCallum JD 3rd, Scott RD. Duplication of medial erosion in unicompartmental knee arthroplasties. *J Bone Joint Surg Br* 1995;77:726–728.

42. Sisto DJ, et al. Unicompartment arthroplasty for osteoarthrosis of the knee. *Clin Orthop* 1993;286:149–153.

43. Simmons S, et al. Proprioception after unicondylar knee arthroplasty versus total knee arthroplasty. *Clin Orthop* 1996;331:179–184.

44. Berger RA, et al. Unicompartmental knee arthroplasty. Clinical experience at 6- to 10-year followup. *Clin Orthop* 1999;367:50–60.

45. Squire MW, et al. Unicompartmental knee replacement. A minimum 15 year followup study. *Clin Orthop* 1999;367:61–72.

46. Marmor L. Unicompartmental knee arthroplasty. Ten- to 13-year follow-up study. *Clin Orthop* 1988;226:14–20.

47. Marmor L. Lateral compartment arthroplasty of the knee. *Clin Orthop* 1984;186:115–121.

48. Ohdera T, Tokunaga J, Kobayashi A. Unicompartmental knee arthroplasty for lateral gonarthrosis: midterm results. *J Arthroplasty* 2001;16:196–200.

49. Ranawat CS, Insall J, Shine J. Duo-condylar knee arthroplasty: Hospital for Special Surgery design. *Clin Orthop* 1976;120:76–82.

50. Ansari S, Newman S, Ackroyd C. Lateral compartment arthroplasty. Proceedings of the 63rd Annual Meeting of the American Academy of Orthopaedic Surgeons; Atlanta; 1996.

51. Gunther T, et al. Lateral unicompartmental arthroplasty with Oxford meniscal knee. *Knee* 1996;3:33–39.

52. Wang CJ, Walker PS. Rotatory laxity of the human knee joint. *J Bone Joint Surg Am* 1974;56:161–170.

53. Sokoloff RM, Farooki S, Resnick D. Spontaneous osteonecrosis of the knee associated with ipsilateral tibial plateau stress fracture: report of two patients and review of the literature. *Skeletal Radiol* 2001;30:53–56.

54. Lotke PA, Battish R, Nelson CL. Treatment of osteonecrosis of the knee. *Instr Course Lect* 2001;50:483–488.

55. Mont MA, et al. Atraumatic osteonecrosis of the knee. *J Bone Joint Surg Am* 2000;82:1279–1290.

56. Ecker ML, Lotke PA. Spontaneous osteonecrosis of the knee. *J Am Acad Orthop Surg* 1994;2:173–178.

57. Potter TA, Weinfeld MS, Thomas WH. Arthroplasty of the knee in rheumatoid arthritis and osteoarthritis. A follow-up study after implantation of the McKeever and MacIntosh prostheses. *J Bone Joint Surg Am* 1972;54:1–24.

58. MacIntosh DL, Hunter GA. The use of the hemiarthroplasty prosthesis for advanced osteoarthritis and rheumatoid arthritis of the knee. *J Bone Joint Surg Br* 1972;54:244–255.

59. MacIntosh D. Arthroplasty of the knee in rheumatoid arthritis. *J Bone Joint Surg Br* 1966;48:179.

60. Swanson AB, et al. Unicompartmental and bicompartmental arthroplasty of the knee with a finned metal tibial-plateau implant. *J Bone Joint Surg Am* 1985;67:1175–1182.

61. Kay NR, Martins HD. The MacIntosh tibial plateau hemiprosthesis for the rheumatoid knee. *J Bone Joint Surg Br* 1972;54:256–262.

62. Robertsson O, et al. Knee arthroplasty in rheumatoid arthritis. A report from the Swedish Knee Arthroplasty Register on 4,381 primary operations 1985–1995. *Acta Orthop Scand* 1997;68:545–553.

63. Bengtson S, Knutson K. The infected knee arthroplasty. A 6-year follow-up of 357 cases. *Acta Orthop Scand* 1991;62:301–311.

64. Marmor L. Unicompartmental and total knee arthroplasty. *Clin Orthop* 1985;192:75–81.

65. Rand JA, Ilstrup DM. Survivorship analysis of total knee arthroplasty. Cumulative rates of survival of 9200 total knee arthroplasties. *J Bone Joint Surg Am* 1991;73:397–409.

66. Laurencin CT, et al. Unicompartmental versus total knee arthroplasty in the same patient. A comparative study. *Clin Orthop* 1991;273:151–156.

67. Rudan JF, Simurda MA. High tibial osteotomy. A prospective clinical and roentgenographic review. *Clin Orthop* 1990;255:251–256.

68. Yasuda K, et al. A ten- to 15-year follow-up observation of high tibial osteotomy in medial compartment osteoarthrosis. *Clin Orthop* 1992;282:186–195.

69. Matthews LS, et al. Proximal tibial osteotomy. Factors that influence the duration of satisfactory function. *Clin Orthop* 1988;229:193–200.

70. Weale AE, Newman JH. Unicompartmental arthroplasty and high tibial osteotomy for osteoarthrosis of the knee. A comparative study with a 12- to 17-year follow-up period. *Clin Orthop* 1994;302:134–137.

71. Stukenborg-Colsman C, et al. High tibial osteotomy versus unicompartmental joint replacement in unicompartmental knee joint osteoarthritis: 7-10-year follow-up prospective randomised study. *Knee* 2001;8:187–194.

72. Insall JN, et al. Rationale of the Knee Society clinical rating system. *Clin Orthop* 1989;248:13–14.

73. Rees JL, et al. Medial unicompartmental arthroplasty after failed high tibial osteotomy. *J Bone Joint Surg Br* 2001;83:1034–1036.

74. Cameron HU, Jung YB. A comparison of unicompartmental knee replacement with total knee replacement. *Orthop Rev* 1988;17:983–988.

75. Cobb A, Kozinn S, Scott R. Unicondylar or total knee replacement: patient preferences. *J Bone Joint Surg Br* 1990;72:166.

76. Newman JH, Ackroyd CE, Shah NA. Unicompartmental or total knee replacement? Five-year results of a prospective, randomised trial of 102 osteoarthritic knees with unicompartmental arthritis. *J Bone Joint Surg Br* 1998;80:862–865.

77. Ryd L, Karrholm J, Ahlvin P. Knee scoring systems in gonarthrosis. Evaluation of interobserver variability and the envelope of bias. Score Assessment Group. *Acta Orthop Scand* 1997;68:41–45.

78. Weale AE, et al. The length of the patellar tendon after unicompartmental and total knee replacement. *J Bone Joint Surg Br* 1999;81:790–795.

79. Kald A, et al. Surgical outcome and cost-minimisation-analyses of laparoscopic and open hernia repair: a randomised prospective trial with one year follow up. *Eur J Surg* 1997;163:505–510.

80. Liem MS, et al. Comparison of conventional anterior surgery and laparoscopic surgery for inguinal-hernia repair. *N Engl J Med* 1997;336:1541–1547.

81. Repicci J, Eberle R. Minimally invasive surgical technique for unicondylar knee arthroplasty. *J South Orthop Soc* 1999;8:20.

82. Price AJ, et al. Rapid recovery after Oxford unicompartmental arthroplasty through a short incision. *J Arthroplasty* 2001;16:970–976.

83. Robertsson O, et al. Use of unicompartmental instead of tricompartmental prostheses for unicompartmental arthrosis in the knee is a cost-effective alternative. 15,437 primary tricompartmental prostheses were compared with 10,624 primary medial or lateral unicompartmental prostheses. *Acta Orthop Scand* 1999;70:170–175.

84. Emerson RH Jr., Potter T. The use of the McKeever metallic hemiarthroplasty for unicompartmental arthritis. *J Bone Joint Surg Am* 1985;67:208–212.

85. Scott RD, et al. McKeever metallic hemiarthroplasty of the knee in unicompartmental degenerative arthritis. Long-term clinical follow-up and current indications. *J Bone Joint Surg Am* 1985;67:203–207.

86. Olsen NJ, Ejsted R, Krogh P. St Georg modular knee prosthesis. A two-and-a-half to six-year follow-up. *J Bone Joint Surg Br* 1986;68:787–890.

87. Tabor OB Jr., Tabor OB. Unicompartmental arthroplasty: a long-term follow-up study. *J Arthroplasty* 1998;13:373–379.

88. Palmer SH, Morrison PJ, Ross AC. Early catastrophic tibial component wear after unicompartmental knee arthroplasty. *Clin Orthop* 1998;350:143–148.

89. Argenson JN, O'Connor JJ. Polyethylene wear in meniscal knee replacement. A one to nine-year retrieval analysis of the Oxford knee. *J Bone Joint Surg Br* 1992;74:228–232.

90. Psychoyios V, et al. Wear of congruent meniscal bearings in unicompartmental knee arthroplasty: a retrieval study of 16 specimens. *J Bone Joint Surg Br* 1998;80:976–982.

91. Ivarsson I, Gillquist J. The strain distribution in the upper tibia after insertion of two different unicompartmental prostheses. *Clin Orthop* 1992;(279):194–200.

92. Riebel GD, et al. Early failure of the femoral component in unicompartmental knee arthroplasty. *J Arthroplasty* 1995;10:615–621.

93. Lindstrand A, Stenstrom A, Lewold S. Multicenter study of unicompartmental knee revision. PCA, Marmor, and St Georg compared in 3,777 cases of arthrosis. *Acta Orthop Scand* 1992;63:256–259.

94. Hodge WA, Chandler HP. Unicompartmental knee replacement: a comparison of constrained and unconstrained designs. *J Bone Joint Surg Am* 1992;74:877–883.

95. Romanowski M, Repicci J. Eight year follow up on minimally invasive unicondylar arthroplasty. Presented at: American Academy of Orthopaedic Surgeons; Dallas; 2002.

96. Ahlback S. Osteoarthrosis of the knee. A radiographic investigation. *Acta Radiol Diagn (Stockh)* 1968;277(Suppl):7–72.

97. Padgett DE, Stern SH, Insall JN. Revision total knee arthroplasty for failed unicompartmental replacement. *J Bone Joint Surg Am* 1991;73:186–190.

98. McAuley JP, Engh GA, Ammeen DJ. Revision of failed unicompartmental knee arthroplasty. *Clin Orthop* 2001;392:279–282.

99. Weinstein JN, Andriacchi TP, Galante J. Factors influencing walking and stairclimbing following unicompartmental knee arthroplasty. *J Arthroplasty* 1986;1:109–115.

100. Lewold S, et al. Revision of unicompartmental knee arthroplasty: outcome in 1,135 cases from the Swedish Knee Arthroplasty study. *Acta Orthop Scand* 1998;69:469–474.

101. Bartel DL, Bicknell VL, Wright TM. The effect of conformity, thickness, and material on stresses in ultra-high molecular weight components for total joint replacement. *J Bone Joint Surg Am* 1986;68:1041–1051.

102. Bartel DL, et al. Stresses in polyethylene components of contemporary total knee replacements. *Clin Orthop* 1995;317:76–82.

103. Blunn GW, et al. Polyethylene wear in unicondylar knee prostheses. 106 retrieved Marmor, PCA, and St Georg tibial components compared. *Acta Orthop Scand* 1992;63:247–255.

104. Rostoker W, Galante JO. Contact pressure dependence of wear rates of ultra high molecular weight polyethylene. *J Biomed Mater Res* 1979;13:957–964.

105. Bartley RE, et al. Polyethylene wear in unicompartmental knee arthroplasty. *Clin Orthop* 1994;299:18–24.

106. Miskovsky C, Whiteside LA, White SE. The cemented unicondylar knee arthroplasty. An in vitro comparison of three cement techniques. *Clin Orthop* 1992;284:215–220.

107. Bartel DL, et al. Performance of the tibial component in total knee replacement. *J Bone Joint Surg Am* 1982;64:1026–1033.

108. Walker PS, et al. Fixation of tibial components of knee prostheses. *J Bone Joint Surg Am* 1981;63:258–267.

109. Hyldahl HC, et al. Does metal backing improve fixation of tibial component in unicondylar knee arthroplasty? A randomized radiostereometric analysis. *J Arthroplasty* 2001;16:174–179.

110. Rougraff BT, Heck DA, Gibson AE. A comparison of tricompartmental and unicompartmental arthroplasty for the treatment of gonarthrosis. *Clin Orthop* 1991;273:157–164.

111. Dennis BD, et al. In vivo three-dimensional determination of kinematics for subjects with a normal knee or a unicompartmental or total knee replacement. *J Bone Joint Surg Am* 2002;83(Suppl 2):104–105.

CHAPTER 77

Posterior Cruciate Ligament Retention in Total Knee Replacement

Creg A. Carpenter and Thomas S. Thornhill

Surgeons continue to debate the merits of posterior cruciate ligament (PCL) retention and substitution in total knee replacement (TKR). Proponents of PCL retention point to superior range of motion, strength, stability, and durability as reasons to spare the ligament in TKR (1). With similar enthusiasm, advocates of PCL substitution argue that resection eases exposure and correction of deformity, decreases polyethylene wear, and provides reliable sagittal plane stability (2). Recent studies of both systems demonstrate the long-term durability of PCL substitution and retention (Table 1) (3–10). This chapter reviews the anatomy and kinematics of the knee as they relate to the PCL. The evolution of cruciate-retaining designs, current controversies of the PCL in TKR, and the authors' reasoning for and technique of PCL-retaining TKR are discussed.

POSTERIOR CRUCIATE LIGAMENT ANATOMY

The PCL runs in a slightly oblique direction from the lateral aspect of the medial femoral condyle to the lateral aspect of the posterior intercondylar area of the tibia (Fig. 1). The tibial insertion flares out for a distance of 2 cm below the articular surface. The broad, distal insertion makes PCL retention and balance during TKR feasible. Two anatomically inseparable bands comprise the PCL. A large anterolateral band tightens in flexion, and a smaller posteromedial band tightens in extension (11). The anterior cruciate ligament (ACL) crosses in front of the PCL, running from the medial aspect of the lateral femoral condyle to the medial aspect of the anterior intercondylar area of the tibia. The synovium covers the anterior surface of the PCL and then fans out laterally onto the surface of the capsule (12). Inflammatory arthritides such as rheumatoid arthritis often spare the PCL because the synovium does not surround the ligament, making it an extrasynovial structure. In contrast, patients with rheumatoid arthritis often lack an ACL, as it is entirely surrounded by synovium.

KNEE KINEMATICS PERTAINING TO THE POSTERIOR CRUCIATE LIGAMENT

Bony contours provide little inherent stability to the knee. The lateral tibial plateau is convex in the sagittal and coronal planes. The medial tibial plateau is slightly larger than the lateral plateau and concave in both planes. Muscles, ligaments, and capsule combine to provide knee stability. Studies of sequential

TABLE 1. *Long-term follow-up to cruciate-retaining total knee replacement*

Study	Prosthesis	Manufacturer	No. of patients/knees	Average follow-up (yr)	Mean age (yr)	Osteoarthritis (%)	Rheumatoid arthritis (%)	10-Yr survivorship	Infection (%)	Radiographic lucent lines (%)	Instability (%)	Reoperation/revision other than infection (%)
Dennis et al. (27)	Posterior cruciate condylar	Howmedica	35/42	11	62.8	50	50	N/A	0	75	2.3	4.7
Schai et al. (28)	Press-Fit Condylar	Johnson & Johnson	122/155	10.5	68	62	33	90	1.2	Tibia 16 Femur 3 Patella 3	0	13.5
Berger et al. (3)	Miller-Galante II	Zimmer	92/109	9	72	94.4	4.6	100	2.8	Tibia 13 Femur 11 Patella 1.4	0	1.8
Parker et al. (7)	Miller-Galante I	Zimmer	67/67	12.8	66	100	0	90	6	N/A	0	52
Gill and Joshi (5)	Kinematic condylar	Howmedica	177/216	10.1	68	88	11	98.2	1	Femur 4.5 Tibia 8.3 Patella 4	0.5	3
Buechel et al. (4)	Low Contact Stress (LCS) meniscal bearing	DePuy Orthopaedics	116/140	12.3	65	89	6.5	100	0.7	Femur 0 Tibia 6.6 Patella 0	0.7	5.7
Ritter et al. (9)	Anatomic Graduated Components	Biomet	3,054/4,583	N/A	70.4	87	N/A	98	1.3	N/A	N/A	N/A
Sextro et al. (10)	Kinematic condylar	Howmedica	118/168	15.7	65.2	64.9	31	96.5	1.2	N/A	0.6	7.7

N/A, not available

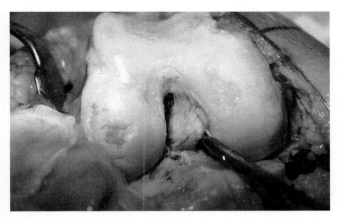

FIG. 1. Dissection of the posterior cruciate ligament during total knee replacement. Note the robust nature of the posterior cruciate ligament passing from the lateral aspect of the inter-condylar notch to the posterior tibia.

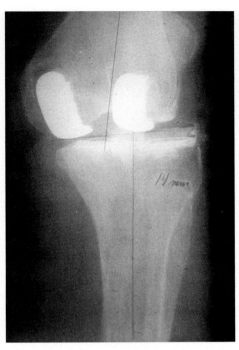

FIG. 2. Early resurfacing total knee replacement (Marmor) demonstrating lateral subluxation of the tibia on the femur.

sectioning of the PCL reveal that in isolation the ligament has a limited role in providing varus/valgus and rotational stability (13). The PCL plays a large role in preventing anterior/posterior translation of the tibia relative to the femur. Prosthetic designs must account for this stability through prosthetic geometry, a post-and-cam mechanism, or PCL retention.

A combination of rolling, sliding, and rotation occurs in normal knee motion. The synchrony of these motions depends on the articular contours of the tibia and femur, menisci, capsular structures and an intact ACL/PCL in the nondiseased native knee. During the first 30 degrees of knee flexion motion occurs predominantly from rolling of the tibial and femoral surfaces relative to one another. As the knee further flexes, tightening of the PCL leads to sliding at the articular interface. This sliding, also referred to as *femoral rollback*, prevents impingement of the posterior surface of the tibia and femur during maximal flexion and allows flexion of approximately 140 degrees in the nondiseased knee. The convex lateral tibial plateau allows more sliding than the more conforming, concave surface of the medial plateau. This creates an obligatory internal rotation of the tibia relative to the femur with knee flexion. Femoral rollback also lengthens the moment arm and improves the direction of pull of the quadriceps, which increases the strength of the quadriceps as the knee flexes (14).

EVOLUTION OF THE CRUCIATE-RETAINING TOTAL KNEE REPLACEMENT

In the early 1970s, many different prosthetic knee designs were being used. Early hinge designs suffered many early and late complications, including infection and loosening, which made their routine use unacceptable. Early resurfacing knee replacements included the polycentric (1970), modular (1972), UCI (1972), McKeever (1960), Geometric (1971), and Duocondylar (1973). These surface replacement designs relied on intact native ligaments and capsule to provide knee stability. These prostheses consisted of medial and/or lateral polyethylene tibial components that were separate or connected by a small bar. Early techniques preserved both cruciate ligaments

and made no provision for the patellofemoral joint. The conformity of the articulation of early total knee arthroplasties varied based on the designer's philosophy. Less conforming articulations attempted to simulate normal knee rollback and motion (polycentric and Duocondylar). Other designs focused on stability and provided more congruent femoral and tibial articular surfaces (Geometric). Problems of tibial subsidence and loosening, patellofemoral pain, and lateral subluxation of the tibia on the femur complicated these early designs (Fig. 2) (15–18).

Modern total knee designs reflect the lessons learned from the shortcomings of early resurfacing knee replacements. These include a one-piece metal condylar femoral component with a trochlear flange, a one-piece metal-backed or all-polyethylene tibial component, and selective resurfacing of the patella with an all-polyethylene component. From these early condylar designs emerged two schools of thought, namely, preservation or sacrifice of the PCL. The latter school, recognizing limited flexion in early cruciate-sacrificing designs and the advantage of femoral rollback and improved patellofemoral mechanics, evolved into cruciate substitution by the addition of a central polyethylene eminence on the tibial component. This eminence engaged in mid-flexion (60 to 80 degrees) to achieve these goals.

Advocates of cruciate sacrifice/substitution developed the total condylar prosthesis in 1973 in response to their experience with the Duocondylar TKR (Fig. 3) (19). This design provided a femoral component with an anterior femoral flange and allowed patellar resurfacing. The tibial component was a one-piece all-polyethylene component that necessitated sacrifice of the PCL. The total condylar prosthesis proved durable and gave reliable results (20,21). Limitations of this prosthesis related to range of motion and posterior subluxation of the tibia relative to the femur. To overcome these shortcomings, the posterior stabilized total knee was introduced in 1978. These devices possess

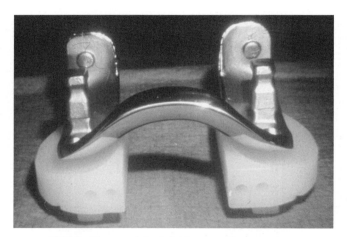

FIG. 3. Duocondylar total knee replacement.

built in posterior constraint and achieved femoral rollback by a post-and-cam mechanism. Numerous authors have subsequently reported excellent results with posterior stabilized designs (22).

Over the same time frame, advocates of cruciate-retaining designs of TKR grew as a result of the limitations these surgeons experienced with the Duocondylar, McKeever, Modular, and other early knee replacements (15,23). One example of an early PCL-retaining design, the Duo-Patellar, evolved from experience with the Duocondylar TKR. Implantation of the Duo-Patellar prosthesis at the Robert Breck Brigham Hospital began in 1974 (24). The femoral component provided an anterior flange to facilitate patellar tracking. The initial tibial component consisted of separate medial and lateral tibial pieces and

allowed for ACL and PCL retention. The tibial contour changed from flat in the sagittal plane to a curved surface to increase articular constraint. The Duo-Patellar was redesigned in 1978 to a one-piece tibial component with a stem to better distribute weightbearing forces (Fig. 4) (25). This tibial component mandated sacrifice of the ACL but maintained a cutout for preservation of the PCL.

Over the next 7 years, gradual refinement of the femoral, tibial, and patellar components occurred and the Duo-Patellar evolved into Robert Breck Brigham Hospital and Kinematic total knee systems (26). The goals of these prostheses were to increase range of motion, improve fixation of the tibial component, and maintain the overall excellent clinical results of the previous designs. The trochlear groove of the femoral component was deepened and aligned in 7 degrees of valgus to improve patellar tracking. In 1980, the tibial component changed to a metal-backed design and reverted to a flattened surface in the sagittal plane to allow rollback. Femoral and tibial intramedullary stems were made available for situations of bone deficiency. Experience with the Kinematic total knee continued the clinical success of previous designs and taught valuable lessons on axial alignment, component position, and cementing technique (18,27).

Advocates of cruciate retention remained concerned about a kinematic conflict if a conforming polyethylene surface directed motion antagonistic to the strong intact PCL. Moreover, cruciate tension was variable and difficult to match with tibiofemoral conformity. This concern led to the development of flat-on-flat cruciate-sparing designs. Unfortunately, these designs did not compensate for the abduction/adduction moments during gait and caused edge loading and polyethylene wear. Additionally, if the PCL was too tight there was abnormal rollback and posterior polyethylene wear; if the PCL was too loose, random contact

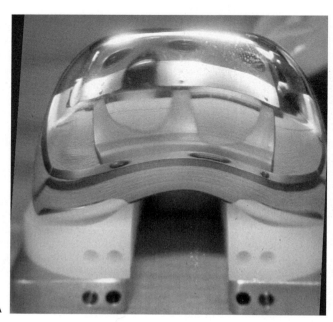

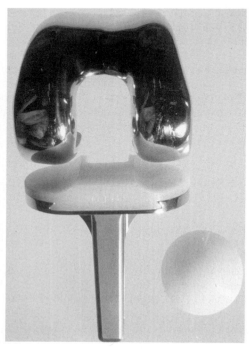

FIG. 4. A: Duo-Patellar total knee replacement. **B:** Design change with one-piece, stemmed tibial component.

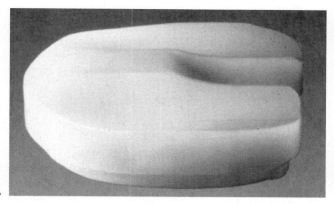 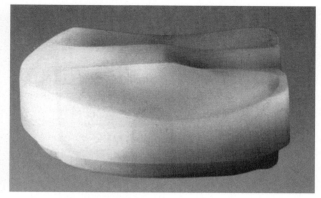

FIG. 5. A: Posterior-lipped polyethylene insert. **B:** Curved polyethylene insert.

leading to abnormal shear stresses and even paradoxic roll forward occurred during flexion.

Recognizing the concerns of kinematic conflict and the problems of flat-on-flat designs, a new direction to cruciate retention was introduced. The Press-Fit Condylar (PFC) design incorporated different tibial contact patterns (posterior-lipped and curved) to accommodate for different cruciate tensions (Fig. 5). Balancing the PCL by recession from either the tibia or femur allowed cruciate retention while accommodating sufficient conformity to allow low contact stress. In a series of patients from our institution who had posterior cruciate–retaining TKR with the PFC system, Schai et al. found no tibial or femoral loosening at a minimum of 10-year follow-up (28). Similarly, Buehler et al. had 98.7% survivorship with posterior cruciate retention with the PFC system at 9-year follow-up (29). The PFC modular cruciate-substituting design was introduced, thus coupling the PCL-retention and PCL-substituting philosophies. In 1996, the PFC Sigma design was introduced as a merged philosophy to allow smooth transition between cruciate retention and substitution, expand revision capabilities, and eliminate gamma-radiated polyethylene sterilized in air.

CURRENT CONTROVERSIES IN POSTERIOR CRUCIATE LIGAMENT–RETAINING AND POSTERIOR CRUCIATE LIGAMENT– SUBSTITUTING TOTAL KNEE REPLACEMENT

Rollback and Kinematics

Neither the cruciate-retaining nor cruciate-substituting knee can reproduce the kinematics of the normal knee. In fact, the unique aspects of the knee with the material properties of the articular cartilage, the cruciate ligaments, and the medial and lateral menisci confer very different properties than seen in metal-to-plastic condylar designs. Meniscal-bearing and rotating-platform knees attempt to more closely mimic normal knees but fall short of this goal. Most meniscal-bearing designs demonstrate paradoxic motion, whereas rotating-platform designs rotate about a fixed central axis rather than accomplishing the complex motion that occurs in the normal knee. It was originally believed that with proper conformity or mobile bearing designs, normal kinematics could be achieved.

Recent fluoroscopic and gait laboratory data have contrasted with these early beliefs (30–32). Fluoroscopic studies demonstrate that cruciate-retaining and cruciate-substituting designs fail to reproduce normal rollback. Strain-gauge studies also demonstrate the inability of TKR to reproduce normal ligament strain behavior (33). As these studies would predict, clinical comparisons show little difference in range of motion achieved in either design (34–38). Similarly, difference in quadriceps efficiency and stair-climbing ability also appears equivocal in cruciate-retaining and cruciate-substituting devices (39,40). Excellent clinical results and range of motion can be achieved with the use of recession to balance the PCL in conjunction with more conforming polyethylene inserts (41–44).

At the present time, clinical and laboratory data fail to produce a clear advantage for PCL retention or substitution with regard to achieving femoral rollback or quadriceps function. Both designs produce predictable functional range of motion and clinical results.

Wear and Loosening

In the past, proponents of cruciate retention have argued that an intact PCL would decrease wear and loosening. The native PCL would theoretically act to absorb shear forces (1). If this biologic structure for absorption was lost, the anterior-posterior shear forces would reroute through the metal-polyethylene and bone-cement interface, leading to a higher rate of wear and loosening.

Reports of excessive polyethylene wear in the literature focusing on cruciate-retaining designs contrast with this theoretical benefit of PCL retention (45–47). Most of these cases of polyethylene failure, however, involve flat-on-flat articulations subject to edge loading and high contact stresses if the PCL is not properly balanced (48,49). These failures also occurred at a time in the evolution of TKR in which thin tibial inserts with heat-pressed polyethylene were used.

More conforming articulations in conjunction with retention of the PCL have not had this high rate of wear (27,50). Improved polyethylene and focus on balancing the PCL should minimize these wear failures in cruciate-retaining designs (42,43). Polyethylene wear has not proved to be a major problem in cruciate-substituting designs in long-term follow-up (22). Aseptic loosening is an uncommon phenomenon in cruciate-sacrificing, cruciate-sparing, and cruciate-substituting designs in long-term follow-up (50–52). Retention or substitution of the PCL as a solution to preventing or decreasing wear and loosening in TKR remains unproved.

Proprioception

Retention of mechanoreceptors within the PCL has been used as an argument to retain the PCL. Theoretically this could improve knee proprioception and provide a more "normal-feeling" knee. Most authors agree that arthritic conditions lead to histologic changes within the ligament and significantly alter proprioception (53,54). The hope that total knee arthroplasty could restore normal joint proprioception is unrealistic. Attempts to evaluate proprioception in knee arthroplasty patients reveal improvement in proprioception after implantation. These studies, however, do not indicate a clear advantage for cruciate-retaining or cruciate-substituting designs with regard to proprioception (34,55,56).

Stability

Retention of the PCL provides anteroposterior stability for the knee. Less conforming polyethylene inserts used in conjunction with PCL retention require an intact PCL to provide this stability. Numerous authors report either flexion or extension instability if the PCL is not properly balanced or late rupture occurs (57–60). This is a rare complication even in the rheumatoid patient (61,62). Cruciate-substituting knee replacement relies on a post-and-cam mechanism to provide anterior and posterior stability. This design requires careful balancing of the flexion and extension gaps to prevent dislocation of the post. Moreover, cam engagement can lead to peg wear or back-sided wear in metal-backed tibial components (63,64). Regardless of the design used for TKR, careful balancing of the soft tissues is required to avoid these pitfalls. Both cruciate-retaining and cruciate-substituting designs of TKR provide reliable stability in the sagittal plane if properly balanced.

AUTHORS' ARGUMENTS FOR POSTERIOR CRUCIATE LIGAMENT RETENTION

Balancing Flexion and Extension Gaps

Advocates of PCL substitution argue that resecting the PCL eases exposure and facilitates balancing the flexion and extension spaces (65). In our experience, the PCL acts as a tether for the flexion space. If the PCL is resected, only the posterior capsule balances the flexion space. The posterior capsule is subject to late attenuation. Retaining the tether of the PCL eases balance of the flexion space and prevents attenuation of the posterior capsule and subsequent late instability or peg wear.

The broad, long medial collateral ligament running from the femur to the tibia tethers the medial side of the knee. In contrast, the lateral side of the knee is restrained by the less robust, round lateral collateral ligament running from the femur to the fibula. The PCL helps balance these disparate structures, serving as a checkrein to the lateral aspect of the medial compartment of the knee.

Bone Sparing

We submit that PCL retention is bone sparing, which eases management of the femur in the revision setting. Retaining the PCL allows one to retain the intercondylar bone. If the PCL is resected, the flexion gap increases. The surgeon must resect a commensurate increase in distal femur to balance this increased flexion gap. Thus, the amount of distal femur that must be resected in a PCL-retaining TKR is less than in a substituting design.

Patellar Clunk and Post Dislocation

The PCL provides anterior and posterior stability in cruciate-retaining designs. In contrast, a post-and-cam mechanism affords stability in this plane in cruciate-substituting TKR. This post may dislocate in the improperly balanced knee (66,67).

The complication of patellar clunk is also associated with cruciate-substituting designs of TKR (68). Although more recent designs limit these complications, the use of cruciate-retaining TKR avoids these problems altogether without adversely affecting patellar tracking. Recent reports of TKR with PCL retention have a very low rate of patellofemoral complications with a low incidence of lateral release (3,5,7,9,10,29).

Ease of Management of Supracondylar Femur Fractures

Fractures of the distal femur above a TKR are an uncommon but difficult-to-treat complication (69,70). With PCL-sparing TKR it is easier to manage a supracondylar femur fracture. Intramedullary nailing of these fractures is easy without the closed box present in cruciate-substituting designs. Recent innovations with supracondylar rods, however, have eased this problem.

Avoidance of Peg Wear and Fracture

Recent studies have shown peg wear can be a problem in poorly balanced cruciate-substituting knees (63,64). If the soft tissues are not balanced in flexion, the anterior translocation of the femur is stopped by the polyethylene eminence, leading to posterior peg wear. If the posterior capsule is not tightened, or if the tibial component is significantly sloped posteriorly, component hyperextension will occur, leading to anterior peg wear. Moreover, any rotational mismatch or increased rotation between the components due to soft tissue balance can lead to rotational peg wear and fracture. Any of these constraining forces will also lead to back-sided wear when metal-backed tibial components are used.

Assessing differences in back-sided wear between cruciate-retaining and cruciate-substituting designs is difficult. Very few studies address the issue of back-sided wear, and confounding variables make comparisons of different systems impossible. In Schai and colleague's follow-up at 10 years with the PFC cruciate-retaining design, however, no osteolysis was noted (28).

SURGICAL TECHNIQUE

Retaining the PCL does not pose a hindrance to operative exposure. A vertical midline incision is made, extending from the distal femur to just medial to the tibial tubercle, followed

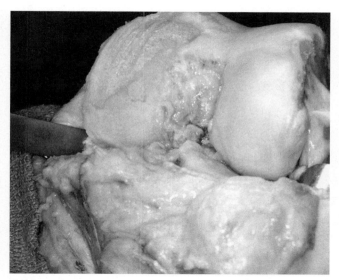

FIG. 6. An osteotome is passed beneath the medial collateral ligament and into the semimembranosus bursa for medial dissection.

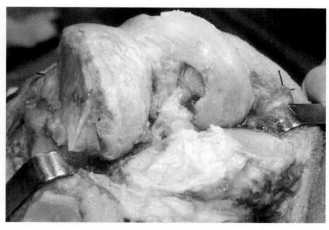

FIG. 7. Excellent exposure for bony cuts of the femoral and tibial surfaces with the posterior cruciate ligament intact is obtained after release of the patellofemoral ligaments, medial dissection, anterior cruciate ligament resection, and removal of remnant menisci.

by a median parapatellar incision in the capsule. Before flexing the knee and everting the patella, all fibers of the patellofemoral ligament are incised. With the knee flexed 90 degrees and the patella everted, the ACL and anterior horns of the menisci are resected. Next, a medial subperiosteal dissection of the soft tissues of the proximal tibia using sharp dissection or a curved osteotome directed beneath the ligament at the joint line into the semimembranosus bursa is undertaken (Fig. 6). The medial dissection is tailored to the degree and type of deformity. A larger, more extensive dissection is performed for varus deformity, with minimal dissection performed for valgus deformity. This medial dissection combined with resection of any ACL remnant allows the proximal tibia to be externally rotated and dislocated anterior to the femur, aiding exposure and relaxation of the patellar tendon. Next, the posterior horns of the menisci are removed, and a PCL retractor facilitates displacing the tibia anteriorly. This sequence provides excellent exposure for the bony cuts whether the tibia or femur is initially prepared (Fig. 7).

With PCL-retaining designs, it is not important whether the tibia or femur is cut first as long as measured resection with restoration of the native joint line is performed. For the tibial cut, a central reference point of the proximal tibia is marked at the junction of the medial one-third and lateral two-thirds of the patellar tendon for rotational alignment. Although optional, a triangular or square bony block is outlined with an osteotome anterior to the PCL to protect the ligament during tibial resection. The PCL inserts distally on the tibia so that proximal tibial resection is possible without injuring the ligament. The proximal cut is made to retain as much proximal tibia as possible, cutting to a depth equal to the anticipated thickness of the prosthetic tibial component with a few degrees of posterior slope in the sagittal plane. The largest tibial component without overhang is used.

An intramedullary guide is used for the femoral bony cut, typically in 5 to 7 degrees of valgus. Valgus knees are cut in no more than 5 degrees of femoral valgus. Care is taken to ensure

the anterior femoral cortex is not notched. Cuts are again based on anatomic considerations, with every attempt made to restore the joint line. The distal cut falls just distal to the PCL insertion on the lateral aspect of the medial femoral condyle. In the varus knee the distal cut will leave an intact bridge between the medial and lateral condylar resections. In contrast, the distal cut in the valgus knee usually leaves independent medial and lateral condylar resections due to the deficient lateral femoral condyle. Rotational alignment of the femoral component is based on a combination of the epicondylar axis, anteroposterior axis (Whitesides line), the posterior femoral condyles, and our previous tibial cut (71,72). Great care must be taken in the valgus knee, as referencing off of the deficient posterolateral femoral condyle will cause a relative internal rotation of the femoral component, adversely affecting patellar tracking.

Patellar thickness is assessed and the patella resurfaced with a thickness of polyethylene equivalent to the amount of bone

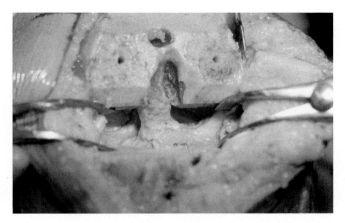

FIG. 8. Before trial reduction, laminar spreaders can be used to tension the medial and lateral soft tissues to assess balance in both flexion and extension.

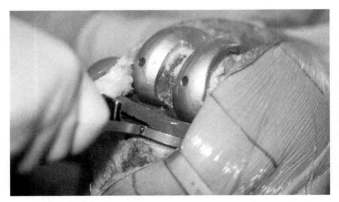

FIG 9. Pull-out/lift-off test. In 90 degrees of flexion, the surgeon should not be able to pull out the tibial tray and there should be no lift-off of the anterior tibial tray.

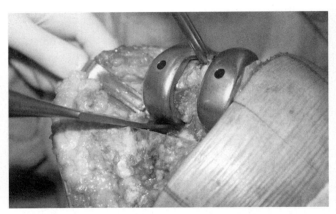

FIG. 11. Excision of posterior condylar osteophytes using a curved osteotome.

resected. A patellar cutting guide or freehand technique may be used for this cut. The patellar cut should pass through the chondral-osseous junction both medially and laterally with complete resection of the medial and lateral facets. Proximally the cut passes just superficial to the quadriceps insertion and distally passes through the nose of the patella. No remnant cartilage should remain after adequate patellar resection.

With the trial components in place, a trial reduction is performed (Fig. 8). The collateral ligaments should balance on both the medial and lateral sides through a full range of motion. Medial tightness is relieved by further subperiosteal dissection of the superficial medial collateral ligament when necessary. The iliotibial band is initially released with the knee in full extension in a pie crust fashion for lateral tightness. Although rarely necessary, further lateral release is achieved by subperiosteal dissection of the lateral structures off of the epicondyle.

In many knees, the PCL will need to be recessed to accommodate a more conforming tibial polyethylene insert to increase contact area. Alternatively, some systems provide less conforming inserts suitable for low-demand patients, obviating the need for PCL recession. An initial release is achieved by peeling the PCL attachment off of the retained tibial spine or removing the tibial spine at the level of the tibial cut. After this initial release, PCL tension is checked with the knee flexed 90 degrees. In this position, the

femoral component should articulate with the middle one-third of the polyethylene on the medial side of the knee. If the PCL is too tight and excessive rollback occurs, the posterior lip of the tibial insert riding on the posterior femoral condyle will cause the anterior aspect of the tibial tray to lift off the tibia as the knee is flexed

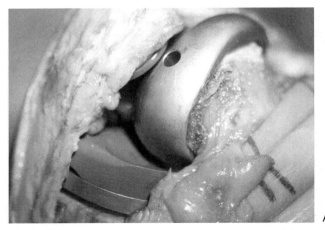

A

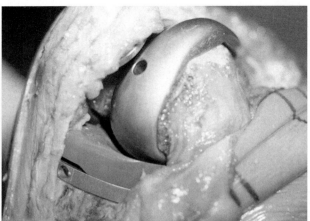

B

FIG. 12. A: Excessive femoral rollback and lift-off of the anterior tibial tray occur if the posterior cruciate ligament is too tight. B: After posterior cruciate ligament recession and removal of osteophytes, there is normal rollback and no anterior lift-off.

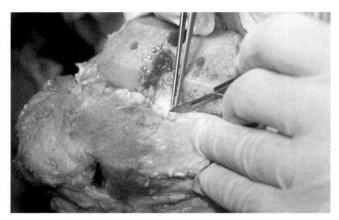

FIG. 10. An excessively tight posterior cruciate ligament is released from the posterior tibia.

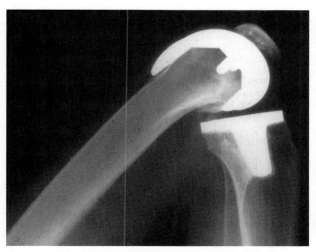

FIG. 13. This radiograph of a cruciate-retaining total knee replacement after posterior cruciate ligament recession demonstrates flexion.

(73). To ensure that the PCL and flexion gap are tight enough, the surgeon should not be able to pull out the tibial tray with its handle in place at 90 degrees of flexion (Fig. 9) (74). The surgeon can also palpate the PCL with the components in place and the ligament should be compressible but not excessively taught and rigid.

If the PCL remains tight after the initial release, the ligament can be further released from the posterior aspect of the tibia (Fig. 10) (1,44). Alternatively, the ligament may be released from the distal femoral attachment to selectively release tight bundles (usually the lateral bundle) (18). If lift-off continues in spite of these releases and the ligament is not too tight to palpation, impingement may occur between the posterior lip of the polyethylene insert and retained posterior femoral osteophytes (Fig. 11). These osteophytes should be excised (Fig. 12).

Patellar tracking is observed without the medial capsule sutured or clamped. As the knee flexes, the patella should remain within the trochlea without manual stabilization—"no touch technique" (18). Good contact between the medial facet of the patella and medial femoral condyle should be maintained as the knee is flexed. If the patella dislocates, subluxates, or tilts laterally, a lateral release should be performed. This release is performed with the knee extended with slight valgus stress. The synovium and lateral retinaculum are incised in a longitudinal fashion from the joint line extending superiorly proximal to the patella. The lateral superior genicular vessels are identified at the inferior margin of the vastus lateralis and protected during the release.

After assessment of medial/lateral balance, PCL tension, and patellar tracking, all bony surfaces are irrigated with pulsatile lavage and dried. Cementing is performed in the sequence of tibia followed by the femur. The knee is then extended, with the final polyethylene insert in place. With the knee in extension for compression on the tibial and femoral components, the patellar component is cemented in place. The senior author inserts the real polyethylene at the time of cementing. With a lipped insert and proper tensioning in flexion, insertion of the real polyethylene component after cementing of the tibial tray and femoral component would not be possible. A careful inspection for loose cement and debris is undertaken and the tourniquet released. After careful hemostasis and thorough irrigation, the knee is closed with the capsule, subcutaneous layers, and skin layers closed independently over Hemovac drains (Fig. 13).

CONCLUSION

The published results of PCL-retaining and PCL-substituting TKR are identical. During the 1980s, PCL-retaining designs kept poor company with flat-on-flat tibial articulations, metal-backed patellae, indiscriminate uncemented fixation, and heat-pressed polyethylene (28,47,58,75). These factors, combined with techniques that stressed bone cuts while ignoring important soft tissues, led to the misconception that PCL substitution was superior to PCL retention. Current techniques with proper soft tissue balancing, PCL recession as necessary, and use of a curved polyethylene insert yield excellent long-term clinical results.

REFERENCES

1. Barnes CL, Sledge CB. Total knee arthroplasty with posterior cruciate ligament retention designs. In: Insall JN, Windsor RE, Scott WN, eds. *Surgery of the knee*, 2nd ed. New York: Churchill Livingstone, 1993:815–827.
2. Freeman MAR, Railton GT. Should the posterior cruciate ligament be retained or resected in condylar nonmeniscal knee arthroplasty: the case for resection. *J Arthroplasty* 1988;3:83.
3. Berger RA, Rosenberg AG, Barden RM, et al. Long-term followup of the Miller-Galante total knee replacement. *Clin Orthop* 2001;388:58–67.
4. Buechel FF Sr, Buechel FF Jr, Pappas MJ. Twenty year evaluation of meniscal bearing and rotating platform knee replacements. *Clin Orthop* 2001;388:41–50.
5. Gill GS, Joshi AB. Long-term results of Kinematic Condylar knee replacement. *J Bone Joint Surg Br* 2001;83:355–358.
6. Laskin RS. The Genesis total knee prosthesis: a ten year followup study. *Clin Orthop* 2001;388:95–102.
7. Parker DA, Rorabeck CH, Bourne RB. Long-term followup of cementless versus hybrid fixation for total knee arthroplasty. *Clin Orthop* 2001;388:68–76.
8. Pavone V, Boettner F, Fickert S, et al. Total condylar knee arthroplasty: a long term followup. *Clin Orthop* 2001;388:18–25.
9. Ritter MA, Berend ME, Meding JB, et al. Long term followup of anatomic graduated components posterior cruciate-retaining total knee replacement. *Clin Orthop* 2001;388:51–57.
10. Sextro GS, Berry DJ, Rand JA. Total knee arthroplasty using cruciate retaining kinematic condylar prosthesis. *Clin Orthop* 2001;388:33–40.
11. Grigis FG, Marshall JL, Monajem ARS. The cruciate ligaments of the knee. *Clin Orthop* 1975;106:216–231.
12. Williams PL, Warwick R, eds. *Gray's anatomy*, 36th ed. Philadelphia: WB Saunders, 1980.
13. Gollehan DL, Torzilli PA, Warren RF. The role of the posterolateral and cruciate ligaments in the stability of the knee: a biomechanical study. *J Bone Joint Surg Am* 1987;69:233–242.
14. Andriacchi TP, Galante JO. Retention of the posterior cruciate in total knee arthroplasty. *J Arthroplasty* 1988;3(Suppl):S13–S19.
15. Ewald FC, Scott RD, Thomas WH, et al. The importance of intercondylar stability in knee arthroplasty: comparison of McKeever, modular and duo-condylar types. *J Bone Joint Surg Am* 1975;57:1033.
16. Gunston FH, MacKenzie RJ. Complications of polycentric knee arthroplasty. *Clin Orthop* 1976;120:11.
17. Ilstrup DM, Coventry MB, Skolnick MD. A statistical evaluation of geometric total knee arthroplasties. *Clin Orthop* 1976;120:27.
18. Scott RD, Volatile TB. Twelve years' experience with posterior cruciate retaining total knee arthroplasty. *Clin Orthop* 1986;205:100–107.
19. Ranawat CS, Insall J, Shine J. Duocondylar knee arthroplasty: hospital for special surgery design. *Clin Orthop* 1976;120:76.
20. Ranawat CS, Flynn WF, Saddler S, et al. Long-term results of the total condylar knee arthroplasty: a 15 year survivorship study. *Clin Orthop* 1993;286:94–102.
21. Vince KG, Insall JN, Kelly MA. The total condylar prosthesis: 10-

to 12-year results of a cemented knee replacement. *J Bone Joint Surg Br* 1989;71:793–797.

22. Colizza WA, Insall JN, Scuderi GR. The posterior stabilized total knee prosthesis: assessment of polyethylene damage and osteolysis after a ten year-minimum follow-up. *J Bone Joint Surg Am* 1995;77: 1713–1720.
23. Sledge CB, et al. Two-year follow-up of the Duocondylar total knee replacement. *Orthop Trans* 1978;2:193.
24. Thomas WH. Duopatellar total knee arthroplasty. *Orthop Trans* 1980;4:329.
25. Scott RD. Duopatellar total knee replacement: the Brigham experience. *Orthop Clin North Am* 1982;13:89–102.
26. Ewald FC, Jacobs MA, Miegel RE, et al. Kinematic total knee replacement. *J Bone Joint Surg Am* 1984;66:1032–1040.
27. Dennis DA, Clayton ML, O'Donnel S, et al. Posterior cruciate condylar total knee arthroplasty. *Clin Orthop* 1992;281:168–176.
28. Schai PA, Thornhill TS, Scott RD. Total knee arthroplasty with the PFC system. *J Bone Joint Surg Br* 1998;80:850–858.
29. Buehler KO, Venn-Watson E, D'Lima DD, et al. The press-fit condylar total knee system: 8- to 10-year results with posterior cruciate retaining design. *J Arthroplasty* 2000;15:698–701.
30. Banks SA, Markovich GD, Hodge WA. In vivo kinematics of cruciate retaining and substituting knee arthroplasties. *J Arthroplasty* 1997;12:297–304.
31. Dennis DA, Komistek RD, Colwell CE, et al. In vivo anteroposterior femorotibial translation of total knee arthroplasty: a multicenter analysis. *Clin Orthop* 1998;356:47–57.
32. Stiehl JB, Komistek RD, Dennis DA, et al. Fluoroscopic analysis of kinematics after posterior cruciate-retaining knee arthroplasty *J Bone Joint Surg Br* 1995;77:884–889.
33. Incavo SJ, Johnson CC, Beynnon BD, et al. Posterior cruciate ligament strain biomechanics in total knee arthroplasty. *Clin Orthop* 1994;309:88–93.
34. Becker MW, Insall JN, Faris PM. Bilateral total knee arthroplasty. *Clin Orthop* 1991;271:122–124.
35. Dorr LD, Ochsner JL, Gronley J. Functional comparison of posterior cruciate-retained versus cruciate-sacrificed total knee arthroplasty. *Clin Orthop* 1988;236:36–43.
36. Hirsch HS, Lotke PA, Morrison LD. The posterior cruciate ligament in total knee surgery. *Clin Orthop* 1994;309:64–68.
37. Pereira DS, Jaffe FF, Ortiguera C. Posterior cruciate ligament sparing versus posterior cruciate ligament sacrificing arthroplasty. *J Arthroplasty* 1998;13:138–144.
38. Udomkiat P, Meng B, Dorr LD, et al. Functional comparison of posterior cruciate retention and substitution knee replacement. *Clin Orthop* 2000;378:192–201.
39. Schoji H, Wolf A, Packard S, et al. Cruciate retained and excised total knee arthroplasty. *Clin Orthop* 1994;305:218–222.
40. Wilson SA, McCann PD, Gotlin RS, et al. Comprehensive gait analysis in posterior-stabilized knee arthroplasty. *J Arthroplasty* 1996;11:359–367.
41. Arima J, Whiteside LA, Martin JW, et al. Effect of partial release of the posterior cruciate ligament in total knee arthroplasty. *Clin Orthop* 1998;353:194–202.
42. Ritter MA, Faris PM, Keating EM. Posterior cruciate ligament balancing during total knee arthroplasty. *J Arthroplasty* 1988;3:323–326.
43. Scott RD, Thornhill TS. Posterior cruciate supplementing total knee replacement using conforming inserts and cruciate recession. *Clin Orthop* 1994;309:146–149.
44. Worland RL, Jessup DE, Johnson J. Posterior cruciate recession in total knee arthroplasty. *J Arthroplasty* 1997;12:70–73.
45. Landy MM, Walker PS. Wear of ultrahigh molecular weight polyethylene in cruciate ligament-retaining total knee arthroplasty: a case study. *J Arthroplasty* 1993;8:439–446.
46. Stiehl JB, Komistek RD, Dennis DA. Detrimental kinematics of a flat on flat total condylar knee arthroplasty. *Clin Orthop* 1999;365:139–148.
47. Swany MR, Scott RD. Posterior polyethylene wear in posterior cruciate ligament retaining total knee arthroplasty. *J Arthroplasty* 1993;8:439–446.
48. Blunn GW, Walker PS, Joshi A, et al. The dominance of cyclic sliding in producing wear in total knee replacements. *Clin Orthop* 1991;273:254–260.
49. Wright TM, Rimnac CM, Stulberg SD, et al. Wear of polyethylene in total joint replacement: observations from retrieved PCA knee implants. *Clin Orthop* 1992;276:126–134.
50. Ritter MA, Herbst SA, Keating EM, et al. Long term survival analysis of a posterior cruciate retaining total condylar total knee arthroplasty. *Clin Orthop* 1994;309:136–145.
51. Malkani AL, Rand JA, Bryan RS, et al. Total knee arthroplasty with the kinematic condylar prosthesis: a ten-year follow-up study. *J Bone Joint Surg Am* 1995;77:423–431.
52. Rand JA, Ilstrup DM. Survivorship analysis of total knee arthroplasty: cumulative rates of survival of 9200 total knee arthroplasties. *J Bone Joint Surg Am* 1991;73:397–409.
53. Kleinbert FA, Bryk E, Evangelista J, et al. Histologic comparison of posterior cruciate ligaments from arthritic and age-matched knee specimens. *J Arthroplasty* 1996;11:726–731.
54. Koralewicz LM, Engh GA. Comparison of proprioception in arthritic and age-matched normal knees. *J Bone Joint Surg Am* 2000;82:1582–1588.
55. Simmons S, Lephart S, Rubash HE, et al. Proprioception following total knee arthroplasty with and without the posterior cruciate ligament. *J Arthroplasty* 1996;11:763–768.
56. Warren PJ, Olanlokun TK, Cobb AG, et al. Proprioception after knee arthroplasty: the influence of prosthetic design. *Clin Orthop* 1993;297:182–187.
57. Dejour D, Deschamps G, Garotta L, et al. Laxity in posterior cruciate sparing and posterior stabilized total knee prostheses. *Clin Orthop* 1999;364:182–193.
58. Laskin RS, O'Flynn HM. Total knee replacement with posterior cruciate ligament retention in rheumatoid arthritis. *Clin Orthop* 1997;345:24–28.
59. Matsuda S, Miura H, Nagamine R, et al. Knee stability in posterior cruciate ligament retaining total knee arthroplasty. *Clin Orthop* 1999;366:169–173.
60. Pagnano MW, Hanssen AD, Lewallen DG, et al. Flexion instability after primary posterior cruciate retaining total knee arthroplasty. *Clin Orthop* 1998;356:39–46.
61. Gill GS, Joshi AB. Long term results of retention of the posterior cruciate ligament in total knee replacements in rheumatoid arthritis. *J Bone Joint Surg Br* 2001;83:510–512.
62. Schai PA, Scott RD, Thornhill TS. Total knee arthroplasty with posterior cruciate retention in patients with rheumatoid arthritis. *Clin Orthop* 1999;367:96–106.
63. Mikulak SA, Mahoney OM, dela Rosa MA. Loosening and osteolysis with press fit condylar posterior cruciate substituting total knee replacement. *J Bone Joint Surg Am* 2001;83:398–403.
64. Puloski SK, McCalden RW, MacDonald SJ. Tibial post wear in posterior stabilized total knee arthroplasty. An unrecognized source of polyethylene debris. *J Bone Joint Surg Am* 2001;83:390–397.
65. Laskin RS. Total knee replacement with posterior cruciate ligament retention in patients with a fixed varus deformity. *Clin Orthop* 1996;331:29–34.
66. Lombardi AV, Mallory TH, Vaughn BK, et al. Dislocation following primary posterior stabilized total knee arthroplasty. *J Arthroplasty* 1993;8:633–639.
67. Sharkey PF, Hozack WJ, Booth RE, et al. Posterior dislocation of total knee arthroplasty. *Clin Orthop* 1992;278:128–133.
68. Beight JL, Yao B, Hozack WJ. The patellar "clunk" syndrome after posterior stabilized total knee arthroplasty. *Clin Orthop* 1994;299:139–142.
69. Aaron RK, Scott RD. Supracondylar fracture of the femur after total knee arthroplasty. *Clin Orthop* 1987;219:136–139
70. Healy WL, Siliski JM, Incavo SJ. Operative treatment of distal femoral fractures proximal to total knee replacements. *J Bone Joint Surg Am* 1993;75:27–34.
71. Berger RA, Rubash HE, Seel MJ, et al. Determining the rotational alignment of the femoral component in total knee arthroplasty using the epicondylar axis. *Clin Orthop* 1993;286:40–47.
72. Whiteside LA, Arima J. The anteroposterior axis for femoral rotational alignment in valgus total knee arthroplasty. *Clin Orthop* 1995;321:168–172.
73. Chmell MJ, Scott RD. Balancing the posterior cruciate ligament during cruciate-retaining total knee arthroplasty: description of the P.O.L.O. test. *J Orthop Tech* 1996;4:12–15.
74. Scott RD. Ligament releases. *Orthopedics* 1994;17:883–885.
75. Bartel DL, Burstein AH, Toda MD, et al. The effect of conformity and plastic thickness on contact stresses in metal-backed plastic implants. *J Biomech Eng* 1985;107:193.

CHAPTER 78

Posterior Stabilization in Total Knee Arthroplasty

Kelly G. Vince, Michel Malo, and Peter J. Thadani

PERSONAL STATEMENT

There is a strong bias in this chapter favoring cruciate-substituting or "posterior stabilized" designs. This bias originated with the influence of John Insall, who trained the senior author. These ideas have been passed on to younger colleagues who collaborated on the chapter. Although we acknowledge some excellent results that have been reported with cruciate-retaining devices (1), there have also been significant failures (2).

It is our belief that the posterior cruciate ligament (PCL) is abnormal in most arthritic knees (3), that it functions poorly in the absence of the anterior cruciate ligament (ACL), and that it is difficult to balance. We believe that femoral rollback so long promised with PCL retention does not occur. Over many hundreds of cases, irrespective of deformity, we believe that acknowledging the inherent mechanical quality of knee arthroplasty surgery, and so using a mechanical device (70,71), will yield more reproducibly good and durable clinical results for our patients.

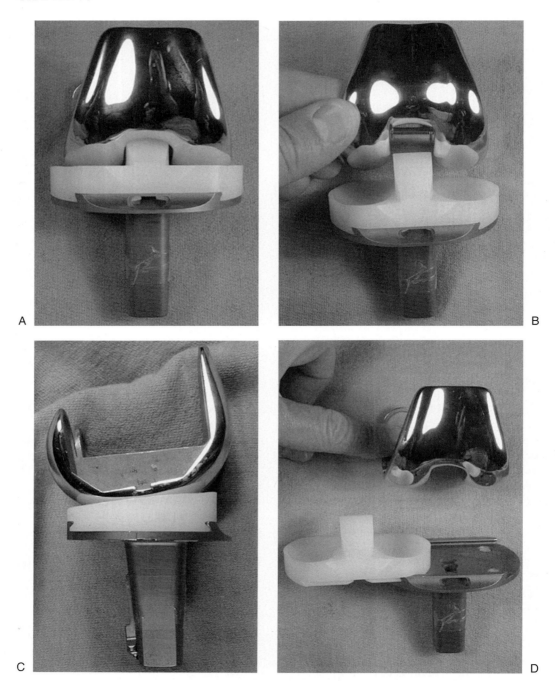

FIG. 1. The Insall-Burstein II posterior stabilized knee prosthesis. **A:** Frontal view in extension. Note that hyperextension would bring the anterior edge of the femoral trochlea against the anterior aspect of the tibial spine. **B:** Frontal view showing the spine-and-cam mechanism. The femoral components are symmetric, neither right- nor left-sided. **C:** Lateral view. Note that posterior tibial slope has been built into the component. **D:** The final version of the Insall-Burstein II prosthesis was modular and introduced in 1998. The locking mechanism required full medial exposure of the knee to slide the polyethylene tray in from the side.

The potential of the posterior stabilized concept has been neither fully understood nor completely exhausted. Mechanical stabilization will probably enable patients to flex their knees maximally and so kneel and squat. Similarly, some unanticipated cases of wear and osteolysis have emerged with posterior stabilized implants that are probably related to materials more than design.

INTRODUCTION

Knee arthroplasty design and surgical technique evolved slowly from the 1950s and 1960s, when two radically different approaches prevailed: hinges and interpositional arthroplasties. The early condylar-type resurfacing arthroplasties (polycentric and Geomedic) were implanted without regard for either cruciate ligament, but eventually there arose a controversy over the importance of the ACL and PCL (70).

With the exception of the Townley (4,5) and Cloutier (6) knee prostheses, virtually all knee arthroplasties required the removal of the ACL. It was difficult to accommodate both ligaments and still have room for a sufficiently large and strong implant. In addition, maintaining both ligaments and performing an arthroplasty was technically challenging and often led to poor motion. Eventually, the cruciate debate focused on what to do with the PCL (7). Surgeons at the Robert B. Brigham Hospital, in Boston, championed the preservation of the PCL. Surgeons and engineers from the Hospital for Special Surgery (HSS), in New York, disagreed, having been influenced by Michael Freeman from the Imperial College London Hospital (United Kingdom), who argued that the PCL often contributed to deformity and should be excised to correct deformity (8). The first successful knee prosthesis to provide mechanical posterior stabilization was the Insall-Burstein posterior stabilized (IBPS) implant. The 1978 version was available with an all-polyethylene tibial component. There followed two major versions: a nonmodular, metal-backed tibia and then a modular metal-backed implant (Fig. 1) (9). This chapter focuses on the IBPS designs but acknowledges innovations that have bee introduced with the NexGen knee system. In addition, other surgeons have developed versions of posterior stabilized implants that are described here when there is research literature that helps us learn from the experience of the design.

The debate over the PCL has evolved but not disappeared over three decades. This evolution has paralleled general improvements in our understanding of knee replacement surgery and implant design implants. Careful study of the details of long-term clinical results may clarify just how the posterior stabilized mechanism contributes to knee replacement function and durability.

DESIGN CONCEPT—WHAT IS A POSTERIOR STABILIZED KNEE PROSTHESIS?

Before the Posterior Stabilized Prosthesis— Cruciate Sacrificing

Before posterior stabilization there were "cruciate-sacrificing" implants. These condylar knee replacements (not hinged devices) included the Imperial College London Hospital implant (8,10) and the immediate predecessor to the IBPS at the HSS, the Total Condylar (11). The surgical technique included removal of the ACL and PCL. Stability depended on conformity of the tibial-femoral articular geometry in conjunction with the collateral ligaments by a mechanism that was referred to as the "uphill principle" (12). The uphill principle describes stability that results from tightening of the collateral ligaments as the femoral component tries to ride up and out of the conforming tibial "well." With greater excursion of the femur, the collateral ligaments tighten and stabilize the joint (Fig. 2). This, introduced with the Total Condylar prosthesis (1973) (13), is attributed to the engineer Peter Walker and depended heavily on equal tension in the flexion and extension gaps to ensure stability. The femoral component was intended to stay generally in the center of the tibial well, regardless of knee flexion. Femoral rollback was not intended; in fact, it was inhibited by the design.

Increased conformity has emerged recently (but not been widely acknowledged) as a common stabilizing mechanism in many cruciate-retaining arthroplasties. As flat tibial surfaces accelerated polyethylene wear, greater conformity was reintroduced to the tibial-femoral articulation. Inevitably, the old problem of "kinematic conflict" reappeared, whereby preservation of the PCL with a more conforming articulation sometimes led to tightness and pain (Fig. 3) (14).

The solution to kinematic conflict became to recess the cruciate ligament when undue tension was present in the arthroplasty (15). Clinical evaluations such as the pull-out/lift-off test have been described to guide surgeons as to when the ligament should be recessed. Arima and others concluded from a cadaver study that partial release could improve knee flexion but that complete release caused unfavorable anteroposterior laxity in their prosthesis (16). To what extent the release of the PCL from either its femoral or tibial attachment represents defunctionalizing of the ligament or effective cruciate sacrifice has not been elaborated. Many cruciate-retaining designs, with greater articular conformity and a released posterior cruciate ligament, have become much like the old total condylar.

Insall-Burstein Posterior Stabilized Knee Prosthesis

The first posterior stabilized knee prosthesis was the IBPS arthroplasty, developed in 1978 at the HSS. It was conceived as a way to remove the PCL and (a) correct deformity, (b) reproduce femoral rollback, (c) ensure stability in flexion, and (d) facilitate flexion. It should be understood that the significant clinical success of the IBPS prosthesis was not exclusively the result of posterior stabilization. The implant was developed by experienced individuals who had extraordinary surgical and engineering expertise for the era. Many features to the design, in addition to the spine-and-cam mechanism, contributed to its success. In other words, one could not expect to improve an existing knee arthroplasty design by simply adding a spine-and-cam mechanism. In addition, not all spine-and-cam mechanisms are the same. Some are significantly inferior to the IBPS, and others have been designed as improvements to the original.

The first attempts at posterior stabilization did not succeed. Several decades ago, surgeons excised the PCL to correct deformity. This was generally a sound approach but some cases were complicated by instability with the simple Total Condylar prosthesis. The short-lived Total Condylar II was an attempt at mechanical stabilization, and it probably failed as a result of a hyperextension stop (69). John Insall and Al Burstein eventually developed a spine-and-cam mechanism that prevented posterior tibial dislocation and reproduced femoral rollback. The tibial spine was sloped posteriorly to avoid impingement on the anterior femoral component.

The phenomenon of rollback translates the extensor mechanism anteriorly and so increases extensor mechanism power. It also helps the posterior tibia from impinging against the posterior femur. Despite the advantages of mechanical rollback, normal human rollback is more complex: It involves rotation of the tibia and the femur with more rollback on the lateral side (Fig. 4).

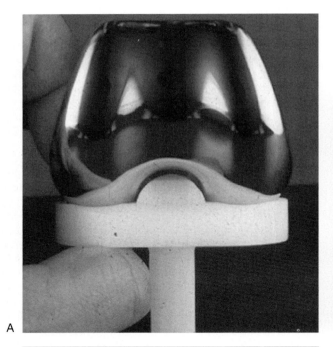

A

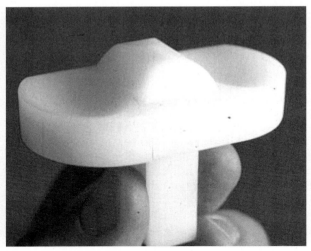

B

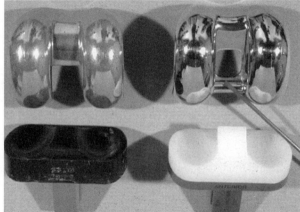

C

FIG. 2. A: Front view of the total condylar knee prosthesis. This was the first cruciate-sacrificing design from the Hospital for Special Surgery in New York. It was the immediate forerunner to the Insall-Burstein posterior stabilized prosthesis. Note the rounded femoral condyles and conforming articular polyethylene. This reduces edge loading. **B:** Total condylar tibial component. Note the conforming wells of the medial and lateral articular surface that provide the "uphill principle" of stability. There is no "posterior cutout" for the posterior cruciate ligament. **C:** The Insall-Burstein posterior stabilized prosthesis developed from the total condylar, with the addition of the spine-and-cam mechanism to prevent posterior tibial dislocation and also to enhance rollback. The total condylar prosthesis is seen on the left, with the black-colored, carbon-impregnated "poly II" (carbon fiber reinforced polyethylene).

Stability was at times difficult to achieve after correction of severe deformity that included excision of the PCL. The knee could be made stable in extension with thicker tibial inserts or with a hinge when collateral insufficiency was severe. Problems in flexion resulted when the flexion gap was much larger than the extension gap. This was particularly common after patellectomy, to the point where absence of the patella was regarded as a contraindication to cruciate-sacrificing designs such as the Total Condylar (11). The posterior stabilized was specifically designed to prevent posterior dislocation of the tibia while the knee was flexed because of this problem with the Total Condylar. Posterior tibial dislocations were not experienced with the first group of posterior stabilized implants, an improvement over the Total Condylar (17,18).

Posterior stabilization was also intended to increase flexion, as the arthroplasty could be left slightly more lax in flexion without fear of posterior dislocation. The average flexion initially reported for Total Condylar implants was approximately 90 degrees (19).

The improved flexion of approximately 115 degrees with the Insall-Burstein posterior stabilized I (IBPS I) prosthesis is largely attributed to the spine-and-cam mechanism (17). It should be noted, however, that the single most important factor predicting postarthroplasty flexion is preoperative flexion and that the pathology in the early Total Condylar implants was probably more severe with greater stiffness. In addition, as surgical technique undoubtedly improved with time, there may have been several factors to explain the improved flexion. Ranawat's experience with the Total Condylar averaged 99 degrees of flexion (20).

Finally, it should be understood that the IBPS prosthesis was never intended to be a "constrained implant" that relied on the implant for stability. None of the IBPS designs provided constraint to varus or valgus forces; this was a feature of constrained implants such as the total condylar 3 and constrained condylar implants. Stability to varus and valgus with an IBPS prosthesis means that medial and lateral collateral ligaments must be intact and balanced, that mechanical limb alignment must be restored to the range of neutral, and that the size of the flexion and extension gaps must be

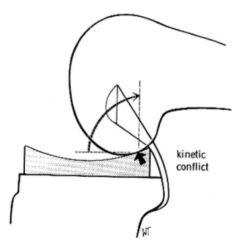

FIG. 3. Schematic lateral view of knee demonstrating how cruciate retention and conforming polyethylene lead to "conflict." The knee cannot roll back, and stiffness, wear, or loosening result. (From Insall JN, ed. *Surgery of the knee*. New York: Churchill Livingstone, 1984, with permission.)

equal. The IBPS prosthesis was never intended as nor did it function as a substitute for precise surgical technique (Fig. 5).

No Edge Loading in the Insall-Burstein Posterior Stabilized Prosthesis

The IBPS prosthesis, as stated previously, has always been more than just a spine-and-cam mechanism. When either the

Total Condylar or IBPS implants are viewed from the front, the conforming, rounded contour between the femur and the tibia is apparent (Fig. 6). This aspect of the design was originally intended to eliminate "edge loading," a deleterious situation that results from the inevitable varus or valgus forces that induce lift-off in one compartment and compression in the other. In this situation, a contoured articulation will maintain a larger area of surface contact and that contact will occur farther from the edge of the tibial bone. The converse will be true for flatter femoral components, where the edge of the component becomes a contact point and a fulcrum. The contact area is smaller and is located close to the edge of the tibia, where catastrophic wear and loosening will be initiated (21). The rounded contours of the IBPS components increase contact areas and therefore diminish point loading and wear.

How Does a Posterior Stabilized Prosthesis Work? The Spine-and-Cam Mechanism

Purists believe that the only true posterior stabilized implants are those with spine-and-cam mechanisms; ultrapurists contend that only those that evolved from the original Insall-Burstein concept should be called "posterior stabilized." Some implants currently available are promoted as posterior stabilized when in fact they feature only a higher anterior lip that prevents the tibia from dislocating behind the femoral condyle. This will enhance stability but not provide rollback.

The IBPS prosthesis was developed in an era where hard lessons had been learned from hinged arthroplasties in terms of high loosening rates, frequent breakage, and difficult, if not impossible revision surgery. Accordingly, the spine-and-cam mechanism was designed to engage only after approximately

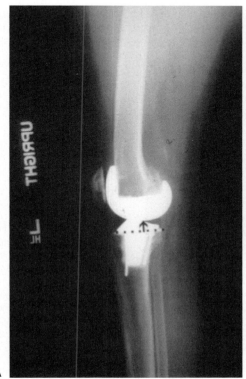

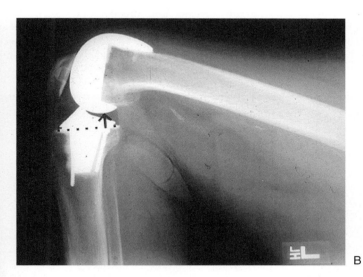

FIG. 4. A: Insall-Burstein I posterior stabilized knee prosthesis in extension. Note contact point of femur on tibia (*arrow*). **B:** As the knee flexes, the contact point moves posteriorly. This motion is ensured by the spine-and-cam mechanism. The more complex rotational feature of this "rollback" is not accommodated with this spine-and-cam mechanism.

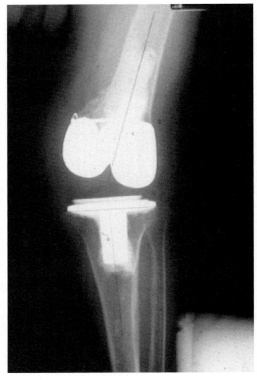

FIG. 5. Unstable Insall-Burstein posterior stabilized knee prosthesis. This prosthesis requires intact and balanced collateral ligaments to function. In this patient without a reliable medial collateral ligament, the Insall-Burstein II posterior stabilized knee arthroplasty is unstable. A constrained implant will be required.

70 degrees of flexion; from full extension until this point the arthroplasty functioned according to the uphill principle of increased conformity between the tibia and the femur. The femoral cam of the IBPS initially engages the lowest part of the tibia spine. As flexion proceeds, the femoral cam climbs up the tibial spine. This was not considered a limitation in an era when the maximum anticipated flexion was approximately 120 degrees (Fig. 7).

Other stabilized knee prostheses developed as the role of posterior stabilization evolved after 1978. Many surgeons, following Insall's lead, adopted the implant for virtually all primary knee replacements. Others resorted to posterior stabilization only in difficult situations, where there was either an increased risk of instability or when extensive releases were required to correct deformity. Laskin recommended the IBPS replacement, specifically in cases of significant deformity or stiffness (22). As individual knee prostheses were incorporated into "knee replacement systems," it became necessary for each manufacturer to provide "posterior stabilized" capability in their system. A variety of mechanisms were introduced, some as innovation and some to circumvent patents, such as the one that covered the original Insall-Burstein design.

Advantages of Posterior Stabilization

Issue of Femoral Rollback

Knee replacement surgery is a relatively crude mechanical reconstruction of a complex biologic joint. In general, attempts to reconstitute anatomy have been successful. At some point, however, the mechanical nature of the implant must be acknowledged. For example, the anatomy of the PCL is determined genetically as is the articular geometry. The relationship between the two then evolves in utero and through childhood and adolescence. It is deranged by arthritis and then completely disrupted by arthroplasty surgery. It is difficult to see how a surgeon can expect to implant a manufactured device composed of metal and plastic into the human knee and expect this geometry to function as precisely as the original anatomy. Joint line and femoral rollback are two examples of functional anatomy that

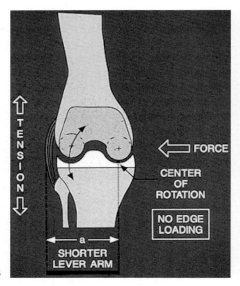
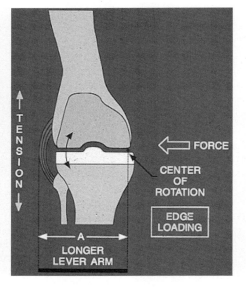

A,B

FIG. 6. A: Schematic diagram of knee prosthesis with rounded condyles when viewed from the front. The contact points between the femur and tibia are close to the midline and so avoid "edge loading." **B:** By contrast, femurs that are flat-on-flat tibial polyethylene in the presence of a varus or valgus load will edge load. This has been the cause of wear and loosening.

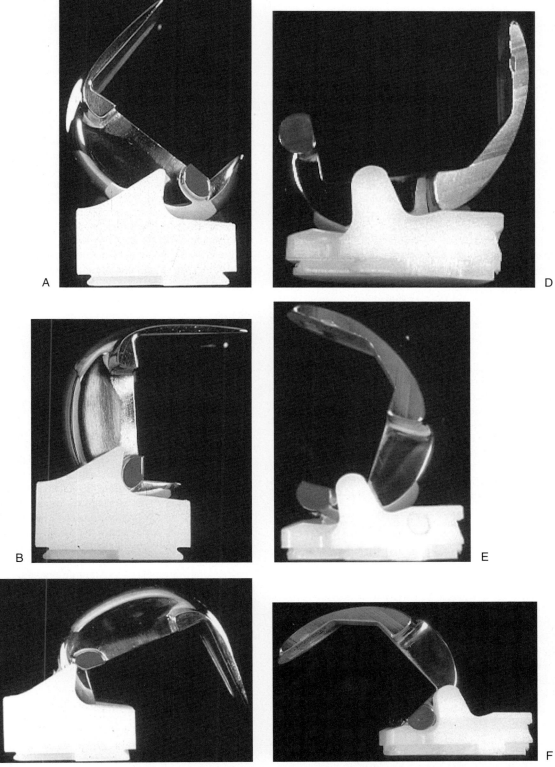

FIG. 7. Cross sections of Insall-Burstein prostheses. **A:** The spine and cam do not engage until 60 to 70 degrees of flexion. Until that point, the arthroplasty is completely nonconstrained. **B:** The femoral cam engages the tibial spine initially at a point low down on the spine. **C:** As maximal flexion is achieved, the cam rides up to the top of the tibial spine and risks dislocation. **D:** The spine and cam still do not engage before 60 to 70 degrees of flexion. **E:** The initial contact point is relatively high on the tibial spine. **F:** With deeper flexion, the cam rides down to a lower, more stable position on the tibial spine.

are difficult to reproduce. Posterior stabilized implants are less sensitive to alterations in joint line and more likely to reproduce femoral rollback.

Normal femoral rollback is a precise and still poorly understood aspect of knee function. The magnitude of rollback has been measured from magnetic resonance imaging scans in 10 normal subjects by Todo and associates in Osaka, Japan. They observed posterior rollback on the medial femoral condyle of 1.9 mm (± 0.8 mm) and 2.3 mm (± 0.5 mm) on the lateral side. The results may be different for the loaded or weightbearing knee, but there has been a consistent observation of asymmetric rollback, indicating internal rotation of the tibia under the flexing femoral condyle (23).

There is general agreement that the lateral femoral condyle rolls back farther than the medial, although the magnitude described by Todo et al. seems conservative. In another study from Japan, five healthy male volunteers had Kirschner wires implanted in their tibias. This method is accurate (if painful) and demonstrated internal external rotation from full extension to 60 degrees of flexion of 10.6 degrees (± 2.8 degrees) representing the screw home mechanism. These investigators also described rollback of 5.2 mm (± 1.7 mm) without specifying which compartment (24).

Until recently, surgeons argued about rollback and how best to achieve it without any means to measure if and to what extent it occurred. Stiehl et al. (25) applied a sophisticated computerized imaging technology to knee arthroplasty research. They evaluated the videofluoroscopy of 64 human knee arthroplasty subjects as they squatted and flexed the loaded knee. At full extension, the mean contact point of the normal and posterior stabilized implanted femurs was anterior to the tibial midpoint in the sagittal plane. In flexion, the posterior stabilized femur rolled back posteriorly, similar to normal knees. The posterior cruciate–retaining knees contacted the tibia posteriorly in extension and translated anteriorly in a substantial number of cases. This was the first direct demonstration of the unpredictability of femoral rollback with cruciate retention.

In a multicenter evaluation of 72 subjects whose surgeries had been performed by five clinicians, videofluoroscopy demonstrated that the lateral femoral condyle rolled back from full extension to 90 degrees of flexion in 100% of posterior cruciate–substituting designs. This desired rollback was observed in 51.6% of cruciate-retaining implants with posterior-lipped tibial inserts (these would be expected to limit rollback as a means to limit wear of the posterior polyethylene) and 58.3% of curved inserts. The degree of posterior femoral rollback for the specific implant design that had been studied was less than would be expected in healthy subjects with intact ligaments. There was frequent and abnormal anterior translation observed in posterior cruciate–retaining arthroplasties that these investigators believed might contribute to premature polyethylene wear (25a).

Conventional radiographic analysis of cruciate-retaining arthroplasties demonstrated no femoral rollback in one cruciate-retaining prosthesis studied by Kim and colleagues at Yale (26). They measured difference in the distances between the contact points of the knees in full extension and in 90 degrees of flexion (rollback distance) with an average posterior translation of –0.2 mm, ranging from –12.7 to +716 mm. This is essentially unpredictable motion, deleterious to polyethylene wear resistance and to the extensor mechanism.

Femoral rollback can be designed into a posterior stabilized implant. In this way engineers can determine and control where the femur will contact the tibia and at what degree of flexion. The articular polyethylene will be made thicker presumably in these areas. As mechanical as posterior stabilized rollback might seem, however, surgical technique can have an influence. Piazza and colleagues (27), working at Northwestern University, in Chicago, used a computer simulation to reveal that even small amounts of posterior tilt in the tibial component limited the interaction of the spine and cam. This study predicted contact of the spine and cam 18 degrees sooner during flexion when the IBPS component had been tilted only 5 degrees.

Finally, the concept of posterior stabilization allows engineers, if not surgeons, to control rollback in a way that will mimic more normal knee function. Walker and Sathasivam (28) developed a theoretical model for posterior stabilization with an intercondylar guide that would produce anterior-posterior motion that was more normal throughout knee flexion, remembering that the spine-and-cam mechanism of the IBPS engages only in later flexion.

Not only does mechanical substitution of PCL function result in greater and more predictable femoral rollback, this rollback has been shown to reduce loads on the patella femoral joint (29). This effect also helps identify which factors are most likely to explain the incidence of patellar fractures that used to be observed in the Insall-Burstein prosthesis.

More Mechanical, Less Sensitive to Anatomic Variation—The Joint Line

The posterior stabilized implant acknowledges the mechanical nature of arthroplasty surgery. The prosthesis is less sensitive to alterations in anatomy and in fact benefits from some of them. Emodi and colleagues (30) evaluated the effect of joint line elevation on knee arthroplasty function, recognizing that small changes of the joint line position significantly altered PCL strain and knee kinematics. When the joint line cannot be restored accurately (and there are little data to confirm just how much latitude there may be), these investigators strongly suggest a posterior cruciate–substituting implant.

In a cadaver study, Mahoney and associates (31) at Baylor College in Texas concluded that in the majority of cases, it is not possible to restore normal ligament loading with knee flexion while maintaining acceptable varus/valgus stability of the knee. After implanting cruciate-retaining knee prostheses in eight cadaveric knees and instrumenting the PCL with strain gauges, they discovered that normal PCL strain levels were produced in only 37% of joints. When a cruciate-retaining implant was used, femoral rollback decreased by 36% on average, and this was associated with a 15% loss of extensor efficiency. When the PCL was cut, rollback decreased by 70% and extensor efficiency by 19%. Cruciate substitution was better, but not perfect, in that rollback decreased by 12%, with an 11% decrease in extensor efficiency.

Cruciate Sacrifice—More Space for Polyethylene

When the PCL is removed, the joint opens slightly, on the order of a few millimeters. This enables the insertion of articular polyethylene that is thicker and more durable. Two studies con-

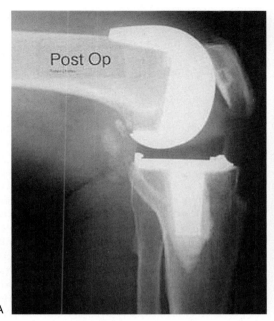
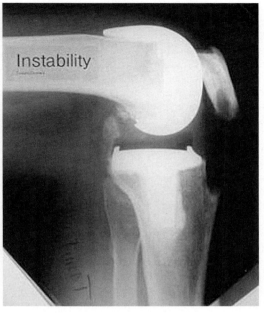

FIG. 8. A: Lateral radiograph of a "reduced" or normally articulating Insall-Burstein II posterior stabilized knee arthroplasty. Note the femoral rollback position, which has the advantage of pushing the tibial tubercle farther anteriorly, thus increasing the moment arm of the extensor mechanism. **B:** Lateral radiograph of a dislocated spine-and-cam mechanism, which means that the knee joint itself is subluxed. This patient cannot extend the knee, which is locked. The problem can be easily solved without surgery by hyperflexing the knee and then applying an anterior "drawer" maneuver to the proximal tibia.

firm that this effect is greater in flexion than it is in extension (32,33). Leaving the knee more lax in flexion is advantageous: Flexion will be easier. Proponents of cruciate retention condemn this approach, arguing that additional distal femoral bone may need to be resected to accommodate the thicker polyethylene that stabilizes the knee in flexion (33). This elevates the joint line. What they fail to recognize is that posterior stabilized arthroplasties are relatively insensitive to small alterations in the height of the joint line because it is the cruciate ligament function itself that suffers from joint line migration. In addition, once this effect is appreciated, instruments can be calibrated to position bone cuts and the component accordingly.

Greater Flexion?

To what extent is the posterior stabilized knee prosthesis capable of giving patients greater flexion when preoperative flexion has long been recognized as the most significant factor in determining postarthroplasty motion? Certainly, if a surgeon selects the most deformed knees for a posterior stabilized implant we might expect to see worse motion.

Some believe, however, that reproduction of femoral rollback as well as the ability to leave the knee more loose in flexion without fearing dislocation will lead to superior motion. Schurman and associates (34) at Stanford studied 13 preoperative and four postoperative variables on 164 Insall-Burstein posterior stabilized (IBPS II) prostheses. They concluded that preoperative flexion, flexion arc, tibiofemoral angle, extensor lag, diagnosis, and age were preoperative variables that led to better motion. Until pathology can be controlled the contention that the posterior stabilized mechanism can provide better flexion will remain controversial.

Paul Lotke, who originally trained at the HSS when Insall was on the faculty, published a report with Hirsch and Morrison concluding that preserving the PCL does not consistently lead to improved functional range of motion. They studied 242 consecutive primary total knee arthroplasties, in one of three groups. Group I had 77 Press-Fit Condylar knee replacements in which the PCL was completely released from its tibial attachment. Group II had 80 of the same prostheses with an intact PCL, and group III had 85 posterior cruciate–substituting IBPS II implants. The first two groups averaged 103 and 104 degrees of flexion, respectively, and the IBPS had 112 degrees ($p = .001$) (35).

Dennis and coworkers (35a) evaluated range of motion after total knee arthroplasty with their unique videofluoroscopy technique. They found that although passive nonweightbearing flexion was similar among cruciate-retaining and cruciate-substituting arthroplasties and although flexion decreased for all groups in the weightbearing situation, posterior stabilized arthroplasties demonstrated greater flexion than posterior cruciate–retaining arthroplasties in the weightbearing situation.

Drawbacks to the Insall-Burstein Posterior Stabilized Device Spine-and-Cam Mechanism—Dislocated Spine-and-Cam Mechanism

As increasingly deep flexion was experienced with knee replacements, there were cases of the tibial spine riding underneath the femoral cam with subluxation of the flexed knee and painful locking of the joint (Fig. 8) (36). This complication resulted from surgical technique, the basic IBPS spine-and-cam mechanism, and some apparently minor design modifications that were made in 1989 when the modular IBPS II prosthesis was introduced. Concurrent with the introduction of modularity to the IBPS I, there were new instruments and changes to the location and size of the spine. The original instruments included a "tenser device" so that soft tissues were balanced first and the limb was aligned as a product of ligamentous balance. If the soft tissue releases were inadequate (or excessive), the alignment was then off also. The newer Dunn-Bertin instruments were based on intramedullary guides that established the angle of bone resection as a product of what was necessary to achieve a neutral mechanical axis of the limb. Soft tissue releases were then performed to stabilize the joint, with the correct alignment ensured. However, the newer instruments did not require that flexion and extension gaps be formally balanced as they had been with the original instruments. If the flexion gap was somewhat more lax than the extension gap, as sometimes happened, the tibial polyethylene might be selected that allowed full stable extension with neither recurvatum nor flexion contracture. This meant laxity in flexion, which had the advantage of facilitating motion, with the risk of dislocation. Dislocation, it might be reasoned, would be prevented by the spine-and-cam mechanism.

However, the tibial spine had been moved 2 mm farther posteriorly by the engineers (ostensibly to increase rollback and flexion) at the same time that the height of the tibial spine was reduced by 2 mm (to decrease its bulk). The combination of new instruments, aggressive surgical technique to make the knee looser in flexion, and design modifications to increase femoral rollback and to reduce the tibial spine led to dislocations. The dislocations occurred clinically when the seated patient hyperflexed the knee and loaded it by trying to rise and had the tibia externally rotated with a foot around the chair leg. Although these dislocations could be reduced easily by hyperflexing the joint with some sedation, it was very difficult to replicate the dislocation in surgery at the time of polyethylene tibial component revision. Unusual loading of the joint in uncommon positions was necessary. Reengineering the tibial spine by restoring the height and anterior posterior position virtually eliminated this complication. The lesson with respect to arthroplasty design is simple: Sometimes very small changes, on the order of millimeters, can result in catastrophic complications. Not all spine-and-cam mechanisms are the same.

These design modifications were evaluated quantitatively by Delp and Kocmond (37) with a computer simulation. They compared the mechanism from the Insall-Burstein I with the original, problematic Insall-Burstein II mechanism, along with the revised Insall-Burstein II device. They found that the most stable position for the IBPS mechanism was in 70 degrees of flexion. The maximum flexion on the computer simulation for the device that in clinical practice suffered the most dislocations was 125 degrees, compared with 115 degrees for the original design and 117 for the revised implant.

Clinical investigation of the problem by Lombardi and colleagues in Columbus, Ohio (37a), identified a significantly higher incidence of posterior dislocation in the first version of the Insall-Burstein II than either the Insall-Burstein I or the later, modified Insall-Burstein II. Having considered 3,032 knee replacements, they found that the only variable that differed between control and study groups was the degree of flexion, with an average of 118 degrees in knees that dislocated and 105 degrees in those that did not. This is very consistent with our own experience. Hossain and colleagues (37b) reported three

dislocations in 1,500 modified IBPS II prostheses, demonstrating a 0.2% incidence of the complication despite the modifications made to the design. In this setting, the complication is invariably related to surgical technique.

Posterior dislocation of the posterior stabilized knee prosthesis does not usually jeopardize the limb. However, one case was reported from Hong Kong in which a compartment syndrome with muscle necrosis occurred. The epidural anesthesia presumably masked the pain. Contrary to the recommendation of these surgeons, we do not believe that epidural anesthesia is contraindicated in complex knee arthroplasty (38).

Flexion instability is not unique to posterior stabilized knee prostheses. Surgeons at the Mayo Clinic reported their experience with 25 painful cruciate-retaining knee replacements that were revised for posterior instability in flexion. Nineteen of 22 that were revised to posterior stabilized implants were improved markedly, as was one of three who were treated with polyethylene exchange only. The point should be highlighted here that the solution to flexion instability is not simply posterior stabilization, but rather manipulation of the flexion and extension gaps to stabilize the joint (39). Ochsner et al. (40) reported two cases of posterior dislocation of a posterior stabilized knee replacement other than the IBPS.

Drawbacks to the Insall-Burstein Posterior Stabilized Device Spine-and-Cam Mechanism—Patellar Fractures

The anterior-posterior dimensions and shape of the femoral component tended to be full to accommodate the spine-and-cam mechanism in the IBPS prosthesis. This pushed the patella anteriorly and presumably increased forces, which may have been responsible for a relatively higher rate of patellar fractures. In ten cadaver knee specimens Matsuda et al. (41), working with Whiteside in St. Louis, demonstrated significantly higher contact stresses in the unresurfaced patella when compared with the normal knee throughout the flexion arc for several implants including the IBPS. They noted that in flexion exceeding 105 degrees, patellofemoral contact occurred in two small patches. These investigators seemed to conclude that the forces could be normalized by extending the trochlear groove farther posteriorly and were less concerned with the anterior prominence of the component.

Mechanical "stops" to hyperextension can be a very damaging mode of constraint in knee arthroplasty design. Although some surgeons argue that hinges with hyperextension stops are essential in the correction of recurvatum deformities, there is no benefit to such constraint in prosthesis intended for general use. The tibial spine will ultimately impinge on the anterior edge of the femoral component in several circumstances:

1. The design of the femoral component includes a trochlear groove that extends farther posteriorly, so much that it comes close to the tibial spine.
2. The knee hyperextends pathologically.
3. The components are implanted with excessive posterior tibial slope or femoral component flexion such that the components are relatively hyperextended when the knee joint itself is normally fully extended (Fig. 9).

Hyperextension with the polyethylene striking the femur will soon break the tibial spine off. The original IBPS implant

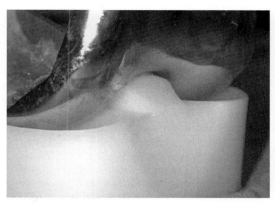
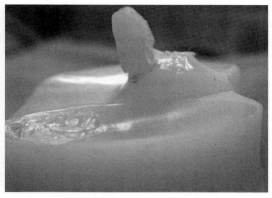

A   B

FIG. 9. A: Relative hyperextension of components can occur when the patient hyperextends the knee, owing to quadriceps weakness (e.g., in a polio patient), in the presence of lax posterior structures, or when the femoral components have been implanted with relative flexion on the femoral side or with increased posterior slope on the tibial side. In this case, laxity and hyperextension brought the anterior femur against the tibial spine. **B:** Chronic hyperextension led to fracture of the tibial spine with an increase in clinical instability in this patient.

avoided this complication with a femoral trochlear groove that simply did not extend very far posteriorly along the track of the patella. This can lead to other problems, specifically "patellar clunk."

Lachiewicz and colleagues at the University of North Carolina concluded that many patellar complications with the IBPS could be avoided by a careful surgical technique (42). They studied 118 arthroplasties at 2 to 8 years and found that no knee required reoperation for the patellofemoral joint. Mean flexion of 112 degrees was comparable to other studies with this device, and they had no cases of patellar clunk syndrome and no subluxations. There were three (2.5%) patellar fractures treated without surgery. Even this small number of fractures might be expected to improve with changes to the femoral prosthesis.

They concluded that the total patellofemoral complication rate in their series was 4.2%. This is superior to the 11% that has generally been described, of which 7% are usually fractures. In this relatively short-term study, however, the reconstructions were performed at a later era when subtleties of femoral component rotation have been better understood. This would be expected to improve the patellar complication rate.

Drawbacks to the Insall-Burstein Posterior Stabilized Device—Intercondylar Distal Femur Fracture

Intraoperative fractures of the femoral condyles have been reported specifically with the IBPS prosthesis. Lombardi and colleagues (43) compared their experience with 898 IBPS implants with 532 posterior stabilized devices from another manufacturer. Although they caused 40 (1 in 22 cases) intercondylar fractures with the IBPS, they had one such fracture with the new product. They attributed this improvement to a measuring device used to confirm the width of the intercondylar notch resection. This complication is related directly to surgical technique and whether the surgeon holds the saw blade parallel to the cutting instrument. A measuring device could easily be made for any implant system and should be for surgeons who are experiencing this type of problem with their techniques.

Drawbacks to the Insall-Burstein Posterior Stabilized Device Spine-and-Cam Mechanism—Patellar Clunk

Deeper flexion was not originally anticipated for the IBPS and led in rare situations, as we have seen, to dislocation of the spine-and-cam mechanism (Fig. 10). Similarly, deeper flexion also enabled the quadriceps tendon to extend beyond the trochlear groove of the femoral component. If the anterior edge of

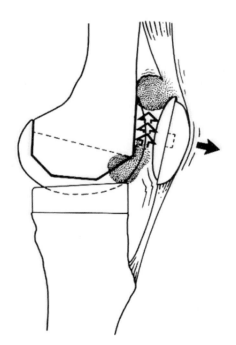

FIG. 10. Patellar clunk. When a lump of scar has formed on the deep surface of the quadriceps tendon, it may catch in the leading edge of the femoral trochlear groove. As the patient extends the knee against resistance, this must escape from the intercondylar group, which it does with a loud and sometimes painful clunk.

the femoral component terminates abruptly, synovium or scar residing on the tendon falls into the intercondylar groove. If this has occurred, the same tissue must ride up out of the intercondylar area and "jump" back up onto the femoral trochlea as the patient extends the knee. Within a few months after the arthroplasty, the offending (or offended) tissue hypertrophies and becomes rubbery. This creates the painful and noisy complication that has been described as "patellar clunk." This scar can be effectively removed arthroscopically. Recurrence is unlikely if the removal is complete (44,45).

The design features responsible for the patellar clunk are a proud (prominent anteriorly) and short (does not extend far along the patellar articulation) patellar articulation. They result from accommodating the bulk of the spine-and-cam mechanism inside the knee and yet preventing impingement on the anterior tibial spine in relative hyperextension. Both were later addressed by reducing the size of the mechanism and locating it farther posteriorly in the joint.

Drawbacks to the Insall-Burstein Posterior Stabilized Device Spine-and-Cam Mechanism—Tibial Spine Wear and Breakage

Surgeons in Croatia reported one case of recurrent dislocation of a posterior stabilized knee prosthesis in a series of 136 implants (46). Their patient had Parkinson's disease and developed the problem 9 months after surgery. At revision surgery they found breakage of the spine mechanism as the cause of instability. We have also seen this but in association with recurvatum deformity in a patient with spinal stenosis and quadriceps weakness. These patients typically walk with a back-kneed gait that may cause the edge of the trochlear flange to impinge against the tibia spine and eventually to fracture it off. It is difficult to understand how simple wear would result in this problem within a year of surgery.

There has been a recent focus on the spine-and-cam mechanism in some posterior stabilized prostheses as a source of wear debris. Mikulak and associates (46a) from Orthopedic Hospital in Los Angeles reported unanticipated aseptic loosening and osteolysis with the posterior stabilized model of the Press-Fit Condylar implant. They found that 16 of 557 (2.9%) had been revised for osteolysis from 37 to 89 months after surgery. Retrieval analysis demonstrated damage to the lateral and medial walls of the tibial spine. There was also damage to the inferior surface of the articular polyethylene inserts.

Similar findings were published in the same issue of *Journal of Bone and Joint Surgery* by Puloski and associates from the University of Western Ontario (47). Their study, by contrast, was a retrieval analysis of a variety of failed posterior stabilized implants. Wear was quantified on the tibial posts of all retrievals, including those revised for infection. They were unable to conclude that this wear mode was responsible for the failures but cautioned that the interaction between the spine and cam is not an "innocuous articulation."

Why Is the Insall-Burstein Posterior Stabilized Device Associated with Low Rates of Catastrophic Wear?

Is there some inherent characteristic of either the IBPS or posterior stabilized implants in general to explain claims that they are more resistant to polyethylene wear? As wear emerged as a major cause of failure in knee arthroplasty surgery over the last decades, some surgeons began to identify accelerated wear with cruciate-retaining implants, hypothesizing that, for a number of reasons, posterior stabilization was inherently more durable. Many factors affect wear rates: (a) polyethylene quality, preparation, and sterilization; (b) articular conformity and point loading; (c) polyethylene thickness as a result of design and surgical technique; (d) kinematics of femoral motion over the surface of the tibia; (e) patient activity; (f) access of polyethylene debris to the interface as a result of component design; and (g) surgical technique and restoration of stability and alignment. Some of these are independent of posterior stabilization; some are the direct result of it. For example, if a posterior stabilized implant is manufactured with uniformly high-molecular-weight polyethylene and is compared with a cruciate-retaining device manufactured with poor-quality polyethylene, one will see higher failure rates in the cruciate-retaining device (Fig. 11). Polyethylene as a variable is independent of design. By comparison, excision of the PCL tends to open the joint slightly and will permit a slightly thicker polyethylene inset. Thicker is generally better than thinner, and so if all other variables were equal, the posterior stabilized device would in this case yield superior results.

Not all polyethylene particles are equally damaging to the joint. Hirakawa from Yokohama in Japan and associates from The Cleveland Clinic evaluated particles in tissues surrounding 75 retrieved failed knee replacements (48). Two out of four groups studied had fewer particles, smaller particles, and less surface damage. These were implants with either more conforming articulations or PCL-resected implants. The two other groups were both cruciate-retaining prostheses. Larger particle sizes might be expected in devices known to suffer catastrophic failure such as the heat-pressed porous-coated anatomic implant. Smaller particle size tends to be associated with osteolysis. The fact that osteolysis has not generally been associated with the IBPS I implant may be related to the smaller volume of particles.

Finite element analysis confirms that stresses and strains in polyethylene are better managed in designs that have more conforming articulations and thicker polyethylene, general characteristics of the IBPS (49). Surgeons have argued that so-called flat-on-flat articulations, where the femoral component is flat from medial to lateral, are a perfect solution to the problem of conformity because the shapes match perfectly. Although edge loading is clearly a risk with this type of design, it also seems that the calculated values for maximum contact stress, von Mises stress, and von Mises strains are the least for curved-on-curved models (49). It should be noted that Don Bartel of the engineering faculty at Cornell University has long collaborated with the surgical and bioengineering staff at Cornell's HSS in Manhattan. This collaboration has influenced the knee designs that originated from the HSS (50–52).

How Has the Cruciate Ligament Controversy Evolved?

The controversy over the PCL in knee arthroplasty originated in unsubstantiated conjecture and evolved into tired saws. Some of the earliest claims and concerns do, however, merit review. Proponents of cruciate-retaining devices at one time predicted the early demise of posterior stabilized devices resulting from increased constraint, predicting that the interface shear stresses inherent in more conforming articulations would lead to loosen-

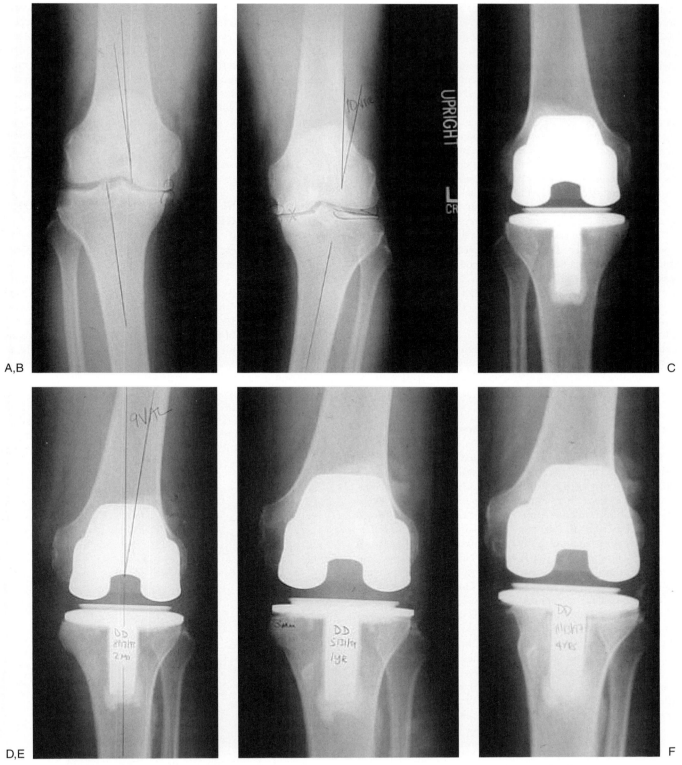

FIG. 11. A, B: Male patient aged 75 years who underwent bilateral total knee arthroplasty under the same anesthesia with cemented Insall-Burstein II posterior stabilized prostheses. **C, D:** Within the first year, both arthroplasties were well fixed with correction of varus deformity and good stability. The patient was without pain and enjoyed excellent function. **E:** Left knee arthroplasty at 1 year demonstrates early loss of bone on the medial tibial plateau. The component is not loose, and patient remains active. **F:** Left knee arthroplasty at 4 years, with tibial loosening and extensive osteolysis. Revision was required, and at that time no deterioration had occurred clinically or radiographically in the right knee.

ing. This happened with neither the total condylar nor the posterior stabilized designs (53).

By contrast, the PCL was intended to stabilize the joint without stressing the fixation interface. To avoid "kinematic conflict" (where either the PCL or the articular geometry—but not both—should dictate kinematics), almost all conformity in the tibial polyethylene was abandoned. This allowed the PCL to guide rollback unfettered. In its extreme form, the earliest uncemented implants featured virtually flat tibias so as not to jeopardize the new fixation technology. Flat tibial components were less expensive to manufacture, were less susceptible to malrotation, and permitted interchangeability of femoral and tibial component sizes. Despite these advantages, flat polyethylene has been abandoned because of catastrophic polyethylene wear. Conformity was reintroduced to cruciate-retaining devices, but the issue of kinematic conflict was resolved by "balancing" or recessing the PCL.

There was also the claim that without a functioning PCL, there could be no femoral rollback and consequently only limited flexion. Femoral rollback does not occur reproducibly, however, with conventional cruciate-retaining devices (25a). Ironically, posterior stabilized devices roll back mechanically and reproducibly, with good flexion. This rollback is engineered into the spine-and-cam mechanism such that the contact between the femur and tibia can be predicted, designed, and controlled. The polyethylene can accordingly be made thicker in these regions. By contrast, late instability occurs in cruciate-retaining devices as the result of unpredictable rollback (or "rollforward") and progressive polyethylene wear (2).

Other "Posterior Stabilized" Prostheses

Knee implants have been developed and promoted as "posterior stabilized" that either have a spine-and-cam mechanism that differs from the IBPS prosthesis or that have no such mechanism at all (54,55). In a short-term comparison of such a "deep-dished" tibial implant with a non-IBPS posterior stabilized implant, Laskin et al. (54) concluded that there was no difference in results, including flexion, which averaged approximately 116 degrees in both groups. This would argue that femoral rollback has no advantage in knee arthroplasty surgery or that the Genesis II prosthesis with its modular posterior stabilized implant did not replicate rollback. The appeal of a dished tibia over a spine-and-cam mechanism is obvious: Manufacturers need not provide a posterior stabilized femoral component, the surgeon need not remove bone from the femoral intercondylar notch, and patents can be circumvented.

There are few long-term reports on posterior stabilized implants other than the IBPS. Laskin (56), originally at the Long Island Jewish Hospital, in New York, but reporting now at the HSS, published 10-year results of the Genesis knee with both posterior cruciate–retaining and posterior cruciate–substituting versions. Those knees with greater deformity were selected for the posterior stabilized device and yet the functional results and durability were similar in both groups.

GAIT STUDIES

Some gait studies have suggested that cruciate-sacrificing arthroplasties function less well than cruciate-retaining devices,

especially on stair climbing (53). With data from a gait laboratory at the Insall-Scott-Kelly Institute in New York, researchers concluded—after evaluating 16 patients with IBPS II implants and comparing them with 32 age-matched controls—that there was no significant difference between the groups during stair ascent. The contention is that the persistent gait abnormalities of patients with posterior stabilized implants are comparable to those of patients with cruciate-retaining implants and superior to those with cruciate-sacrificing implants such as the Total Condylar (57,58). Given that the spine-and-cam mechanism tends to engage only at approximately 70 degrees of flexion, would it really be expected to enhance stair climbing?

CLINICAL RESULTS FROM THE HOSPITAL FOR SPECIAL SURGERY

One of the largest studies completed by Insall and associates compared the failure rates of several types of cruciate-retaining arthroplasties. All yielded excellent long-term results. The oldest implant, the all-polyethylene, non–posterior stabilized total condylar was implanted in 215 patients and had a "21 year success rate of 98.10%." Similarly, the all-polyethylene posterior stabilized had a "14 year success rate of 98.10%." Surgeons must be careful not to necessarily extrapolate these results to groups of patients who are younger and more active. Bear in mind that in most 10-year evaluations of knee replacements in the literature, approximately 30% of the original cohort will have died (9).

However, when results from a group of 114 younger (aged 22 to 55 years, mean of 51), active patients who had knee replacements with the IBPS prosthesis were studied the results were

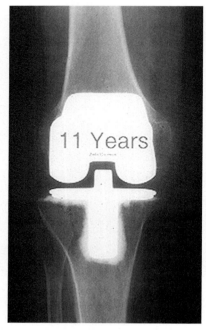

FIG 12. Eleven-year result of the Insall-Burstein metal-backed but nonmodular tibial component. This bone-cement interface is without radiolucencies and is typical of the patients in this study.

surprisingly good. Granted, with an average age of 51 years, this group is not likely to have the life expectancy nor the activity level of the average 30-year-old patient. Nonetheless, there were but seven reoperations in the entire group, for a predicted survivorship of 87% at 18 years. These results exceed general expectations of knee arthroplasty longevity and tend to dispel the belief that posterior stabilized replacements are likely to have higher failure rates due to constraint.

CLINICAL RESULTS NOT FROM THE HOSPITAL FOR SPECIAL SURGERY

The IBPS prosthesis, used extensively around the globe, was introduced in 1978 with an all-polyethylene tibial component. This has been referred to as the *IBPS I* prosthesis, and it became available within several years with a nonmodular, metal-backed tibia (Fig. 12). Aglietti and coworkers, who trained with Insall during the development of the total condylar replacement, reviewed their results at a minimum of 10 years with 99 posterior stabilized prostheses. Thirty-nine knees were in patients who had died before the 10-year follow-up and four were removed or revised, leaving 56 knees for evaluation at an average of 12 years. There were 58% excellent, 25% good, 7% fair, and 10% poor results. Knee flexion averaged 106 degrees. Of the six (10%) failures, four were attributable to aseptic component loosening; none were attributable to polyethylene wear. With revision as the end point, 10-year survivorship was 92% (59).

One of the first overseas long-term follow-up studies was published by Nafei et al. in 1993 (60). One hundred thirty-eight knees were observed at an average of 10 years (range of 9 to 11 years). HSS scores were excellent or good in 86%, fair in 8%, and poor in 6%. The "crude prosthetic survival rate" was 98%, with two failures secondary to deep prosthetic infection. Average range of motion was reported to be 104 degrees.

Li et al. (61) from the Royal National Orthopedic Hospital, in Stanmore, England, reported their experience with an Insall-Burstein II prosthesis in 1999. Of 146 knees, 94 were reviewed at a mean of 10 years. HSS scores were excellent or good in 79%, fair in 14%, and poor in 7%. The average Knee Society score was 87. Knee flexion improved from an average of 88 degrees preoperatively to 100 degrees after arthroplasty, considerably less than has been expected from this device. The 10-year survivorship was 92.3% using revision as the end point, and there were nine failures. In this series, the authors reported that "anterior knee pain was a significant problem."

CLINICAL RESULTS IN SPECIFIC PATHOLOGIC SITUATIONS

Aglietti et al. (62) evaluated the performance of the IBPS prosthesis specifically in 67 knees with valgus deformity. The results were rated as excellent in 53%, good in 39%, fair in 6% and poor in 2%. A patellofemoral clunk was present in three (6%) knees and the mechanical axis had been restored to within 5 degrees of neutral in only 88% of cases. There were four failures: aseptic loosening, lateral instability, deep infection, and recurrent patellar dislocation. The results of this same group with the IBPS prosthesis in patients with rheumatoid disease were also reliably good at 5 to 13 years after surgery (62).

The knee with a prior patellectomy suffered unacceptably high rates of posterior tibial dislocation in flexion with the Total Condylar prosthesis, and this was one of the motivations for developing the IBPS implant. Paletta and Laskin (62a) evaluated the results of knee replacement surgery after patellectomy. They concluded that IBPS patients had better scores for pain and function than did those with the (nonposterior stabilized) cruciate-sacrificing Total Condylar I. All patients could ascend stairs reciprocally and four patients lacked 5 to 20 degrees of active extension. Interestingly, the longer the interval between the arthroplasty and the assessment, the better the score. This last point goes against the general trend at longer intervals in which knee scores decline with advancing age. Cameron and colleagues in Toronto (63) described 16 patients with a prior patellectomy for whom they selected a non-IBPS posterior stabilized implant and concluded that these patients did well on stair climbing and had 69% good or excellent functional results.

Most surgeons worry about the durability of knee arthroplasty in obese patients. Griffin, working with Insall and colleagues, evaluated results of knee replacement using cemented posterior stabilized implants in 165 knees 10 years after surgery. Functional scores were comparable to nonobese arthroplasty patients and revision rates were no higher (64). The real challenge in the obese patient is the difficult surgical exposure. Wound problems seem to occur with a greater frequency in obese patients (65).

PERSONAL RESULTS

Insall-Burstein I

Long-term experience with posterior stabilized total knee arthroplasty has been documented from other institutions as well. We reviewed our results of the metal-backed posterior stabilized prosthesis at a minimum of 10 years. One hundred total knee arthroplasties were performed in 86 consecutive patients by the senior author. Thirty-six were in patients who had died and two were in patients who were infirm. Of the remaining 62 knees, 54 were directly evaluated and eight by phone at an average of 10.8 years. No patients were lost. At latest follow-up, 64% were rated as excellent, 18% as good, 7% as fair, and 11% as poor, which included six failures. Flexion averaged 111 degrees. Excluding the failures, the average Knee Society clinical score was 91.6. Of the six failures, two were secondary to sepsis, two secondary to nonspecific pain, one secondary to patellar wear and fracture, and one because of aseptic tibial component loosening. Polyethylene wear was specifically examined in this study, and no implant demonstrated significant polyethylene wear or failure. There were seven patellar fractures—four required additional surgery, and the remaining three were asymptomatic and discovered incidentally at routine follow-up. Using revision as the end point, 12-year survivorship averaged 92% (66).

Insall-Burstein II

The modular IBPS II prosthesis was introduced in 1989 with modifications to the patellofemoral articulation and the posterior stabilized mechanism that increased femoral rollback and theoretically flexion. As we have seen, this device was more susceptible to posterior dislocation at higher flexion. We followed 100 of these, whose surgeries were performed consecutively,

TABLE 1. *Comparison of Insall-Burstein I and Insall-Burstein II complications*

	Insall-Burstein I	Insall-Burstein II
Treatment of patellar fractures		
Asymptomatic-healed	3	0
Patellar component revisions	2	1
Revision total knee replacement	1	0
Patellectomy	1	1
Total	7	2
Reoperations (not revisions)		
Patellar component revisions	2	1
Patellar component removal	1	0
Patellectomy/fracture	1	1
Spine-and-cam dislocation	0	3
Polyethylene dissociation	0	1
Patellar clunk	0	6
Total	4	12
Revisions		
Sepsis (early)	2	1
Sepsis (late)	0	1
Tibial-femoral instability	0	2
Loosening	1	0
Osteolysis	0	1
Stiff	0	1
Patellar wear	1	0
Total	4	6

prospectively. Fifty-one knees were evaluated at 10 or more years with Knee Society scores and radiographs; 14 were evaluated by phone. An additional six knees required revision and 29 were in patients who died. None were lost. Complete revision surgery was performed for instability (two knees), sepsis (two), loosening from osteolysis (one), and stiffness (one). Twelve patients required reoperations without revision of the tibia and femoral components: patellar revision for loosening (one), patellectomy for fracture (one), polyethylene exchange for dislocation of the spine-and-cam mechanism (three) and for dissociation (one), and arthroscopic resection of scar from the quadriceps tendon in six (patellar clunk).

These two groups were definitely different from each other (Table 1). There was no incidence of osteolysis leading to loosening in the nonmodular Insall-Burstein I prostheses that had been manufactured from molded polyethylene. One case occurred in the Insall-Burstein II. The problem of patellar fractures was decreased significantly in the Insall-Burstein II group probably as a result of smoothing the anterior trochlear groove. However, new problems arose with the Insall-Burstein II, in large part due to changes in the spine-and-cam mechanism as well as the instruments. Tibial-femoral dislocation, not seen in the Insall-Burstein I with tensor instruments, occurred in three Insall-Burstein II prostheses.

DESIGN ENHANCEMENTS

Deep Flexion

The knee joint behaves differently as the knee is flexed maximally, as in kneeling and squatting activities. This has been a logical area for physiologic investigation and prosthetic development, considering that for many years knee arthroplasty was considered an inappropriate intervention in cultures where people kneel for meals or prayer.

Cooke and associates in Saudi Arabia concluded—based on a radiographic study—that in very deep flexion the lateral femoral condyle rolled farther over the medial aspect of the lateral tibial plateau. Contact of the medial femoral condyle occurred more anteriorly but still in the posterior part of the plateau. This asymmetric rolling indicated some internal rotation of the tibia, a motion that has not been anticipated in most arthroplasty designs, certainly not in early posterior stabilized implants (67).

Mobile Bearing Hi Flex

Mobile bearing technology has not by itself ensured physiologic rollback, as was once hoped. In a videofluoroscopy study of ten patients with a mobile bearing cruciate-retaining implant, many exhibited rollforward. This effect was clearly not intended and is deleterious to extensor mechanism function as well as wear resistance. In addition, only half of the mobile bearings had some movement, whereas the others remained fixed (68). It would seem that mobile bearings, in the usual range of knee arthroplasty flexion, serve to correct surgical errors of implantation at the time of surgery. However, in deep flexion, as the tibia must rotate to accommodate the maximum position, the mobile bearing may prove necessary for optimum flexion.

REFERENCES

1. Schai PA, Thornhill TS, et al. Total knee arthroplasty with the PFC system. Results at a minimum of ten years and survivorship analysis. *J Bone Joint Surg Br* 1998;80:850–858.
2. Feng EL, Stulberg SD, et al. Progressive subluxation and polyethylene wear in total knee replacements with flat articular surfaces. *Clin Orthop* 1994;299:60–71.
3. Kleinbart FA, Bryk E, et al. Histologic comparison of posterior cruciate ligaments from arthritic and age-matched knee specimens. *J Arthroplasty* 1996;11:726–731.
4. Mallory TH, Smalley D, et al. Townley anatomic total knee arthroplasty using total tibial component with cruciate release. *Clin Orthop* 1982;169:197–201.
5. Townley CO. The anatomic total knee resurfacing arthroplasty. *Clin Orthop* 1985;192:82–96.
6. Cloutier JM, Sabouret P, et al. Total knee arthroplasty with retention of both cruciate ligaments. A nine to eleven-year follow-up study. *J Bone Joint Surg Am* 1999;81:697–702.
7. Scott RD. Duopatellar total knee replacement: the Brigham experience. *Orthop Clin North Am* 1982;13:89–102.
8. Freeman MA, Sculco T, et al. Replacement of the severely damaged arthritic knee by the ICLH (Freeman-Swanson) arthroplasty. *J Bone Joint Surg Br* 1977;59:64–71.
9. Font-Rodriguez DE, Scuderi GR, et al. Survivorship of cemented total knee arthroplasty. *Clin Orthop* 1997;345:79–86.
10. Moreland JR, Thomas RJ, et al. ICLH replacement of the knee: 1977 and 1978. *Clin Orthop* 1979;145:47–59.
11. Vince KG, Insall JN, et al. The total condylar prosthesis. 10- to 12-year results of a cemented knee replacement. *J Bone Joint Surg Br* 1989;71:793–797.
12. Walker PS, Masse Y. Principles of condylar replacement knee prosthesis design. *Acta Orthop Belg* 1973;39:151–163.
13. Insall J, Ranawat CS, et al. Total condylar knee replacement: preliminary report. *Clin Orthop* 1976;00(120):149–154.
14. Insall J. *Surgery of the knee.* Edinburgh: Churchill Livingstone, 1984.
15. Scott RD, Thornhill TS. Posterior cruciate supplementing total knee replacement using conforming inserts and cruciate recession. Effect on range of motion and radiolucent lines. *Clin Orthop* 1994;309:146–149.
16. Arima J, Whiteside LA, et al. Effect of partial release of the posterior cruciate ligament in total knee arthroplasty. *Clin Orthop* 1998;353:194–202.

17. Insall JN, Lachiewicz PF, et al. The posterior stabilized condylar prosthesis: a modification of the total condylar design. Two to four-year clinical experience. *J Bone Joint Surg Am* 1982;64:1317–1323.

18. Scott WN, Rubinstein M. Posterior stabilized knee arthroplasty. Six years' experience. *Clin Orthop* 1986;205:138–145.

19. Insall J, Scott WN, et al. The total condylar knee prosthesis. A report of two hundred and twenty cases. *J Bone Joint Surg Am* 1979;61:173–180.

20. Ranawat CS, Boachie-Adjei O. Survivorship analysis and results of total condylar knee arthroplasty. Eight- to 11-year follow-up period. *Clin Orthop* 1988;226:6–13.

21. Goldberg VM, Henderson BT. The Freeman-Swanson ICLH total knee arthroplasty. Complications and problems. *J Bone Joint Surg Am* 1980;62:1338–1344.

22. Laskin RS. The Insall Award. Total knee replacement with posterior cruciate ligament retention in patients with a fixed varus deformity. *Clin Orthop* 1996;331:29–34.

23. Todo S, Kadoya Y, et al. Anteroposterior and rotational movement of femur during knee flexion. *Clin Orthop* 1999;362:162–170.

24. Ishii Y, Terajima K, et al. Three-dimensional kinematics of the human knee with intracortical pin fixation. *Clin Orthop* 1997;343:144–150.

25. Stiehl JB, Komistek RD. Fluoroscopic analysis of kinematics after posterior-cruciate-retaining knee arthroplasty. *J Bone Joint Surg Br* 1995;77:884–889.

25a. Dennis DA, Komistek RD. In vivo anteroposterior femorotibial translation of total knee arthroplasty: a multicenter analysis. *Clin Orthop* 1998;356:47–57.

26. Kim H, Pelker RR, et al. Rollback in posterior cruciate ligament-retaining total knee arthroplasty. A radiographic analysis. *J Arthroplasty* 1997;12:553–561.

27. Piazza SJ, Delp SL, et al. Posterior tilting of the tibial component decreases femoral rollback in posterior-substituting knee replacement: a computer simulation study. *J Orthop Res* 1998;16:264–270.

28. Walker PS, Sathasivam S. Controlling the motion of total knee replacements using intercondylar guide surfaces. *J Orthop Res* 2000;18:48–55.

29. Churchill DL, Incavo SJ, et al. The influence of femoral rollback on patellofemoral contact loads in total knee arthroplasty. *J Arthroplasty* 2001;16:909–918.

30. Emodi GJ, Callaghan JJ, et al. Posterior cruciate ligament function following total knee arthroplasty: the effect of joint line elevation. *Iowa Orthop J* 1999;19:82–92.

31. Mahoney OM, Noble PC, et al. Posterior cruciate function following total knee arthroplasty. A biomechanical study. *J Arthroplasty* 1994;9:569–578.

32. Kadoya Y, Kobayashi A, et al. Effects of posterior cruciate ligament resection on the tibiofemoral joint gap. *Clin Orthop* 2001;391:210–217.

33. Mihalko WM, Krackow KA. Posterior cruciate ligament effects on the flexion space in total knee arthroplasty. *Clin Orthop* 1999;360:243–250.

34. Schurman DJ, Matityahu A, et al. Prediction of postoperative knee flexion in Insall-Burstein II total knee arthroplasty. *Clin Orthop* 1998;353:175–184.

35. Hirsch HS, Lotke PA, et al. The posterior cruciate ligament in total knee surgery. Save, sacrifice, or substitute? *Clin Orthop* 1994;309:64–68.

35a. Dennis DA, Komistek RD, et al. Range of motion after total knee arthroplasty: the effect of implant design and weight-bearing conditions. *J Arthroplasty* 1998;13:748–752.

36. Galinat BJ, Vernace JV, et al. Dislocation of the posterior stabilized total knee arthroplasty. A report of two cases. *J Arthroplasty* 1988;3:363–367.

37. Delp SL, Kocmond JH, et al. Tradeoffs between motion and stability in posterior substituting knee arthroplasty design. *J Biomech* 1995;28:1155–1166.

37a. Lombardi AV Jr, Mallory TH, Vaughn BK, et al. Dislocation following primary posterior-stabilized total knee arthroplasty. *J Arthroplasty* 1993;8:633–639.

37b. Hossain S, Ayeko C, Anwar M, et al. Dislocation of Insall-Burstein II modified total knee arthroplasty. *J Arthroplasty* 2001;16:233–235.

38. Tang WM, Chiu KY. Silent compartment syndrome complicating total knee arthroplasty: continuous epidural anesthesia masked the pain. *J Arthroplasty* 2000;15:241–243.

39. Pagnano MW, Hanssen AD, et al. Flexion instability after primary posterior cruciate retaining total knee arthroplasty. *Clin Orthop* 1998;356:39–46.

40. Ochsner JL, Kostman WC, Dodson M. Posterior dislocation of a posterior stabilized total knee arthroplasty. A report of two cases. *Am J Orthop* 1996;25:310–312.

41. Matsuda S, Ishinishi T, et al. Contact stresses with an unresurfaced patella in total knee arthroplasty: the effect of femoral component design. *Orthopedics* 2000;23:213–218.

42. Larson CM, Lachiewicz PF. Patellofemoral complications with the Insall-Burstein II posterior-stabilized total knee arthroplasty. *J Arthroplasty* 1999;14:288–292.

43. Lombardi AV Jr, Mallory TH, et al. Intercondylar distal femoral fracture. An unreported complication of posterior-stabilized total knee arthroplasty. *J Arthroplasty* 1995;10:643–650.

44. Beight JL, Yao B, et al. The patellar clunk syndrome after posterior stabilized total knee arthroplasty. *Clin Orthop* 1994;299:139–142.

45. Lucas TS, DeLuca PF, et al. Arthroscopic treatment of patellar clunk. *Clin Orthop* 1999;367:226–229.

46. Erceg M, Maricevic A. Recurrent posterior dislocation following primary posterior-stabilized total knee arthroplasty. *Croat Med J* 2000;41:207–209.

46a. Mikulak SA, Mahoney OM, dela Rosa MA, et al. Loosening and osteolysis with the press-fit condylar posterior-cruciate-substituting total knee replacement. *J Bone Joint Surg Am* 2001;83-A:398–403.

47. Puloski SK, McCalden RW, et al. Tibial post wear in posterior stabilized total knee arthroplasty. An unrecognized source of polyethylene debris. *J Bone Joint Surg Am* 2001;83:390–397.

48. Hirakawa K, Bauer TW, et al. Relationship between wear debris particles and polyethylene surface damage in primary total knee arthroplasty. *J Arthroplasty* 1999;14:165–171.

49. Bartel DL, Rawlinson JJ, et al. Stresses in polyethylene components of contemporary total knee replacements. *Clin Orthop* 1995;317:76–82.

50. Bartel DL, Burstein AH, et al. Performance of the tibial component in total knee replacement. *J Bone Joint Surg Am* 1982;64:1026–1033.

51. Bartel DL, Bicknell VL, et al. The effect of conformity, thickness, and material on stresses in ultra-high molecular weight components for total joint replacement. *J Bone Joint Surg Am* 1986;68:1041–1051.

52. Wright TM, Bartel DL. The problem of surface damage in polyethylene total knee components. *Clin Orthop* 1986;205:67–74.

53. Andriacchi TP, Galante JO. Retention of the posterior cruciate in total knee arthroplasty. *J Arthroplasty* 1988;3(Suppl):S13–19.

54. Laskin RS, Maruyama Y, et al. Deep-dish congruent tibial component use in total knee arthroplasty: a randomized prospective study. *Clin Orthop* 2000;380:36–44.

55. Hofmann AA, Tkach TK, et al. Posterior stabilization in total knee arthroplasty with use of an ultracongruent polyethylene insert. *J Arthroplasty* 2000;15:576–583.

56. Laskin RS. The Genesis total knee prosthesis: a 10-year followup study. *Clin Orthop* 2001;388:95–102.

57. Wilson SA, McCann PD, et al. Comprehensive gait analysis in posterior-stabilized knee arthroplasty. *J Arthroplasty* 1996;11:359–367.

58. Bolanos AA, Colizza WA, et al. A comparison of isokinetic strength testing and gait analysis in patients with posterior cruciate-retaining and substituting knee arthroplasties. *J Arthroplasty* 1998;13:906–915.

59. Aglietti P, Buzzi R, et al. The Insall-Burstein total knee replacement in osteoarthritis: a 10-year minimum follow-up. *J Arthroplasty* 1999;14:560–565.

60. Nafei A, Kristensen O, et al. Total condylar arthroplasty for gonarthrosis. A prospective 10-year study of 138 primary cases. *Acta Orthop Scand* 1993;64:421–427.

61. Li PL, Zamora J, et al. The results at ten years of the Insall-Burstein II total knee replacement. Clinical, radiological and survivorship studies. *J Bone Joint Surg Br* 1999;81:647–653.

62. Aglietti P, Buzzi R, et al. Insall-Burstein posterior-stabilized knee prosthesis in rheumatoid arthritis. *J Arthroplasty* 1995;10:217–225.

62a. Paletta GA Jr., Laskin RS. Total knee arthroplasty after a previous patellectomy. *J Bone Joint Surg Am* 1995;77:1708–1712.

63. Cameron HU, Hu C, et al. Posterior stabilized knee prosthesis for total knee replacement in patients with prior patellectomy. *Can J Surg* 1996;39:469–473.

64. Griffin FM, Scuderi GR, et al. Total knee arthroplasty in patients who were obese with 10 years followup. *Clin Orthop* 1998;356:28–33.

65. Winiarsky R, Barth P, et al. Total knee arthroplasty in morbidly obese patients. *J Bone Joint Surg Am* 1998;80:1770–1774.

66. Thadani PJ, Vince KG, et al. Ten- to 12-year followup of the Insall-Burstein I total knee prosthesis. *Clin Orthop* 2000;380:17–29.

67. Hefzy MS, Kelly BP, et al. Kinematics of the knee joint in deep flexion: a radiographic assessment. *Med Eng Phys* 1998;20:302–307.

68. Stiehl JB, Dennis DA, et al. In vivo kinematic analysis of a mobile bearing total knee prosthesis. *Clin Orthop* 1997;345:60–66.

69. Insall J, Tria AJ. The Total Condylar II Knee Prosthesis. *Orthop Trans* 1979;3:300–301.

70. Vince K, ed. *Evolution of total knee arthroplasty.* St. Louis: Mosby, 1993.

71. Vince KG. Principles of condylar knee arthroplasty: issues evolving. *Instr Course Lect* 1993;42:315–324.

CHAPTER 79

Mobile Bearing Knee Replacement

Frederick F. Buechel

HISTORY AND DEVELOPMENT OF MOBILE BEARINGS

The need for mobile bearings in knee replacement developed after analysis of failed fixed bearing knee replacements. Significant component loosing was seen in early fixed-hinge devices (1) and congruent fixed bearing nonhinged devices (2) in less than 2 years of active use. Incongruent knee replacements that were developed to avoid loosening problems were plagued with wear-related problems in less than 5 years (3,4). Modular fixed bearing polyethylene inserts were developed to allow intraoperative adjustment of component stability, but their locking mechanisms created a new source of wear debris that compounded the existing wear problems (5).

It was established that congruity without mobility and mobility without congruity were flawed design concepts that caused premature loosening or excessive wear. Congruity with mobility has become the ideal stress and movement concept to minimize loosening and wear problems. That is to say, mobile bearings without locking mechanisms represent the most effective way to avoid the identified problems seen with fixed bearing knee designs over the past three decades.

The kinematic tibiofemoral motion requirements dictate the use of spherical upper tibial bearing surfaces and a flat under surface to accommodate the variety of movements in the most congruent way. The Oxford meniscal knee (6) uses matching spherical surfaces for the femoral component and the upper meniscal bearing surface and a flat surface to match a flat tibial component.

This preferred geometry appears to work well as a medial unicompartmental replacement (7) but has had dislocation problems in other applications (8). These problems most likely are caused by a larger than normal single radius of curvature of the femoral component, which under the pull of the posterior cruciate ligament (PCL) in flexion moves the bearing too far posteriorly (Fig. 1).

A design solution to the Oxford problem in the presence of cruciate ligaments is seen in the low contact stress (LCS) femoral component (9), which uses the same spherical surface of revolution in the medial-lateral plane but decreases the radius of curvature from extension to flexion, thus maintaining full-area contact on the upper meniscal bearing surface from 0 to 45 degrees, where walking loads are encountered, and maintaining at least spherical line contact at deeper flexion angles (Fig. 2). This surface geometry allows a more central femoral component position in flexion by reducing the PCL tension, which tends to pull the femur posteriorly when overstretched (Fig. 3). Another design solution to prevent meniscal bearing dislocation is the use of radial tracks on the LCS tibial components. These tracks allow axial rotation and controlled anteroposterior translation, which impedes direct dislocation by means of the cruciate bone bridge posteriorly and the patellar tendon anteriorly (Fig. 4). When com-

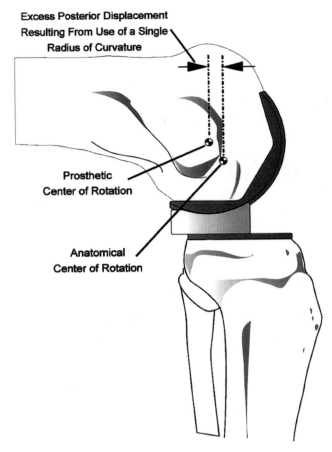

FIG. 1. Excessive posterior bearing displacement due to the use of a single radius of curvature of the femoral component.

bined with stable flexion and extension gaps at surgery, the LCS meniscal bearings can be safely used when both cruciate ligaments are intact or if only the PCL is intact (Fig. 5).

In the event of a nonfunctional or absent PCL, central stability with the ability to axially rotate is essential. Long-term survivor-

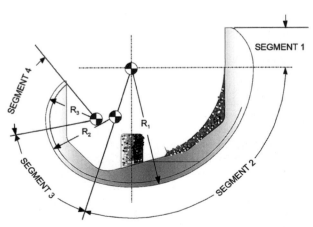

FIG. 2. Decreasing radius (R) of curvature of low contact stress femoral component.

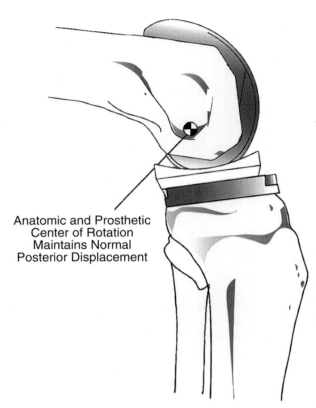

FIG. 3. Maintenance of central position of bearing using decreasing radius of curvature.

ship studies have demonstrated that a centrally stabilized total condylar knee replacement is predicted to last for 15 years in more than 90% of cases when used in elderly patients with low loading demands (10,11). These important studies prove that cruciate function is not essential for successful long-term fixation and function in low-demand situations.

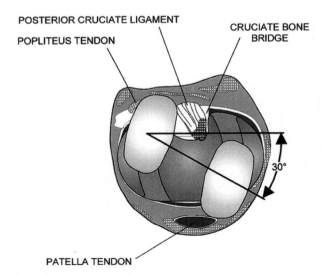

FIG. 4. Soft tissues and radial tracks limit bearing motion, preventing bearing dislocation during normal activities.

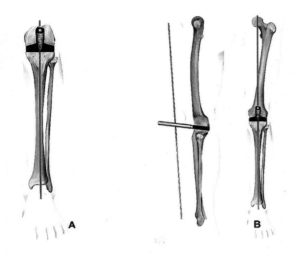

FIG. 5. Use of a spacer block to check the resection gaps during flexion **(A)** and extension **(B)** to ensure that they are equivalent.

Because wear increases as the loads and demands increase, it seems most appropriate to use the proven fixation and central stabilizing concepts of the total condylar device and provide a more wear-resistant and dislocation-resistant bearing surface to achieve better long-term survivorship and reduce wear-related failures. These concepts led to the development of a rotating-platform total knee device that uses the same spherical surface geometry as the meniscal bearings (Fig. 6).

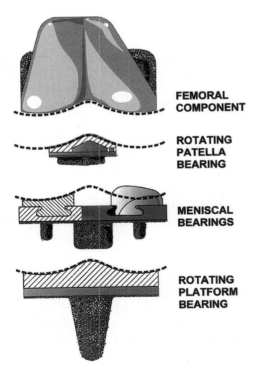

FIG. 6. Same common generating curve used for all bearing surfaces.

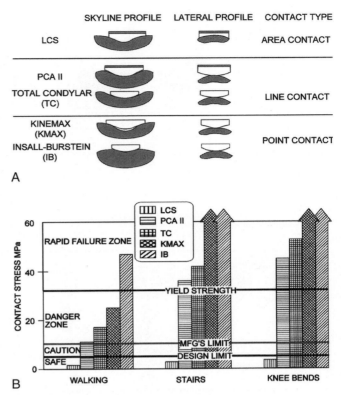

FIG. 7. A: Surface geometry of varying patellar designs at 30 degrees of flexion and **(B)** contact stress of varying patellar designs. LCS, low contact stress; MFG, manufacturer; MPa, megapascal; PCA, porous-coated anatomic.

The patellofemoral design process, like the tibiofemoral design process, seeks to provide proper motion and maintain contact stresses below the ideal 5 megapascals (MPa) during walking, stair climbing, and deep-knee bending (12). Button or nonrotating anatomic-type patellar replacements suffer from either point or line contact stresses or from overconstraint. High contact stress will cause early wear failure (13), whereas overconstraint will cause early loosening failure (14). For these reasons, a rotating bearing patellar replacement was developed to maintain spherical area contact on the medial and lateral facets while congruently matching the surface of revolution of the deep sulcus femoral groove. Rotating bearing patellar replacement of the LCS design greatly improves on the contact stress seen in other design configurations (Fig. 7) (12).

EVOLUTION OF THE NEW JERSEY LOW CONTACT STRESS MOBILE BEARING KNEE

The first mobile bearing application was seen in shoulder replacement in which two eccentrically placed spherical elements improved the range of motion over simple ball-and-socket systems. These "floating-socket" (15) bearings were developed in 1974 and used clinically from 1975 to 1979, when less constrained shoulder implants were developed (16).

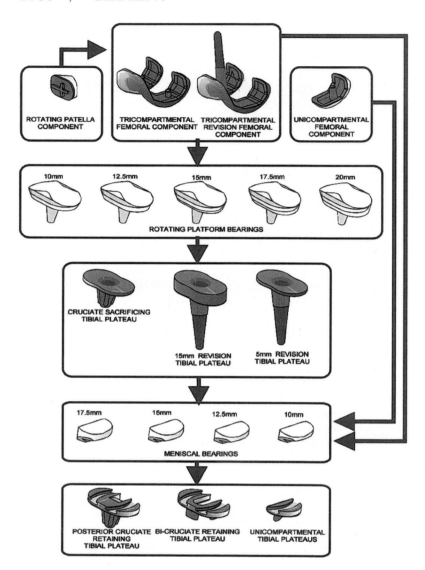

FIG. 8. New Jersey low contact stress knee system.

Later, knee (9) and ankle (17) bearings were developed using similar concepts.

The first complete systems approach to total knee replacement (TKR) using meniscal bearings was developed in 1977 and reported in 1986 (18). Unicompartmental, bicompartmental, and tricompartmental disease was managed with a variety of primary and revision components that allowed retention of both cruciate ligaments, only the posterior cruciate, or no cruciate ligaments. Additionally, the first metal-backed, rotating bearing patellar replacement was developed in 1977 to provide mobility with congruity in patellofemoral articulation. This New Jersey LCS total knee system, initially used with cement in 1977, was expanded to noncemented use in 1981 with the availability of sintered-bead porous coating (19) and remains the only knee system in the United States to have undergone formal U.S. Food and Drug Administration Investigational Device Exemption (FDA-IDE) clinical trials in both cemented and cementless appli-

cations before being released for general clinical use (Fig. 8) (20–23).

COMPONENT SURFACE GEOMETRY REQUIREMENTS

Surface congruence is essential to improve wear life in ultra-high molecular weight polyethylene bearings, especially in major repetitive load-bearing activities, such as walking, which generates loads of 2.5 times body weight, and stair climbing, which can generate loads of eight times body weight. Aside from direct compressive loading, however, the tibiofemoral bearings must be able to accommodate flexion of 155 degrees, varus-valgus movements of 10 degrees, axial rotation of 30 degrees, and anteroposterior translation of 15 mm when the cruciate ligaments are retained. The patellofemoral articulation is also loaded mainly in compression and needs to accommodate

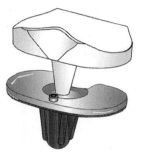
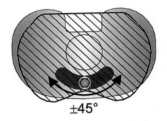

±45°

FIG. 9. Rotating-platform tibial component with rotational stop.

similar flexion to 155 degrees, axial rotation of 6 degrees, and the ability to tilt laterally and medially in the femoral groove without dislocating or rubbing on an edge.

RECENT MOBILE BEARING ADVANCES

Since 1977, the basic design philosophy of the LCS knee has remained unchanged and the articulating surface geometries continue in their original form. However, problems of meniscal bearing and rotating platform bearing dislocation have prompted a review of design parameters to evaluate alternative concepts to reduce the number of these complications, even though small.

Rotating Platform with Rotational Stop Tibial Component

In cases of flexion instability and the absence of cruciate ligaments, rotating-platform dislocation has occurred, especially in revision situations (24). The addition of a rotational stop pin that

allows 90 degrees of axial rotation has helped to eliminate this problem (Fig. 9). Introduced in 1991, this important modification has virtually eliminated dislocations in a consecutive series of 130 primary and multiply operated knees followed over a 10-year period without causing loosening or increasing wear (Fig. 10). The most important use has been in revising chronically unstable rotating platforms (25) to regain stability and function without the need for an intercondylar post (Fig. 11).

Universal Anteroposterior Glide Meniscal Bearing Tibial Component

Axial malposition of meniscal bearing tibial components have been responsible for cantilever bending/fractures and dislocations in posterior cruciate–retaining (PCR) LCS meniscal bearing knee replacement (26). Rotation beyond 30 degrees can allow standard meniscal bearings to overhang or dislocate from their tracks on the tibial component. A single meniscal bearing on a rotatable control arm that allows normal anteroposterior gliding motion with PCL retention has been designed to potentially eliminate meniscal bearing dislocation and fracture problems (Fig. 12). Designed in 1989 and clinically introduced in 1991, this anteroposterior glide meniscal bearing device has a tibial component tray that is compatible with a rotating platform, making it a universal tibial component for cruciate retention or cruciate sacrifice (Fig. 13). Additionally, this tray can accept a removable stop pin for cases in which flexion instability may be improved when using a rotating platform (Fig. 14).

Three-Peg Rotating Bearing Patella Component

Technical difficulties have been encountered in preparing the cruciate-fixturing fin channels for the rotating bearing patella component. Although not insurmountable, these difficulties,

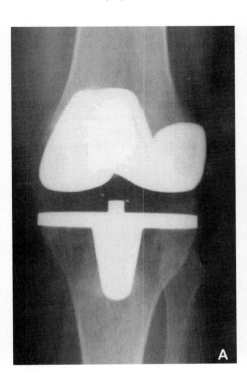
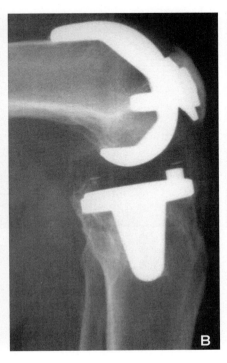

FIG. 10. A: Anteroposterior radiograph of a well-functioning cementless left rotational stop rotating platform total knee replacement after 7 years in an active 89-year-old osteoarthritic female. **B:** Lateral radiograph of the same knee.

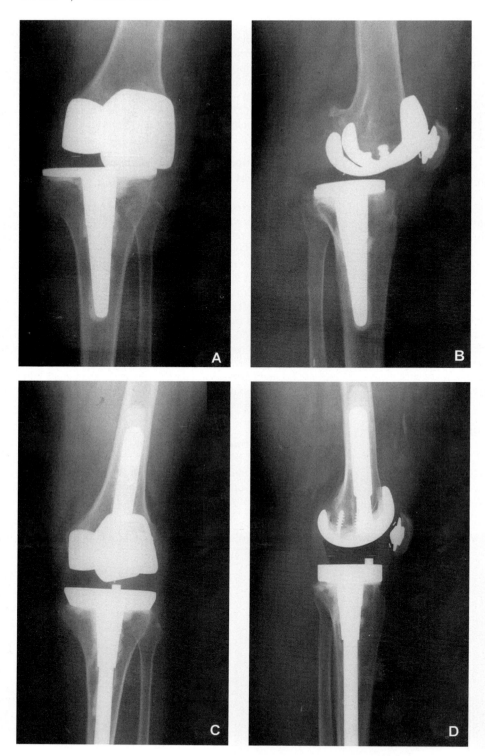

FIG. 11. A: Anteroposterior radiograph of a 69-year-old obese woman demonstrating a deep dish rotating platform bearing that is disengaged completely from the lateral compartment and is only held in the medial compartment, causing a marked valgus alignment. **B:** Lateral radiograph of the same knee as in **A**. **C:** Anteroposterior radiograph 1 year and 4 months after revision demonstrating stable alignment and fixation of a deep dish rotating platform with rotational stop. **D:** Lateral radiograph of the same knee as in **C**.

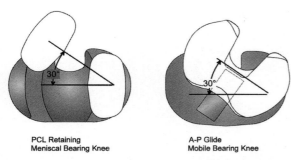

FIG. 12. A: Meniscal bearing device at 30 degrees rotation allows dislocation of bearing. **B:** Anteroposterior (A-P) glide device at 30 degrees rotation remains stable without bearing dislocation. PCL, posterior cruciate ligament.

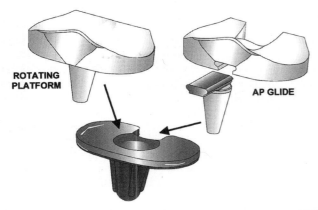

FIG. 13. Universal tibial tray accepts anteroposterior (AP) glide or rotating platform bearings.

which usually involve prolonged use of a high-speed burr in sclerotic bone, are time-consuming, aggravating, and annoying to the surgeon and support staff. To simplify the fixation preparation, a three-peg template has been developed, which uses a stop drill for quick and easy fabrication of the three fixation

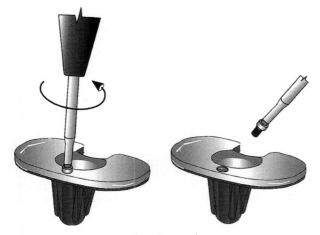

FIG. 14. Removable rotational stop pin.

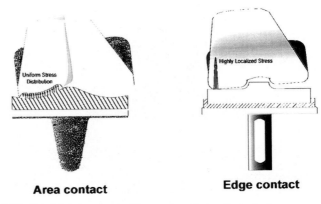

FIG. 15. Maintenance of congruent contact during varus-valgus condylar lift-off with a spherical anterior bearing design versus a horizontal straight design.

holes. Developed in 1995, this technique has improved the surgical speed of implantation of the patellar component, with no reported compromise in fixation or function of the implant.

WEAR PROPERTIES OF MOBILE BEARINGS AND FIXED BEARINGS

Examination of retrieved tibiofemoral and patellofemoral bearing surfaces has demonstrated a high clinical wear rate in nonconforming fixed bearing knee replacements, especially in combination with poor quality polyethylene and gamma radiation in air sterilization (5,27–30). Similar retrieval analyses of meniscal bearings, rotating-platform bearings, and rotating patellar bearings demonstrated significantly less wear than with fixed bearings (20). Although mobile bearings allow reduced contact stress, they can be overloaded to failure by excessive weight, excessive activity, malalignment, or a combination of these factors. However, by their nature, spherically surfaced mobile bearings accommodate malalignment without overload more easily than fixed bearings. Whether the overall knee alignment is in neutral (5 degrees valgus) or not, the spherical bearing surface always sees congruent contact with the femoral component as compared with a flat-on-flat bearing surface that becomes overloading during normal condylar lift-off (Fig. 15).

FIXATION OF MOBILE BEARINGS

The use of methylmethacrylate bone cement was the initial adjunctive method of bony attachment for the first LCS unicompartmental meniscal bearing device used in 1977 (18) and for subsequent bicompartmental and tricompartmental devices.

The tibial fixation surface of the LCS unicompartmental knee replacement has a flat tibial loading plate and a short-angled stem to resist tipping and shear loads. Bicruciate-retaining LCS tibial components use three short fixation fins for anchorage, whereas PCR LCS meniscal bearing and LCS rotating-platform tibial components use a short, conical metaphyseal fixation stem centered in the proximal tibia. All femoral components use shallow cement-locking pockets and centralized femoral fixation pegs.

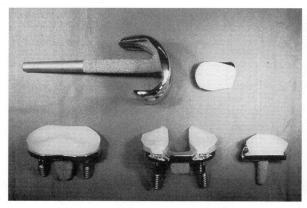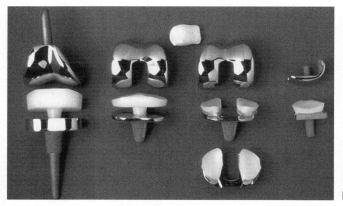

FIG. 16. A: Porous-coated low contact stress knee replacements with adjunctive 6.5-mm cancellous screw fixation, early 1981. **B:** Porous-coated low contact stress knee replacements without screw fixation, late 1981.

The rotating bearing patellar replacement uses cruciform fin geometry for fixation. This geometry reinforces the thin metal plate against torsional failure and reinforces the patellar remnant against fractures while engaging the patellar bone stock sufficiently to prevent loosening.

Cementless fixation with sintered-bead cobalt-chromium-molybdenum porous coating on the cobalt-chromium-molybdenum substrate using the same articulating and fixation geometries was first used clinically in early 1981. Bicruciate retaining and rotating-platform tibial components were developed with four screw holes and spherical seats. These implants used 6.5-mm cancellous bone screws to augment fixation (Fig. 16A).

Concerns over fretting corrosion, screw breakage, osteolysis, and potential neurovascular injuries from screw penetration led the developers away from screw fixation later in the same year. These early concerns are now complications that have been documented by several authors in other cementless knee devices (27,30,31).

Press-fit non–screw-fixed mobile bearing knee replacements with porous coating have been in successful clinical use since 1981 (Fig. 16B). Twenty-year rotating-platform studies have demonstrated a 99.4% overall fixation survivorship with these devices.

CLINICAL APPLICATION OF MOBILE BEARINGS

Unicompartmental Knee Replacement

Unicompartmental meniscal bearings are well adapted for knee replacement because they allow retention of both cruciate ligaments and allow the normal forward and backward translational movement of the femur on the tibia as well as axial rotation and varus-valgus movement with excellent congruity of the bearing surfaces. The Oxford meniscal bearing unicompartmental device has had excellent success when used as a medial unicompartmental replacement (7) but has functioned less consistently as a lateral compartment replacement because of significant dislocation problems (8).

The cementless LCS unicompartmental knee replacement was approved by the FDA Orthopaedic Advisory Panel in August 1991 and released for general use by the FDA in November 1992 after successful completion of an FDA-IDE clinical trial. Good or excellent results using a strict knee scoring scale (32) were seen in 98.4% of 122 patients followed for 2 to 6 years (mean of 3.3 years). One bearing fractured after trauma, and one tibial component loosened in a patient with posttraumatic osteoporotic bone deficiency. Progressive disease in the opposite knee compartment was an additional cause for revision. Such disorders represent current failure mechanisms for this device and are now considered contraindications.

Unicompartmental Oxford meniscal bearings showed a minimal wear rate of 0.03 mm per year, attesting to the concept of increased congruity decreases the wear rate. (33) Survivorship of the cemented device was 98% at 10 years in the developer's series (34) and 90% at 5 years in a National Swedish Arthroplasty study. Bearing dislocation was the major problem leading to failure in both studies.

Bicompartmental Knee Replacement

The articulating geometry of the femoral component is critical to the success or failure of the patellar component. A bispherical, continuous-surface-of-revolution femoral groove matching a bispherical congruently tracking patellar component will provide for a long service life for the patellar bearing. This same femoral groove can match the anatomic patellar geometry and can allow retention of the natural patella, with highly predictable results (35). No difference has been reported between bicompartmental (retention of natural patella) and tricompartmental (replaced patella) knee replacements, using the unique femoral groove of the LCS design (35), in a 10-year clinical series of 52 patients in whom one patella was replaced and the other patella was retained, as reported by Keblish et al. (36).

Such predictability can allow patellar retention in patients such as farmers or laborers who require repetitive squatting loads that may increase patellar component wear. Additionally, patellar retention in conditions such as patella infera, patella alta, or hypoplasia can facilitate central tracking without fear of early knee replacement failure (37). Finally, those patients with previous patellectomies can undergo a patellar tendon bone grafting (Fig. 17) (38) and enjoy a well-functioning bicompartmental replacement with improvement in both quadriceps leverage and tibiofemoral dislocation resistance.

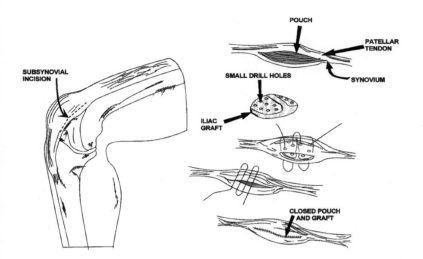

FIG. 17. Technique for patellar tendon bone grafting in the previously patellectomized knee.

Tricompartmental Knee Replacement

Retaining both viable cruciate ligaments as a concept is appealing because normal knee kinematics depends on the anterior-posterior translation of the femur on the tibia, which is under the direct control of these intact structures (39). Ligament loads greater than body weight have been recorded for all knee ligaments.

Thus, in theory at least, in the absence of each ligament structure, these loads would need to be carried by the remaining ligaments and perhaps transferred to the prosthesis itself. As such, retention of all load-bearing ligaments would be ideal if normal kinematic knee motion were allowed. Based on these concepts, the bicruciate-retaining, LCS meniscal bearing knee replacement was developed and successfully tested in FDA-IDE clinical trials (20).

The use of three fixation fins rather than a central conical peg has led to a greater incidence of tibial component loosening with this device than with central conical peg devices (40). Also, reports from Hamelynck (41) in Holland indicate that loosening of these tri-finned components is increased in patients with previous high tibial osteotomies or proximal tibial fractures. Such conditions appear to alter blood flow and impede osseointegration in cementless bicruciate-retaining knees and as such remain contraindications to their cementless use. Additionally, early or late rupture of the anterior cruciate ligament (ACL) degrades the arthroplasty to the level of an ACL-deficient knee in many cases and raises doubts as to whether ACL retention should be attempted in other than circumstances of youth, good bone stock, and a perfect ACL, which is a rare situation at best (9).

The overall failure rate of bicruciate-retaining, meniscal bearing TKR as a result of fracture, dislocation, or bearing wear-through has been two out of 34 cemented TKRs, or 5.8%, and four out of 59 cementless TKRs, or 6.7%, in a series of primary and multiply-operated knee replacements followed for 0.2 to 21 years (mean of 8.8 years). One undersized, cemented tibial component loosened after 2 years and one cemented tibial component loosened secondary to trauma after 6.6 years. One cementless post–high tibial osteotomy tibial component loosened after 5 months. The survivorship of these primary, cemented, bicruciate-retaining meniscal bearing TKRs using an end point of revision of any component was 72% at 18 years. The primary cementless bicruciate survivorship was 81.2% at 18 years.

Retention of the PCL has been reported to improve quadriceps leverage, increase extension torque, and improve flexion over cruciate-sacrificing designs (42). In fixed bearings, this increased motion and function are related to increased posterior rollback or rollforward on the incongruent tibial bearing surface, which increases wear over cruciate-sacrificing, fixed bearing designs (43). A meniscal bearing device potentially allows more congruent rollback or rollforward in flexion to improve wear resistance over fixed bearing designs.

The Oxford meniscal knee, however, functioned poorly with only an intact PCL. Therefore, the Oxford knee device developers did not recommend using the Oxford device in any ACL-deficient knee and cautioned against the use of any meniscal bearing (7) device in the absence of the ACL. The significant dislocation rate of 9.3% reported in 1990 for use of rotating-platform and PCR LCS knee replacements would tend to support this concept (44). However, as was pointed out in rebuttal to that report (45), meniscal or rotating bearings require adequate control of the flexion and extension gaps during surgery to maintain contact stability of the prosthesis. Thus, failure to maintain flexion and extension gap stability will compromise the results of any mobile bearing knee replacement, whether both, one, or no cruciate ligaments are preserved.

The successful FDA-IDE cementless clinical trial of the PCR meniscal bearing LCS knee replacement documented the ability to retain only the PCL and maintain long-term stability and function with a meniscal bearing device (21).

Tibial component subluxations and dislocations were seen in knees with poor flexion stability and were noted to be technique-related rather than implant-related. Early or late PCL instability remains a concern for this arthroplasty. Intraoperative diligence to avoid any release of this ligament attachment is desirable, and if PCL compromise is noted, replacement to a centrally stabilized rotating platform is advisable for long-term stability and function.

The overall failure rate of cementless PCR meniscal bearing TKR as a result of fracture, dislocation, or bearing wear-through has been six out of 140 TKRs, or 4.3%, in a series of primary and multiply operated knee replacements followed for 0.25 to 16 years (mean of 8.9 years). No loosening of any component was seen. The survivorship of these primary cementless PCR meniscal bearing knee replacements using revision as an end

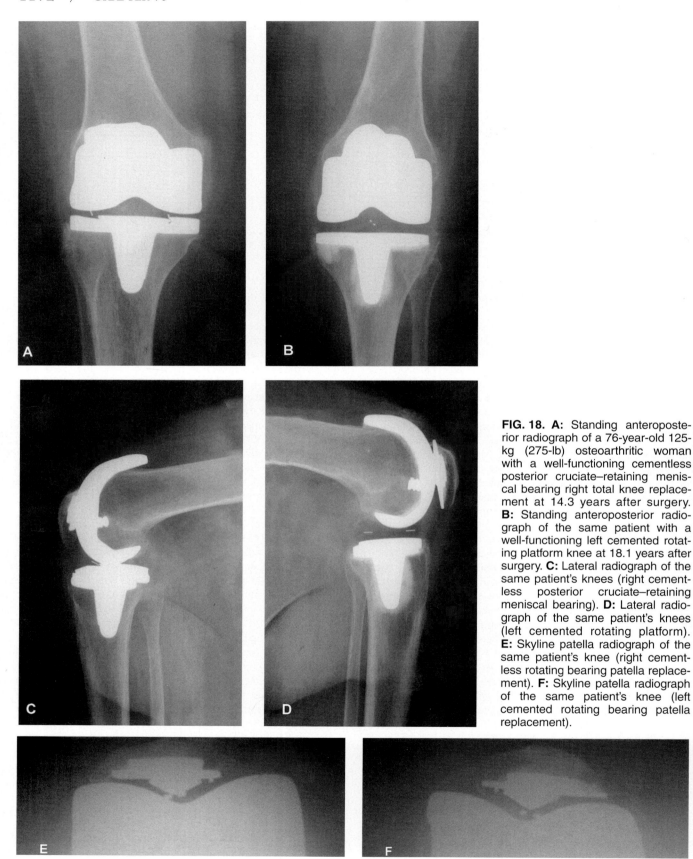

FIG. 18. A: Standing anteroposterior radiograph of a 76-year-old 125-kg (275-lb) osteoarthritic woman with a well-functioning cementless posterior cruciate–retaining meniscal bearing right total knee replacement at 14.3 years after surgery. **B:** Standing anteroposterior radiograph of the same patient with a well-functioning left cemented rotating platform knee at 18.1 years after surgery. **C:** Lateral radiograph of the same patient's knees (right cementless posterior cruciate–retaining meniscal bearing). **D:** Lateral radiograph of the same patient's knees (left cemented rotating platform). **E:** Skyline patella radiograph of the same patient's knee (right cementless rotating bearing patella replacement). **F:** Skyline patella radiograph of the same patient's knee (left cemented rotating bearing patella replacement).

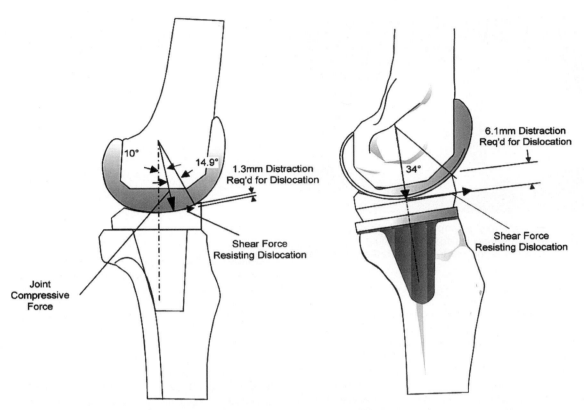

FIG. 19. Comparison of total condylar and original low contact stress rotating-platform articulating geometries in the lateral plane.

point was 83% at 16 years (46). A similar study by Jordan et al. (47) demonstrated a 94.6% survivorship of PCR cementless meniscal bearing knee replacements at 8 years, with 3.6% revised because of meniscal bearing wear or dislocation. Sanchez-Sotelo et al. reported on 83 PCR cementless meniscal bearing TKRs at 4 to 8 years follow-up (mean of 5.2 years), documenting two meniscal bearing dislocations but no wear or loosening problems (48). A long-term radiograph of a right cementless PCR meniscal bearing device is shown in an obese patient with bilateral knee replacements in Figures 18A to 18C.

Cruciate sacrifice is often desirable in certain conditions, such as fixed flexion, fixed valgus, and some severe fixed varus deformities. It is often unavoidable in conditions in which significant trauma, rheumatoid arthritis, or inflammatory arthritis has destroyed these structures. In such cases, a centrally stabilized device with long-term fixation and excellent wear properties would be most desirable. The cemented total condylar knee replacement has been used in such cases of elderly patients over a 10- to 15-year period, with exceptionally good results and reported 90% survivorship, using revision as an end point (11).

Considering these results to represent the standard for future design comparisons, any cemented or cementless cruciate-sacrificing design should demonstrate at least a 90% 10-year survivorship and have contact stresses less than the total condylar device to merit any attention (49). Additionally, because total condylar range of motion was considered to be only fair (85 to 95 degrees) and dislocations fairly frequent, any new design should improve on motion and dislocation resistance.

The LCS rotating-platform knee replacement represents an improvement over the total condylar device in concept and in clinical performance. Conceptually, the deeper engagement of the rotatable, spherically congruent surfaces allows lower contact stresses during normal walking, namely 25 MPa for total condylar and 4.9 MPa for LCS (50). This deeper engagement also improves dislocation resistance over the total condylar device (Fig. 19). The LCS device uses a conical central tibial component stem that approximates the successful total condylar stem. Thus, similar fixation is achieved with rotational relief of shear stresses to tibial fixation with the rotating-platform design.

FDA-IDE clinical trials have demonstrated long-term safety and efficacy of the rotating-platform in a wide variety of primary and multiply operated cases in both cemented and cementless applications. The FDA Orthopaedic Advisory Panel recommended approval of the cemented rotating-platform device in 1984 (20) and the cementless device in 1991 (23), making the rotating-platform the first and, currently, the only total knee device in the United States to be approved for both cemented and cementless applications.

The overall failure rate of rotating-platform TKRs as a result of bearing dislocation has been two out of 64 cemented TKRs, or 3.1%, and two out of 169 cementless TKRs, or 1.2%, in a series of primary and multiply operated knee replacements followed for 0.25 to 19.5 years (mean of 7.5 years) in cemented cases and 0.25 to 19.0 years (mean of 8 years) in cementless cases. Two cementless rotating-platform bearings (1.2%) devel-

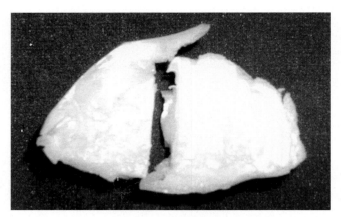

FIG. 20. The dominant mechanisms of mechanical failure are wear-through of the bearing on the lateral facet and transverse bearing fractures of the gamma irradiated-in-air meniscal bearings.

oped severe wear, requiring revision in multiply operated cases; no fractured bearings were seen in either group. One tibial component loosening and one femoral component loosening (3.2%) were seen in the cemented rotating-platform group; and one tibial component loosening (0.6%) was seen in a multiply operated post–high tibial osteotomy patient in the cementless group. The survivorship of these primary cemented rotating-platform knee replacements using revision as an end point was 97.7% at 20 years (46). The primary cementless rotating-platform survivorship was 98.3% at 18 years (46). In two independent studies, Sorrells (51) reported 94.7% cementless rotating-platform survivorship at 11 years, whereas Callaghan et al. (52) reported 100% cemented rotating-platform survivorship at 12 years. A long-term radiograph of a left cemented rotating-platform device is shown in Figures 18D to 18F.

Rotating Bearing Patella Replacement

Failures of the rotating bearing patella have been rare and usually associated with displaced patellar fractures, malposition, subluxation, or excessive, repetitive hyperflexion loads.

The overall complications of rotating bearing patellar replacements that required revision surgery in 515 knees originally followed for 6 months to 11 years (53) and now followed for 8 to 19 years (mean of 12.5 years) were five of 515, or 0.97%. Wear-through of the bearing on the lateral facet and transverse bearing fractures have been the dominant mechanisms of mechanical failure (Fig. 20). These have been associated with unrecognized poor-quality polyethylene and gamma radiation oxidation, which has also negatively affected the tibial bearings of the past two decades.

REVISION TOTAL KNEE REPLACEMENT

Aseptic failed knee replacement surgery is usually accompanied by a loss of bone stock and a loss of the cruciate ligaments. In such cases, a centrally stabilized rotating-platform device with intramedullary stems can be used to successfully salvage a wide variety of complex pathologies (54). These stems can be fixed to the femoral or tibial components or be modular constructs with the ability to increase or decrease diameter as well as length, similar to that found in current revision hip replacements (55).

Attention to surgical technique, with regard to flexion-extension stability as well as varus-valgus ligamentous balancing, remains crucial to revision success. In 5.8% of 86 revision rotating platform cases, persistent instability continued to be a problem, requiring a thicker rotating bearing, the use of a total condylar III (56) or a rotating-hinge design achieve acceptable stability. Currently, most of these instability problems have been eliminated by use of the rotational stop device (25).

FUTURE DIRECTIONS OF MOBILE BEARING KNEE REPLACEMENT

Meniscal bearings represent the logical approach for future development of human knee joint replacements (57). This fact is supported by long-term survivorship and contact-stress studies, which favor mobile bearings over fixed bearings in a wide variety of clinical applications varying from unicompartmental to tricompartmental arthroplasty (5,7,9,12,40,58–63). It is important to explore alternative bearing geometries (57) and biomaterials, such as wear-resistant titanium nitride ceramic coatings and more durable polyethylene bearings, to optimize future designs. However, be wary of intercondylar posts and excessive mechanical stops that may contribute to increased wear or loosening. Such designs need to be clinically proved before being universally accepted.

In the meantime, bearing exchange techniques are currently available to maintain well-fixed metallic components while replacing worn or broken bearings with improved polyethylene that has been gas sterilized to enhance future wear properties. Such techniques allow extended performance of currently available mobile bearing devices with same-day or overnight-stay surgery. Patient acceptance of elective bearing exchange surgery over the past 5 years has been extremely favorable, with patients reporting less pain and faster recovery than they experienced after their original primary knee replacement procedure.

Future mobile bearing knee designs should continue to provide these important features of wear resistance and bearing exchangeability to maintain optimal knee function for a maximum duration with a minimum of surgical intervention.

REFERENCES

1. Rand JA, Chao EY, Stauffer RN. Kinematic rotating hinge total knee arthroplasty. *J Bone Joint Surg Am* 1987;69:489–497.
2. Riley D, Woodyard JE. Long term results of Geomedic total knee replacement. *J Bone Joint Surg Br* 1985;67:548–550.
3. Lewallen DG, Bryan RS, Peterson LF. Polycentric total knee arthroplasty: a 10-year followup study. *J Bone Joint Surg Am* 1984;66:1211–1218.
4. Collier JP, Mayor MB, McNamara JL, et al. Analysis of the failure of 122 polyethylene inserts from uncemented tibial knee components. *Clin Orthop* 1991;273:232–242.
5. Engh GA, Dwyer DA, Hanes CK. Polyethylene wear of metal-backed tibial components in total and unicompartmental knee prosthesis. *J Bone Joint Surg Br* 1992;74:9–17.
6. Goodfellow J, O'Connor J. The mechanics of the knee and prosthesis design. *J Bone Joint Surg Br* 1978;60:358–368.

7. Carr AJ, Keyes C, Miller RK, et al. Medial unicompartmental arthroplasty: a survival study of the Oxford meniscal knee. *Clin Orthop* 1993;295:205–213.

8. Goodfellow JW, O'Connor JS. Clinical results of the Oxford knee surface arthroplasty of the tibio-femoral joint with a meniscal bearing prosthesis. *Clin Orthop* 1986;205:21–42.

9. Buechel FF, Pappas MJ. New Jersey LCS Knee Replacement System: 10 year evaluation of meniscal bearings. *Orthop Clin North Am* 1989;20:147–177.

10. Ranawat CS, Flynn WF, Saddler S, et al. Long-term results of the total condylar knee arthroplasty. A 15-year survivorship study. *Clin Orthop* 1993;286:94–102.

11. Scuderi GR, Insall JN, Windsor RE. Survivorship of cemented knee replacements. *J Bone Joint Surg Br* 1989;71:798–803.

12. Buechel FF, Pappas MJ, Makris G. Evaluation of contact stress in metal-backed patellar replacements: a predictor of survivorship. *Clin Orthop* 1991;273:190–197.

13. Wright TM, Timnac CM, Stulberg SD, et al. Wear of polyethylene in total joint replacements. Observations of retrieved PCA knee implants. *Clin Orthop* 1992;276:126–134.

14. Bourne RB, Goodfellow JW, O'Connor JJ. A functional analysis of various knee arthroplasties. *Trans Orthop Res* 1978;156.

15. Buechel FF, Pappas MJ, DePalma AF. Floating-socket total shoulder replacement: anatomical, biomechanical and surgical rationale. *J Biomed Mater Res* 1978;12:89–114.

16. Buechel-Pappas total shoulder system implants and instruments. South Orange, NJ: Endotec, 1992.

17. Buechel FF. Total ankle replacement—state of the art. In: Jahas MH, ed. *Disorders of the foot and ankle: surgical and medical management.* Philadelphia: WB Saunders, 1991:2671–2687.

18. Buechel FF, Pappas MJ. The New Jersey Low-Contact-Stress Knee Replacement System: biomechanical rationale and review of the first 123 cemented cases. *Arch Orthop Trauma Surg* 1986;105:197–204.

19. Pilliar PM, Cameron UH, Welsh RP, et al. Radiographic and morphologic studies of load-bearing porous-surfaced structured implants. *Clin Orthop* 1981;156:249–257.

20. Buechel FF, Pappas MJ. *New Jersey integrated total knee replacement system: biomechanical analysis and clinical evaluation of 918 cases.* U.S. Food and Drug Administration panel presentation; Silver Spring, MD; July 11, 1984.

21. Buechel FF, Pappas MJ. *New Jersey LCS posterior cruciate retaining total knee replacement: clinical, radiographic, statistical, and survivorship analyses of 395 cement-less cases performed by 13 surgeons.* U.S. Food and Drug Administration panel presentation; Rockville, MD; June 1, 1990.

22. Buechel FF, Pappas MJ. *New Jersey LCS unicompartmental knee replacement: clinical, radiographic, statistical and survivorship analyses of 106 cementless cases performed by 7 surgeons.* U.S. Food and Drug Administration panel presentation; Rockville, MD; Aug. 16, 1991.

23. Buechel FF, Sorrels B, Pappas MJ. *New Jersey Rotating Platform total knee replacement: clinical, radiographic, statistical, and survivorship analyses of 346 cases performed by 16 surgeons.* U.S. Food and Drug Administration panel presentation; Gaithersburg, MD; Nov. 22, 1991.

24. Buechel FF. Cementless meniscal bearing knee arthroplaasty: 7- to 12-year outcome analysis. *Orthopedics* 1994;17:833–836.

25. Buechel FF. Recurrent LCS rotating platform dislocation in revision total knee replacement: mechanism, management and report to two cases. *Orthopaedics* 2002 (in press).

26. Weaver JK, Derkash RS, Greenwald AS. Difficulties with bearing dislocation and breakage using a movable bearing total knee replacement system. *Clin Orthop* 1993;290:244–252.

27. Collier JP, Mayor MB, Surprenant VA, et al. The biomechanical problems of polyethylene as a bearing surface. *Clin Orthop* 1990;261:107–113.

28. Bohl JR, Bohl WR, Postak PD, et al. The effects of shelf life on clinical outcome for gamma sterilized polyethylene tibial component. *Clin Orthop* 1999;367:28–38.

29. Landy M, Walker PA. Wear in condylar replacement knees. A 10 year follow-up. *Trans Orthop Res Soc* 1985;10:96.

30. Peter PC, Engh GA, Dwyer KA. Osteolysis after total knee arthroplasty without cement. *J Bone Joint Surg Am* 1992;74:864–876.

31. Schatzker J, Home JG, Sumner-Smith G. The effect of movement on the holding power of screws in bone. *Clin Orthop* 1975;111:257–262.

32. Buechel FF. A simplified evaluation system for the rating of knee function. *Orthop Rev* 1982;11:97–101.

33. Psychoyios V, Crawford RW, O'Connor JJ, et al. Wear of congruent meniscal bearings in unicompartmental knee. *J Bone Joint Surg Br* 1998;80:970–982.

34. Murray DW, Goodfellow JW, O'Connor JJ. The Oxford medial unicompartmental arthroplasty: a ten-year survival study. *J Bone Joint Surg Br* 1998;80:983–989.

35. Buechel FF, Pappas MJ. New Jersey Meniscal Bearing Knee [July 27, 1982, patent no. 4,340,1978].

36. Keblish PA, Varma AK, Greenwald AS. Patellar resurfacing or retention in total knee arthroplasty. A prospective study of patients with bilateral replacements. *J Bone Joint Surg Br* 1994;76:930–937.

37. Buechel FF. Treatment of the patella in revision total knee surgery using a rotating-bearing patellar replacement. *Orthop Rev Suppl* 1990;75–82.

38. Buechel FF. Patella tendon bone grafting for patellectomized patients undergoing knee replacement. *Clin Orthop* 1991;271:72–78.

39. Tria AJ, Klein KS. *An illustrated guide to the knee.* New York: Churchill Livingstone, 1992.

40. Buechel FF, Pappas MJ. Long-term survivorship analysis of cruciate sparing versus cruciate sacrificing knee prostheses using meniscal bearings. *Clin Orthop* 1990;260:162–169.

41. Hamelynck KJ. The total knee prosthesis: indications and complications. *Ned Tijdschr Geneeskd* 1998;142:2030–2034.

42. Ochsner JL, Gonley J. Functional comparison of posterior cruciate-retaining versus cruciate sacrificed total knee arthroplasty. *Clin Orthop* 1988;236:36–43.

43. Ewald FC, Jacobs MA, Miegel RE, et al. Kinematic total knee replacement. *J Bone Joint Surg Am* 1984;66:1032–1040.

44. Bert JM. Dislocation/subluxation of meniscal bearing elements after New Jersey low-contact stress total knee arthroplasty. *Clin Orthop* 1990;254:211–217.

45. Buechel FF. New Jersey low-contact-stress (LCS) knee replacement system [letter, comment]. *Clin Orthop* 1991;264:309–311.

46. Buechel FF Sr., Buechel FF Jr., Pappas MJ, et al. Twenty-year evaluation of meniscal bearing and rotating platform knee replacements. *Clin Orthop* 2001;388:41–50.

47. Jordan LR, Olivio JL, Voorhorst PE. Survivorship analysis of cementless meniscal bearing total knee arthroplasty. *Clin Orthop* 1997;338:119–123.

48. Sanchez-Sotelo J, Ordonez JM, Prats SB, et al. Results and complications of the low contact stress knee prosthesis. *J Arthroplasty* 1999;14:815–821.

49. Buechel FF, Pappas MJ, Greenwald AS. Use of survivorship and contact stress analyses to predict the long term efficacy of new generation joint replacement designs: a model for FDA device evaluation. *Orthop Rev* 1991;20:50–55.

50. Pappas MJ, Makris G, Buechel FF. Biomaterials and clinical applications: evaluation of contact stresses in metal-plastic knee replacements. In: Pizzoferrato PG, ed. *Biomaterials for hard tissue applications.* Amsterdam: Elsevier, 1987:259–264.

51. Sorrells RB. The rotating platform mobile bearing TKA. *Orthopaedics* 1996;19:793–796.

52. Callaghan JJ, Squire MW, Goetz DD, et al. Cemented rotating-platform total knee replacement. *J Bone Joint Surg Am* 2000;82:705–711.

53. Buechel FF, Rosa RA, Pappas MJ. A metal backed, rotating-bearing patellar prosthesis to lower contact stress: an 11-year clinical study. *Clin Orthop* 1969;248:34–49.

54. Buechel FF. Knee arthroplasty in post-traumatic arthritis. *J Arthroplasty* 2002;17:63–68.

55. Schramm M, Wirtz DC, Holzwarth U, et al. The Morse taper junction in modular hip replacement—a biomechanical and retrieval analysis. *Biomed Tech* 2000;45:105–109.

56. Hohl WM, Crawfurd E, Zelicof SB, et al. The Total Condylar III prosthesis in complex knee reconstruction. *Clin Orthop* 1991;273:91–97.

57. Callaghan JJ, Insall JN, Greenwald AS, et al. Mobile-bearing knee replacement concepts and results. *J Bone Joint Surg Am* 2000;82:1020–1041.

58. Bartel DL, Bicknell VL, Wright TM. The effect of conformity,

thickness, and material on stress on ultra-high molecular weight polyethylene components for total joint replacement. *J Bone Joint Surg Am* 1986;68:1041–1051.

59. Huang CH. Clinical results of the New Jersey Low Contact Stress knee arthroplasty with two to five years follow-up. *J Orthop Surg* 1991;8:295–303.

60. Huson A, Spoor CW, Verbout AJ. A model of the human knee derived from kinematic principles and its relevance for endoprosthesis design. *Acta Morphol Neerl Scand* 1989;270:45–55.

61. Moran CC, Pinder IM, Lees TA, et al. Survivorship analysis of the uncemented porous coated anatomic knee replacement. *J Bone Joint Surg Am* 1991;73:848–857.

62. Nielsen PT, Hansen EB, Rechnagel K. Cementless total knee arthroplasty in unselected cases of osteoarthritis and rheumatoid arthritis: a 3 year follow-up study of 103 cases. *J Arthroplasty* 1992;7:137–143.

63. Schlepckow P. Three dimensional kinematics of total knee replacement systems. *Arch Orthop Trauma Surg* 1992;3:204–209.

CHAPTER 80

Constrained Total Knee Replacement

David G. Nazarian and Robert E. Booth, Jr.

Knee arthroplasty, which had its beginnings as early as the nineteenth century, has enjoyed nearly continuous improvement in success (1,26,35,52,58). The excellent results of this procedure are due to the dual advancements in surgical technique and in prosthetic technology. Early interpositional designs failed to allow for the complexities of natural knee motion, although they provided appropriate stability through the natural contours of the osteochondral surfaces (2). Stability was initially achieved with the development of highly constrained rigid-hinge devices (Fig. 1). These designs restricted rotation and translation of the implant and allowed flexion and extension in only one plane (3,4). Although devices of this linked design provided immediate relief, surgeons were confronted with an extremely high rate of complication and failure (5–8,10,12–20). The restricted rotation and translation of these rigid hinges transfer significant stresses to the prosthesis-cement-bone interfaces because the soft tissues provide no-load dampening effect. Devices such as the Walldius hinge ultimately failed because of loosening, bone loss, and patellofemoral complications (Fig. 2). Early flawed designs contributed to the understanding of knee joint mechanics and its multidimensional nature. The evolution of the understanding of knee kinematics and of constraint, conformity, and motion has allowed surgeons to develop more advanced prosthetic devices with improved clinical results. The lack of rotation allowed in a rigid-hinge design was overcome by the development of rotating-hinge devices such as the spherocentric knee prosthesis. These devices have been improved by availability of additional sizing options, modularity, and a more durable linkage.

Simultaneously, other nonlinked knee designs were being introduced into clinical practice. Resurfacing arthroplasty devices such as the Duocondylar knee became popular. They were followed by the development of the cruciate-sacrificing total condylar design. The problem inherent in these cruciate-sacrificing implants was the potential for tibiofemoral dislocation. This led to the development and advancement of the posterior cruciate ligament (PCL)–sparing and PCL-substituting knees. Subluxation of these articulations was resisted by the PCL or by a post-and-cam mechanism. These knees however, require competence of the collateral ligaments for appropriate stability and function.

The introduction of the semiconstrained category of components such as the constrained condylar knee addressed situations involving collateral ligament attenuation in knees with marked coronal plane deformity or revision surgery. The increased popularity of these semiconstrained prosthetic knees has significantly reduced the need for the highly constrained linked designs.

CHOICE OF A DESIGN

Perioperative Evaluation

As the design of prosthetic devices continues to advance, the surgeon remains the ultimate arbiter of which device may best serve each particular patient. Careful preoperative evaluation of the condition and deformity of the knee helps the physician choose the device that is most appropriate. The two most important criteria in this evaluation are the condition of the soft tissue constraints and the condition of the bone available for implant support. The assessment of the soft tissue envelope involves an evaluation of the PCL and the collateral ligaments. The PCL is best examined with the knee flexed to 90 degrees, whereas the collateral ligaments should be assessed with the knee in both full extension and at 90 degrees of flexion. One may also assess collateral ligament competence after induction of anesthesia for primary and revision arthroplasty. Furthermore, stress radiographs can be performed to help distinguish ligamentous incompetence from bone deficiencies. Although preoperative planning is essential to a well-performed procedure, the surgeon's ability

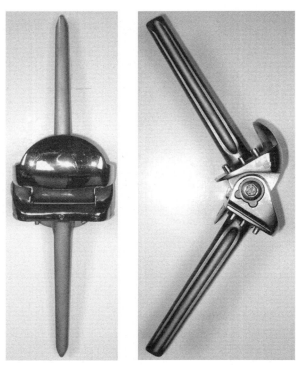

A,B

FIG. 1. Front **(A)** and side **(B)** views of a nonrotating rigid-hinge device designed for intramedullary cement fixation.

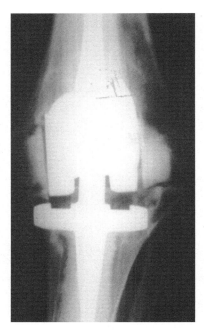

FIG. 2. Anteroposterior radiograph of a loose rigid-hinge device at 3.4 years after surgery.

to adapt to intraoperative discoveries ultimately helps ensure success of the arthroplasty.

Constraint in Total Knee Arthroplasty

The amount of constraint provided by the soft tissue envelope most often guides the decision in prosthetic device selection (Fig. 3). Total knee implants are designed with a varying degree of inherent constraint within the femoral tibial articulation (9). The implant that provides the least amount of mechanical constraint that will achieve a stable knee is often the device recommended for use (9,25,68). The less intrinsically constrained the device used, the lower the amount of force transmission to the implant-cement-bone interfaces. The more highly constrained devices spare the soft tissue envelope from absorbing the multiplanar forces around the knee. A simplified classification system of prosthetic knees separates these devices into two types: surface replacement and constrained design.

Surface replacement devices are further subdivided into PCL-sacrificing, PCL-substituting, and PCL-retaining designs. The cruciate-sacrificing total condylar knee was the forerunner of the modern total knee design. This device gained sagittal plane stability through a curved tibial articular surface, whereas coronal plane stability was achieved with a median intercondylar eminence (38–42). The conforming tibial and femoral surfaces of this design have mistakenly led some to link the terms *conformity* and *constraint*. Conformity occurs when the tibial and femoral surfaces have similar radii of curvature. Constraint, however, is provided by the prosthetic surface contours and the periarticular soft tissues (78). A curved tibial articular surface may provide constraint in the sagittal plane but may lack ideal surface conformity.

A greater understanding of knee kinematics led to the development of PCL-substituting and -retaining designs. The cruciate-retaining prostheses were imagined to more closely replicate knee kinematics, and they relied on the PCL to provide increased stability and femoral rollback (26,30–33,36,37) (Fig. 4). These devices have traditionally had a more flattened and therefore less constrained articulation to allow for femoral rollback. This round-on-flat design, however, may create greater point contact stress areas with higher polyethylene wear (70).

The cruciate-substituting devices were designed with greater tibial contouring (Fig. 5). These devices achieve sagittal plane stability and femoral rollback with a spine-on-cam mechanism. This cam mechanism provides no resistance to rotational or angular forces in the coronal (varus-valgus) plane, however, and relies solely on the collateral ligaments for stability in this regard. The cruciate-substituting and -retaining designs have had similar success regarding patient outcomes and implant survivability (26–29,31,34,43–46). Many surgeons feel that the posterior stabilized designs are more useful because the issue of cruciate ligament balancing is eliminated, whereas others maintain that PCL retention provides improved knee kinematics. Thus, the decision as to which of these devices to implant is based largely on surgical training, experience, and the amount of knee deformity (32,33,36,37).

Because the total condylar and posterior stabilized designs rely on appropriate collateral ligament tensioning, soft tissue laxity may lead to postoperative dislocations (49–51).

SEMICONSTRAINED DEVICES

The most constrained of the unlinked devices is the semiconstrained component such as the Zimmer constrained condylar knee or the Total Condylar III (Johnson & Johnson, Raynham,

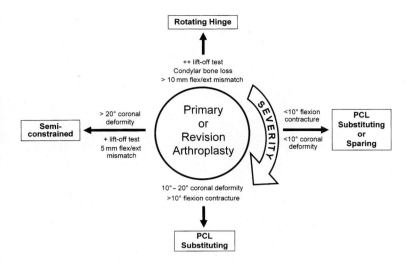

FIG. 3. Algorithm for choosing the level of constraint needed in primary or revision arthroplasty. +, positive result; ++ strongly positive result; ext, extension; flex, flexion; PCL, posterior cruciate ligament.

MA) (Fig. 6) (21–25,47,48,53,67). These devices are designed with intimately fitting cam-in-spine mechanisms that are broader and more elevated than in a posterior stabilized knee (74,77). These devices allow less than 2 degrees of internal or external rotation and 1.25 degrees of varus-valgus motion. In addition, these devices more effectively resist component dislocation

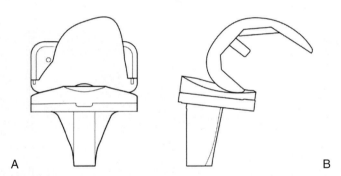

FIG. 4. Frontal **(A)** and side **(B)** views of NexGen posterior cruciate–retaining device showing minimal tibial femoral articular constraint.

because of the higher "jump distance" (distance above which the cam must travel before dissociating from the tibial spine) (Fig. 7). These more highly constrained devices are used in both primary and revision situations when there is partial collateral ligament incompetence or imbalance of the flexion extension gaps, or, less commonly, when an extensor mechanism allograft has been placed (74). The components are modular with augments and stem extensions available for both femoral and tibial bone deficiencies. The greater inherent constraint in the semiconstrained devices may transmit more significant shear forces into the bone-cement-prosthesis interfaces. Several reports have therefore recommended the simultaneous use of intramedullary stems to distribute these forces broadly into the periprosthetic bone and ensure adequate component alignment (59,65,66,69). The authors recommend the use of stem extensions when bone deficiencies require augments or allograft or for protection of the tibia when extensor allografting or tibial tubercle osteotomy is performed. There are favorable results with the use of both cemented and cementless stems (66). Bourne and Finlay showed that use of a 70-mm cementless stem decreases axial loads by 23% in a cadaveric study (69). Although some authors have found a higher loosening rate with the use of cementless stems, others advocate the use of these stems because the revision of a

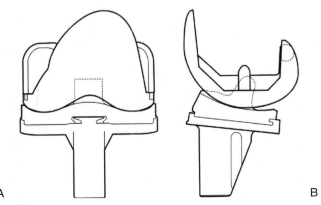

FIG. 5. Frontal **(A)** and side **(B)** views of posterior cruciate–substituting device with post-and-cam mechanism (NexGen posterior stabilized knee).

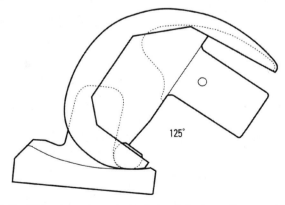

FIG. 6. Side view of semiconstrained device with more highly captured post-and-cam mechanism (NexGen constrained condylar knee).

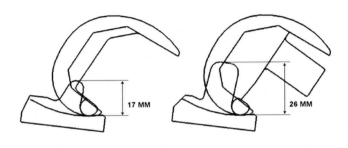

FIG. 7. Example of the different "jump distances" between a posterior stabilized and constrained condylar knee (Zimmer NexGen devices). LPS, Legacy posterior stabilized; LCCK, Legacy constrained condylar knee.

cemented stem presents a formidable surgical challenge. Of additional note, if the constrained condylar knee femoral component is used because of a bone deficiency but the collateral ligaments remain competent, a modular posterior stabilized tibial insert can be used. This replicates the less constrained posterior stabilized knee and is recommended by the authors in both primary and revision arthroplasty. If the medial collateral ligament is partially attenuated, the surgeon may place the arthroplasty in 3 to 4 degrees of valgus rather than 5 to 7 degrees. This transfers the mechanical axis to a more medial than normal position and therefore subjects the medial collateral ligament to less strain. The disadvantage of this technique is the potential for increased shear forces on the implant interfaces.

Semiconstrained devices have enjoyed excellent clinical success in both difficult primary and revision arthroplasty. Easley et al. reported on the use of the constrained condylar knee in 44 arthritic valgus knees with an average 7.8 year follow-up (67). These patients enjoyed an average postoperative knee score of 89.6 points with no cases of radiographically detected loosening, prosthetic failure, or flexion instability. In one study of revision arthroplasty, the survivorship of the constrained condylar knee device was 98% at 7 years, with 80% of the patients obtaining a good or excellent result at this duration (11,74). Several series, however, do report a 70% incidence of radiolucent lines. These lines tended not to be progressive and do not correlate with radiographically determined failure. Trousdale et al. have reported the longest study of a semiconstrained device, with 80% of the Total Condylar III knees in place at an average of 15.3 years of follow-up (79).

LINKED PROSTHESES

Walldius designed the first fixed hinged prosthesis for primary total knee arthroplasty in 1953 (17). Poor results were observed with these devices because of loosening, infection, and patellofemoral problems (14,19). The lack of rotational freedom transmitted significant shear stresses to the bone-prosthesis interface. Metal-on-metal articulation also led to significant particulate debris, which may have contributed to the high infection rates. Furthermore, the rotational limitation of this device disallowed normal patellofemoral mechanics with an unacceptable level of patellofemoral subluxation. Therefore, the use of these arthroplasty devices has since been abandoned.

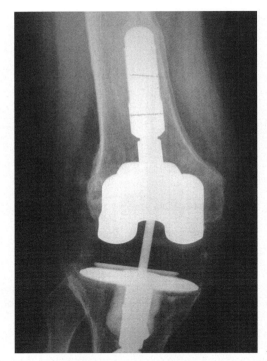

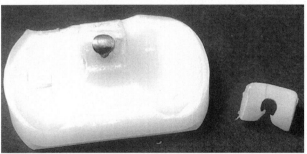

FIG. 8. A: Anteroposterior radiography of a semiconstrained knee with failure of the post-and-cam mechanism. **B:** Retrieved tibial insert from a semiconstrained device with a sheared tibial post.

The results with the use of the semiconstrained device when complete medial collateral ligament deficiency exists are less than satisfactory (21,22). Persistent instability of the knee may result because in a semiconstrained device the tibial spine alone is unable to overcome the significant rotational forces at the knee. The spine may therefore spin out of the constrained cam or may plastically deform until it is rendered incompetent (Fig. 8).

Situations in which there is a complete loss of the collateral ligaments with a very large flexion space, severe compromise of periarticular bone from fracture, or loss of the extensor mechanism necessitate the use of a rotating-hinge device (54–57,60–64). These devices have a metal-on-polyethylene axle bearing that allows internal and external rotation (Fig. 9).

The first generation of these devices used adapted ball and socket joints that allowed multiplanar motion with varus-valgus laxity and axial rotation (71,76). Despite the increased motion, these prostheses also were associated with a high rate of infection, loosening, and component fracture. Initially, the short-term results using the Kinematic rotating-hinge knee were also char-

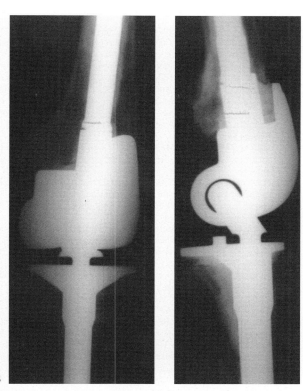

A,B

FIG. 9. Anteroposterior **(A)** and lateral **(B)** radiographic views of a rotating-hinge knee design (Finn knee).

acterized by similar rates of infection and loosening (55). Biomechanical analyses of the Kinematic rotating-hinge knee, however, showed levels of torsional stiffness and rotatory laxity similar to those of a normal knee (72). Understanding of the reasons for these high complication rates has led to improvement in the design of these prostheses. The shallow femoral groove was deepened, the all-polyethylene tibia was replaced with a metal-backed component, modular stems and augments were added, and the tibial femoral articulation was improved (73).

Lombardi reported short-term results on the use of 113 rotating-hinge devices for revision knee surgery and found a 5% incidence of femoral loosening (70). In a series reported by Springer et al., the all-cemented Kinematic rotating-hinge prosthesis was associated with relatively high rates of infection (14.5%), patellar instability (13%), component breakage (10%), and aseptic loosening in 69 knees (63). The results for revision knee arthroplasty using the S-ROM rotating-hinge device compared favorably with those for a group of less severely affected knees revised using a semiconstrained device, as reported by Barrack et al. (75). These authors further noted in a follow-up study that a group of 23 knees implanted with a rotating-hinge device exhibited no cases of loosening, one case of patellar instability, and no infections with an average 58 months of follow-up (64). The device was fixed with cement at the metaphyseal and bone surfaces, while cementless intramedullary stems filled the diaphyses. The success of this implant was attributed, in part, to the use of these canal-filling stems, which help ensure proper component alignment and prevent pathologic forces on the bone, implant, or interfaces. It is difficult to compare studies of these devices directly because of the heterogeneous nature of

the involved patients. Despite the emergence of improved results with these devices, it must be emphatically stated that a rotating-hinge knee arthroplasty device should be used only when a semiconstrained implant or allograft prosthetic composite will not adequately address a patient's soft tissue or bone deficiency.

SURGICAL TECHNIQUES

Once the preoperative assessment is completed, the surgeon should have available prosthetic devices with an appropriate level of inherent constraint. In primary arthroplasty, most minimally deformed knees can be treated with either a cruciate-sparing or cruciate-substituting design. Native knees that preoperatively have greater than a 10-degree flexion contracture or a 15-degree coronal plane deformity usually require significant recession of the PCL. Thus, these knees are often best treated with a cruciate-substituting design.

The authors use a posterior stabilized knee in most primary and revision situations. It is recommended, however, that a semiconstrained device always be available if the medial collateral ligament is felt to be partially incompetent during the procedure. The procession of steps should follow a readily repeatable sequence. The authors expose the knee through a median parapatellar approach, evert the patella, elevate the deep but not the superficial fibers of the medial collateral ligament, and dislocate the tibial femoral articulation. The tibia is cut at a 90-degree coronal angle and, in revision arthroplasty, this cut is performed after component and cement removal. A flat tibial surface later serves as a foundation for the remainder of the arthroplasty.

In primary arthroplasty, femoral rotation is determined by ligamentous tensioning in flexion, and the flexion gap is measured with calibrated spacer blocks. The distal femoral cut is performed to create a neutral mechanical axis and to equilibrate the extension gap with the flexion gap. After placement of the trial components, the knee should be tight without lift-off at 90 degrees of flexion and with 1 to 2 mm of play while at 0 degrees extension. The flexion tightness can be tested with a lift-off test. In this test the surgeon places his or her forearm under the patient's femur and lifts while using the opposite hand to stabilize the patient's foot on the operating table. There should be no lift-off of the components with approximately 30 lb of force (Fig. 10). If significant lift-off (more than 3 to 5 mm) occurs, then use of either a larger tibial spacer or a semiconstrained device is recommended.

In revision arthroplasty, after the femoral component and cement are removed, the appropriate component rotation is determined by finding the epicondylar axis. The level of the joint line can be determined by using the fibular head, the medial epicondyle, or the remaining meniscal scar. The femur is usually reconstructed with a posterior stabilized or constrained condylar knee. Stems, augments, and allograft are used to reconstruct a femur with significant bone deficiency. Once the femur is reconstructed, the flexion space is determined by trial placement of a posterior stabilized tibial insert, and the lift-off test is performed. The extension gap is equalized with the flexion gap by posterior capsular release or manipulation of the femoral position in space. Significant flexion lift-off, asymmetry of the flexion and extension gaps, or varus-valgus laxity (of more than 5 mm) requires the use of a semiconstrained tibial insert.

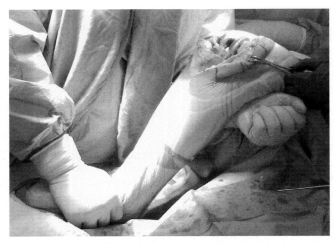

FIG. 10. Intraoperative lift-off test with knee in 90 degrees of flexion and 30-lb force exerted under patient's femur.

A rotating-hinge device is recommended when there is severe asymmetry of the flexion and extension gaps, complete incompetence of the medial collateral ligament, or severe loss of the femoral condyles. This rare salvage situation occurs with a frequency of 0.6% at the author's institution. These linked devices secure the knee with very large flexion and extension spaces. Implantation of a hinged knee involves maintaining an idealized notion of the knee, because many anatomic landmarks no longer remain. Femoral rotation can be based on the linea aspera when the condyles are not present, and tibial alignment is based on the position of the tibial tubercle. Adequate external rotation helps avoid patellofemoral subluxation. Although there is a polyethylene stop to prevent hyperextension, it is recommended that one fill the extension space with femoral augments or tibial polyethylene to avoid significant stress on this stop mechanism. Fixation of the device should be augmented with cement, and it is still a matter of debate as to whether the stems should be cemented or cementless. With the ever-expanding number of knee arthroplasties performed each year, the number of revision procedures and cases of ligamentous incompetence consequently will also grow. Therefore, the arthroplasty surgeon should be familiar with and prepared for the use of all levels of device constraint in primary, revision, and salvage procedures.

REFERENCES

1. Ferguson W. Excision of the knee joint: recovery with a false joint and a useful limb. *Med Times Gaz* 1861;1:601.
2. Oglesby JW, Wilson FC. The evolution of knee arthroplasty. *Clin Orthop* 984;186:96–103.
3. Jones GB. Arthroplasty of the knee by the Walldius prosthesis. *J Bone Joint Surg Br* 1968;50(3):505–510.
4. Merryweather R, Jones GB. Total knee replacement: the Walldius arthroplasty. *Orthop Clin North Am* 1973;4(2):585–596.
5. Phillips RS. Shiers' arthroplasty of the knee. *Clin Orthop* 1973;94:122–127.
6. Bargar WL, Cracchiolo A, Amstutz HC. Results with the constrained total knee prosthesis in treating severely disabled patients and patients with failed total knee replacements. *J Bone Joint Surg Am* 1980;65(4):504–512.
7. Cameron HU, Jung YB. Hinged total knee replacement: indications and results. *Can J Surg* 1990;33(1):53–57.
8. Cameron HU, Hu C, Vyamont D. Hinge total knee replacement revisited. *Can J Surg* 1997;40:278–283.
9. Cuckler JM. Revision total knee arthroplasty: how much constraint is necessary? *Orthopedics* 1995;18:932–936.
10. Deburge A, Guepar. Guepar hinge prosthesis: complications and results with two years' follow-up. *Clin Orthop* 1976;120:47–53.
11. Ewald FC. The Knee Society total knee arthroplasty roentgenographic evaluation and scoring system. *Clin Orthop* 1989;248:9–12.
12. Freeman PA. Walldius arthroplasty: a review of 80 cases. *Clin Orthop* 973;94:85–91.
13. Grimer RJ, Karpinski MRK, Edwards AN. The long-term results of Stanmore total knee replacements. *J Bone Joint Surg Br* 1984;66(1):55–62.
14. Habermann ET, Deutsch SC, Rovere GD. Knee arthroplasty with the use of the Walldius total knee prosthesis. *Clin Orthop* 1972;94:72–84.
15. Hui FC, Fitzgerald RHI Jr. Hinged total knee arthroplasty. *J Bone Joint Surg Am* 1980;62(4):513–519.
16. Jones EC, Insall JN, Inglis AE, et al. GUEPAR knee arthroplasty results and late complications. *Clin Orthop* 1979;140:145–152.
17. Jones GB. Total knee replacement—the Walldius hinge. *Clin Orthop* 1973;94:50–57.
18. Karpinsky MRK, Grimer RJ. Hinged knee replacement revision arthroplasty. *Clin Orthop* 1987;220:185–191.
19. Phillips H, Taylor JG. The Walldius hinge arthroplasty. *J Bone Joint Surg Br* 1975;57(1):59–62.
20. Wilson FC, Ventors GC. Results of knee replacement with the Walldius and Geometric prostheses. *J Bone Joint Surg Br* 1980;62(4):497–503.
21. Donaldson WF, Sculco TP, Insall JN, et al. Total Condylar III knee prosthesis. Long-term follow up study. *Clin Orthop* 1988:226:21–28.
22. Hohl WM, Crawford E, Zelicof SB, et al. The Total Condylar III prostheses in complex knee reconstruction. *Clin Orthop* 1991:273:91–97.
23. Sculco TP. Total Condylar III prosthesis in ligament instability. *Orthop Clin North Am* 1989:20(2):221–226.
24. Chotivivhit AL, Cracchiolo AD, Chow GH, et al. Total knee arthroplasty using the Total Condylar III knee prosthesis. *J Arthroplasty* 1991;6(4):341–350.
25. Vince KG. Revision knee arthroplasty technique. *Instr Course Lect* 1993;42:325–339.
26. Scott RD, Volatile TB. Twelve years experience with posterior cruciate retaining total knee arthroplasty. *Clin Orthop* 1986:206:100–107.
27. Scuderi GR, Insall JN, Windsor RE, et al. Survivorship of cemented knee replacements. *J Bone Joint Surg Br* 1989;71:798–803.
28. Stern SH, Insall JN. Posterior stabilized prosthesis. Results after follow up of 9 to 12 years. *J Bone Joint Surg Am* 1992;74:980–986.
29. Aglietti P, Buzzi R. Posteriorly stabilized total-condylar knee replacement: 3-8 years follow up of 85 knees. *J Bone Joint Surg Br* 1988;70(2):211–216.
30. Andriacchi TP, Galante JO. Retention of the posterior cruciate in total knee arthroplasty. *J Arthroplasty* 1988;3[Suppl]:S13–S19.
31. Dorr LD, Ochsner JL, Gronley J, et al. Functional comparison of posterior cruciate-retained versus cruciate-sacrificed total knee arthroplasty. *Clin Orthop* 1988;236:36–43.
32. Freeman MAR, Railton GT. Should the posterior cruciate ligament be retained or resected in condylar nonmeniscal knee arthroplasty? The case for resection. *J Arthroplasty* 1988;3[Suppl]:S3–S12.
33. Corces A, Lotke PA, Williams JL. Strain characteristics of the posterior cruciate ligament in total knee replacement. Paper presented at: 56th Annual Meeting of the American Academy of Orthopaedic Surgeons; February 9–14, 1989; Las Vegas.
34. Insall JN, et al. A comparison of four models of total knee replacement prosthesis. *J Bone Joint Surg Am* 1976;58:754–765.
35. Rand JA, Illstrup DM. Survivorship analysis of total knee arthroplasty. *J Bone Joint Surg Am* 1991;73:397–409.
36. Alexiades M, Scuderi G, Vigorita V, et al. A histologic study of the posterior cruciate ligament in the arthritic knee. *Am J Knee Surg* 1989;2(3):153–159.
37. Dorr LD, Scott RD, Ranawat CS. Importance of retention of the posterior cruciate ligament. In: Ranawat CS, ed. *Total condylar knee arthroplasty.* New York: Springer-Verlag, 1985:197–202.
38. Freeman MAR. A 3 to 5 year follow-up of the Freeman-Swanson arthroplasty of the knee. *J Bone Joint Surg Br* 1977;59:64–71.
39. Freeman MAR, Todd RC, Bamert P, et al. ICLH arthroplasty of the knee: 1968–1978. *J Bone Joint Surg Br* 1978;60:339–344.

40. Gallannaugh C. The Attenborough and Gallannaugh knee prostheses for total knee arthroplasty. A comparison and survival analysis. *Clin Orthop* 1992:281:177–188.

41. Insall TN, Scott WN, Ranawat CS. The total condylar knee prosthesis: a report of 220 cases. *J Bone Joint Surg Am* 1979:61:173

42. Insall JN, Hood RW, Flawn LB, et al. The total condylar knee prosthesis in gonarthrosis: a 5–9 year follow-up of the first 100 consecutive replacements. *J Bone Joint Surg Am* 1983;65:619.

43. Insall JN, Lachiewics PF, Burstein AH. The posterior stabilized condylar prosthesis: a modification of the total condylar design. Two to 4 year clinical experience. *J Bone Joint Surg Am* 1982;64:1317–1323.

44. Scuderi GR, Insall JN. The posterior stabilized knee prosthesis. *Orthop Clin North Am* 1989;20(1):71–78.

45. Vince KG, Kelly M, Insall JN. Posterior stabilized knee prosthesis: follow-up at 5–8 years. *Orthop Trans* 1988:12:157.

46. Scott WN, Rubenstein M, Scuderi G. Results after knee replacement with a posterior cruciate substitutive prosthesis. *J Bone Joint Surg Am* 1989;70:1163–1173.

47. Kavoulus CH, Faris PM, Ritter MA, et al. The Total Condylar III knee prosthesis in elderly patients. *J Arthroplasty* 1991;6(1):39–43.

48. Kraay M, Goldberg VM, Figgie MP, et al. Technical factors influencing the results of Total Condylar III knee arthroplasty. *Am J Knee Surg* 1988:1(2):125–133.

49. Lombardi AV, Mallory TH, Vaughn BK, et al. Dislocation following primary posterior stabilized total knee arthroplasty. *J Arthroplasty* 1993;8(6):633–639.

50. Sharkey PF, Hozack WJ, Booth RE, et al. Posterior dislocation of the total knee arthroplasty. *Clin Orthop* 1992:278:128–133.

51. Striplin DB, Robinson RP. Posterior dislocation of the Insall/Burstein II posterior stabilized total knee prosthesis. *Am J Knee Surg* 1992:5(2):79–83.

52. Krakow KA, ed. *The technique of total knee arthroplasty.* St. Louis: Mosby, 1990.

53. Lombardi AV, Mallory TH, Vaughn BK, et al. The Total Condylar III prosthesis in complex primary total knee arthroplasty: a 3 to 10 year clinical and radiographic evaluation. Paper presented at: Ninth Combined Meeting of the Orthopaedic Associations of the English-speaking World; June 1992; Toronto.

54. Sim FK, Chao EYS. Prosthetic replacement of the knee and large segment of the femur or tibia. *J Bone Joint Surg Am* 1979;61(6):887–892.

55. Rand JA, Chao EYS, Stauffer RN. Kinematic rotating hinge total knee arthroplasty. *J Bone Joint Surg Am* 1987;69(4):489–497.

56. DiGioia AM, Rubash HE. Periprosthetic fractures after total knee arthroplasty. *Clin Orthop* 1991;271:135–142.

57. Kraay MJ, Goldberg VM, Figgie MP, et al. Distal femoral replacement with allograft/prosthetic reconstruction of supracondylar fractures in patients with total knee arthroplasty. *J Arthroplasty* 1992; 7(1):7–16.

58. Gill GS, Mills DM. Ten to 16 year follow-up of cemented total knee arthroplasties. Paper presented at: Second Annual Meeting of the Association for Arthritic Hip and Knee Surgery; November 13–15, 1992; Dallas.

59. Murray PB, Rand JA, Hanssen AD. Cemented long-stem revision total knee arthroplasty. *Clin Orthop* 1994;309:116–123.

60. Shaw JA, Balcorn W, Greer III RB. Total knee arthroplasty using the kinematic rotating hinge prosthesis. *Orthopedics* 1989;12:647–654.

61. Walker PS, Emerson R, Potter T, et al. The kinematic rotating hinge: biomechanics and clinical application. *Orthop Clin North Am* 1982; 13:187–199.

62. Westrich GH, Mollano AV, Sculco TP, et al. Rotating hinge total knee arthroplasty in severely affected knees. *Clin Orthop* 2000;379:195–208.

63. Springer BD, Hanssen AD, Sim FH, et al. The kinematic rotating hinge prosthesis for complex knee arthroplasty. *Clin Orthop* 2001;392:283–291.

64. Barrack RL. Evolution of the rotating hinge for complex total knee arthroplasty. *Clin Orthop* 2001;392:292–299.

65. Vince KG, Lang W. Revision knee arthroplasty: the limits of press fit, medullary fixation. *Clin Orthop* 1995;317:172.

66. Bertin KC, Freeman MAR, Samuelson KM, et al. Stemmed revision arthroplasty for aseptic loosening of total knee replacement. *J Bone Joint Surg Br* 1985;67:242.

67. Easley ME, Insall JN, Scuderi GR, et al. Primary constrained condylar knee arthroplasty for the arthritic valgus knee. *Clin Orthop* 2000;380:58–64.

68. Edwards E, Miller J, Chan KH. The effect of postoperative collateral ligament laxity in total knee arthroplasty. *Clin Orthop* 1988;236:44–51.

69. Bourne RB, Finlay JB. The influence of tibial component intramedullary stems and implant-cortex contact on the strain distribution of the proximal tibia following total knee arthroplasty: an in vitro study. *Clin Orthop* 1986;208:95–99.

70. Lombardi AV, Mallory TH, Fada RA, et al. An algorithm for the posterior cruciate ligament in total knee arthroplasty. *Clin Orthop* 2001;392:75–87.

71. Murray DG, Wilde AH, Werner F, et al. Herbert total knee prosthesis. *J Bone Joint Surg Am* 1977;59:1026.

72. Kabo JM, Yang RS, Dorey FJ, et al. In vivo rotational stability of the kinematic rotating hinge knee prosthesis. *Clin Orthop* 1997;336:166.

73. Finn HA, Golden D, Kneisl JA, et al. The Finn Knee: rotating hinge replacement of the knee preliminary report of new design. In: Brown KLB, ed. *Complications of limb salvage: prevention, management and outcome.* Montreal: ISOLS, 1991:413.

74. Hartford JM, Goodman SB, Schurman DJ, et al. Complex primary and revision total knee arthroplasty using the condylar constrained prosthesis: an average 5-year follow-up. *J Arthroplasty* 1998;13:380–387.

75. Barrack RL, Lyons TR, Ingraham RQ, et al. The use of a modular rotating hinge component in salvage revision total knee arthroplasty. *J Arthroplasty* 2000;15:858–866.

76. Matthews LS, Goldstein SA, Kolowich PA, et al. Spherocentric arthroplasty of the knee: a long-term and final follow-up evaluation. *Clin Orthop* 1986;205:58.

77. Haas SB, Insall JN, Montgomery W III, et al. Revision total knee arthroplasty with use of modular components with stems inserted without cement. *J Bone Joint Surg Am* 1995;77:1700.

78. Scuderi GR. Revision total knee arthroplasty: how much constraint is enough? *Clin Orthop* 2001;392:300–305.

79. Trousdale RT, Beckenbaugh JP, Pagnano MW. 15 year results of the Total Condylar III implant in revision total knee arthroplasty. In: *Proceedings of the Sixty-Eighth Annual Meeting of the American Academy of Orthopaedic Surgeons, San Francisco.* Rosemont, IL: American Academy of Orthopaedic Surgeons, 2001:585.

CHAPTER 81

Osseous Deficiencies in Total Knee Replacement and Revision: Femur

Daniel P. Hoeffel and Harry E. Rubash

Complex primary and revision total knee arthroplasty can pose several surgical challenges. The surgeon must often address bone loss, component malposition, ligamentous laxity, and component instability. These factors account for reported complication rates as high as 30% (1). Surgical decisions regarding the use of bone grafts, component augmentation, axial and rotational alignment, and femoral stems must be properly addressed to achieve consistently successful outcomes. This requires an understanding of normal knee kinematics, total knee arthroplasty mechanics, and the mechanisms that contribute to total knee arthroplasty failure. The goal is to achieve a femoral construct that has osseous and ligamentous stability with proper alignment.

Preservation of bone stock with judicious use of bone graft, modular augments, and intramedullary stems is the key to achieving mechanical stability and favorable kinematics. A systematic approach encompassing preoperative assessment, implant removal, bone deficiency assessment, and femoral reconstruction is presented.

PREOPERATIVE ASSESSMENT

Preoperative assessment allows the surgeon to establish the mechanism of failure of the implants, determine ligamentous stability, estimate bone loss, and plan a subsequent reconstruction. The mechanism of failure often can be determined through the evaluation of serial radiographs. Common causes of failure include aseptic loosening, infection, tibiofemoral instability, wear, osteolysis, and patellofemoral instability (2,3). Revision arthroplasty must correct factors that led to failure of the primary arthroplasty.

The assessment involves examination of the patient to determine skin integrity and viability, range of motion, stability, extensor mechanism competency, and the presence or absence of contracture. Laboratory tests include erythrocyte sedimentation rate, C-reactive protein level, and possibly fluid aspiration with culture to differentiate septic from aseptic loosening (4,5).

In most instances, preoperative radiographs are the major source of information regarding the mechanism of failure and bone loss. Recommended views include standing anteroposterior, lateral, Merchant, and standing full-length views of the bilateral lower extremities. Fluoroscopically guided spot views can also be obtained to better evaluate the status of the bone-cement or bone-implant interface (6).

When radiographs of failed implants are evaluated, one should keep in mind that bone loss usually exceeds the radiographic estimation. This is especially true in the case of osteolysis, in which the remaining bone is often of such poor quality as to be structurally incompetent; when it is adequately débrided, a much larger defect than predicted must be reconstructed.

In addition, one should be suspicious of the distal femoral interface and the posterior condylar interface, as these are the most common sites for interface loosening and subsequent bone loss with currently used condylar designs. Osseous defects tend to be larger in hinged implants, stemmed implants, and posterior cruciate–substituting designs. A thorough preoperative assessment provides the information needed to plan the reconstruction. Modular augments, intramedullary stems, particulate bone graft, and structural bone graft can then be used rationally in the femoral reconstruction.

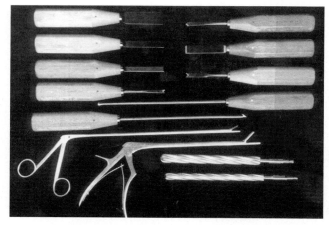

FIG. 1. Specialized knee revision instrumentation can be used to aid component and cement removal. (Courtesy Johnson & Johnson Orthopedics.)

IMPLANT REMOVAL

Removal of the femoral implant should begin at the anterior femoral interface with a Gigli saw or reciprocating saw. Once the implant-bone or cement-bone interface is exposed, the anterior interface is disrupted and the medial and lateral condyles then are freed with osteotomes. The posterior femoral condyles can be released with the Gigli saw. The femoral notch interfaces are then released with curved and straight osteotomes or, rarely, high-speed burrs. If a well-fixed stemmed femoral component is present, the stem may require transection at its junction with the condylar portion of the implant. Metal cutting burrs used with saline irrigation or sterile gel lubrication allow division of the stem from the intercondylar box while minimizing debris scatter. Femoral hip revision instruments or specialized cemented knee revision instruments may be used to remove the remaining stem and cement from the intramedullary canal (Fig. 1). Femoral windows can be used to directly remove adherent cement.

It is critical that the manufacturer and design of the components to be removed be known preoperatively so that design-specific disassembly or removal tools are available. Universal femoral extraction devices are available to grasp various implants and facilitate removal. Judicious use of these devices is recommended, however, as overly aggressive blows or incomplete disruption of the prosthesis bone interface may result in removal of the prosthesis with a condyle or the entire distal femur attached. If osteotomes are used to lever against the condyles, the cancellous bone of the distal femur will be crushed, which results in a larger osseous defect. The authors frequently use high-speed burrs and ultrasonic devices to facilitate removal of the residual cement in the metaphyseal-diaphyseal region while maintaining bony integrity (2,3,7,8).

OSSEOUS DEFECT ASSESSMENT AND CLASSIFICATION

Bone deficiency is assessed after component removal of the prosthesis. Three aspects should be assessed: the volume of the defects, the locations of deficiencies, and the quality of remaining bone stock. Several classifications have been developed to stratify bone loss and guide reconstruction (9–11).

The Massachusetts General Hospital femoral defect classification system separates osseous defects into major and minor

TABLE 1. *Massachusetts General Hospital femoral defect classification system for total knee arthroplasty and treatment algorithm*

Classification
Minor
Below the level of the epicondyles
Volume <1 cm³
Contained: No cortical bone loss, cancellous defects only
Uncontained: Cortical loss resulting in lack of support of a portion of the implant
Major
Defects are at or above the level of the epicondyles
Volume >1 cm³
Contained: No cortical bone loss, cancellous defects only
Uncontained: Cortical loss resulting in lack of support of a portion of the implant or condylar fracture

Treatment algorithm

Defect type	Minor	Major
Contained	Particulate graft Cement Implants: CR or PS ± stem	Bulk allograft Femoral head allograft Implants: PS with stem, possible constrained condylar
Uncontained	Augments Structural graft Cement or particulate graft if <5 mm fill and varus/valgus stable Implants: PS with stem	Augments Condylar allograft Bicondylar allograft Distal femoral allograft Implants: Constrained condylar with long stem or hinged device

CR, cruciate-retaining design; PS, posterior cruciate–substituting design.

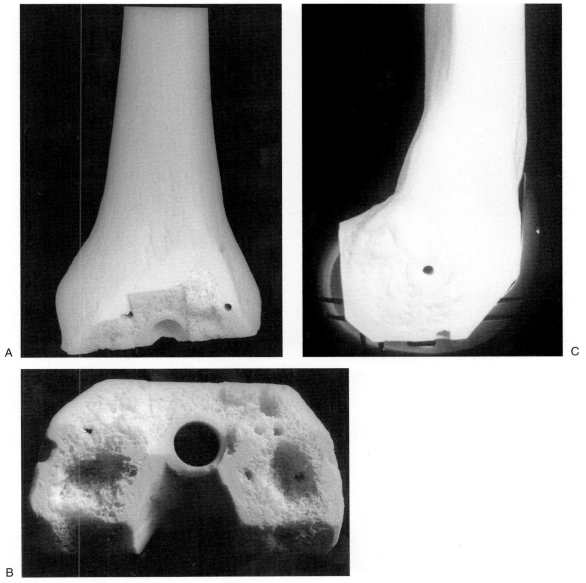

FIG. 2. In the Massachusetts General Hospital femoral defect classification system for total knee arthroplasty, defects are classified as major or minor based on the size of the defects and whether they are above or below the level of the epicondyles. Additional classification is based on containment of the defect (contained or uncontained). This results in four classes of defects. **A:** Shown here is a minor contained defect of the left femur. Anteroposterior view showing no loss of cortical support. **B:** *En fosse* view of the left femur with minor contained defect according to the Massachusetts General Hospital femoral defect classification system. Cancellous bone loss is located below the level of the epicondyles. **C:** Reconstruction of a minor contained defect can be performed using standard cruciate-retaining or posterior cruciate–substituting components without augments. Particulate bone graft or cement may be used to fill defects.

categories and then further into contained or uncontained defects (Table 1, Fig. 2) (10).

Minor defects are less than 1 cm³ and are below the level of the epicondyles. The epicondyles are in continuity with the metaphysis. Major defects are either larger than 1 cm³ or are located above the level of the epicondyles. Defects are then subclassified into contained or uncontained types. Contained defects have cancellous bone loss only. No significant cortical loss is present. Uncontained defects have cortical bone loss that

results in lack of support for a portion of the implant. Condylar dissociations are categorized as uncontained (10).

Minor contained defects (Fig. 2) are treated with particulate bone graft or cement. Primary total knee arthroplasty implants are generally used; intramedullary stems are rarely needed. The authors prefer to use posterior stabilized implants. Minor uncontained defects (Fig. 3) can be treated with particulate bone graft or cement if there is 5 mm or less of fill and the implant is axially and rotationally stable. In most cases, structural bone

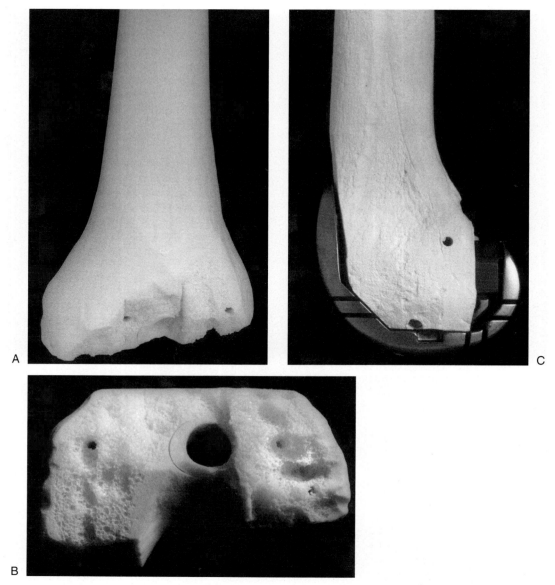

FIG. 3. A: Minor uncontained defect. Minimal bone loss is seen on the anteroposterior view of the distal femur. **B:** Minor uncontained defect, *en fosse* view. Bone loss in this example is confined mainly to the lateral posterior condyle. **C:** Minor uncontained defect of **A** and **B** with a posterior augment used for reconstruction. The anterior bone loss in this case could be filled with cement.

grafting or modular augments are needed for stable reconstruction. Rotational and axial stability can be enhanced with the use of an intramedullary stem. Intramedullary stems also load-share the stresses on any bone graft used for reconstruction. Major contained lesions (Fig. 4) are reconstructed with the use of femoral head allograft or large bulk allografts. These grafts lend structural support in addition to providing an osteoconductive substrate for incorporation. The authors use a posterior stabilized implant in these cases. The degree of constraint is dictated by ligamentous stability.

Major uncontained defects (Fig. 5) present complex technical challenges. Condylar or bicondylar allografts may be required. The most severe deficiencies may necessitate the use of a whole distal femoral allograft. Augments are used as indicated (Fig. 6).

These reconstructions are performed using a constrained condylar device with an intramedullary stem or a hinged prosthesis (Table 1).

The Anderson Orthopaedic Research Institute bone defect classification (15) divides femoral osseous deficits into three types based on the radiographic status of the metaphyseal bone of the distal femur and proximal tibia (9,12,13). The metaphyseal region is defined as bone distal to the femoral epicondyles on the femur and proximal to the tibial tubercle for tibial defects. Femoral defects are denoted with an F; tibial defects are denoted with a T. Subdivision into types 1, 2, and 3 is then performed. Only femoral defects are discussed here (Fig. 7).

Type 1 femoral defects have intact metaphyseal bone with structurally sound cancellous bone and no component subsid-

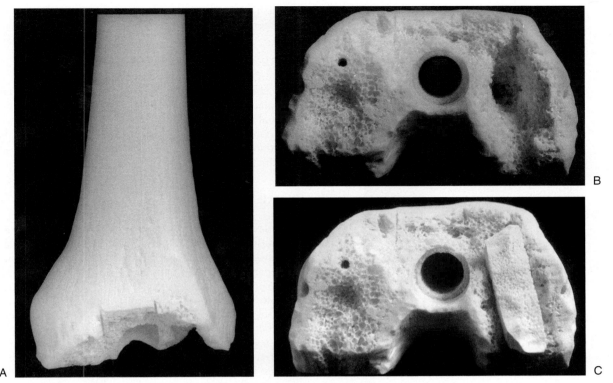

FIG. 4. A: Major contained defect. The contained nature of the defect implies minimal to no loss of cortical structural support as seen in the anteroposterior view. **B, C:** *En fosse* views of a major contained defect. Cancellous bone loss is greater than 1 cm³ and extends proximal to the epicondyles. Structural allograft can be used for reconstruction of the major contained defect.

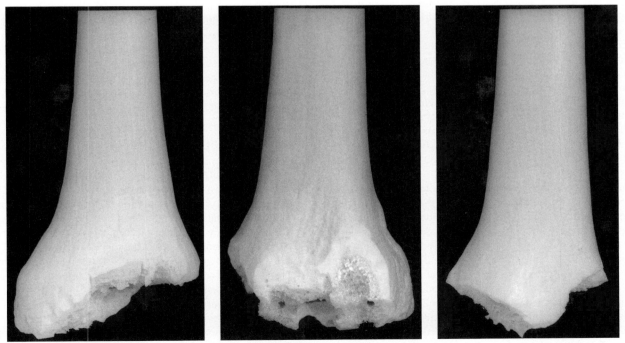

FIG. 5. A: Major uncontained defect has three subtypes—lateral condylar, medial condylar, and bicondylar. Cortical and cancellous bone loss is extensive in this class, necessitating the use of large posterior and distal augments or allograft femoral heads. Shown is a major uncontained lateral condylar defect. **B:** Medial condylar subtype of major uncontained defect. **C:** Bicondylar subtype of major uncontained defects. This subtype may require whole distal femoral allografts for reconstruction.

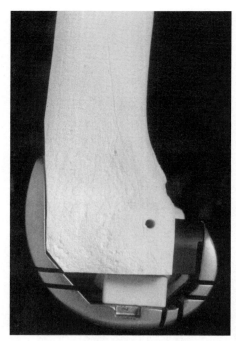

FIG. 6. Reconstruction of a major uncontained defect of the lateral femoral condyle using distal and posterior augments.

ence. The remaining cancellous bone is firm to manual compression. Type 2 defects have component subsidence or joint-line elevation with damaged cancellous bone. Osseous defects, if present, are small and distal to the epicondyles. Type 3 defects have deficient metaphyseal bone. Bone damage has occurred at or above the level of the epicondyles with subsidence of the femoral component to that level.

Engh and Ammeen (12) have stated that type 1 defects are smaller than 1 cm³ and should not require femoral augments, structural bone graft, or cement fill. Type 2 defects are larger than 1 cm³ and may require femoral augments, particulate graft, or cement fill to restore alignment and an anatomic joint line. Type 3 defects require structural grafting in the form of femoral head allografting or composite distal femoral allografting. Modular stems should be used with type 2 and 3 defects, and also with type 1 defects with poor cancellous bone stock.

Rand (11) presented an osseous defect classification based on three criteria: symmetry, location, and extent. Symmetric defects are often seen with tibial subsidence in which both condyles show even depression. Femoral defects are frequently asymmetric as the implant falls into varus or valgus depending on which condyle is more severely affected by bone loss. Location is simply based on the site of femoral involvement—anterior, posterior, or distal. The extent of bone loss is determined after implant removal and preliminary bone cuts are completed. Subdivisions are minimal, moderate, extensive, and cavitary. The cavitary category is further subdivided into defects having an intact or deficient peripheral rim.

Ghazavi and colleagues (15) have proposed a system for classification of defects. The initial differentiation is between contained and uncontained defects. The uncontained defects are then subdivided into circumferential and noncircumferential.

Each of these subdivisions is then categorized as smaller or larger than 3 cm in size.

SURGICAL RECONSTRUCTION

The goal of femoral reconstruction is the restoration and maintenance of femoral alignment. This involves restoration of axial alignment, rotational alignment, and the joint line. Cement augmentation, modular augmentation, bone grafting, and intramedullary stem use are methods by which these goals are achieved.

Axial Alignment

Several authors have reported a correlation between clinical results and prosthesis alignment (16–18). The relationship between the distal femoral cutting block and the intramedullary alignment device (usually 5 to 7 degrees valgus) reestablishes the correct axial alignment (19,20) (Fig. 8). The proposed cut, however, may not remove bone from both condyles. In these cases, a flat bony surface is created only on one condyle. The deficient condyle may require trimming to allow the placement of augments or bone graft. The cut femoral surface provides a reference line that is parallel and often proximal to the desired joint line. Augmentation of both condyles will move the reconstructed joint line to an appropriate level. If the medial collateral ligament is functionally incompetent, the femur should be cut in slightly less than the usual 5 to 7 degrees valgus. A relative varus alignment of the mechanical axis protects an incompetent medial collateral ligament.

A second method for axial alignment involves the use of revision systems with cutting slots in the trial components (Figs. 9A and B). The cutting slots correspond to the modular augments available in the revision system. The intramedullary stem of the trial serves to re-create the axial alignment. The trial stem is advanced until bone is encountered and pinned in place. The bone cuts are performed through the slots on the trial component. Augments are then added to one or both condyles to restore the joint line (Fig. 9C).

Rotational Alignment

Rotational alignment is crucial for patellofemoral mechanics and the balancing of flexion and extension gaps (16,17,21–23). Internal rotation of the femoral component can result in poor patellar tracking, subluxation, patellar clunk, increased patellar component wear, and anterior knee pain.

Rotational landmarks and reference lines are used to guide femoral component placement. Several anatomic references have been described (21,22,24,25). The posterior condylar line, surgical epicondylar axis, and Whiteside axis (26) are commonly used in primary total knee arthroplasty for femoral alignment. At revision surgery, however, the posterior condyles generally are not available for visual reference because of their resection at the index arthroplasty. In nearly all cases of revision, additional bone loss has occurred about the condyles and obscures distal femoral anatomy. Similarly, the previous anterior and distal resection of the femur limits the use of the Whiteside axis in the revision setting.

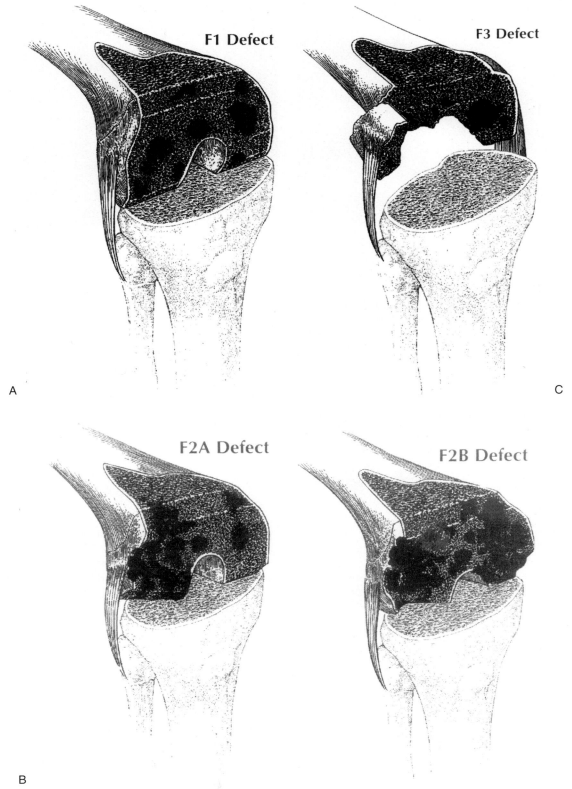

FIG. 7. A: Anderson Orthopaedic Research Institute (AORI) type F1 defect showing minimal bone loss involving only the metaphysis of the femur. **B:** AORI type F2 defects with bone loss involving cancellous support below the levels of the epicondyles. **C:** AORI type F3 defect showing severe bone loss in the metaphysis and above the levels of the epicondyles. The epicondyles may be fractured or absent secondary to bone resorption.

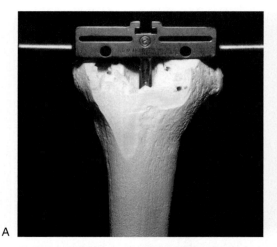

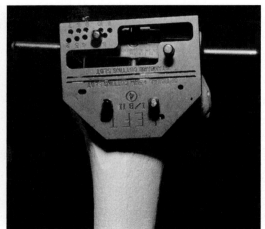

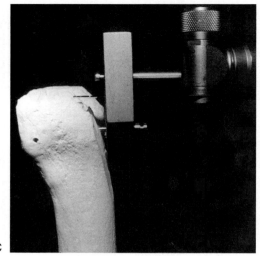

FIG. 8. A: When an intramedullary-based system is used, the intramedullary guide is inserted until it seats against bone. **B:** After rotational alignment is checked, the distal cutting guide is applied in appropriate axial alignment, and the saw is used to establish a stable bony surface. This surface is parallel and proximal to the desired joint line. Care must be taken to avoid elevating the joint line. **C:** Bone may be resected from the less involved condyle to create a flat surface parallel to the desired joint line. Distal augments are added to bring the femoral component distal to reestablish an appropriate level for the joint line.

The surgical epicondylar axis is defined by a line connecting the peak of the lateral epicondyles and the sulcus between the two prominences of the medial epicondyles (Figs. 10 and 11). It most consistently re-creates a balanced flexion space at primary total knee arthroplasty and is available in nearly all revision cases (22,27). The posterior condylar line connects the posterior-most points on the medial and lateral condyles when the femur is viewed in flexion. Berger et al. (22) determined normal values for the relationship between the surgical epicondylar axis and the posterior condylar line. The surgical epicondylar axis was on average 3.5 degrees externally rotated with respect to the posterior condylar line in males and 0.3 degree externally rotated in females.

Joint-Line Restoration

An anatomic joint line should be restored at the time of revision surgery. In the femoral revision setting, the use of distal femoral augments or bone graft should be adjusted to reestablish an appropriate joint line. Alteration of the joint line severely alters patellofemoral mechanics and tibiofemoral kinematics. Patellar baja in severe cases may result in impingement of the patella on the tibial implant. Patella alta increases the patellar strains and risk of subluxation (28–30). Midflexion instability

also may result. Midflexion instability is present when the knee is stable in extension and flexion but unstable within the arc of motion, usually within the 30- to 60-degree range. This phenomenon is a result of tight posterior structures providing stability in extension and at 90 degrees flexion. The collateral ligaments are not competent in these cases, and the knee is unstable unless in full extension or 90 degrees flexion (11,31).

The femoral epicondyles serve as useful landmarks for reconstruction of the joint line. The lateral epicondyle lies 2.0 to 2.5 cm proximal to the joint line in the normal knee (32,33). A secondary landmark for the level of the joint line is present if remnants of the meniscal rim remain. Some surgeons use the inferior pole of the patella as a landmark to guide placement of the joint line. This technique works well if preoperative radiographs of the contralateral knee are available for comparison. The reconstructed joint line can be placed at the same level as the native knee. Intraoperatively the knee should be in extension and the patellar tendon taut when measuring from the inferior pole of the patella. The surgeon must be aware of the presence of patella baja or patella alta, which can result in inaccurate joint-line placement with this technique.

The effect of joint-line restoration after revision arthroplasty on clinical outcome has been reported. Partington et al. (34) compared joint-line position at three time points: before arthroplasty, after primary arthroplasty, and after revision

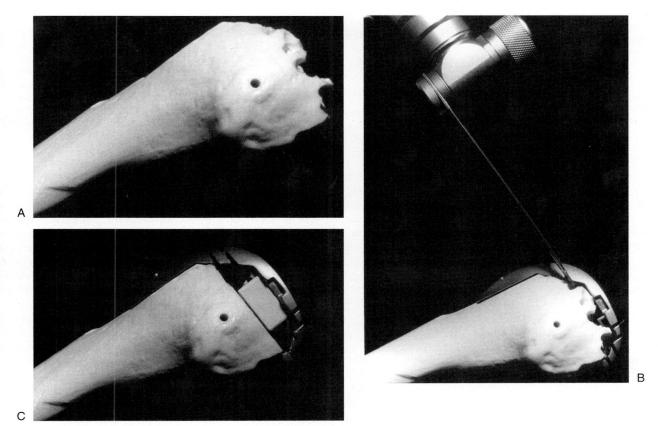

FIG. 9. A: Lateral view of minor uncontained defect. **B, C:** Photographs showing the use of slotted trials with cutting guides. The intramedullary stem on the trial restores appropriate axial alignment (5 to 7 degrees valgus). The trial is inserted to a depth that restores the level of the joint line, and the appropriate cutting slots are used to trim irregular bony prominences. A stable base for reconstruction with metal augments is thereby established.

arthroplasty. One hundred seven revision knee arthroplasties were performed in 99 patients. Joint-line position was determined by the technique described by Figgie et al. (17). Compared to the preoperative state, 1% of the primary arthroplasties and 79% of the revisions had elevation of the joint line. Elevations greater than 8 mm were associated with lower Knee Society clinical rating scores (35) at an average follow-up of 3.7 years. Femurs that had distal augments applied had an average elevation of 10 mm. Those without augments averaged 7 mm of elevation. More frequent and aggressive use of distal augments to better restore the anatomic joint line was recommended. The finding of greater joint-line elevation despite the use of augments indicates that larger augments than expected should be considered, because the common error remains joint-line elevation.

Reconstruction of Bony Defects

Cementing of Bone Defects

In selected cases, cement or cement with screw augmentation may be used to fill bony voids (36). Cement filling alone is an acceptable option for femoral reconstruction when one or both of the distal condyles do not have flush contact with the trial component, yet the chamfer cuts are providing stability and are

flush with the trial component. The trial component must be stable to varus and valgus stressing. The current authors prefer the use of metal augments to the distal femur if the defect is larger than 2 mm.

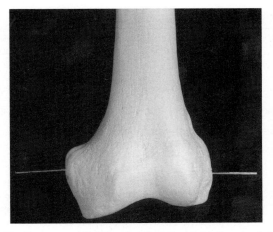

FIG. 10. Bone model with pins inserted into the medial and lateral epicondyles. Note that the medial epicondyle sits more proximal to the joint line than the lateral epicondyle.

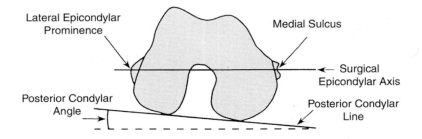

FIG. 11. Surgical epicondylar axis and posterior condylar line. The surgical epicondylar axis serves as a consistent and reproducible reference for rotational alignment in revision total knee arthroplasty. (From Berger RA, Rubash HE, Seel MJ, et al. Determining the rotational alignment of the femoral component in total knee arthroplasty using the epicondylar axis. *Clin Orthop* 1993;286:40–47, with permission.)

Scott (36,37) reported the use of a screw-cement construct to confer stability when the femoral chamfer cuts do not provide stability and one distal femoral condyle is deficient. A titanium screw is left proud in the distal femoral condyle to reinforce the cement and support the deficient condyle. Biomechanical testing of this technique for a tibial wedge defect reconstruction found it to have 30% less deflection than cement alone (38). However, metal augmentation is a preferred method of reconstruction in these cases.

Augments

Modular augmentation of the femoral component in revision knee arthroplasty fills bony defects with biomechanically stable fixation. Augments allow the surgeon to create ligamentous stability by adjusting flexion and extension spaces. The anatomic joint line can also be restored with distal augmentation. The use of augments has become a preferred method to correct isolated and complex defects that previously would have required a custom prosthesis, large cement volumes, or significant bone grafting (36,39).

As described earlier, bone loss on the femur is often on the posterior or distal surfaces; therefore, posterior and distal augments are the most frequently used. Restoration of the anterior, posterior, and mediolateral dimensions of the femur in conjunction with a nearly anatomic joint line results in balanced soft tissues with ligamentous stability throughout the range of motion (31).

The effects of augments on flexion and extension spaces are similar to those encountered in primary arthroplasty. The extension space is affected by the status of the distal femur. Augmentation of the distal femur decreases the extension space and lowers the joint line. Augmentation of the posterior condyles may decrease the flexion space if it translates the femoral component posteriorly. It should be noted that the use of a posterior augment on the lateral condyle will externally rotate the femoral component. Bone loss on the tibia affects the extension and the flexion spaces equally (31).

When components with augments are trialed, the size and symmetry of the flexion and extension spaces are evaluated along with ligamentous stability in flexion and extension (Table 2). Laxity in extension with stability in flexion indicates that the extension gap is too large and that distal femoral augments are needed (11). Stability in extension with laxity in flexion signifies an excessive flexion space. A larger femoral component or larger posterior augmentation should be considered to effectively move the femoral component posterior. Laxity in the flexion and extension spaces should prompt a reassessment of the integrity of the collateral ligaments. If they are in continuity, then an evaluation of the joint line is required. If the joint line is elevated, distal and posterior femoral augmentation should be used to lower the joint line while simultaneously decreasing the flexion and extension spaces. If the joint line is depressed because of tibial bone loss, tibial augments or a thicker tibial tray should be added. Many cases are dictated by the amount of bone available for fixation, and a combination of femoral and tibial adjustments is necessary.

TABLE 2. *Assessment and treatment of flexion and extension spaces*

Flexion space	Extension space		
	Tight	Stable	Loose
Tight	Use thinner polyethylene insert. Resect more tibia.	Offset stem to move femoral component anteriorly. Use smaller femoral component. Use distal femoral augment and thinner polyethylene insert.	Offset stem to move femoral component anteriorly and thicker tibial insert. Use smaller femoral component and thicker tibial insert.
Stable	Resect more distal femur.	No changes necessary.	Add distal femoral augments.
Loose	Resect more distal femur and offset stem to move femoral component posteriorly and posterior femoral augments. Resect more distal femur and use thicker tibial insert. Resect more distal femur and use larger femoral component and posterior femoral augments.	Offset stem to move femoral component posteriorly and posterior femoral augments. Resect more distal femur and use thicker tibial insert. Use larger femoral component and posterior femoral augments.	Use thicker tibial insert.

Biomechanical testing of augments and wedges has focused on tibial defects with few data on femoral augments (38,40–42). Brooks et al. (38) analyzed five different techniques for reconstruction of medial tibial plateau bony defects in cadaveric specimens (38). Cement alone, cement with screw augmentation, polymethylmethacrylate wedge, metal wedge, and a custom one-piece prosthesis were tested under axial and varus directed loads. In comparison to cement alone, axial loading of the cement with screw augmentation showed 30% less deflection, polymethylmethacrylate wedge showed 68% less deflection, metal wedge showed 83% less deflection, and the custom implant showed 91% less deflection. Compared with cement alone, the metal wedge augments were more stable in both axial and varus loading.

Chen and Krackow studied the effect of defect shape on the stability of tibial reconstruction. Step-shaped reconstructions of the tibia have been shown to provide more rigid support than wedge reconstructions (40). The stepped augments exhibited decreased shear forces at the augment-cement interface and the cement-bone interface.

In a clinical follow-up study, Brand et al. (43) reviewed 22 revision knee arthroplasties using cemented tibial wedges at an average of 37 months. Twenty-seven percent of the wedges had nonprogressive radiolucencies less than 1 mm at the wedge-cement interface. There were no instances of component loosening and no subsequent revisions.

Bone Grafting

The use of bone graft for femoral component revision can be subdivided into three categories (44–46). Particulate graft usually fills small defects less than 1 cm^3. Structural allograft often is used for defects larger than 1 cm^3. Defects with extensive cortical bone loss or condylar discontinuity may require composite distal femoral allografting.

Whiteside and Bicalho (47) reported on biopsy specimens obtained at the time of revision surgery in patients who had received morselized allograft at the time of revision knee arthroplasty. The specimens showed vascular ingrowth into the allograft with new osteoid overlying the allograft trabeculae. Sixty-two patients received at least 30 mL of particulate allograft to treat bony defects. Rigid intramedullary stem fixation and rim seating of the implants was achieved in every case. Fourteen patients (22%) underwent revision surgery for various complications. Only two patients (3%) had loose implants.

Structural bone grafting in the setting of knee revision has good results at short- to medium-term follow-up. Parks and Engh (48) examined radiographs and histologic specimens retrieved from nine total knee arthroplasties that had structural grafting. The grafts had been *in situ* for an average of 41 months. All grafts were intact without collapse. There was no development of radiolucent lines and no component loosening. Histologic sections showed callus formation at the cortical margins of the allograft. There was no trabecular collapse, but no revascularization of allograft was evident. Clearing the allograft cartilage and subchondral plate was felt to be critical for ingrowth, as areas of residual subchondral plate lacked host ingrowth. The long-term results of structural allografting have yet to be reported.

Engh et al. (49) also reviewed their clinical experience using stemmed components and allograft. In a group of 30 patients

with 35 allografts, 13 patients had femoral implants with stems (four cemented stems, nine uncemented stems). At an average follow-up of 50 months, 87% good to excellent results were reported in the entire cohort. No grafts had collapsed and no revisions had been performed. No patient had evidence of graft resorption or progressive radiolucent lines at the graft-prosthesis junction on radiograph. No osteolytic lesions were observed around a component supported by graft. None of the cemented femoral components showed subsidence. Three press-fit femoral components did show subsidence.

The authors support the use of cemented components with uncemented canal-filling femoral stems when using allograft to allow axial loading at the graft-host junction, which possibly enhances graft-host union. The stem acts as a "load-sharing" device and possibly protects the allograft from microfracture and subsequent propagation with collapse.

Whole Allograft Reconstructions

Stockley et al. (50) reported on 32 allografts used to augment 20 total knee arthroplasties. The average follow-up was 4.2 years. Eighteen surgeries were revision arthroplasties. Femoral reconstruction used bulk allograft in 12 patients. Seven of the 12 bulk allografts were complete distal femurs. The complete distal femurs were cemented to the prosthesis. There were three reoperations. All reoperations were for infection. One femoral bulk allograft fractured in the supracondylar region but healed with nonoperative treatment. All remaining grafts united to host bone.

Tsahakis et al. (51) reviewed 13 distal femoral allografts. Six whole distal femurs and seven distal and posterior condyles were used for reconstruction of large uncontained defects. By 1 year, all allografts had achieved incorporation or union to host bone. No collapse had occurred. There were no cases of sepsis.

Mow and Weidel (52) reviewed their results in 15 patients with structural allograft used in total knee revisions. Seven femurs required allografting. Three prostheses were press-fit to allograft and host. Four were cemented to allograft and press-fit to host. All allografts united to host bone. There were no fractures, subsidences, or osteolysis at an average 47-month follow-up. One femoral component had a nonprogressive radiolucent line. No patient underwent revision surgery for a femoral component complication.

Harris et al. (53) performed a clinical and radiographic review of 14 patients treated with prosthesis allograft composites (six tibias and eight femurs). The average follow-up was 43 months. Thirteen of 14 patients had good to excellent clinical results. One patient underwent two subsequent revision surgeries for component failure. Excluding the graft in this patient, all grafts united to host bone. There were no progressive radiolucent lines at the allograft-prosthesis junction. No prosthesis had changed position. There were six complications in four patients: One was a deep infection and one was a vascular injury, which was repaired. The current authors use large bulk allograft when there is loss of one or both condyles, or when a large contained defect is present in which a large femoral head allograft can be placed to give stability to the reconstruction. A distal femoral allograft rarely is necessary but can be used in the setting of massive metaphyseal and diaphyseal bone loss with no native bone stock available for reconstruction. If the stem of the component does not cross the host-graft junction adequately or if the host-graft

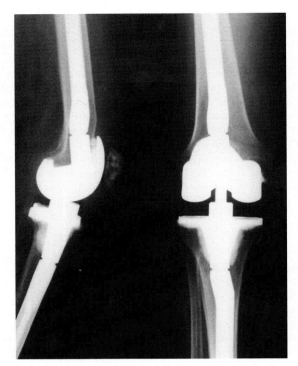

FIG. 12. Offset femoral stems can be helpful in balancing the flexion and extension spaces and allowing for versatility in component position relative to the intramedullary canal. In this case, the offset femoral stem translates the femoral component posteriorly. This tightens the flexion space but leaves the extension space unchanged. (Radiographs courtesy of Kim Bertin, MD, Salt Lake City, UT.)

junction is unstable, then cerclage wiring, single plating, and in most cases double plating of the femur are indicated.

Intramedullary Stem Use

The use of stems at revision surgery confers stability to the reconstruction through fixation and load transfer from the components into diaphyseal bone. Correct axial alignment is also reproduced. As with metal augments, nearly all biomechanical testing of stems has been performed on the tibia, with the rationale carried over to femoral reconstruction. Brooks et al. (38) determined that a 70-mm stem used in the tibia bears 23% to 38% of an applied axial load. Bourne and Finlay (54) also examined stem loading in the tibia. Strain distributions for 37.5-mm, 50.0-mm, and 150-mm stems were measured. Use of the stems resulted in stress shielding of the proximal tibia. The distance of the shielding essentially was equivalent to the length of the stem. These investigators expressed concern that the stress shielding may result in bony resorption and late component failure.

Offset stems have been introduced to address instances in which the medial-lateral or anteroposterior position of the implant is not appropriate because of malalignment in the distal femur. When large press-fit stems are used, the position of the femoral implant is dictated by the axis of the distal femur. The stems are modular and allow for shifting of the condyles relative to the stem in both the medial-lateral and anteroposterior directions. Offset stems also may be used to help adjust the flexion

and extension spaces (Fig. 12). The flexion space is increased if the stem shifts the femoral component anteriorly. Conversely, a posterior shift decreases the flexion space (Table 2).

The use of stems for revision can be divided into two categories, the cemented and uncemented techniques. One proposed advantage of the uncemented technique is easier removal of components and debris should a subsequent revision be necessary (55). Disadvantages can be encountered in the setting of femoral shaft obliquity because of a healed fracture or a previous osteotomy. Passage of a large canal-filling stem can be difficult if not impossible (31).

Bertin et al. (56) followed 53 revisions performed for aseptic loosening for a range of 6 to 48 months. All revisions used minimally constrained implants with smooth uncemented stems on the femur, tibia, or both. Of the 45 patients reviewed at final follow-up, 91% had satisfactory relief of pain. Arc of motion was greater than 90 degrees in 84% of patients. Seventy-six percent of the femoral components had a radiolucent zone less than 2 mm. No radiolucent zone progressed. No component subsided. Cortical hypertrophy at the stem tip occurred with 2 of the 34 stemmed femoral components.

Haas et al. (55) reported on 76 revisions using uncemented fluted intramedullary stems. Sixty-seven knees had complete follow-up at an average of 3.5 years. Twenty-three femurs had modular augments applied. Good to excellent clinical results were observed in 84% of the revisions. Six of the 67 knees (9%) had a second revision due to prosthesis failure. Fifty-seven posterior stabilized and 19 constrained condylar devices were implanted. There was no difference in clinical outcomes between patients receiving the two component designs. Eighty-one percent of patients had more than 90 degrees of flexion. Of the femoral components, 33% had radiolucent lines, only one of which was progressive. The most common location for these lines on the femur was anterior.

Vince and Long (57) reviewed the results of press-fit intramedullary fixation in 44 revision knee arthroplasties at 2 to 6 years of follow-up. All components had cement fixation of the cut bone surfaces. Thirteen knees were reconstructed using constrained condylar devices. Three of the 13 patients (23%) with the constrained condylar devices underwent revision surgery or were awaiting revision surgery for loosening. All three patients had initial revision surgery for infection. These investigators suggest that the press-fit stem technique may not provide adequate fixation for the constrained condylar implant when bone quality is poor.

Murray et al. (58) reported on 38 knees that had femoral revision with the use of cemented long stem implants. Two femoral components showed a radiolucent line on postoperative radiographs. One femoral implant was considered loose at 8-year follow-up because of a complete radiolucent line about the femoral stem and the component. Three other femoral components developed incomplete radiolucent lines in the follow-up period. No patient had revision surgery for loosening.

Femoral reconstruction in the presence of osseous defects requires the surgeon to recall the basic objectives of all condylar knee arthroplasties. One must achieve ligamentous balance, biomechanically stable fixation, and proper alignment. These objectives are met in the revision setting through the use of augments, bone graft, and intramedullary stems, while using anatomic landmarks to restore the joint line as well as axial and rotational alignment. A systematic approach to addressing and correcting bony and biomechanical deficiencies gives the greatest probability of a successful long-term outcome.

REFERENCES

1. Elia EA, Lotke PA. Results of revision total knee arthroplasty associated with significant bone loss. *Clin Orthop* 1991;271:114–121.
2. Bourne RB, Crawford HA. Principles of revision total knee arthroplasty. *Orthop Clin North Am* 1998;29(2):331–337.
3. Bryan RS, Rand JA. Revision total knee arthroplasty. *Clin Orthop* 1982;170:116–122.
4. Spangehl MJ, Masri BA, O'Connell JX, et al. Prospective analysis of preoperative and intraoperative investigations for the diagnosis of infection at the sites of two hundred and two revision total hip arthroplasties. *J Bone Joint Surg Am* 1999;81(5):672–683.
5. Spangehl MJ, Younger AS, Masri BA, et al. Diagnosis of infection following total hip arthroplasty. *Instr Course Lect* 1998;47:285–295.
6. Mintz AD, Pilkington CA, Howie DW. A comparison of plain and fluoroscopically guided radiographs in the assessment of arthroplasty of the knee. *J Bone Joint Surg Am* 1989;71(9):1343–1347.
7. Insall JN, Dethmers DA. Revision of total knee arthroplasty. *Clin Orthop* 1982;170:123–130.
8. Whiteside LA. Cementless revision total knee arthroplasty. *Clin Orthop* 1993;286:160–167.
9. Engh GA, Ammeen DJ. Classification and preoperative radiographic evaluation: knee. *Orthop Clin North Am* 1998;29(2):205–217.
10. Hoeffel DP, Rubash HE. Revision total knee arthroplasty: current rationale and techniques for femoral component revision. *Clin Orthop* 2000;380:116–132.
11. Rand JA. Bone deficiency in total knee arthroplasty. Use of metal wedge augmentation. *Clin Orthop* 1991;271:63–71.
12. Engh GA, Ammeen DJ. Bone loss with revision total knee arthroplasty: defect classification and alternatives for reconstruction. *Instr Course Lect* 1999;48:167–175.
13. Engh GA, Parks NL. The management of bone defects in revision total knee arthroplasty. *Instr Course Lect* 1997;46:227–236.
14. Reference deleted in text.
15. Ghazavi MT, Stockley I, Yee G, et al. Reconstruction of massive bone defects with allograft in revision total knee arthroplasty. *J Bone Joint Surg Am* 1997;79(1):17–25.
16. Berger RA, Crossett LS, Jacobs JJ, et al. Malrotation causing patellofemoral complications after total knee arthroplasty. *Clin Orthop* 1998;356:144–153.
17. Figgie HE, Goldberg VM, Heiple KG, et al. The influence of tibial-patellofemoral location on function of the knee in patients with the posterior stabilized condylar knee prosthesis. *J Bone Joint Surg Am* 1986;68(7):1035–1040.
18. Lotke PA, Ecker ML. Influence of positioning of prosthesis in total knee replacement. *J Bone Joint Surg Am* 1977;59(1):77–79.
19. Reed SC, Gollish J. The accuracy of femoral intramedullary guides in total knee arthroplasty. *J Arthroplasty* 1997;12(6):677–682.
20. Ries MD. Endosteal referencing in revision total knee arthroplasty. *J Arthroplasty* 1998;13(1):85–91.
21. Anouchi YS, Whiteside LA, Kaiser AD, et al. The effects of axial rotational alignment of the femoral component on knee stability and patellar tracking in total knee arthroplasty demonstrated on autopsy specimens. *Clin Orthop* 1993;287:170–177.
22. Berger RA, Rubash HE, Seel MJ, et al. Determining the rotational alignment of the femoral component in total knee arthroplasty using the epicondylar axis. *Clin Orthop* 1993;286:40–47.
23. Mantas JP, Bloebaum RD, Skedros JG, et al. Implications of reference axes used for rotational alignment of the femoral component in primary and revision knee arthroplasty [see comments]. *J Arthroplasty* 1992;7(4):531–535.
24. Eckhoff DG, Metzger RG, Vandewalle MV. Malrotation associated with implant alignment technique in total knee arthroplasty. *Clin Orthop* 1995;321:28–31.
25. Yoshioka Y, Siu D, Cooke TD. The anatomy and functional axes of the femur. *J Bone Joint Surg Am* 1987;69(6):873–880.
26. Whiteside LA, Arima J. The anteroposterior axis for femoral rotational alignment in valgus total knee arthroplasty. *Clin Orthop* 1995;321:168–172.
27. Olcott CW, Scott RD. The Ranawat Award. Femoral component rotation during total knee arthroplasty. *Clin Orthop* 1999;367:39–42.
28. Insall J, Goldberg V, Salvati E. Recurrent dislocation and the high-riding patella. *Clin Orthop* 1972;88:67–69.
29. Singerman R, Davy DT, Goldberg VM. Effects of patella alta and patella infera on patellofemoral contact forces. *J Biomech* 1994;27(8):1059–1065.
30. Singerman R, Heiple KG, Davy DT, et al. Effect of tibial component position on patellar strain following total knee arthroplasty. *J Arthroplasty* 1995;10(5):651–656.
31. Rand JA. Modular augments in revision total knee arthroplasty. *Orthop Clin North Am* 1998;29(2):347–353.
32. Rand JA. Revision total knee arthroplasty for aseptic loosening. In: Lotke PA, ed. *Master techniques in orthopaedic surgery, knee arthroplasty.* New York: Raven Press, 1995:206.
33. Scuderi GR, Mann JW. Cement fixation techniques for revision total knee arthroplasty. In: Lotke PA, Garino JP, eds. *Revision total knee arthroplasty.* Philadelphia: Lippincott–Raven Publishers, 1999: 304–305.
34. Partington PF, Sawhney J, Rorabeck CH, et al. Joint line restoration after revision total knee arthroplasty. *Clin Orthop* 1999;367:165–171.
35. Insall JN, Dorr LD, Scott RD, et al. Rationale of the Knee Society clinical rating system. *Clin Orthop* 1989;248:13–14.
36. Scott RD. Bone loss: prosthetic and augmentation method. *Orthopedics* 1995;18(9):923–926.
37. Scott RD. Revision total knee arthroplasty. *Clin Orthop* 1988;226: 65–77.
38. Brooks PJ, Walker PS, Scott RD. Tibial component fixation in deficient tibial bone stock. *Clin Orthop* 1984;184:302–308.
39. Dennis DA. Repairing minor bone defects: augmentation and autograft. *Orthopedics* 1998;21(9):1036–1038.
40. Chen F, Krackow KA. Management of tibial defects in total knee arthroplasty. A biomechanical study. *Clin Orthop* 1994;305:249–257.
41. Fehring TK, Peindl RD, Humble RS, et al. Modular tibial augmentations in total knee arthroplasty. *Clin Orthop* 1996;327:207–217.
42. Rand JA. Augmentation of a total knee arthroplasty with a modular metal wedge. A case report. *J Bone Joint Surg Am* 1995;77(2):266–268.
43. Brand MG, Daley RJ, Ewald FC, et al. Tibial tray augmentation with modular metal wedges for tibial bone stock deficiency. *Clin Orthop* 1989;248:71–79.
44. Dennis DA. Structural allografting in revision total knee arthroplasty. *Orthopedics* 1994;17(9):849–851.
45. Sculco TP, Choi JC. The role and results of bone grafting in revision total knee replacement. *Orthop Clin North Am* 1998;29(2):339–346.
46. Whiteside LA. Morselized allografting in revision total knee arthroplasty. *Orthopedics* 1998;21(9):1041–1043.
47. Whiteside LA, Bicalho PS. Radiologic and histologic analysis of morselized allograft in revision total knee replacement. *Clin Orthop* 1998;357:149–156.
48. Parks NL, Engh GA. The Ranawat Award. Histology of nine structural bone grafts used in total knee arthroplasty. *Clin Orthop* 1997;345:17–23.
49. Engh GA, Herzwurm PJ, Parks NL. Treatment of major defects of bone with bulk allografts and stemmed components during total knee arthroplasty. *J Bone Joint Surg Am* 1997;79(7):1030–1039.
50. Stockley I, McAuley JP, Gross AE. Allograft reconstruction in total knee arthroplasty. *J Bone Joint Surg Br* 1992;74(3):393–397.
51. Tsahakis PJ, Beaver WB, Brick GW. Technique and results of allograft reconstruction in revision total knee arthroplasty. *Clin Orthop* 1994;303:86–94.
52. Mow CS, Wiedel JD. Structural allografting in revision total knee arthroplasty. *J Arthroplasty* 1996;11(3):235–241.
53. Harris AI, Poddar S, Gitelis S, et al. Arthroplasty with a composite of an allograft and a prosthesis for knees with severe deficiency of bone. *J Bone Joint Surg Am* 1995;77(3):373–386.
54. Bourne RB, Finlay JB. The influence of tibial component intramedullary stems and implant-cortex contact on the strain distribution of the proximal tibia following total knee arthroplasty. An in vitro study. *Clin Orthop* 1986;208:95–99.
55. Haas SB, Insall JN, Montgomery W, et al. Revision total knee arthroplasty with use of modular components with stems inserted without cement. *J Bone Joint Surg Am* 1995;77(11):1700–1707.
56. Bertin KC, Freeman MA, Samuelson KM, et al. Stemmed revision arthroplasty for aseptic loosening of total knee replacement. *J Bone Joint Surg Br* 1985;67(2):242–248.
57. Vince KG, Long W. Revision knee arthroplasty. The limits of press fit medullary fixation. *Clin Orthop* 1995;317:172–177.
58. Murray PB, Rand JA, Hanssen AD. Cemented long-stem revision total knee arthroplasty. *Clin Orthop* 1994;309:116–123.

CHAPTER 82

Osseous Defects in Total Knee Arthroplasty: Tibia

Kevin M. Terefenko, James P. McAuley, and Gerard A. Engh

Bone loss in the setting of total knee arthroplasty is most commonly encountered during revision situations. Chronic fixed angular deformities about the knee, however, can cause osseous defects that must be addressed during primary procedures. Chronic instability due to articular cartilage loss, patellofemoral subluxation, meniscal injury, or ligament damage can lead to bone loss about the knee. These bony deficiencies are most commonly seen on the tibial side and are fairly consistent in their location.

Bone loss on the medial tibial plateau can result in varus deformities (Fig. 1), which are more common among men than women. Because the bone of the medial femoral condyle is stronger than that of the medial tibia, defects in femoral bone stock rarely occur in conjunction with those of the proximal tibia (1). Medial tibial bone loss leads to contracture of the medial collateral ligament, the posterior medial capsule, the pes anserinus, and the semimembranosus. In addition, the status of the anterior cruciate ligament (ACL) can influence the location and character of bone deficiency. Harman et al. (2) have shown that varus knees with intact or attenuated ACLs demonstrate bone loss on the middle to anterior aspect of the plateau, whereas varus knees with ACL deficiencies show more posterior bone loss. Therefore, chronic ACL deficiency in association with long-standing varus deformity can lead to erosion of the tibial plateau on the posteromedial cortical rim.

Valgus deformity (Fig. 2), more frequent among women, results from lateral femoral bone loss and progressive contracture of the lateral structures (1). These structures include the lateral collateral ligament, the posterior lateral capsule, the popliteus, the iliotibial band, and the biceps femoris. Bone loss commonly occurs just posterior to the center of the lateral tibial plateau, regardless of the status of the ACL (2). Most commonly, the resulting defect is a central cavitary defect, although erosion of bone from the posterolateral cortical rim can occur with advanced disease.

RADIOGRAPHIC EVALUATION

Adequate radiographs are necessary to assess bone loss, accurately define the amount of angular deformity, and plan the surgical procedure. The authors recommend acquiring multiple 14- by 17-in. radiographs with the knee centered on the film (3). Radiographic views should include a standard anteroposterior weightbearing view with the knee in maximal extension (Fig. 3). When the patient is able, a single-leg-stance view is best. If the patient has a valgus deformity, an anteroposterior weightbearing view with the knee flexed 30 degrees (Fig. 4) is most useful for assessing lateral compartment collapse and bone loss. A radiograph of a valgus knee in full extension does not show the true collapse of the lateral compartment, because tension in the medial collateral ligament holds the lateral compartment open (3). In addition, a lateral radiograph (Fig. 5) with the knee flexed to 90 degrees is recommended. To better assess the extent of bone deficiency, magnification markers are useful on this radiograph. To obtain a true lateral radiograph, the x-ray technician should take care that the ankle, knee, and hip rest flat against the table. A true lateral radiograph is particularly helpful in assessing posterior cortical bone loss and evaluating the slope of the tibia. This radiograph also may identify excessive femoral rollback, which indicates contracture of the posterior cruciate ligament (Fig. 6).

Genu varum

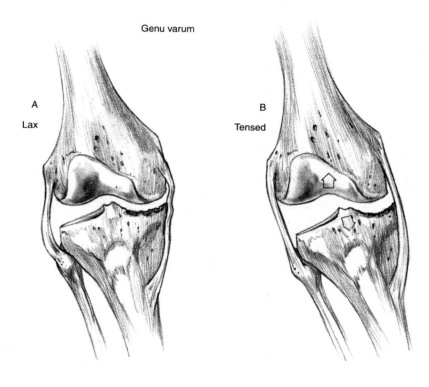

FIG. 1. A, B: Bone loss on the medial tibial plateau can result in varus deformity. (From Scuderi GR, Insall JN. Fixed varus and valgus deformities. In: Lotke PA, ed. *Knee arthroplasty.* New York: Raven Press, 1995:112, with permission.)

Genu valgum

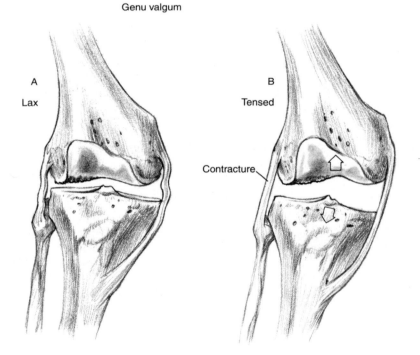

FIG. 2. A, B: Valgus deformity results from lateral femoral bone loss and progressive contracture of the lateral structures. (From Scuderi GR, Insall JN. Fixed varus and valgus deformities. In: Lotke PA, ed. *Knee arthroplasty.* New York: Raven Press, 1995:113, with permission.)

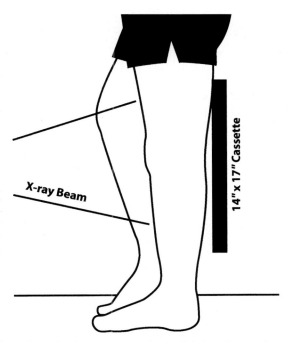

FIG. 3. Standard anteroposterior weightbearing radiograph with the knee in maximal extension. (From Engh GA. *Preoperative planning for total knee arthroplasty.* Alexandria, VA: Anderson Orthopaedic Institute, 1998:14, with permission.)

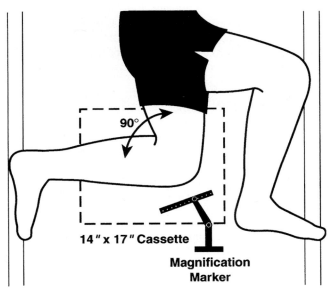

FIG. 5. Table-down lateral radiograph with the knee flexed to 90 degrees. (From Engh GA. *Preoperative planning for total knee arthroplasty.* Alexandria, VA: Anderson Orthopaedic Institute, 1998:15, with permission.)

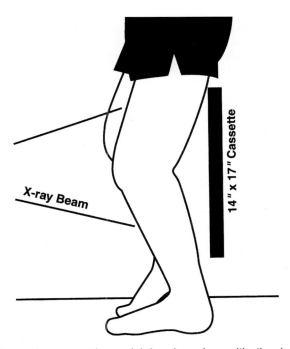

FIG. 4. Anteroposterior weightbearing view with the knee flexed 30 degrees is helpful in evaluating bone loss associated with valgus deformities. (From Engh GA. *Preoperative planning for total knee arthroplasty.* Alexandria, VA: Anderson Orthopaedic Institute, 1998:14, with permission.)

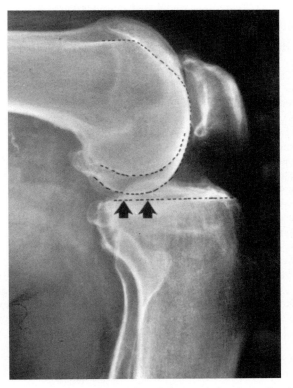

FIG. 6. Increased femoral rollback (*arrows*) due to contracted posterior cruciate ligament evident on a true lateral radiograph. (From Engh GA. *Preoperative planning for total knee arthroplasty.* Alexandria, VA: Anderson Orthopaedic Institute, 1998:15, with permission.)

To measure the size of the defect radiographically, a line is drawn along the lowest point of bone loss on the periphery of the tibial plateau, perpendicular to the midline of the tibia. The defect depth is defined as the distance between this line and the contralateral unaffected tibial plateau (4).

CLASSIFICATION OF BONE DEFICIENCY

To discuss the evaluation and management of bone deficiency in total knee arthroplasty, a common classification system must be referenced. Rand proposed a system to quantify tibial bone loss encountered during primary total knee arthroplasty (4). In this system, bone deficiency is estimated after the initial tibial or femoral bone cuts are made. As seen in Table 1, the defect is classified as minimal (I), moderate (II), extensive (III), or massive cavitary (IV). A minimal defect comprises less than 50% of a single plateau and has a depth of less than 5 mm. A moderate defect comprises 50% to 70% of a single plateau with a depth ranging from 5 to 10 mm. To be classified as extensive, a defect must comprise 70% to 90% of a plateau and have a depth of 10 mm or more. Finally, a massive cavitary defect comprises more than 90% of a single plateau, and the category is subdivided into defects with intact peripheral rims (IV-a) and defects with deficient peripheral rims (IV-b). This basic classification is referenced throughout this chapter as a means of helping the surgeon develop a working algorithm for managing bone deficiency of the tibia during primary total knee arthroplasty.

SURGICAL PLANNING AND TECHNIQUES

Despite bone deficiency, one should adhere to standard principles for performing total knee arthroplasty. As always, soft tissue balancing should be assessed carefully and corrected as necessary. The amount of bone resection should be no more than 6 to 8 mm on the medial side and 10 mm on the lateral side (5). The surgeon must resist the urge to resect additional bone from the tibia in an attempt to eliminate the defect. This is important for three reasons. First, as the distance from the subchondral bone surface increases, the cancellous bone of the proximal tibia becomes weaker (6). Second, as the distance from the normal joint line increases, the cross-sectional area of the tibia decreases and appropriate component sizing becomes difficult (7). Third, resections greater than 1 cm from the lateral tibial plateau disrupt capsular attachments and create lateral side laxity.

Management of bone deficiency during total knee arthroplasty depends on the extent of the defect. Methods of managing bone loss include (a) methylmethacrylate augmentation alone, (b) methylmethacrylate augmentation reinforced with screws,

TABLE 1. *Defect classification*

Defect type	% Involvement of single plateau	Defect depth (mm)
Minimal (I)	<50	<5
Moderate (II)	50–70	5–10
Extensive (III)	70–90	>10
Massive cavitary (IV)	>90	—

(c) metal wedge augmentation, (d) the use of custom prostheses, and (e) bone grafting.

Methylmethacrylate Augmentation Alone

After appropriate resection of proximal tibial bone, minimal defects (type I measuring 3 to 5 mm) may remain. With this technique, residual sclerotic bone should be identified and fenestrated, using a small drill bit to allow ingress of cement. Small minimal deficiencies, whether central or peripheral, then can be filled with cement, provided the bone stock is adequate for tibial tray stability. For larger minimal defects, Lotke et al. recommended slightly shifting the tibial tray away from the defect with a corresponding shifting of the femoral component (8). This process reduces the deficient area and allows for more complete bony support of the component.

Because of the difficulty in maintaining pressurization during cement polymerization, radiolucent lines are often seen at the cement-bone interface after this procedure (5,8,9). Although Lotke et al. noted radiolucent lines in 43 of 59 patients treated with this technique, only 1 patient experienced treatment failure because of progressive loosening of the prosthesis (8). The authors concluded that no correlation existed between the presence of radiolucencies and the patient's clinical symptoms.

Lotke has reported success with this technique in defects up to 25 mm in depth, provided that the defect encompasses less than 50% of the hemiplateau, and the bone is adequate to support the implant. Despite this success, many would agree that this procedure should be reserved for minimal defects (5,10).

Methylmethacrylate Reinforced with Screws

Screw augmentation of the cement may be necessary in situations in which the bony defect might compromise the stability of the tibial tray (for instance, the tray rocks with slight manual pressure). Ritter first described this technique and advocated it for moderate (type II) or extensive (type III) defects (greater than 5 mm in depth) (11). The technique involves using 35-mm stainless steel cancellous bone screws to support the tibial tray. After appropriate débridement of the defect and drilling of the sclerotic bone, the screws are seated into the defect until they are just below the surface of the tibial resection. Next, the screws should be threaded to a level at which their heads are surrounded by cement. The number of screws varies, based on the size of the defect. Mechanical testing in the laboratory has brought the effectiveness of this construct into question (12). However, in a series of 25 patients treated with this technique and followed for more than 7 years, Ritter et al. saw no evidence of cement failure or loosening of the prostheses or screws (13). As with cement alone, there were radiolucencies at the cement-bone interface, but they were not progressive.

Modular Metal Wedge Augmentation

In 1984, Brooks et al. examined proximal tibial defects in cadaveric specimens (12). The authors evaluated the mechanical stability of the following constructs: cement augmentation, cement augmentation with screw reinforcement, metal wedges, and custom prostheses. Their analysis revealed that custom pros-

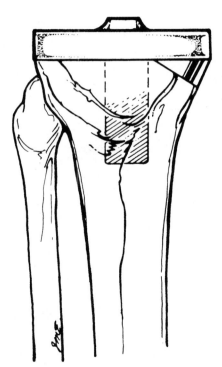

FIG. 7. Moderate bone loss can be managed with a small modular wedge. (From Dorr LD. Management of bone defects. In: Rand JA, ed. *Total knee arthroplasty.* New York: Raven Press, 1993:315, with permission.)

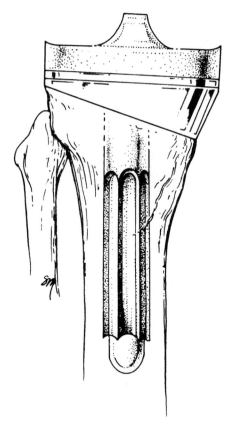

FIG. 8. More extensive bone loss may require large custom wedge augmentation. (From Dorr LD. Management of bone defects. In: Rand JA, ed. *Total knee arthroplasty.* New York: Raven Press, 1993:315, with permission.)

theses were far superior to cement augmentation (with or without screws) in their ability to resist deflection when loaded axially or with a varus load. Metal wedges resisted deflection nearly as well as the custom components and therefore were considered acceptable alternatives. In large part, this study led to more widespread use of custom wedges to fill bone defects in primary and revision situations (4). Although today's modular wedges are available in a variety of sizes (Figs. 7 and 8), their use often requires additional resection of bone to ensure a proper fit. The components are easily assembled intraoperatively and can be fastened to the tibial tray with cement or with screw fixation.

Numerous authors have shared their experiences with wedge augmentation over the past two decades (4,14,15). Brand et al. reviewed the use of wedges in 17 primary knee arthroplasties (14). At a mean follow-up of 36 months, 16% were noted to have radiolucent lines measuring less than 1 mm at the cement-bone interface beneath the wedge. No radiolucent lines were progressive, however, and no components were revised. In follow-up to Rand's initial series (4), Pagnano et al. described the mid-term results of wedge augmentation in 24 primary total knees (15). At a mean follow-up of 5.6 years, the authors reported radiolucencies beneath the wedge in 13 patients. Again, the radiolucencies were not progressive, and no revisions were necessary for tibial component loosening. Patient satisfaction was high in both series. In both studies, the authors recommended the use of wedges in treating elderly patients with moderate to extensive defects (5 to 15 mm).

The use of augmented stems with modular metal wedges continues to be controversial. Although normally used during revi-

sion knee arthroplasty when wedge augmentation is required, stems may not be necessary in the primary setting (4,15).

Custom Implants

Custom one-piece tibial prostheses can be used instead of tibial trays with modular metal wedges. In elderly patients with severe defects, these implants may be a viable option when there is concern about bone graft. Opponents contend that these components are costly and require extensive time to process and manufacture. Furthermore, exact fit is difficult to obtain based on radiographic evaluation alone. However, current three-dimensional computed tomographic reconstruction techniques may provide data to more accurately determine the size and shape of the bone defect, so that a prosthesis can be manufactured that will reconstruct the deficiency. Still, a burr must often be used to contour the defect to facilitate fitting the prosthesis.

Limited experience is reported in the literature regarding augmented integral all-polyethylene tibial components. Jeffery et al. reported on 26 knees in which the Denham prosthesis was used (16). This implant features 15-degree and 30-degree augments built into the undersurface of the polyethylene tibial component. Using a rongeur, the surgeon can trim this polyethylene augment to fit the defect, thereby preserving bone stock. At a

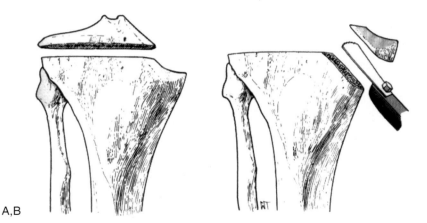

A,B

FIG. 9. With the Sculco technique, after a standard proximal tibial resection is made **(A)**, an oblique cut is used to expose cancellous bone beneath the eroded medial tibia **(B)**. (From Windor RE, Insall JN, Sculco TP. Bone grafting of tibial defects in primary and revision total knee arthroplasty. *Clin Orthop* 1986;205:132–137, with permission.)

median follow-up of 8 years, the authors reported no evidence of loosening.

Bone Grafting

Autologous bone grafting has been shown to be an effective method of addressing moderate (type II), extensive (type III), and cavitary (types IV-a and IV-b) defects during primary and revision procedures (10,17,18). During primary arthroplasty, bone usually is taken locally from the distal or posterior condylar resections. When a posterior-stabilized prosthesis is used, ample bone graft also can be obtained from the intercondylar bony resection. On rare occasions, autologous graft may need to be harvested from the iliac crest. Autologous bone graft should be of good quality and free of osteoarthritic cysts (19). Should revision surgery be necessary, many authors advocate the use of bone grafting in young patients in an attempt to preserve bone stock (1,9). The procedure, however, has been associated with high rates of graft union in elderly patients as well (5,7,9,10).

Basic principles of bone grafting must be followed when tibial defects are grafted. To promote graft union, sclerotic bone must be débrided appropriately, and a viable bleeding cancellous bed should be exposed. To ensure proper fit, the graft must be prepared meticulously. It then must be fixed in a stable manner at the host-graft interface to prevent micromotion. The anatomic alignment of the limb should be corrected to 5 to 9 degrees of valgus to prevent overload and subsequent collapse of the graft. It also is important to prevent collapse or resorption of unstressed graft by completely covering the exposed graft with the tibial component. The use of a metal tibial tray is recommended, because the tray more evenly distributes load to the proximal tibia.

Advantages of autogenous grafting over other techniques include preservation of bone stock, cost effectiveness, and the ease of harvesting bone. Moreover, when grafting is done properly, load transfer to the underlying tibia is more physiologic than with metal custom or augmented components or large cement columns (20). Furthermore, there are no inherent risks

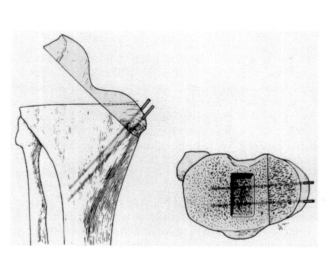

FIG. 10. Distal femoral or posterior condylar bone graft is placed into the defect and temporarily fixed with Kirschner wires. (From Windor RE, Insall JN, Sculco TP. Bone grafting of tibial defects in primary and revision total knee arthroplasty. *Clin Orthop* 1986;205:132–137, with permission.)

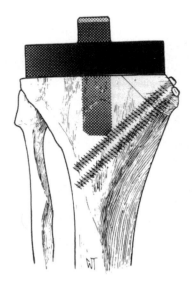

FIG. 11. Cannulated cancellous screws are threaded over Kirschner wires, and the tibial tray is cemented into position. (From Windor RE, Insall JN, Sculco TP. Bone grafting of tibial defects in primary and revision total knee arthroplasty. *Clin Orthop* 1986;205:132–137, with permission.)

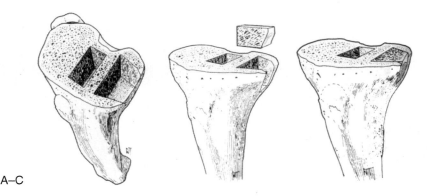

A–C

FIG. 12. In the Insall technique, a surgeon creates a rectangular or trapezoidal defect with a burr **(A)**. Next, a bone graft block is fashioned to fit this defect **(B)**. This graft is tapped into place to ensure a self-locking fit **(C)**. (From Windor RE, Insall JN, Sculco TP. Bone grafting of tibial defects in primary and revision total knee arthroplasty. *Clin Orthop* 1986;205:132–137, with permission.)

of disease transmission, as seen with allograft bone. Disadvantages to autogenous bone grafting include the possibility of graft nonunion, collapse, or fragmentation (21).

Numerous methods of tibial bone grafting have been described in the literature; however, the most commonly used have been those of Sculco and Insall. The Sculco technique (7) is useful for peripheral lesions, whereas the Insall technique (22) can be used for either central or peripheral lesions.

With the Sculco technique, a standard proximal 5-mm resection is done (Fig. 9). A saw is used to remove sclerotic bone in the defect and expose an oblique cancellous bone bed to accept the graft. Distal femoral or posterior condylar bone graft is then placed into the defect and the excess is removed with a saw (Fig. 10). The graft is temporarily held in place with Kirschner wires, which are later replaced with cancellous screws (Fig. 11). When the prosthesis is cemented into place, it is important to prevent cement from entering the interface between graft and native bone.

Insall described a technique that used self-locking dowel fixation, which eliminated the need for screw fixation. The surgeon creates a rectangular or trapezoidal defect using a burr. Then a bone graft block is fashioned to fit this defect and tapped into place to ensure a snug fit (Fig. 12). When the defect is peripheral, the widest base of the trapezoid should be located centrally to lock the graft in place. This technique allows axial compressive forces but prevents shear forces from disrupting the graft or preventing union. Based on the size of the grafted defect, weightbearing may be limited postoperatively. With small lesions, routine postoperative rehabilitation can be followed, with weightbearing permitted as tolerated. When larger grafts have been used to reconstruct more extensive bone deficiency, weightbearing can be protected for up to 3 to 4 months.

Results described in the literature using allografting techniques have been encouraging, with high rates of graft union and patient satisfaction (9,10,16,17,23). The few observed failures resulted from lack of restoration of proper limb alignment and from improper preparation of the sclerotic bony bed.

CONCLUSION

Angular deformity about the knee results in asymmetric bone loss primarily on the tibia. While addressing these deformities during primary total knee arthroplasty, the surgeon must resist the temptation to resect excess bone to eliminate the defect. Resection more than 5 mm from the proximal tibia places higher loads on weaker cancellous bone and potentially contributes to

collapse of the bone and loosening of the prosthesis. After standard tibial resection has been performed, numerous techniques exist to deal with residual bone deficiency. For minimal defects, the authors recommend cement augmentation, cement augmentation reinforced with screws, or autologous bone grafting (Table 1). Moderate and extensive defects can be managed with metal wedge augmentation, custom implants, or a variety of bone-grafting techniques. Cavitary defects require extensive bone grafting and may necessitate the use of allograft bone. The specific technique used is based on the size and location of the lesion, as well as the experience of the surgeon. When they are used in the proper setting, excellent results can be obtained with any of these techniques.

REFERENCES

1. Scuderi GR, Insall JN. Fixed varus and valgus deformities. In: Lotke PA, ed. Knee arthroplasty. New York: Raven Press, 1995:111–127.
2. Harman MK, Markovich GD, Banks SA, et al. Wear patterns on tibial plateaus from varus and valgus osteoarthritic knees. *Clin Orthop* 1998;352:149–158.
3. Engh GA. Preoperative planning for total knee arthroplasty. Alexandria, VA: Anderson Orthopaedic Institute, 1998:14–16.
4. Rand JA. Bone deficiency in total knee arthroplasty: use of metal wedge augmentation. *Clin Orthop* 1991;271:63–71.
5. Dorr LD. Management of bone defects. In: Rand JA, ed. Total knee arthroplasty. New York: Raven Press, 1993:309–317.
6. Harada Y, Wevers HW, Cooke TDV. Distribution of bone strength in the proximal tibia. *J Arthroplasty* 1988;3:167–175.
7. Sculco TP. Bone grafting. In: Lotke PA, ed. Knee arthroplasty. New York: Raven Press, 1995:131–140.
8. Lotke PA, Wong RY, Ecker ML. The use of methylmethacrylate in primary total knee replacements with large tibial defects. *Clin Orthop* 1991;270:288–294.
9. Dorr LD. Bone grafts for bone loss with total knee replacement. *Orthop Clin North Am* 1989;20:179–187.
10. Dorr LD, Ranawat CS, Sculco TA, et al. Bone graft for tibial defects in total knee arthroplasty. *Clin Orthop* 1986;205:153–165.
11. Ritter MA. Screw and cement fixation of large defects in total knee arthroplasty. *J Arthroplasty* 1986;1:125–129.
12. Brooks PJ, Walker PS, Scott RD. Tibial component fixation in deficient tibial bone stock. *Clin Orthop* 1984;184:302–308.
13. Ritter MA, Keating EM, Faris PM. Screw and cement fixation of large defects in total knee arthroplasty: a sequel. *J Arthroplasty* 1993;8:63–65.
14. Brand MG, Daley RJ, Ewald FC, et al. Tibial tray augmentation with modular metal wedges for tibial bone deficiency. *Clin Orthop* 1989;248:71–79.
15. Pagnano MW, Trousdale RT, Rand JA. Tibial wedge augmentation for bone deficiency in total knee arthroplasty: a followup study. *Clin Orthop* 1995;321:151–155.

16. Jeffery RS, Orton MA, Denham RA. Wedged tibial components for total knee arthroplasty. *J Arthroplasty* 1994;9:381–387.
17. Stockley I, McAuley JP, Gross AE. Allograft reconstruction in total knee arthroplasty. *J Bone Joint Surg Br* 1992;74:393–397.
18. Hill RA, Phillips H. Bone grafting in primary uncemented total knee arthroplasty. *J Arthroplasty* 1992;7:25–30.
19. Aglietti P, Buzzi R, Scrobe F. Autologous bone grafting for medial tibial defects in total knee arthroplasty. *J Arthroplasty* 1991;6:287–293.
20. Shrivastava SC, Ahmed AN, Shriazi-Adl A, et al. Effect of cement-bone composite layer and prosthesis geometry on stresses in a prosthetically resurfaced tibia. *J Biomed Mater Res* 1982;16:929–949.
21. Laskin RS. Total knee arthroplasty in the presence of large bony defects of the tibia and marked knee instability. *Clin Orthop* 1989;248:66–70.
22. Windsor RE, Insall JN, Sculco TP. Bone grafting of tibial defects in primary and revision total knee arthroplasty. *Clin Orthop* 1986;205:132–137.
23. Scuderi GS, Insall JN, Haas SB, et al. Inlay autogenic bone grafting of tibial defects in primary total knee arthroplasty. *Clin Orthop* 1989;248:93–97.

CHAPTER 83

Soft Tissue Balancing of the Valgus Knee

Chitranjan S. Ranawat, Douglas S. Holden, Amar S. Ranawat, and Vijay J. Rasquinha

Approximately 10% of patients requiring total knee arthroplasty have a valgus deformity. The correction of the valgus deformity has posed technical challenges and has produced variable clinical results in terms of correction of deformity, stability, and overall results. Valgus deformity may be caused by rheumatoid arthritis, posttraumatic arthritis, osteoarthritis, and metabolic bone disease.

The valgus deformity consists of two components: an element of bone loss, primarily from the lateral femoral condyle and lateral tibial plateau, and a soft tissue contracture consisting of tight lateral structures such as the iliotibial band, lateral collateral ligament, popliteus tendon, posterolateral capsule, and hamstring muscles (1). In this chapter, we describe how the senior author approaches the valgus knee when performing a total knee replacement.

PREOPERATIVE EVALUATION

Clinical Assessment

Preoperatively, the patient is evaluated for weightbearing alignment to determine the true amount of deformity. Any flexion contractures and instability are noted, as are medial and lateral soft tissue laxity. The laxity is graded as type I (less than 5 mm), type II (5 to 10 mm), or type III (more than 10 mm). The majority of valgus knees have medial ligament and capsular stretching in combination with shortening of the posterolateral structures. The exception to this is found in rheumatoid patients who have a valgus knee, along with synovitis.

Radiographic Imaging

Standing anteroposterior, lateral, and sunrise views of the knee, and an anteroposterior view of the pelvis are obtained for all patients. These are evaluated for bony deformity and osteophytes, as well as for the alignment of the ipsilateral hip. The medial soft tissue laxity is noted on the radiographs as well. Any discrepancy between the medial and lateral joint spaces, as well as any disparity between the femoral and tibial alignment, can be assessed on the anteroposterior view. These radiographs are used to determine the bony cuts and the implant size needed.

Templating

Anteroposterior View

1. Draw a vertical line down the center of the femoral and tibial shafts (Fig. 1).
2. On the tibial shaft, draw a perpendicular line to the first line at the level of the more involved tibial plateau (in this case, the lateral plateau). This will be used to give an idea of the tibial resection that will be performed. The relative amount of the bony resection can be determined as well as the ratio of lateral to medial resection.
3. On the femoral side, draw a horizontal line that is in 5 degrees of valgus from the vertical line that was drawn in step 1. This line, passing through the highest point of the intercondylar notch, gives an idea of the bony resection needed from the medial and lateral femoral condyles.

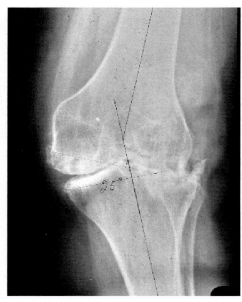

FIG. 1. Preoperative templating on the anteroposterior view helps determine the amount of bony resection required.

Lateral View

1. On the lateral view, identify any posterior osteophytes and outline them with a marker. During the procedure, be certain to remove these osteophytes, as they may hinder the range of motion as well as the soft tissue balance.
2. The lateral view is used for sizing the femoral component, as magnification of the femoral condyle is between 5% and 7% on the anteroposterior view.

PATIENT POSITIONING

After administration of the selected anesthetic agent, the patient is positioned supine on the operative table. A tourniquet is placed on the thigh, and the knee is shaved if necessary. Positioned to align with the level of the tourniquet, a lateral thigh post can help prevent excessive external rotation when the knee is placed in flexion. The knee is then flexed to 85 degrees and a bump is placed under the ipsilateral foot with the knee in this position and is then taped securely to the table. During the procedure, the bump helps maintain the knee in flexion.

SURGICAL TECHNIQUE

Approach and Exposure

After positioning, the extremity is prepared and draped. An Esmarch bandage is used to exsanguinate the limb and the tourniquet is inflated. With the knee flexed to 90 degrees, a long straight midline incision is made starting approximately 12 cm proximal to the superior pole of the patella and continuing an equal distance distal to the inferior pole of the patella. This size of incision is used to decrease skin tension as well as fat necrosis of the underlying soft tissues.

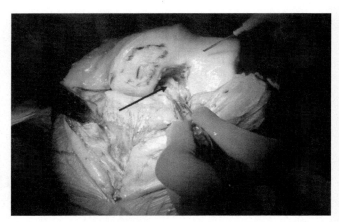

FIG. 2. With the knee flexed, the cruciate ligaments (*arrow*) are removed.

The incision is carried down to the deep fascial layer to expose the quadriceps tendon, vastus medialis oblique, patella, and patella tendon. Undermining of the skin flaps is avoided. The quadriceps tendon is incised 2 to 3 mm lateral to the medial margin of the tendon and carried along the medial margin of the patella (with a 2- to 3-mm slip of tissue left on the patella) and the patella tendon, and subperiosteally 5 cm distal to the superior margin of the tibial tubercle.

The medial soft tissues are released subperiosteally from the proximal tibia using an osteotome or electrocautery to create a small medial sleeve of tissue. The patella is then everted and the knee fully flexed to expose the cruciates and the menisci. Our preference, a posterior stabilized knee, requires release of both cruciates at this point (Fig. 2). The menisci are excised and the tibia is maximally flexed and externally rotated to expose the entire tibial plateau. The knee is stabilized in flexion by placing the foot on the previously installed bump.

Tibial Resection

The malleolar clamp of the tibial alignment guide is positioned just proximal to the malleoli. The platform is raised to the level of the plateau. The lower alignment guide is positioned slightly medial to the midline of the ankle to accommodate the more prominent lateral malleoli. (Bisecting the transmalleolar axis would prejudice a varus cut.) The upper platform is aligned with the medial third of the tibial tubercle and the medial margin of the lateral intercondylar eminence, with the cutting surface placed against the anterior cortex. The exact level of resection varies depending on the patient's preoperatively evaluated deformity and ligamentous laxity.

In varus knees the stylus is positioned on the lateral plateau, and 10 mm is resected from the less involved side (in this case, the lateral side) (11). With a valgus knee, however, we place the stylus on the medial plateau and remove 6 to 8 mm, depending on the amount of deformity and on medial and lateral laxity. Before making the tibial cuts, alignment should be confirmed with the alignment guide. The distal portion of the alignment device should align with the center of the talus on the anteroposterior view. On the lateral view, the alignment rod should run parallel with the tibial crest. Once the cutting jig is

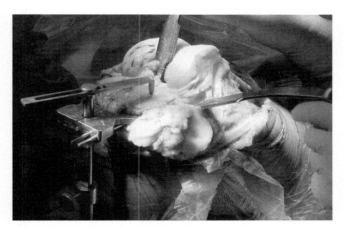

FIG. 3. Measured tibial bone resection is 6 to 10 mm, depending on preoperative templating.

secured in place, the proximal tibial resection is performed (Figs. 3 and 4).

Next, the tibial template is used to determine the size of the tibial tray needed. An alignment rod is used to check the alignment of the cut tibial surface (Fig. 5).

Femoral Resection

The femoral canal is first entered using a gouge to assist in drill passage. The entry point is chosen by first noting the intersection of the patellofemoral and the tibiofemoral articular surfaces on the lateral and medial femoral condyles. Next a line connecting these two points is visualized. Then, the midline of the intercondylar notch is identified and its perpendicular to the first line is marked. The intersection of these two lines is the entry point (Fig. 6). The gouge is used to make a shallow depression for placement of the drill bit. The canal is entered with a drill and the entry point is then enlarged by rotating the drill before sinking the drill completely. If the entry was correct, the drill should not come into contact with the cortices of the femoral shaft.

Next, the intramedullary femoral rod is placed into the hole and the femoral cutting jig is aligned with the distal aspect of the femur. The valgus angle with the appropriate right or left desig-

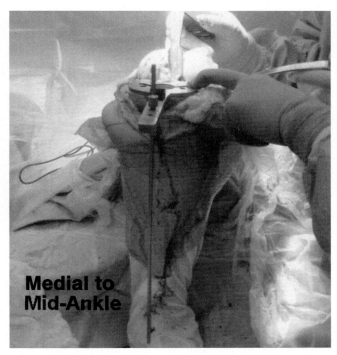

FIG. 5. Alignment of the cut tibial surface is checked with the alignment rod. The rod should pass slightly medial to the midline of the ankle.

nation is set and placed on the front of the locating device. With a valgus knee, we usually set the jig to 3 degrees of valgus to compensate for diaphyseal valgus remodeling that has taken place and to avoid undercorrection.

The cutting block is then rotated until it is perpendicular to the mechanical axis of the tibial cut with the knee in 90 degrees of flexion. The anterior rough cut is made (Fig. 7), and then the distal cut is made according to the system being used (Fig. 8). We usually perform a 10-mm distal resection.

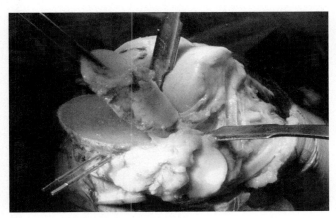

FIG. 4. Resected tibial bone is removed.

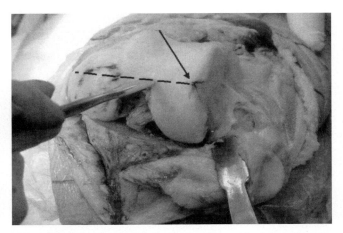

FIG. 6. The entry point for the femoral canal is determined by the intersection of two lines. First, find the intersection of the patellofemoral and tibiofemoral articular surfaces (*arrow*) on each femoral condyle and draw a horizontal line connecting them. Next, draw the midline of the intercondylar notch. Where these two intersect is the entry point.

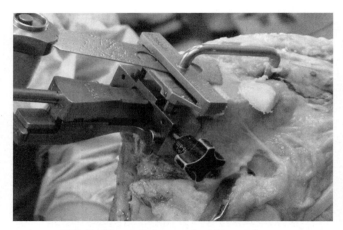

FIG. 7. The anterior rough cut is made.

Evaluation of the Flexion and Extension Gap

Once the distal femoral cut has been made, the knee is placed in full extension and the laminar spreaders are applied centrally to evaluate the gap. The goal is a rectangular extension gap. When the gap is trapezoidal, additional soft tissue balancing is necessary (Figs. 9 through 14). (Bone cuts are not altered to obtain a rectangular gap in extension.)

When blocks are used to assess flexion and extension gaps, a 10-mm-thick spacer block should be used to evaluate the extension gap and an 8-mm-thick block should be used to assess the flexion gap (Figs. 15 through 17). This will compensate for the 2-mm difference between the distal and posterior resection levels.

The flexion gap is likewise evaluated with laminar spreaders and the femoral cutting block is adjusted accordingly to create a rectangular flexion gap via bone cuts (Fig. 18). Alternatively, an 8-mm spacer block may be used to assess the flexion gap (Fig. 19).

Lateral Ligament Release for a Fixed Valgus Deformity

1. Remove peripheral osteophytes.
2. Perform medial and lateral meniscectomy.

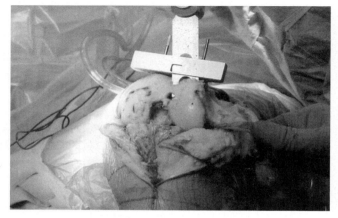

FIG. 8. The distal femoral cuts are made.

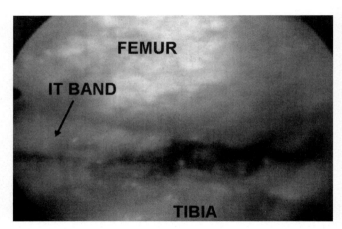

FIG. 9. After assessing the extension gap with laminar spreaders in the valgus knee, a trapezoidal space is noted with marked tightening of the lateral structures. Figure shows a view of the inside of the knee before lateral soft tissue release. Important landmarks are identified. The iliotibial (IT) band is first identified and then the posterolateral capsule.

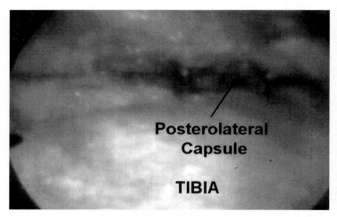

FIG. 10. The posterolateral capsule has been identified. The release is initiated from just lateral to the insertion of the posterior cruciate ligament to the posterior margin of the iliotibial band at the level of the tibial resection.

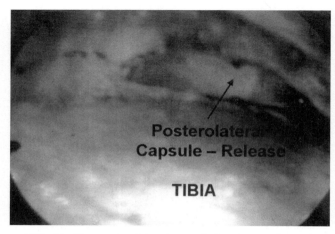

FIG. 11. The posterolateral capsule has been released.

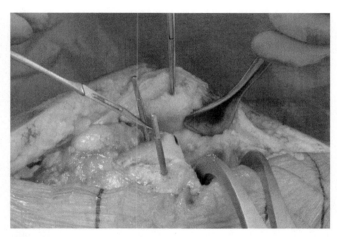

FIG. 12. The extension gap is reassessed with a laminar spreader after posterolateral capsule release.

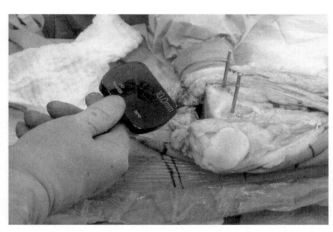

FIG. 15. Alternatively, the extension space can be checked with a 10-mm spacer block.

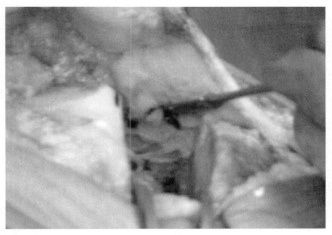

FIG. 13. If further release is necessary at this point, multiple stab incisions are made in the iliotibial band (pie crusting). In most cases, these steps allow for a balanced knee. However, if further release is needed, the popliteus tendon can be released at this point.

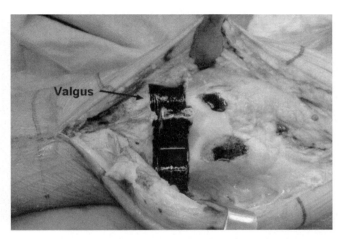

FIG. 16. When the extension gap is checked with the 10-mm spacer block, a valgus stress is first placed, and the amount of medial opening is noted.

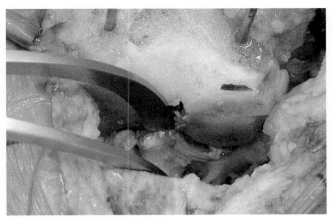

FIG. 14. The extension gap is assessed after final release. Note that the extension space is now square.

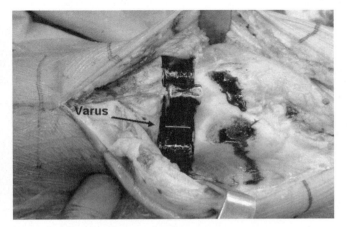

FIG. 17. A varus stress is placed, and the amount of lateral opening is noted. The amount of opening on valgus and varus stress should be equal.

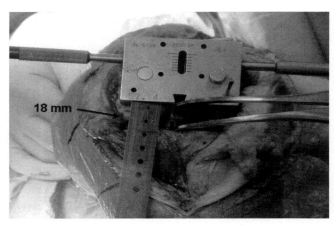

FIG. 18. Laminar spreaders are used to check the flexion gap. The laminar spreaders are placed in the middle of the femoral cutting block and opened. The amount of opening should be equal medially and laterally.

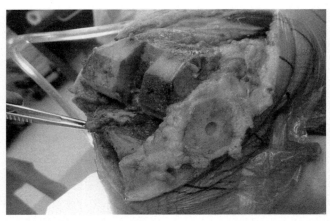

FIG. 20. Soft tissues have been balanced and all bone cuts made. Any soft tissue remaining posteriorly that may hinder placement of the components is removed.

3. Release of the posterolateral capsule is performed with the knee extended and distracted with laminar spreaders. The popliteus is preserved at this point. The release is performed intraarticularly just above the level of the tibial cut using electrocautery transversely from the posterior margin of the iliotibial band to just lateral to the posterior cruciate ligament, which is resected in all cases (Figs. 9 through 14).

4. The iliotibial band is lengthened as necessary from inside with multiple transverse stab incisions a few centimeters above the joint. This is termed the "pie crusting" technique (2).

5. Release of the posterolateral capsule and lengthening of the iliotibial band results in a balanced knee in all but the most severe valgus knees. In these cases, release of the popliteal tendon is performed with electrocautery from within the joint. The release of the lateral collateral ligament has not been necessary with the use of this soft tissue release technique but, as described previously, can be performed as a final step, if needed, from the femoral attachment.

6. The retention of at least one or two of the lateral stabilizers is important for stability. If instability is detected after

releases have been performed, then use of a constrained component is considered.

7. A complete lateral retinacular release has not been necessary with this technique. Instead, patellar tracking is assessed after the trial components are inserted by flexing the knee between 60 and 90 degrees with the tourniquet released. With no external pressure applied to the patella, it should rest in the trochlear groove in contact with the medial and lateral femoral condyles. If the patella is not touching the medial femoral condyle, multiple pie-crusting transverse stab incisions are made on the lateral retinaculum. The lateral superior geniculate artery is identified and preserved whenever possible.

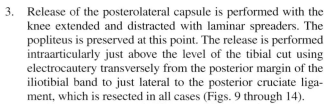

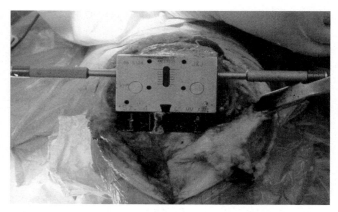

FIG. 19. Alternatively, an 8-mm spacer block may be used to check the flexion gap.

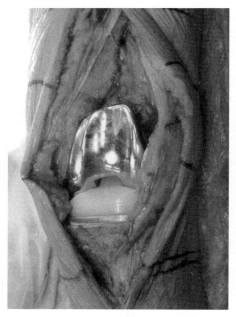

FIG. 21. All components are cemented in place, and the cement is allowed to cure.

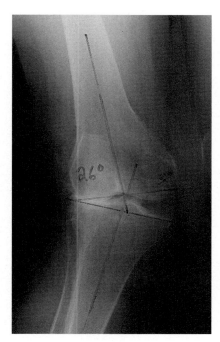

FIG. 22. Preoperative anteroposterior view of a valgus knee.

Once the soft tissues are balanced to give a rectangular gap, the femur is sized and the appropriate cuts made to fit the trial component (Fig. 20).

Once all bony cuts have been made, flexion and extension gaps are again tested with spacer blocks to assess for equal medial and lateral soft tissue tension.

The patella is prepared. Then all trial components are placed and the alignment and soft tissue balance are reassessed by per-

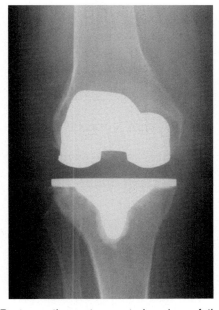

FIG. 23. Postoperative anteroposterior view of the knee in Figure 22 with PFC Sigma posterior stabilized rotating platform prosthesis.

forming a varus and valgus stress and thereby evaluating for equal medial and lateral soft tissue tension. If the tension is satisfactory, the components are cemented into place and the cement is allowed to cure (Fig. 21). The knee is then irrigated, a Hemovac drain placed, and the incision closed. A sterile dressing is placed and the patient is begun on continuous passive motion the first postoperative day, along with physical therapy for ambulation.

POSTOPERATIVE COURSE

The patient is evaluated closely for any signs of peroneal nerve compromise. If any sign of nerve compromise develops, the knee is placed in flexion. If the compromise does not improve, the bandage is then loosened.

Physical therapy and continuous passive motion are initiated on postoperative day 1 after the Hemovac drain has been removed. Patients are progressed to weightbearing as tolerated (Figs. 22 and 23).

RESULTS AND DISCUSSION

Many different surgical techniques and approaches have been described for correcting the valgus knee (4–7,10,12–17). The results are generally good, and excellent long-term function can be expected from a well-balanced knee regardless of the technique used (Table 1). The results are generally inferior and the complication rates are generally higher when correcting valgus deformity, however, than when correcting its varus counterpart (15). This is due, in part, to the technically demanding nature of soft tissue balancing in the valgus knee. This, in turn, has led some surgeons to accept the use of constrained implants when stability could not be achieved with balancing techniques alone. Other surgeons have promoted medial-sided medial collateral ligament–tightening reconstructions or lateral parapatellar approaches to deal with these inherent instabilities (6,7,12,13). It is the senior author's opinion that these techniques are not only unnecessary but also technically difficult, which increases the risk for wound and extensor mechanism complications. The technique described herein was adopted by the senior author in 1985 to reduce the need for constrained implants and reduce the incidence of late instability noted with his earlier technique, originally described in 1979 with the total condylar knee (Figs. 24 through 27) (1,2,9). The technique is simple, reproducible, and enduring.

When this technique was used with the PFC Sigma posterior stabilized total knee system, only 6% of patients with total knee replacements had a mild degree of postoperative mediolateral instability at an average of 7 years follow-up. Regarding intraoperative instability after ligament release, there have been no cases of progressive instability and no cases in which a constrained implant was needed.

In the 2-year period from March 1999 to March 2001, the senior author performed 349 total knee replacements using the PFC Sigma posterior stabilized rotating platform knee system, 45 of which were in valgus knees. Of these 45 valgus knees, 2 (4.4%) required a lateral release, none required a constrained total condylar III prosthesis, and clinically all knees have been stable. Despite other authors' findings in cadaveric studies using this technique (8), we have had no instances of neurovascular injury.

We therefore recommend this technique for the correction of all valgus deformities.

TABLE 1. *Results of total knee replacement for valgus deformity*

Study	Implant	PCL status	TKR (N)	Follow-up (yr)	Results	Complications					
						Instability	Delayed wound healing	Patellofemoral problems	Peroneal nerve palsy	Aseptic loosening	Reoperation
Soft tissue balancing procedures											
Whiteside (4)	Ortholoc	PCL retained	231	6	N/R	None	N/R	None	N/R	N/R	N/R
Miyasaka et al. (2)	TC	PCL sacrificed	108	14	91% survivorship at 13 yr	2%	N/R	2%	None	3%	6%
Aglietti et al. (18)	IB	PCL stabilized	67	6	95% survivorship at 10 yr	2%	3%	6%	None	3%	4%
Karachalios et al. (14)	Kinematic	PCL retained	34[a]	5	85% good/excellent	3%	N/R	12%	N/R	N/R	N/R
Whiteside (5)	Ortholoc	PCL retained	135	6	N/R	1.8%	5%	9%	N/R	N/R	13%
Laurencin et al. (17)	Variable	84% PCL retained	25	5	N/R	4%	4%	4%	4%	None	12%
Stern et al. (15)	Variable	81% PCL stabilized	134	5	91% good/excellent	N/R	N/R	N/R	4%	2%	3%
Insall et al. (10)	TC	PCL sacrificed	90[a]	4	90% good/excellent	2.2%	N/R	N/R	2%	N/R	4%
Medial reconstruction procedures											
Healy et al. (6)	Variable	7 PCL retaining	8	6	100% good/excellent	None	N/R	None	N/R	N/R	0%
Krackow et al. (13)	PCA	PCL retaining	99	5	90% good/excellent	6%	11%	2%	3%	3%	6%
Lateral approach procedures											
Fiddian et al. (7)	PFC	PCL retaining	27	1	100% good/excellent	N/R	7%	None	None	None	0%
Keblish (12)	LCS	74% PCL retaining	53	3	94.3% good/excellent	2%	6%	None	4%	None	4%
Buechel (16)	N/R	N/R	N/R	N/R	N/R	N/R	N/R	N/R	N/R	N/R	N/R

IB, Insall-Burstein; LCS, low contact stress; N/R, not reported; PCA, porous-coated anatomic; PCL, posterior cruciate ligament; PFC, PFC Sigma; TC, total condylar; TKR, total knee replacements.

[a]Subset.

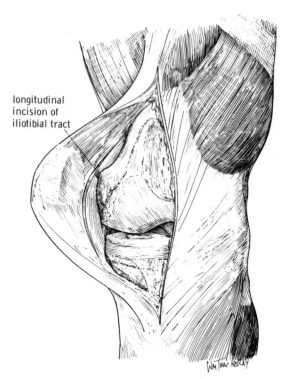

FIG. 24. Technique of soft tissue release performed by the senior author before 1985. With the knee in full extension, the patella is everted and the lateral retinaculum released longitudinally.

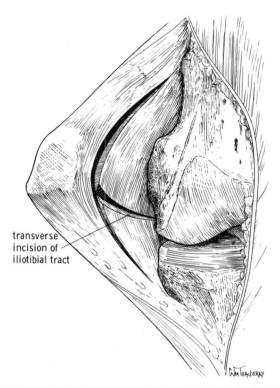

FIG. 25. In the technique used before 1985, the iliotibial band was incised transversely 1 in. above the joint line.

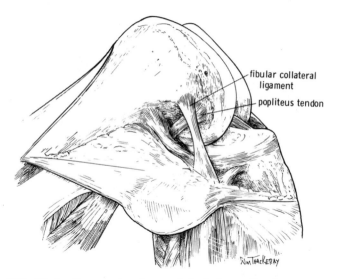

FIG. 26. In the previously used technique, the knee was flexed to 90 degrees with the patella everted laterally. This exposed the femoral attachments of the collateral ligament, popliteus tendon, and posterior capsule.

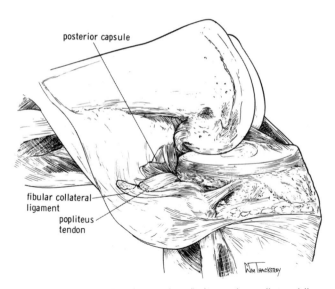

FIG. 27. In the previously used technique, the collateral ligament, popliteus tendon, and posterior capsule were released from the femoral attachments.

REFERENCES

1. Ranawat CS, ed. *Total-condylar knee arthroplasty*. New York: Springer-Verlag, 1985.
2. Miyasaka KC, Ranawat CS, Mullaji A. 10- to 20-year follow-up of total knee arthroplasty for valgus deformities. *Clin Orthop* 1997;345:29.
3. Reference deleted in text.
4. Whiteside LA. Selective ligament release in total knee arthroplasty of the knee in valgus. *Clin Orthop* 1999;367:130.
5. Whiteside LA. Correction of ligament and bone defects in total arthroplasty of the severely valgus knee. *Clin Orthop* 1993;288:234.

6. Healy WL, Iorio R, Lemos DW. Medial reconstruction during total knee arthroplasty for severe valgus deformity. *Clin Orthop* 1998;356:161.

7. Fiddian NJ, Blakeway C, Kumar A. Replacement arthroplasty of the valgus knee. A modified lateral capsular approach with repositioning of vastus lateralis. *J Bone Joint Surg Br* 1998;80:859.

8. Mihalko WM, Krackow KA. Anatomic and biomechanical aspects of pie crusting posterolateral structures for valgus deformity correction in total knee arthroplasty cadaveric study. *J Arthroplasty* 2000;15:347.

9. Ranawat CS, Rose HA, Rich DS. Total condylar knee arthroplasty for valgus and combined valgus-flexion deformity of the knee. *Instr Course Lect* 1984;33:412.

10. Insall JN, Scott WN, Ranawat CS. The total-condylar knee prosthesis. *J Bone Joint Surg Am* 1979;61:173.

11. Scott DS, Thornhill TS, Ranawat CS. *Surgical technique for use with PFC Sigma Knee Systems.* Warsaw, IN: Depuy Orthopedics, 1998.

12. Keblish PA. The lateral approach to the valgus knee. *Clin Orthop* 1991;271:52.

13. Krackow KA, Jones MM, Teeny SM, et al. Primary total knee arthroplasty in patients with fixed valgus deformity. *Clin Orthop* 1991;273:9.

14. Karachalios TH, Sarangi PP, Newman JH. Severe varus and valgus deformity treated by total knee arthroplasty. *J Bone Joint Surg Br* 1994;76:938.

15. Stern SH, Moeckel BH, Insall JN. Total knee arthroplasty in valgus knees. *Clin Orthop* 1991;273:5.

16. Buechel FF. A sequential three-step lateral release for correcting fixed valgus deformities during total knee arthroplasty. *Clin Orthop* 1990;260:170.

17. Laurencin CT, Scott RD, Volatile TB, et al. Total knee replacement in severe valgus deformity. *Am J Knee Surg* 1992;5(3):135.

18. Aglietti P, Buzzi R, Giron F, et al. The Insall-Burstein posterior stabilized total knee replacement in the valgus knee. *Am J Knee Surg* 1996;9(1):8.

CHAPTER 84

Soft Tissue Balancing of the Varus Knee

Richard S. Laskin

A varus deformity is the most common anatomic deformity encountered by surgeons performing knee replacements for patients with advanced arthritis. In some cultures, as in Japan, a varus knee is endemic to the point of being the norm. Of the last 1,000 primary total knee replacements that the author performed for patients with osteoarthritis, 83% of the extremities were in varus. Although it has been suggested that most patients with rheumatoid arthritis have a valgus deformity, over 55% of the author's patients with this disease had a varus deformity as well.

A leg is neutrally aligned (or has a neutral mechanical axis) in the coronal plane when a line drawn from the center of the femoral head to the center of the ankle mortise passes through the center of the knee joint. Because at surgery localization of the femoral head is often difficult and inaccurate (i.e., without preoperative radiographic markers), most surgeons now use a measurement based on the intramedullary canals of the femur and tibia. When this anatomic axis measurement system is used, the range of 4 to 9 degrees of valgus is considered neutral alignment. Any coronal alignment of less than 4 degrees of valgus is considered varus.

TYPES OF VARUS DEFORMITY

Knee deformities in the arthritic patient can be divided into three types. *Flexible* deformities are those that can passively be corrected to a neutral leg alignment. *Fixed* deformities are those that cannot be passively corrected. *Mixed* deformities may be partially correctible but are still partially fixed.

Pain may preclude the examiner from making a proper evaluation as to the nature of a patient's deformity; therefore, the final determination as to whether a deformity is fixed or flexible should be made with the patient under anesthesia. When a large series of patients undergoing knee replacement were evaluated (1), less than one-third of the varus deformities that appeared

fixed preoperatively were indeed fixed when the patient was anesthetized. It was only these fixed deformities that required soft tissue releases. If a surgeon were to erroneously perform a soft tissue release for a varus deformity that was not truly fixed, the outcome would be knee instability.

Many patients with fixed varus deformities have a concomitant inability to fully extend the knee passively. In two groups that we studied over the past 10 years (2), over 75% of all patients with a fixed varus deformity also had a fixed flexion deformity. There was, however, no correlation between the exact magnitude of the varus deformity and the magnitude of the flexion deformity.

CAUSES OF VARUS DEFORMITY

Some patients have a varus deformity of the leg secondary to an angulation of the femoral or tibial shaft at some distance from the knee. This may be the result of a malunited fracture, Paget disease, a congenital deformity (such as Blount disease or fibrous dysplasia), or an underlying metabolic process. Although such deformities must be taken into account when assessing overall leg alignment, this chapter does not deal with these problems but rather with those deformities that exist because of a pathologic process in or immediately adjacent to the knee joint.

The basic intraarticular cause of a varus deformity is an asymmetric loss of articular cartilage or bone that is greater from the medial side than from the lateral side of the knee. Loss of cartilage often occurs from medial overload in a knee with abnormal kinematics. The two most common etiologic conditions are an insufficient anterior cruciate ligament and a prior total meniscectomy (3). Medial overload can also occur in the leg with a varus hip alignment or a bowing of the femoral shaft. The author has seen the problem in two patients after total hip replacement

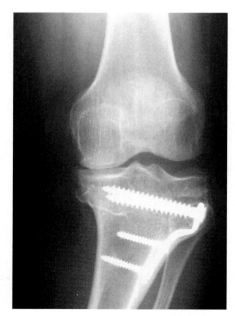

FIG. 1. Varus collapse after osteotomy.

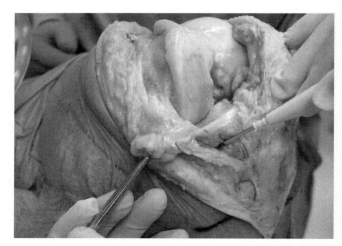

FIG. 2. Elevation of the anteromedial capsule with a cautery.

in which an abnormally high offset prosthesis had been used as well as in patients with a malunited femoral shaft fracture.

The loss of articular cartilage medially leads to increased stress in the underlying bone of the tibial plateau. The initial response is subchondral sclerosis. The increased stiffness of the subchondral bone can lead to increased stresses in the articular cartilage. With time, however, this increased bone adaptation can fail, which leads to microfractures and bony collapse. Furthermore, with loss of cartilage, there can be intrusion of synovial fluid into the bone surface. With subsequent pressurization of the fluid, cystic changes occur. As the cysts collapse, further bone loss can occur.

Improperly performed high tibial osteotomies can also cause bone collapse medially. The most common scenario is an osteotomy that had been performed too close to the joint surface, with subsequent fracture or avascular collapse of the medial tibial plateau fragment (Fig. 1).

Initially, the medial soft tissues in a patient with a varus deformity are relatively normal. In some patients they remain normal, and the deformity remains flexible. In other patients, the soft tissues medially become contracted. It is this contracture—accentuated by peripheral osteophyte formation—that makes the varus deformity fixed.

In the valgus knee there is often an associated hypoplasia or dysgenesis of the posterior and distal aspects of the lateral femoral condyle. This perpetuates (or possibly even is the cause of) the valgus deformity and renders the posterior condylar line ineffective in determining position of the femoral component. This does not appear to occur, however, in the varus knee. Using magnetic resonance imaging, Matsuda et al. (4) evaluated the femoral geometry of 30 normal and 30 varus knees. In the sagittal view, the distal part of the medial condyle was somewhat deformed but not shortened in the varus knees. There was no significant difference in the shape or extent of the posterior portion of the medial femoral condyle when varus knees were compared with knees that were in neutral alignment. In the

transverse view, the transepicondylar axis was positioned at approximately 6 degrees of external rotation relative to the posterior condylar axis in the varus knees and the normal knees. These results suggested that, unlike in valgus knees, there was no hypoplasia of the femoral condyles.

TREATMENT OF INTRAARTICULAR VARUS DEFORMITY

The correction of a varus deformity during a total knee replacement should be gradual and progressive. Overzealous releases can lead to an imbalance of the flexion and extension spaces and postoperative knee instability.

The surgeon should initially ascertain that there truly is a fixed deformity that requires release. If, under anesthesia, the leg can be corrected to neutral alignment, then no soft tissue releases should be performed.

The standard surgical exposure of the knee involves an elevation of the soft tissues from the anteromedial tibial plateau. This elevation begins at the medial border of the patellar tendon insertion and progresses around the medial tibia to the level of the midcoronal plane. Technically this exposure is most easily performed with the knee in flexion and with gradual external rotation of the lower leg (Fig. 2). At this point anteromedial osteophytes are removed. With the knee held in external rotation, a curved periosteal elevator is passed posteriorly to just beyond the midcoronal line (Fig. 3). The author considers this soft tissue elevation to be not a formal release but rather an integral part of the exposure of the knee. To properly visualize the tibial plateau surface, the tibia must be subluxed anterior to the femur. One needs a soft tissue "window" at least the size of the bone to be delivered through it. Forcible attempts to deliver the tibia anteriorly through a soft tissue window that is not at least as wide as the tibia in its midcoronal plane can lead to inadvertent tearing of the medial capsular structures.

At this stage of the operation the surgeon should remove any accessible osteophytes from the medial tibia and medial femoral condyle, as well as any osteophytes anteriorly on the tibia that may be blocking full extension. In the past we had assessed ligamentous balance at this point and then begun our soft tissue

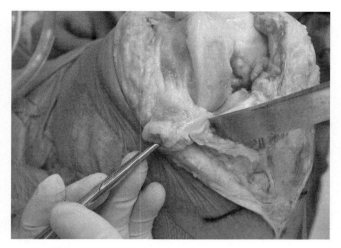

FIG. 3. Use of an elevator posteromedially.

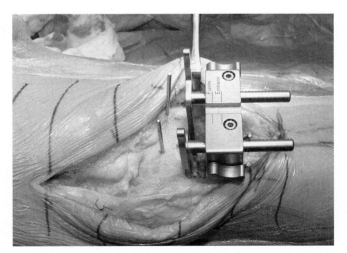

FIG. 5. Measurement of the extensor space with a block.

releases. We have discovered, however, that at this stage of the procedure it is not possible to easily remove those osteophytes that are very posterior on the tibia and femur. Currently, therefore, we defer any decisions about releases and progress to resection of the proximal tibia and distal and posterior femur. Remaining osteophytes are then easily removed. Only at that point can we formally assess ligament balance and evaluate any contractures that may be present.

We have, over the years, used a variety of methods to determine whether or not there is a residual medial contracture. The simplest method involves using laminar spreaders with large flat paddles (Fig. 4). With the knee fully extended, the spreaders are placed between the cut surfaces of the distal femur and proximal tibia. These are extended until a firm end point is obtained. The distance between the cut surfaces is then measured. If there is no contracture, the distances medially and laterally should be equal.

A second method uses spacer blocks (Fig. 5). These blocks, which are available with most implant sets, come in varying thicknesses. They are progressively placed into the extension

space until the space appears filled. The knee is then stressed into varus and valgus. There should be less than 2 mm of gapping, but, more important, any such gapping should be equal medially and laterally.

A third method of determining rectangularity of the extensor space is by using a graduated tensor device. Although, of the three methods described, the tensor method is the most accurate, the sheer bulk of most tensor devices has precluded their widespread use. Recent design changes, however, have made these devices easier to insert and more accurate (Fig. 6).

The basic difficulty with all these methods is determining the "end point." When the author first began performing knee replacement surgery in the early 1970s, it was felt that the knee had to be extremely tight in extension. Bowstringing of the medial and lateral soft tissues was considered optimal. We subsequently learned that such tightness was not optimal and led to an inability to easily achieve flexion. At present, a slight give of less than 2 mm medially and laterally is considered optimal. Obviously gross instability is not to be encouraged.

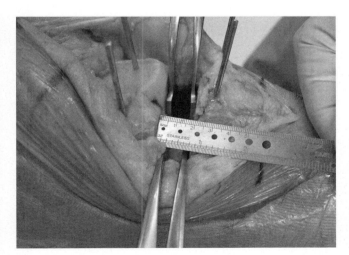

FIG. 4. Measurement of the extensor space with laminar spreaders.

FIG. 6. Measurement of the extensor space with a tensor device.

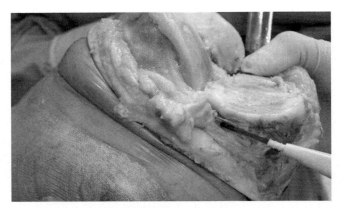

FIG. 7. Release of the semimembranosus muscle.

Computerized surgical navigation methods currently under study may obviate this problem. These systems may rely on intraoperative localization at times in association with either preoperative computerized tomography or preoperative image intensifier images. One system that we have used allows a gradual distraction of the medial and lateral soft tissues with an objective end point of a neutral axis that is not dependent on the surgeon's feel using the laminar spreaders.

If, using one of these methods, it is determined that a fixed varus deformity is present, further releases should be performed in a sequential manner (5). The knee should be externally rotated and the insertion of the semimembranosus tendon on the posteromedial tibia identified (Fig. 7). This insertion is then released. If, using one of the previously described methods, there is now found to be no remaining contracture, no further soft tissue release is required. If a residual contracture still remains, however, the next step should be a release of the posterior cruciate ligament (PCL).

There is obviously some debate among orthopedic surgeons as to whether or not the PCL should be released or retained during total knee replacement surgery. We feel that regardless of the surgeon's particular bias in this regard, release of the ligament should be universal in patients with a severe varus deformity.

In 1995 we reported on the long-term follow-up of patients who had a preoperative varus deformity of more than 15 degrees and who had undergone what was felt to be an adequate medial capsular release without concomitant release of the PCL (6). In these patients, a PCL-retaining prosthesis, either the Tricon-M or the porous coated anatomic, had been used. We compared these patients with a group with a similar varus deformity greater than 15 degrees who had undergone a PCL resection as part of the surgery, with insertion of a posterior stabilized Insall-Burstein prosthesis. We evaluated the patients using the clinical and radiographic parameters of the Knee Society (7). At 10 years after surgery, the deformed knees in which the PCL had been retained had a significantly higher incidence of bone cement radiolucencies in tibial plateau zones I and II, as well as a significantly higher incidence of pain. This group had a lower survivorship and a higher incidence of revision surgery than the PCL-resected group. Their knee scores were lower, as was their flexion arc. We concluded that, in the severely varus knee, the PCL was part of the deformity; complete release of the deformity was not possible without concomitant release of the PCL.

Furthermore, the PCL in the patient with advanced arthritis is not normal. Alexiades et al. (8) and Kleinbart et al. (9) demonstrated that, as the angular deformity increased, the degenerative changes in the PCL increased as well. PCLs taken from patients with advanced arthritis with angular deformities microscopically had large numbers of inclusion bodies and vacuoles. There was a large percentage of fiber fragmentation in the ligament as well. One might reasonably assume that a ligament that had marked deficiency in its fiber architecture would not have normal biomechanical properties, and indeed that was reported by Incavo et al. (10).

The PCL may be released from either its femoral or tibial insertion, or sectioned in its midsubstance. Over the years we have performed all three types of releases. Our present preference is to release the ligament subperiosteally from the back of the proximal tibia, which allows it to retract proximally. This retains the bulk of the ligament posteriorly and avoids excess bleeding from a branch of the middle genicular artery, which is often seen when the ligament is excised completely.

If release of the semimembranosus and PCL is still not sufficient to correct the fixed varus deformity, the next step is a subperiosteal elevation (or recession) of the insertion of the pes anserinus tendons and the superficial medial collateral ligament. This release is not analogous to a transection of the capsule at the joint line, because the capsule is still tethered posteriorly. The subperiosteal elevation can progress distally as far as necessary to effect a complete release medially. The author has not encountered any varus knee deformity that could not be released by this last step.

RESULTS OF SOFT TISSUE RELEASES IN THE VARUS KNEE

In 1987 we reported our experience with follow-up of a series of patients who had undergone a medial capsular recession (1) and who were followed for at least 2 years after surgery. Of the 71 knees in the series, 51 had been followed for at least 4 years, 41 for at least 6 years, and 19 for longer than 10 years.

On follow-up examination at 2 years, all knees were subjected to a varus stress with the knee flexed several degrees. Performing the varus stress in this manner is more accurate then performing the varus stress in full extension, because in full extension the taut posterior capsule can sometimes mask even gross instability. Seventy-three percent of the knees had less than 5 degrees of varus-valgus instability, 25% had 5 to 10 degrees of instability, and only two knees (2%) had greater than 10 degrees of instability. In patients undergoing a total knee replacement *without* a medial capsular recession (i.e., patients who did not have a fixed varus deformity of more than 15 degrees), the comparable varus-valgus stability numbers were 85%, 14%, and 1%, respectively. The differences between the two groups were not statistically significant. These percentages did not change as the patients were followed for longer periods of time. The findings in the patients who had been followed for longer than 10 years were almost identical to their individual findings at 2 years.

There were four patients in our initial series who had undergone a medial capsular recession and who developed significant medial instability. One patient fell 3 months after surgery and tore through the midportion of the medial collateral ligament.

She underwent a semitendinosus transfer; however, the instability recurred. She declined to have any further surgery and had been kept permanently in a brace when she walked. Another patient had both anteroposterior and medial lateral instability noted within the first weeks after surgery. As the normal postoperative swelling abated, this became more obvious and symptomatic. He underwent a revision of his knee surgery with the insertion of a thicker polyethylene component. In retrospect, an insufficiently thick component had been inserted at the time of the first surgery. A third patient with rheumatoid arthritis who had been taking large doses of systemic steroids developed a progressive valgus deformity after surgery. When she underwent revision surgery, the medial capsular flap was noted to be severely attenuated, however, not disrupted. The prosthesis was revised to one with intrinsic constraint. A final patient was diagnosed after surgery as having a neuropathic arthropathy secondary to diabetes mellitus. His knee became gradually unstable and required permanent bracing.

When the medial capsule is recessed, there is an increase in the size of the extension and flexion spaces. If the PCL requires release as well, the flexion space increases even further. In our study, the average thickness of the tibial component used in patients who did not require a capsular recession was 7.5 mm, whereas the thickness in the group with a capsular recession was 12.5 mm. If after releasing a fixed varus deformity the surgeon is only able to insert a thin tibial polyethylene component, most likely the fixed deformity has not been adequately released.

Bone cement radiolucencies were found in 5.7% of the patients who had undergone a medial capsular recession. No lucency was larger than 1 mm in width. The incidence and location of these lucencies (mainly in zones I and IV) were statistically indistinguishable from those seen in patients without a varus deformity who had not undergone a capsular recession. Likewise, the eventual flexion arc in the group that had undergone a medial capsular recession was statistically no different than that seen in the group with a neutrally aligned knee that had not required a capsular recession ($p > .1$).

The author was able to examine the knee of one patient who had previously undergone a medial capsular recession and who had died several years later of unrelated causes. The medial capsular flap was firmly adherent to the underlying bone of the tibia, with the microscopic appearance of Sharpey fibers attaching it to the bone. This case supported our clinical impression that it was not necessary to staple or otherwise suture the recessed capsule back done to bone during initial surgery. Stability is obtained by the thickness of the implants used.

We have recently examined a group of patients who underwent a medial recession during the early 1990s and who were followed for at least 5 years after surgery. Ninety-four percent had no residual varus-valgus instability, and the remaining 6% had mild instability of 5 to 10 degrees. Of interest was one patient who had been maintained long-term on ciprofloxacin by her urologist for a recurrent urinary tract infection. She suffered a rupture of her contralateral quadriceps tendon, her contralateral Achilles tendon, and her rotator cuff, possibly secondary to the detrimental effects of ciprofloxacin on collagen fibrils. Her recessed medial soft tissues continued to function well, however, and she had no instability 6 years after surgery.

An alternative to a medial release for a varus contracture is advancement and tightening of the lateral soft tissues as suggested by Krackow and colleagues (11,12) and Pritsch et al.

(13). The potential disadvantage of these procedures is that motion exercises must be limited until the ligament advancement heals. The result in the two patients in whom the author has personally used this type of procedure has been moderate restriction of flexion.

Engh and Ammeen (14) suggested using a medial epicondylar osteotomy to correct varus deformities in total knee arthroplasties. They felt that, unlike the traditional method of subperiosteal stripping of tibial ligaments, this was an alternative that did not theoretically damage the ligaments (although in our series no damage was seen). Between 1991 and 1996, they performed medial epicondylar osteotomies in 80 patients (93 knees) at the time of primary total knee arthroplasty. At a 2- to 4-year follow-up, no patients had instability. On the Knee Society scale for instability (in which 15 points equals no instability), the mean instability score was 14.2. The Knee Society clinical score was 93 points, compared with a preoperative score of 42 points. The average postoperative femoral-tibial angle was 7 degrees of valgus, improved from a preoperative mean of 6 degrees of varus. The mean postoperative flexion of 110 degrees was not statistically different from that seen in patients who had not undergone an epicondylar osteotomy. Bone union occurred in 54% of the knees and fibrous union occurred in 46%. Focal tenderness, restricted motion, or other symptoms were not associated with fibrous union.

CONCLUSION

Correction of a medial varus contracture can be obtained through a method of gradual releasing of the medial and posteromedial soft tissues. With proper filling of the flexion and extension space, the surgeon can obtain excellent stability that does not deteriorate with time. Capsular recession does not appear to increase the incidence of postoperative flexion contracture or the development of bone cement radiolucencies.

REFERENCES

1. Laskin RS. Medial capsular recession for severe varus deformities. *Clin Orthop* 1987;2:313–316.
2. Laskin RS. The Genesis total knee prosthesis. *Clin Orthop* 2001;388:95–102.
3. Maletius W, Messner K. The effect of partial meniscectomy on the long-term prognosis of knees with localized, severe chondral damage. A twelve- to fifteen-year followup. *Am J Sports Med* 1996;24(3):258–262.
4. Matsuda S, Matsuda H, Miyagi T, et al. Femoral condyle geometry in the normal and varus knee. *Clin Orthop* 1998;349:183–188.
5. Insall JN, Binazzi R, Soudry M, et al. Total knee arthroplasty. *Clin Orthop* 1985;192:13–20.
6. Laskin RS. Total knee replacement with posterior cruciate ligament retention in patients with a fixed varus deformity. *Clin Orthop* 1996;331:29–34.
7. Insall JN, Dorr LD, Scott RD, et al. Rationale of the Knee Society clinical rating system. *Clin Orthop* 1989;248:13–14.
8. Alexiades M, Scuderi G, Vigorita V, et al. A histologic study of the posterior cruciate ligament in the arthritic knee. *Am J Knee Surg* 1989;2:153–159.
9. Kleinbart FA, Bryk E, Evangelista J, et al. Histologic comparison of posterior cruciate ligaments from arthritic age-matched knee specimens. *J Arthroplasty* 1996;11:726–731.
10. Incavo SJ, Johnson CC, Beynnon BD, et al. Posterior cruciate ligament strain biomechanics in total knee arthroplasty. *Clin Orthop* 1994;309:88–93.

11. Krackow W. Chapter IV. In: Hungerford D, Krackow W, Kenna R, eds. *Total knee arthroplasty.* Baltimore: Williams and Wilkins, 1984.

12. Mihalko WM, Krackow KA. Posterior cruciate ligament effects on the flexion space in total knee arthroplasty. *Clin Orthop* 1999;360:243–250.

13. Pritsch M, Fitzgerald RH, Bryan RS. Surgical treatment of ligamentous instability after total knee arthroplasty. *Arch Orthop Trauma Surg* 1984;102:154–160.

14. Engh GA, Ammeen D. Results of total knee arthroplasty with medial epicondylar osteotomy to correct varus deformity. *Clin Orthop* 1999;367:141–148.

CHAPTER 85

Soft Tissue Balancing of the Knee—Flexion

Adolph V. Lombardi, Jr.

Total knee arthroplasty (TKA) is perhaps the most successful orthopedic surgical intervention, as documented by multiple reports (1–38). The correction of deformity and attainment of good alignment have been paramount to the success of these arthroplasties. Advancements in instrumentation have assisted the surgeon in achieving appropriate alignment in both the coronal and sagittal planes by facilitating the osteotomies required in TKA. This technology does not lessen the importance of soft tissue balancing of the knee, however, as functional restoration is fundamentally dependent on such balancing.

Flexion contracture is inherent to the pathophysiology of osteoarthritis and inflammatory arthritis of the knee. In osteoarthritis, such deformity is limited to the soft tissues, with minimal posterior bone involvement. The deformity is more widespread in rheumatoid arthritis, however, and is characterized by significant posterior femoral condylar erosion (39). The inflammatory elements of such diseases lead to the development of effusions that prevent full extension of the knee. Coupled with painful stimuli, these effusions often inhibit range of motion. Other characteristics associated with these disease processes, such as posterior osteophytes, posterior adhesive capsulitis, and contracture of the capsule, cruciate ligaments, and hamstrings, further inhibit full extension of the knee, which leads to the development of a fixed flexion deformity (40). Such fixed flexion contractures affect the gait cycle at the terminal swing stage and also during stance, at the initial contact, midstance, and terminal stance stages, which results in a pathologic gait (41). These alterations in the gait cycle cause inefficient locomotion, resulting in increased energy expenditure. The ensuing flexed posturing of the knee associated with this type of deformity necessitates the increased recruitment of the quadriceps mechanism, which leads to further increased energy expenditure and accelerated fatigue (41,42).

Although the pathophysiology and associated symptoms of fixed flexion deformities are well understood, controversy exists over the decision to fully correct such flexion contractures at the time of the TKA. Dorr states that a 10-degree flexion contracture is acceptable, but no greater contracture is permissible for optimum postoperative function (43). Tanzer and Miller report that knee flexion contractures can significantly improve postoperatively, concluding that complete intraoperative correction is not necessary and that the removal of excess bone adversely affects knee kinematics (44). A more recent study by McPherson et al. lends further support to this opinion (45). Conversely, other authors, including the author of this chapter, argue that full correction of flexion contractures must be performed at the time of surgical intervention and further suggest that optimum correction may be obtained only at the time of surgery (39,42,46,47).

MANAGEMENT OF FLEXION CONTRACTURES— AN ALGORITHMIC APPROACH

The correction of flexion contracture at the time of TKA is dependent on the degree of flexion contracture, surgical technique, and the type of prosthetic device used. It is the author's preference to use pathologic criteria for determination of the fate of the posterior cruciate ligament (PCL) to assist in the decision to use posterior cruciate–retaining (PCR) versus posterior stabilized (PS) devices. The key to successful management of flexion contracture is addressing the contracture by a combination of soft tissue release and bony resection. As in varus or valgus contractures, careful soft tissue release is of paramount importance. Correction of these deformities cannot be performed by bony resection alone. If attention is not paid to care-

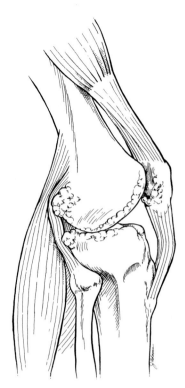

FIG. 1. Grade I flexion deformity represents mild flexion contracture of 15 degrees or less and is the most commonly encountered type in primary total knee arthroplasty. Note the posterior adhesive capsulitis and posterior osteophytes.

ful posterior soft tissue release, then an erroneous distal femoral resection will be performed in an effort to obtain full extension and balanced flexion-extension gaps. This incorrect resection will result in a proximal joint line that leads to midflexion instability and negatively affects the kinematic function of the PCL if it is retained, as well as patellar-femoral kinematics. The two most commonly used techniques for obtaining balanced flexion-extension gaps are the *measured resection technique* and the *variable distal femoral resection technique*, also referred to as the *classic flexion-extension gap balance technique*. In the measured resection technique, the surgeon removes from the distal femur and proximal tibia the amount of bone that is being replaced by the prosthetic device. Therefore, distal femoral resection and posterior femoral condylar resection are equal to the thickness of the metallic femoral component. The proximal tibial resection approximates the thickness of the tibial component. The soft tissues are balanced to obtain stable and symmetrical flexion-extension gaps. Conversely, the variable distal femoral resection technique is based on the appropriate sizing of the femur with respect to the anteroposterior dimension. Posterior femoral condylar resection, therefore, varies as determined by appropriate sizing. The proximal tibial resection is performed to remove approximately 2 mm of bone from the more deficient tibial plateau. These two resections determine the dimension of the flexion gap, with the extension gap created to match these dimensions. If appropriate posterior soft tissue release has not been performed, this technique is more susceptible to erroneous distal femoral resection than the measured resection technique. Hence, a number of surgeons who have traditionally used the variable distal femoral resection technique

now favor a combination technique, referred to as the *modified gap technique*, that attempts to blend the measured resection and the variable distal femoral resection techniques (39).

The author assigns flexion contracture deformities into one of three grades, based on the degree of deformity. Grade I represents mild flexion contractures of 15 degrees or less (Fig. 1). Grade II flexion contractures are of moderate severity, 15 through 30 degrees. Flexion contractures greater than 30 degrees are classified as grade III. Each grade of flexion contracture requires a slightly different surgical approach to soft tissue release, bony resection, and degree of constraint of the prosthetic design. The algorithms depicted in Figure 2 are based on this flexion contracture classification and have been developed by the author as a logical means of dealing with such deformities. The remainder of this chapter describes the detailed surgical procedures involved in treating each grade of contracture.

GRADE I FLEXION CONTRACTURES

The algorithm for treating grade I flexion contractures is illustrated in Figure 2A. For such contractures of 15 degrees or less, the choice of PCR versus PS devices depends on the correctability of the deformity and competency of the PCL.

Measured Resection Technique

The following represents the sequence of steps to be followed when using the measured resection technique in the performance of TKA.

1. Elementary correction of the coronal deformity by appropriate osteophyte removal and soft tissue release is performed.
2. Bony resection of the femur and tibia is achieved using the concept of measured resection with the goal of obtaining appropriate alignment in both the coronal and sagittal planes. Appropriate landmarks determine rotational alignment of the femur and tibia.
3. Overhanging posterior femoral condyle and posterior femoral osteophytes are removed (Figs. 3 and 4).
4. Periosteal stripping of the posterior capsule is performed in an effort to reestablish the posterior recess of the knee. Placing the 0.5-in. curved osteotome between the PCL and the collateral ligament structures facilitates this release (Fig. 5).
5. Trial reduction with implants is carried out in an effort to obtain balance and equal tension in the medial collateral ligament and lateral collateral ligament, appropriate tension of the PCL, and symmetry of the flexion-extension gaps.
6. If these goals have been accomplished, then a PCR device may be implanted (Fig. 6).
7. If there is inequality of the flexion-extension gaps, however, with the extension gap being slightly smaller than the flexion gap, further posterior capsule release must be performed (Fig. 7), along with the resection of an additional 2 mm of distal femoral condyle (Fig. 8). Two millimeters is chosen as it represents the upper level of joint line elevation that may be tolerated by the PCL (Fig. 9). Greater elevation of the distal femoral joint line will significantly alter the kinematic function of the PCL (46,48).
8. On completion of these steps, trial reduction is again performed.

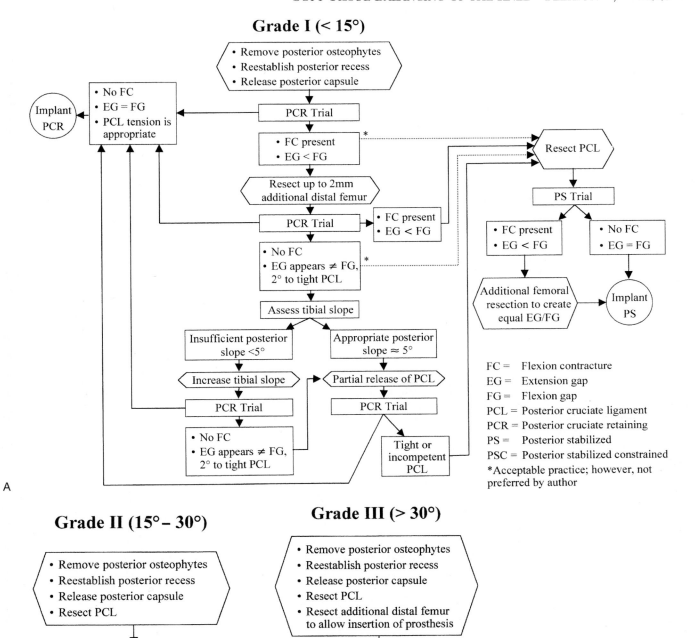

FIG. 2. A: Algorithm for treating grade I flexion contractures. **B:** Algorithm for treating grade II flexion contractures. **C:** Algorithm for treating grade III flexion contractures.

9. If the previously stated goals have been accomplished, PCR implantation ensues.
10. Frequently, asymmetry of the flexion-extension gaps is noted, with the flexion gap appearing somewhat tighter than the extension gap secondary to a tight PCL. If this occurs, the posterior slope of the tibial resection should be evaluated to ensure that it is 5 to 8 degrees. A slight increase of posterior slope may balance the flexion-extension gaps with satisfactory tension in the medial and lateral collateral ligaments and the PCL (Fig. 10).

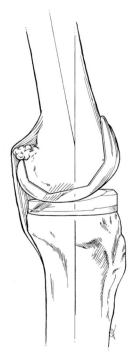

FIG. 3. Note the residual 10-degree flexion contracture. The surgeon has failed to remove the posterior osteophytes that are tenting the posterior capsule, which inhibits the patient from obtaining full extension. In addition, there has been failure to release the posterior capsule.

11. If appropriate posterior slope is present or if an increase in posterior slope does not serve to accomplish balance of the flexion-extension gaps and appropriate tension in the PCL, partial release or recession of the PCL is performed. Three methods of PCL release have been described.
   a. The most common technique involves direct release from the posterior aspect of the proximal tibia and

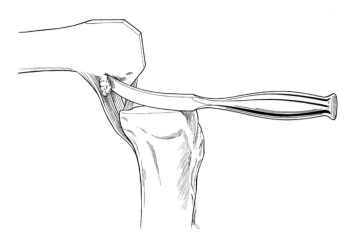

FIG. 4. Appropriate bony resections, meticulous removal of osteophytes, and reestablishment of the posterior recess will correct the majority of grade I flexion contractures. With the knee in flexion, a curved osteotome is used to remove posterior osteophytes.

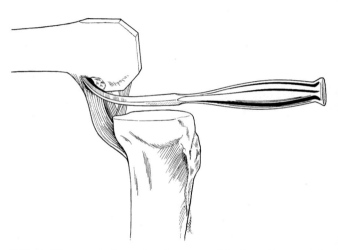

FIG. 5. The posterior adhesive capsulitis is addressed by subperiosteal stripping of the posterior capsule with a curved osteotome, which thereby reestablishes the posterior recess of the knee.

is based on the anatomy of the PCL attachment to the proximal tibia, which spans 2 cm distal to the joint line (48). Because approximately 1 cm of proximal tibia has been removed during the previous steps, approximately 1 cm of attachment remains (Fig. 11).

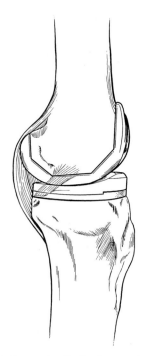

FIG. 6. Note that the patient's flexion contracture has been successfully treated. This has been accomplished in part by appropriate bony resection but, even more important, by attention to removal of posterior femoral osteophytes and release of the posterior capsule.

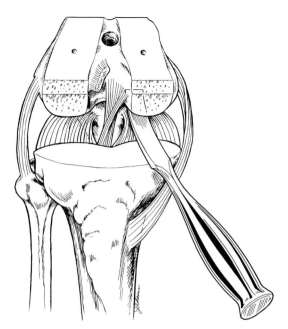

FIG. 7. If a slight flexion contracture exists, further subperiosteal stripping can be performed between the posterior cruciate ligament and the collateral ligament structures using a curved osteotome.

b. A modification of this type of release involves a V-shaped osteotomy of the posterior tibia at the point of attachment of the PCL (Fig. 12). It is stated that the osteotomized bone and PCL will slide on a periosteum sleeve and ultimately reattach at the point of appropriate tension in the PCL (49).

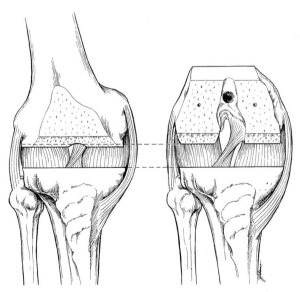

FIG. 8. On occasion, despite meticulous attention to removal of posterior osteophytes and release of the posterior capsule, the extension gap remains smaller than the flexion gap. An additional 2 mm of distal femur can be removed without alteration of the kinematic function of the posterior cruciate ligament.

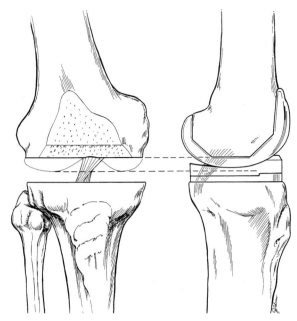

FIG. 9. Two additional millimeters of distal femur have been resected with resultant elevation of the joint line by 2 mm. Full extension of the knee is obtained, and kinematic function of the posterior cruciate ligament is maintained.

c. A third method of release and recession of the PCL involves partial release of the attachment of the PCL on the medial femoral condyle (Fig. 13) (43).
12. Subsequent to release of the PCL, trial reduction with PCR components is performed.
13. If the flexion-extension gap is balanced, a PCR component may be implanted.
14. If the PCL remains too tight or has been rendered incompetent, however, the author recommends progressing to a PS

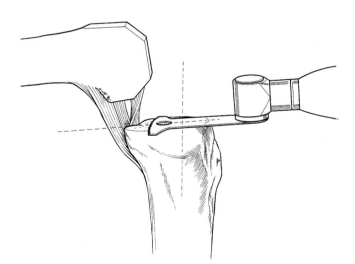

FIG. 10. With preservation of the posterior cruciate ligament, the tibia should be sloped posteriorly 5 to 8 degrees. If tibial resection has not been carried out with posterior slope of 5 to 8 degrees, then adjustment of the slope may assist in balancing the flexion-extension gap.

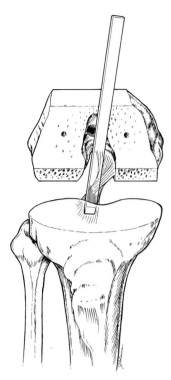

FIG. 11. The posterior cruciate ligament (PCL) attaches to an area 2 cm in length, distal to the tibial articular surface. Eight to 10 mm of tibial bone has been removed, which leaves approximately 1 cm of PCL insertion. In the presence of a tight PCL, an osteotome can be used to perform a partial release of the PCL from the posterior aspect of the tibia.

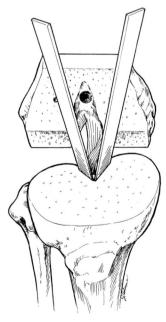

FIG. 12. Release of the posterior cruciate ligament (PCL) can be accomplished by performing a V-shaped osteotomy of the posterior tibia and allowing the PCL to slide on a periosteal sleeve.

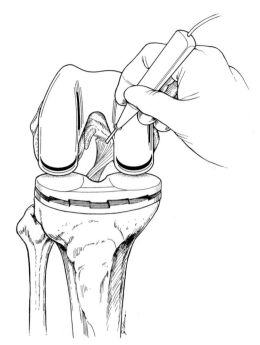

FIG. 13. Note the tension in the posterior cruciate ligament (PCL), which results in excessive rollback of the femur with respect to the tibia. Partial release of the insertional fibers of the PCL on the medial femoral condyle is performed with electrocautery.

device, which should be implanted pending determination by trial reduction of the correction of the flexion contracture and equality of the flexion-extension gaps.

15. If a flexion contracture persists and the extension gap is determined to be less than the flexion gap, additional femoral resection should be performed to equalize the flexion-extension gaps, followed by implantation of a PS device.

Classic Flexion-Extension Gap Balance Technique

If the variable distal femoral resection or classic flexion-extension gap balance technique is chosen, the following sequence of steps is performed.

1. Ligamentous balance in the coronal plane by appropriate soft tissue release from the convex side of the deformity.
2. Proximal tibial resection by removal of approximately 2 mm of bone from the more deficient tibial plateau. If a PCR device is used, a posterior slope of 5 to 8 degrees must also be incorporated. For a PS device, a neutral resection is advised.
3. Anterior and posterior femoral resection based on appropriate sizing of the femoral component.
4. Removal of overhanging posterior femoral condyle and posterior femoral osteophytes.
5. Reestablishment of the posterior recess of the knee with appropriate release of the posterior capsule.
6. Evaluation of the integrity of the PCL, if it is to be retained.
7. Measurement of the flexion gap, which may be performed with either a spacer block or tensor.

8. Distal femoral resection based on the concept of equalizing the flexion gap.
9. Trial reduction to determine ligamentous balance of the medial collateral ligament, lateral collateral ligament, and PCL.
10. Adjustment of ligamentous balance and ultimate implantation of the PCR device, performed according to the previously described steps (see Measured Resection Technique steps 10 through 15 earlier).

When using this technique, the importance of removal of posterior femoral osteophytes, release of the posterior capsule, and reestablishment of the posterior recess of the knee cannot be minimized. If the latter steps are not performed before distal femoral resection, an erroneous resection will result, as the posterior tether will prevent appropriate tensing of the collateral ligaments. Such an error will result in an elevated joint line as well as midflexion laxity and alteration of the kinematics of the patellar-femoral articulation. The amount of bone resection from the distal femur should be measured. Elevation of the joint line will result if this distal femur resection is greater than the thickness of the component. In addition, if this elevation is greater than 2 mm, then a PS device should be used (46,48).

GRADE II FLEXION CONTRACTURES

The method of treating grade II flexion contractures of 15 through 30 degrees is similar to the method for treating grade I flexion contractures. The key difference between the two techniques involves the treatment of the PCL. In a study evaluating the results of PCR versus PS arthroplasties for the treatment of patients with fixed varus deformities and flexion contractures in excess of 15 degrees, Laskin et al. observed postoperative residual flexion contractures of an average of 11 degrees in cases in which the PCL was retained (50). The residual contractures, coupled with the less favorable results in the PCR group than in the PS group, led the authors to recommend PS arthroplasty in cases of significant flexion contractures and associated coronal malalignment. It is also the opinion of the author that the PCL should be sacrificed in cases with grade II flexion contractures and a PS design should be used (51). The algorithm for treatment of grade II flexion contractures of 15 through 30 degrees is summarized in Figure 2B. The sequence of steps varies slightly based on the ligamentous balancing technique selected.

Measured Resection Technique

If the measured resection technique is selected, the following steps are recommended.

1. Appropriate soft tissue release is performed from the convex side of the deformity to establish ligamentous balance in the coronal plane.
2. Proximal tibial resection of 8 to 10 mm from the more intact tibial plateau is performed to restore the tibial joint line.
3. Distal femoral resection is 2 mm thicker than the design to be implanted.
4. Anterior, posterior, chamfer, and intercondylar resections are performed.

5. Overhanging posterior femoral condyle osteophytes and remaining portions of the PCL are débrided from the posterior recess of the knee.
6. The posterior recess of the knee is reestablished via release of the posterior capsule with a curved osteotome.
7. Trial reduction is performed to determine equality and balance of the flexion-extension gaps with concomitant correction of the flexion contracture.
8. If balance and symmetry of the flexion-extension gaps are obtained, then the PS components may be implanted.
9. If flexion contracture persists, however, the author first recommends further release of the posterior capsule from the posterior aspect of the distal femur, followed by trial reduction.
10. In some cases, additional femoral resection is required to obtain full extension.

Classic Flexion-Extension Gap Balance Technique

The sequence of steps is as follows for the classic method of ligamentous balancing.

1. Soft tissue release from the convex side of the deformity to establish appropriate ligamentous balance in the coronal plane.
2. Proximal tibial resection of approximately 2 mm from the more deficient tibial plateau.
3. Anterior and posterior resection as determined by appropriate prosthetic sizing.
4. Transection of the PCL.
5. Removal of overhanging posterior femoral condyle osteophytes and remaining portions of the PCL.
6. Release of the posterior capsule and reestablishment of the posterior recess of the knee with a curved osteotome. The higher the degree of deformity, the more aggressive the posterior capsule release.
7. Measurement and sizing of the flexion gap.
8. Distal femoral resection based on equalizing the flexion gap. As a caveat, the amount of distal femoral resection may appropriately be in excess of 2 to 4 mm of the thickness of the femoral component. However, if it is determined that the distal femoral resection would be more than 4 mm thicker than the femoral component, the author suggests a revisit to the posterior capsule release before performing the distal femoral resection.
9. Completion of distal femoral resections.
10. Trial reduction and implantation of a PS device.

GRADE III FLEXION CONTRACTURES

Grade III flexion contractures are those greater than 30 degrees and typically are seen in patients diagnosed with rheumatoid arthritis. In general, such patients have resorted to the use of a wheelchair for locomotion and are more concerned with pain than with loss of function. As expected, radiographs reveal advanced arthrosis. Due to the severity of the arthrosis and associated contractures, it is extremely difficult, if not impossible, to balance the flexion-extension gaps. Therefore, constrained prostheses should be considered. The key to obtaining full extension is a generous posterior capsule release combined with a gener-

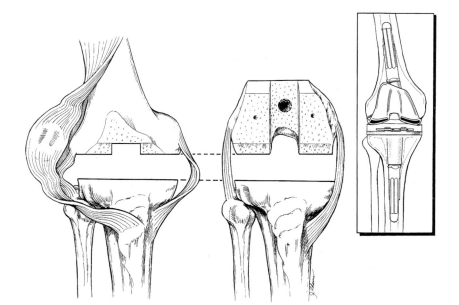

FIG. 14. Grade III contractures are treated with extensive, meticulous removal of posterior osteophytes and release of the posterior capsule. In addition, a generous amount of distal femoral resection is required, which results in a relative laxity of all structures anterior to the midcoronal plane. This is best treated with use of a constrained device.

ous distal femoral resection (Fig. 14). The algorithm demonstrating the correction of this type of deformity is summarized in Figure 2C. The method of dealing with these contractures involves the following steps.

1. Appropriate soft tissue release from the convex side of the deformity to correct coronal alignment.
2. Proximal tibial resection based on a 2 mm resection from the more deficient tibial plateau, unless the deficiency is excessive. If the deficiency is excessive, the resection should be minimized to approximately 10 mm from the more intact tibial plateau.
3. A preliminary distal femoral resection set at 2 mm greater than the thickness of the femoral component.
4. Anterior, posterior, chamfer, and intercondylar resections based on appropriate femoral sizing.
5. Removal of the overhanging posterior femoral condyle and posterior osteophytes.
6. Transection of the PCL.
7. Reestablishment of the posterior recess of the knee via elevation of the posterior capsule combined with release of the gastrocnemius from the posterior aspect of the femur. This release should be generous and extensive, reaching 5 to 6 cm proximal to the joint line.
8. Measurement and sizing of the flexion gap.
9. Adjustment of the extension gap to equalize the flexion gap.
10. Trial reduction and implantation of a PS constrained device.

The degree of ligamentous balance and inequality of the flexion-extension gap determines the level of constraint required. A constrained condylar design should be used if stability may be obtained. However, one should also consider the use of the rotating hinge if gross disparity between the flexion-extension gap and significant ligamentous instability are present. In these severe cases, a redundancy of the extensor mechanism often exists and is best treated by distal and lateral advancement of the vastus medialis obliquus (Fig. 15).

POSTOPERATIVE PHYSICAL THERAPY AND REHABILITATION

Patients presenting with grade I flexion contractures may follow standard postoperative rehabilitation. When patients are treated for grade II and III flexion contractures, however, the postoperative physical therapy and rehabilitation program should be modified accordingly. Although patients in this latter group generally do not have difficulty in obtaining flexion, they often have a problem obtaining and maintaining full

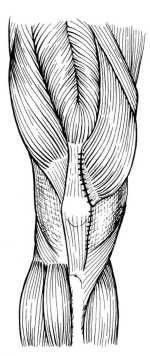

FIG. 15. In combination with the use of a constrained device to treat ligamentous laxity, distal and lateral advancement of the extensor mechanism is performed.

extension. Before TKA, these patients were accustomed to maintaining the affected extremities in a flexed posture and developed gait patterns to accommodate this flexed posture. Postoperatively, the pain stimuli from the arthroplasty and the hematoma within the knee may cause a return to the flexed posture. During the acute postoperative phase, patients will typically insert a pillow underneath the knee, because this is a position of comfort. In addition, these patients will spend a great deal of time postoperatively in a seated position with the knees flexed and will sleep in the fetal position with the knees flexed. The postoperative physical therapy and rehabilitation program must, therefore, aggressively encourage extension of the knee to counteract these natural tendencies to maintain the knee in flexion. Three or four 20-minute sessions of stretching routines are recommended on a daily basis. Furthermore, it is suggested that patients use a night splint for at least the first 6 weeks postoperatively.

Technical Pearls

- Preoperative evaluation of candidates for TKA should include careful assessment of the preoperative flexion contracture, including use of the author's classification system involving three grades of deformity.
- The grade of deformity has a distinct implication on the type of prosthesis that should be used at the time of arthroplasty.
- Correction of flexion contracture in TKA should be addressed by appropriate soft tissue release and bony resection.
- Of paramount importance with respect to soft tissue release is removal of the overhanging posterior femoral condyle and posterior femoral osteophytes. Furthermore, careful subperiosteal release of the posterior capsule from the posterior aspect of the distal femur should be performed before consideration of further distal femoral bony resection.
- If a PCR device is considered, the amount of distal femoral resection should be limited to no more than 2 mm greater than the thickness of the femoral component used, as this will result in an approximately 2 mm elevation of the joint line. Any further elevation of the joint line will alter the kinematic function of the PCL. Therefore, if more than 2 mm of distal femoral resection is required to obtain full extension after meticulous attention to the posterior aspect of the knee, a PS device should be considered.
- A PS device should be considered for grade II flexion contractures between 15 and 30 degrees.
- As flexion contractures greater than 30 degrees are accompanied by extreme difficulty in balancing of flexion-extension gaps, the use of constrained devices should be considered.
- In severe cases of flexion contracture, such as grade III deformities, a redundancy of the extensor mechanism often exists and is best treated by distal and lateral advancement of the vastus medialis obliquus.
- Patients with grades II and III flexion contractures should have a slight modification in their postoperative physical therapy rehabilitation programs to include specific focus on extension exercises. It is also recommended that these patients use a night splint for the first 6 weeks postoperatively.

CONCLUSION

The treatment of flexion contractures follows a logical approach, as summarized by the proposed algorithm illustrated in Figure 2. Grade I flexion contractures are of a mild nature and, therefore, may be treated with PCR devices. In these cases, additional bony resection should be limited to 2 mm to avoid adversely affecting the function of the PCL. PS devices should be used in cases of grade II flexion contractures. In addition to meticulous posterior osteophyte removal and release of the posterior capsule, bony resection of 2 to 6 mm may be necessary to obtain full extension of the knee. Grade III flexion contractures mandate aggressive posterior capsule release and generally considerable bony resection. Therefore, in these deformities, the surgeon should consider the use of constrained devices of either constrained condylar or rotating hinge designs.

REFERENCES

1. Aglietti P, Buzzi R, De Felice R, et al. The Insall-Burstein total knee replacement in osteoarthritis. A 10-year minimum follow-up. *J Arthroplasty* 1999;14(5):560–565.
2. Aglietti P, Buzzi R, Segoni F, et al. Insall-Burstein posterior-stabilized knee prosthesis in rheumatoid arthritis. *J Arthroplasty* 1995;10(2):217–225.
3. Ansari S, Ackroyd CE, Newman JH. Kinematic posterior cruciate ligament-retaining total knee replacements. A 10-year survivorship study of 445 arthroplasties. *Am J Knee Surg* 1998;11(1):9–14.
4. Becker MW, Insall JN, Faris PM. Bilateral total knee arthroplasty. One cruciate retaining and one cruciate substituting. *Clin Orthop* 1991;271:122–124.
5. Bugbee WD, Ammeen DJ, Parks NL, et al. 4- to 10-year results with the anatomic modular total knee. *Clin Orthop* 1998;348:158–165.
6. Callahan CM, Drake BG, Heck DA, et al. Patient outcomes following tricompartmental total knee replacement. A meta-analysis. *JAMA* 1994;271(17):1349–1357.
7. Chmell MJ, Scott RD. Total knee arthroplasty in patients with rheumatoid arthritis. An overview. *Clin Orthop* 1999;366:54–60.
8. Colizza WA, Insall JN, Scuderi GR. The posterior stabilized total knee prosthesis. Assessment of polyethylene damage and osteolysis after a ten-year-minimum follow-up. *J Bone Joint Surg Am* 1995;77(11):1713–1720.
9. Dennis DA, Komistek RD, Stiehl JB, et al. Range of motion after total knee arthroplasty. The effect of implant design and weight-bearing conditions. *J Arthroplasty* 1998;13(7):748–752.
10. Diduch DR, Insall JN, Scott WD, et al. Total knee replacement in young, active patients. *J Bone Joint Surg Am* 1997;79(4):575–582.
11. Dorr LD, Ochsner JL, Gronley J, et al. Functional comparison of posterior cruciate-retained versus cruciate-sacrificed total knee arthroplasty. *Clin Orthop* 1988;236:36–43.
12. Ebert FR, Krackow KA, Lennox DW, et al. Minimum 4-year follow-up of the PCA total knee arthroplasty in rheumatoid patients. *J Arthroplasty* 1992;7(1):101–108.
13. Emmerson KP, Moran CG, Pinder IM. Survivorship analysis of the Kinematic Stabilizer total knee replacement. A 10- to 14-year follow-up. *J Bone Joint Surg Br* 1996;78(3):441–445.
14. Faris PM, Herbst SA, Ritter MA, et al. The effect of preoperative knee deformity on the initial results of cruciate-retaining total knee arthroplasty. *J Arthroplasty* 1992;7(4):527–530.
15. Font-Rodriguez DE, Scuderi GR, Insall JN. Survivorship of cemented total knee arthroplasty. *Clin Orthop* 1997;345:79–86.

16. Hanyu T, Murasawa A, Tojo T. Survivorship analysis of total knee arthroplasty with the kinematic prosthesis in patients who have rheumatoid arthritis. *J Arthroplasty* 1997;12(8):913–919.

17. Huang CH, Lee YM, Liau JJ, et al. Comparison of muscle strength of posterior cruciate-retained versus cruciate-sacrificed total knee arthroplasty. *J Arthroplasty* 1998;13(7):779–783.

18. Insall JN, Lachiewicz PF, Burstein AH. The posterior stabilized condylar prosthesis: a modification of the total condylar design. Two- to four-year clinical experience. *J Bone Joint Surg Am* 1982;64(9):1317–1323.

19. Li PLS, Zamora J, Bentley G. The results at ten years of the Insall-Burstein II total knee replacement. Clinical, radiological and survivorship studies. *J Bone Joint Surg Br* 1999;81(4):647–653.

20. Mahoney OM, Noble PC, Rhoads DD, et al. Posterior cruciate function following total knee arthroplasty. A biomechanical study. *J Arthroplasty* 1994;9(6):569–578.

21. Malkani AL, Rand JA, Bryan RS, et al. Total knee arthroplasty with the kinematic condylar prosthesis. *J Bone Joint Surg Am* 1995;77(3):423–431.

22. Martin SD, McManus JL, Scott RD, et al. Press-fit condylar total knee arthroplasty. 5- to 9-year follow-up evaluation. *J Arthroplasty* 1997;12(6):603–614.

23. Ranawat CS, Luessenhop CP, Rodriguez JA. The press-fit condylar modular total knee system. Four-to-six year results with a posterior-cruciate-substituting design. *J Bone Joint Surg Am* 1997;79(3):342–348.

24. Ranawat CS, Flynn WF, Deshmukh RG. Impact of modern technique on long-term results of total condylar knee arthroplasty. *Clin Orthop* 1994;309:131–135.

25. Ranawat CS, Flynn WF, Saddler S, et al. Long term results of total condylar knee arthroplasty. A 15-year survivorship study. *Clin Orthop* 1993;286:94–102.

26. Rand JA, Ilstrup DM. Survivorship analysis of total knee arthroplasty. Cumulative rates of survival of 9200 total knee arthroplasties. *J Bone Joint Surg Am* 1991;73(3):397–409.

27. Ritter MA, Campbell E, Faris PM, et al. Long-term survival analysis of the posterior cruciate condylar total knee arthroplasty. A 10-year evaluation. *J Arthroplasty* 1989;4(4):293–296.

28. Ritter MA, Herbst SA, Keating EM, et al. Long-term survival analysis of a posterior cruciate-retaining total condylar total knee arthroplasty. *Clin Orthop* 1994;309:136–145.

29. Ritter MA, Gioe TJ, Stringer EA, et al. The posterior cruciate condylar total knee prosthesis. A five year follow-up study. *Clin Orthop* 1984;184:264–269.

30. Rodriguez JA, Saddler S, Edelman S, et al. Long-term results of total knee arthroplasty in class 3 and 4 rheumatoid arthritis. *J Arthroplasty* 1996;11(2):141–145.

31. Schai PA, Scott RD, Thornhill TS. Total knee arthroplasty with posterior cruciate retention in patients with rheumatoid arthritis. *Clin Orthop* 1999;367:96–106.

32. Schai PA, Thornhill TS, Scott RD. Total knee arthroplasty with the PFC system. Results at a minimum of ten years and survivorship analysis. *J Bone Joint Surg Br* 1998;80(5):850–858.

33. Scott RD, Volatile TB. Twelve years' experience with posterior cruciate-retaining total knee arthroplasty. *Clin Orthop* 1986;205:100–107.

34. Scuderi GR, Insall JN, Windsor RE, et al. Survivorship of cemented knee replacements. *J Bone Joint Surg Br* 1989;71(5):798–803.

35. Stern SH, Insall JN. Posterior stabilized prosthesis. Results after follow-up of nine to twelve years. *J Bone Joint Surg Am* 1992;74(7):980–986.

36. Tankersley WS, Hungerford DS. Total knee arthroplasty in the very aged. *Clin Orthop* 1995;316:45–49.

37. Vince KG, Insall JN, Kelly MA. The total condylar prosthesis. 10- to 12-year results of a cemented knee replacement. *J Bone Joint Surg Br* 1989;71(5):793–797.

38. Worland RL, Jessup DE, Johnson J. Posterior cruciate recession in total knee arthroplasty. *J Arthroplasty* 1997;12(1):70–73.

39. Insall JN, Easley ME. Surgical techniques and instrumentation in total knee arthroplasty. In: Insall JN, Scott WN, ed. *Surgery of the knee*, 3rd ed. New York: Churchill Livingstone, 2001:1553–1620.

40. Freeman MAR. The surgical anatomy and pathology of the arthritic knee. In: Freeman MAR, ed. *Arthritis of the knee: clinical features and surgical management*. Berlin: Springer-Verlag, 1980:31–56.

41. Perry J. Pathologic gait. *Instr Course Lect* 1990;39:325–331.

42. Tew M, Forster IW. Effect of knee replacement on flexion deformity. *J Bone Joint Surg Br* 1987;69(3):395–399.

43. Dorr LD. Total knee replacement: from exposure to soft tissue balance. *Orthop Today* 1993;13(11):12–13.

44. Tanzer M, Miller J. The natural history of flexion contracture in total knee arthroplasty. A prospective study. *Clin Orthop* 1989;248:129–134.

45. McPherson EJ, Cushner FD, Schiff CF, et al. Natural history of uncorrected flexion contractures following total knee arthroplasty. *J Arthroplasty* 1994;9(5):499–502.

46. Firestone TP, Krackow KA, Davis JD, et al. The management of fixed flexion contractures during total knee arthroplasty. *Clin Orthop* 1992;284:221–227.

47. Schurman DJ, Parker JN, Ornstein D. Total condylar knee replacement. A study of factors influencing range of motion as late as two years after arthroplasty. *J Bone Joint Surg Am* 1985;67(7):1006–1014.

48. Ritter MA, Faris PM, Keating EM. Posterior cruciate ligament balancing during total knee arthroplasty. *J Arthroplasty* 1988;3(4):323–326.

49. Bugbee WD. How to balance the PCL. Paper presented at: American Academy of Orthopaedic Surgeons course, "Unicondylar, primary and revision total knee arthroplasty: basic techniques and solutions to difficult problems"; October 13–15, 2000; Rosemont, IL.

50. Laskin RS, Rieger M, Schob C, et al. The posterior-stabilized total knee prosthesis in the knee with severe fixed deformity. *Am J Knee Surg* 1988;4(1):199–203.

51. Lombardi AV, Mallory TH, Fada RA, et al. An algorithm for the posterior cruciate ligament in total knee arthroplasty. *Clin Orthop* 2001;392:75–87.

CHAPTER 86

Improving Flexion in Total Knee Arthroplasty

Guoan Li, Steven L. Schule, Shay J. Zayontz, William J. Maloney, and Harry E. Rubash

Total knee arthroplasty (TKA) was initially developed to alleviate pain in cases of severe arthritis of the knee. As the procedure evolved, the long-term success rate in terms of patient satisfaction has improved to in excess of 85% at 10 to 15 years' follow-up (1–8). Yet, the accomplishments achieved in restoration of knee motion and kinematics have not paralleled those in pain relief. Attempts at improving knee flexion after TKA have focused on surgical technique, implant design, and postoperative rehabilitation methods.

The amount of knee flexion has been linked to functional outcome and the activities of daily living (9). Flexion of the knee beyond 90 degrees is essential in many situations, and, therefore, patients whose movement is restricted after TKA may experience disability. An individual typically needs 130 degrees of hip flexion and 111 to 165 degrees of knee flexion to squat and sit cross-legged (10). Squatting and kneeling during prayer may require flexion over 120 degrees (11); stair negotiation and sitting on chairs requires at least 90 degrees of flexion; and the use of a bathtub requires 135 degrees of flexion (12). These functions are also essential for individuals who participate in recreational activities (e.g., gardening and golfing) as part of their daily lives. In questioning patients after TKA, Schai et al. (8) commented that less than half of their patients had the perception that they could kneel easily. Under direct observation, however, all the patients were capable of performing this activity. Patients who felt they were unable to kneel cited fear of harming the prosthesis as the main hindrance. Squatting was possible in only 45% of patients after TKA despite the fact that the study was conducted on Asian patients accustomed to squatting (13).

Contemporary TKA rarely results in knee flexion greater than 120 degrees (Table 1) (14–25). In this chapter, we define high

knee flexion as flexion of more than 120 degrees. Current prosthetic designs and surgical techniques may not be meeting the needs of patients who require high knee flexion for their daily activities.

The range of motion after TKA has an important influence on the overall functional outcome (26). Two commonly used knee scoring systems, the Hospital for Special Surgery and the Knee Society systems, include total range of motion as part of their evaluation (27,28). The Hospital for Special Surgery score allocates 18 points (out of 100) for range of motion—one point for each 8 degrees. The Knee Society score assigns 25 points (out of 100)—one point for every 5 degrees of motion. In an analysis of the Hospital for Special Surgery knee rating scale, Ritter (26) noted that the amount of flexion influenced the overall score, the walking ability score, and the stair-climbing score. The pain score was not influenced by the amount of flexion unless there was a flexion contracture.

Range of flexion after TKA is influenced by preoperative, operative, and postoperative factors. Preoperative factors that have been examined in the literature include range of motion, diagnosis, deformity, age, sex, and weight of the patient (29–37). Intraoperative factors include flexion-extension gap balancing, patella resurfacing and tracking, prosthetic design, management of the posterior cruciate ligament (PCL), component sizing, and wound closure. Postoperative rehabilitation also plays an important role in knee flexion, and issues such as the use of continuous passive motion (CPM) devices need to be considered. In this chapter, we review the biomechanical aspects of knee flexion, prosthesis designs, and various surgical and rehabilitative techniques that impact knee flexion after TKA.

TABLE 1. *Reported range of motion for three types of total knee design*

Study	Follow-up (yr)	Design	No. of knees	Mean flexion (degrees) (range)
Cruciate sacrificing				
Goldberg et al. (17)	9	Total condylar	109	95 (15–115)
Insall et al. (19)	6.5	Total condylar	100	89 (no range reported)
Ranawat et al. (22)	13.2	Total condylar	62	99 (65–120)
Cruciate substituting				
Aglietti et al. (14)	5.5	Insall-Burstein	73	96 (70–120)
Emmerson et al. (16)	12.7	Kinematic stabilizer	109	98 (25–130)
Ranawat et al. (23)	4.8	Press-Fit condylar	125	111 (75–135)
Cruciate retaining				
Dennis et al. (15)	11	Cruciate condylar	42	104 (76–120)
Lee et al. (20)	9	Cruciate condylar	144	106 (no range reported)
Malkani et al. (21)	10	Kinematic condylar	119	105 (±11)
Rosenberg et al. (25)	3.5	Miller-Galante	116	105 (45–140)

FLEXION OF THE NATIVE KNEE

To better understand the limitations of TKA flexion, it is essential to appreciate the factors influencing native knee flexion. Flexion in the nonpathologic knee requires that there be no restriction to flexion (as may occur with posterior osteophytes or a quadriceps contracture) and that the joint remain stable at all positions of knee flexion. These characteristics are brought about by several factors, such as the geometry of the articulating surfaces (including the menisci) and the ligaments and soft tissues about the knee.

Geometry of the Native Knee

To design implants that allow the reconstructed knee to reach the level of flexion seen in the native knee, one must first understand the geometry of the nonpathologic knee that allows for high flexion. Knee flexion is normally limited by the patient's body habitus when the calf contacts the posterior thigh in 150 to 160 degrees of flexion.

The important geometrical features of the distal femur are that the femoral condyles are offset posteriorly relative to the posterior

femoral cortex and have a smaller radius posteriorly than distally (Fig. 1) (38). This anatomical arrangement is crucial in permitting unrestricted flexion by providing a space for the posterior tibial cortex and the intervening soft tissues in the back of the knee. If there were no such offset, the posterior edge of the tibial plateau would impinge on the posterior cortex of the distal femur and the intervening soft tissues (Fig. 1). Hence, an appropriate offset needs to be incorporated into a TKA design so that the posterior condyles are replaced rather than removed or reduced in size. Furthermore, the radii of the medial and lateral femoral condyles are asymmetrical. The lateral condyle has a larger distal radius than the medial side. This may be responsible for some of the axial tibial rotation seen during flexion, because the lateral condyle rolls back faster than the medial side (39).

The posterior surfaces of the femoral condyles are involved in the articulation with the tibia at higher flexion (Fig. 1). The proximal tibia has a posterior slope of 5 to 10 degrees built into the osseous surface (Fig. 2). This posterior slope is vital to femoral rollback of the native knee and is a significant consideration for the reconstructed knee in optimizing flexion. Another important feature of the tibia is that the lateral tibial plateau has a shorter anteroposterior dimension than the medial tibial plateau. This contributes to the observed rolling of the lateral femoral condyle off the plateau surface in high flexion (Fig. 3). In this situation, however, the menisci may play an important role in knee stability by translating posteriorly and effectively "elongating" the tibiofemoral articular surfaces. In high flexion, the lateral femoral condyle thus continues to articulate with the posterior meniscus on the lateral tibial plateau (Fig. 2). Therefore, the geometry of the native knee not only allows high flexion, but also provides intrinsic stability in this position (Fig. 2).

Normal Knee Kinematics at High Flexion

The knee undergoes posterior femoral translation (femoral rollback) as it flexes. The kinematics of the native knee in high flexion has been examined by Hefzy et al. (11) using a radiographic technique, by Nakagawa et al. (40) using magnetic resonance imaging, and by Li et al. (41) using robotic technology. Hefzy and colleagues examined *in vivo* kneeling activities of Middle Eastern subjects, whereas Nakagawa and coworkers measured *in vivo* passive knee flexion in Japanese subjects. Li et al. investigated *in vitro* knee flexion up to 150 degrees using

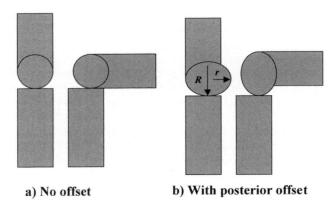

a) No offset **b) With posterior offset**

FIG. 1. Schematic drawings showing the effect of posterior offset of femoral condyles on posterior impingement during knee flexion. With posterior offset, the distal radius (R) is larger than the posterior radius (r).

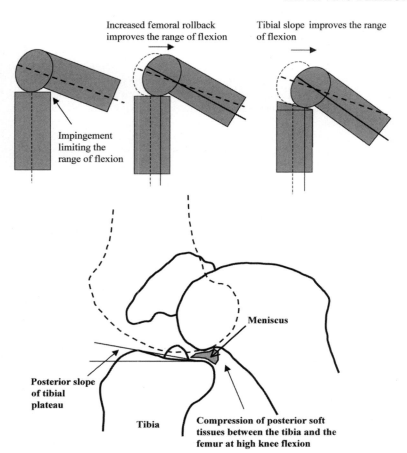

Increased femoral rollback improves the range of flexion

Tibial slope improves the range of flexion

Impingement limiting the range of flexion

Meniscus

Posterior slope of tibial plateau

Tibia

Compression of posterior soft tissues between the tibia and the femur at high knee flexion

FIG. 2. Femoral rollback and posterior tibial slope improve range of flexion of the knee.

cadaveric human knee specimens. These studies showed that, when the knee flexes beyond 135 degrees, the lateral femoral condyle rolls over the posteromedial aspect of the lateral tibial plateau, whereas the medial femoral condyle continues to articulate with the tibial surface. The robotic studies of Li et al. (41) showed that posterior femoral translation (measured at the knee center) could reach a mean of approximately 31 mm at 150 degrees of knee flexion.

Muscle loads affect knee kinematics and are dependent on the flexion angle. For example, quadriceps contraction increases posterior femoral translation (anterior tibial translation) at flexion angles below 60 degrees and thus increases posterior femoral translation. Beyond 60 degrees, the quadriceps contraction causes anterior femoral translation (posterior tibial translation) and reduces posterior femoral translation (41). The *in vitro* robotic study of Li et al. (41), however, demonstrated that the

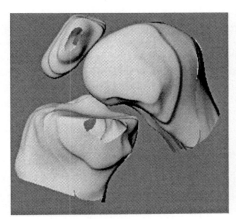

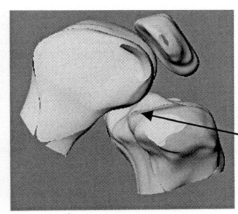

Femoral rolloff

Medial view   **Lateral view**

FIG. 3. Tibiofemoral contact pattern at high flexion of the knee.

muscles have little impact on femoral translation at 150 degrees. This stability is due to the impingement between the posterior aspect of both femur and tibia and the intervening soft tissues, such as the menisci and the posterior capsule (Fig. 2).

Role of the Posterior Cruciate Ligament in Knee Flexion

The anatomy of the PCL has been studied extensively (42–45). Composed of two major bundles, it is 1.5 times larger than the anterior cruciate ligament at the femoral and midsubstance levels, and 1.2 times larger at the tibial insertion (46). The anterior bundle makes up the bulk of the ligament; it is tight in flexion and lax in extension (42,43). The posterior bundle is much smaller, and is tight in extension and lax in flexion.

The PCL has been identified as the primary restraint to posterior tibial translation at all flexion angles over 30 degrees (43,47–51). The PCL is shown to carry significant forces when the knee is subject to a posterior tibial load from full extension to 120 degrees of flexion (52). Isolated loss of the PCL has also been demonstrated to increase posterior laxity from 4 to 7 mm to 10 to 16 mm with a 134-N posterior force from full extension to 120 degrees of flexion (52). An *in vitro* study (53) further confirmed that the PCL also carried increased load beyond 60 degrees of flexion when the knee was under various simulated muscle loads. Isolated loss of the PCL increased posterior tibial translation (reduced posterior femoral translation) when the knee was flexed beyond 60 degrees under muscle loads.

Femoral rollback is essential for knee flexion. This obligatory motion creates a space for the tibia posterior to the femur (complementing the geometrical features discussed earlier) and thus prevents posterior impingement and allows knee flexion (Fig. 2) (41). The PCL-deficient knee is associated with reduced femoral rollback. This phenomenon causes early posterior impingement of the femur and tibia, which limits knee flexion. Understanding these concepts is important for understanding the debate between using a posterior cruciate–retaining or cruciate-substituting TKA prosthesis. Both TKAs were designed to achieve appropriate femoral rollback either with the tension of the PCL or with a cam-spine contact mechanism designed to substitute for the function of the PCL.

FACTORS AFFECTING FLEXION IN TOTAL KNEE ARTHROPLASTY

Preoperative Factors

Preoperative knee flexion is predictive of flexion postoperatively (30,31,33–37). In a large multicenter, prospective study, patients were divided into three groups based on their preoperative range of motion (less than 90 degrees, 91 to 105 degrees, more than 105 degrees). Patients with the least preoperative motion improved the most, whereas those with the best preoperative motion tended to lose motion after surgery. Age, gender, weight, and previous surgery did not show a significant correlation with the postoperative range of motion (29). Another prospective study using multivariate analysis also found that the best predictor of postoperative flexion is preoperative flexion (32). In addition, this study found a correlation between the relative weight of the patient and postoperative flexion. Patients with preoperative flexion of less than 75 degrees gain the most flexion, whereas patients with flexion greater than 100 degrees before surgery tend to retain or lose some motion after surgery. Even though patients with less preoperative motion stand to gain the most motion after TKA, they are also at greatest risk of not attaining the necessary range of motion required for specific activities. These patients should be warned before surgery that, even with a technically sound operation and aggressive physiotherapy, their motion might not exceed 90 to 100 degrees.

Intraoperative Factors

Surgical factors that may influence the range of motion after TKA include careful attention to the soft tissues, accurate flexion and extension gap balancing, implant design and sizing, as well as reconstruction of the patellofemoral joint. The procedure begins with the approach, continues with the soft tissue balancing and osseous cuts, and ends with the closure. Restoring femoral rollback is essential to maximizing flexion after TKA (54). The interaction of each of these with the biomechanical design of the implant generates a multifactorial scenario that determines the final motion of the knee arthroplasty.

Approach

Several studies have looked at the outcome of TKA performed using a median parapatellar, midvastus, and subvastus approach (55,56). Both midvastus and subvastus approaches appear to protect the extensor mechanism and decrease the need for a lateral release. The theoretical benefits of both the subvastus and midvastus approaches are due to the limited disruption of the extensor mechanism. These approaches are not recommended for the obese patient, however, because in such patients it is difficult to sublux the patella during the exposure.

Parentis et al. (57) reported a prospective, randomized study of the midvastus versus the median parapatellar approach. There were no significant differences in range of motion, strength, knee scores, tourniquet time, or proprioception. Another randomized, prospective study by Keating et al. (55) comparing the midvastus and median parapatellar approaches also failed to demonstrate a difference in motion. In a retrospective study of the subvastus and median parapatellar approaches by Matsueda and Gustilo (56), the type of approach once again was not found to influence the range of motion achieved. However, there were fewer knees in the subvastus group that required a lateral release. The choice of surgical approach does not seem to affect the ultimate flexion of the knee but, theoretically, may allow for faster rehabilitation with a more rapid return of flexion. With the available data, a recommendation of a specific approach that will optimize range of motion cannot be made.

Component Geometry

The geometry of the components has a profound bearing on the kinematics of the knee after TKA. The condyles of most femoral components have symmetric profiles in the sagittal plane, the dimensions of which are based on the average sagittal profiles of the medial and lateral femoral condyles of the intact

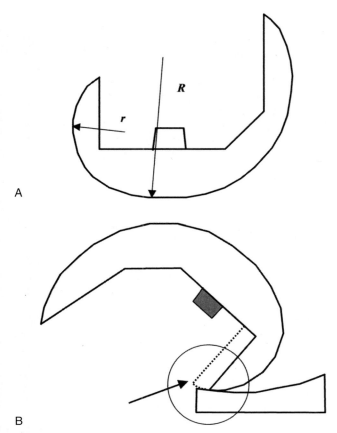

FIG. 4. A: Different radii in distal arc (R) and posterior arc (r) of the femoral component. **B:** Improvement of tibiofemoral contact at high flexion can be achieved by increasing the thickness of the posterior wall of the femoral component (*arrow*).

knee. Some newer designs, however, have a medial-lateral asymmetry that mimics the profiles of medial and lateral femoral condyles of the intact knee to improve axial rotation in early flexion.

Femoral components also exhibit a differential in the radius of curvature between the posterior and distal sections similar to that in the native knee (Fig. 4) (58). The radius of the posterior arc of the femoral condyles is less than the distal arc in the sagittal plane, which thus allows femoral rollback and flexion. When the total condylar knee was modified by changing the center of curvature of the femoral component, the range of motion improved by 10 degrees (59). However, the authors attributed the better postoperative motion to the fact that this group has better preoperative motion. Determining the effectiveness of a new component design is fraught with difficulty due to the multifactorial nature of knee flexion.

Robotic cadaver studies performed in our laboratory have revealed that, if a modern knee prosthesis is flexed beyond 120 degrees, the knee hinges at the posterior-superior tip of the femoral component (Fig. 4). The posterior edge of the polyethylene component may compress the posterior soft tissue against the distal posterior femoral cortex at high flexion. This may limit flexion and can potentially increase polyethylene wear posteriorly due to point loading. This may be overcome by increasing

the thickness of the posterior wall of the femoral component (Fig. 4) (60).

Surgical Technique

Once exposure of the knee has been achieved, there are many other important intraoperative influences on the function of the knee arthroplasty. It is essential to create a symmetrical flexion-extension gap to optimize flexion. This is done through a series of surgical techniques that address ligamentous tension, proper resection of bone, and the use of appropriately sized implants. Factors such as PCL retention, component sizing, osteophyte removal, tibial slope, the patellofemoral joint, and wound closure may all limit knee flexion. Of great importance, however, is the controversy over whether or not to retain the PCL. PCL retention has been stated to have the potential advantage of a better passive range of knee flexion, improved rollback of the femur, and enhanced joint stability (54). Proponents of PCL substitution claim, however, that this surgical procedure is more reliable and that it may improve the range of knee flexion by reliably initiating femoral rollback.

Posterior Cruciate Ligament Retention

The contribution of the PCL to rollback in the TKA has been studied over many years. Walker and Garg (61) showed in a computer simulation that maximum flexion was related to tension in the PCL. During femoral rollback, PCL tension increases. The computer analysis used 15% strain as the maximum tension allowed in the PCL. In the model, when the PCL experiences strain greater than that, the femur rolls back an additional 1 mm and thus reduces the tension on the PCL.

Andriacchi and Galante (54) reported that flexion range after TKA in patients without the PCL is less than in those undergoing a PCL-retention procedure. *In vivo* knee kinematics after TKA have been studied using fluoroscopy. Some investigators (15,62,63) have found that the PCL does not produce a consistent rollback after TKA. Using fresh frozen cadaver knees, however, our laboratory has been able to simulate knee motion and directly compare the kinematics of the normal knee with that of a PCL-retention TKA on the *same* knee, under identical conditions. When the PCL was cut in the TKA and its contribution to rollback accurately measured, it was found that the PCL does restore rollback to 50% of that of the normal knee (64). Rollback was virtually nonexistent, however, without the PCL (Fig. 5). The force in the PCL after TKA was also measured and compared with the PCL forces previously measured in other native knees (65). The results corresponded with our observations on the effects of the PCL on TKA kinematics—that is, the force was present but with a reduced magnitude. *In vivo* studies have also shown that femoral rollback does occur after PCL retention TKA (66). These studies included examination of activities such as walking and stepping up a rise. Although these studies did not compare rollback in the normal knee with their results, our controlled comparison showed that normal rollback is not fully restored and that the PCL has a reduced force.

These results demonstrate that the PCL can be valuable in TKA but beg the question as to why the PCL force decreases (which thereby reduces its influence on kinematics) after a

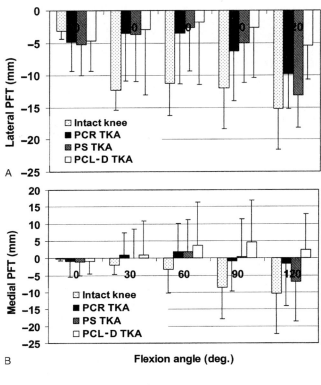

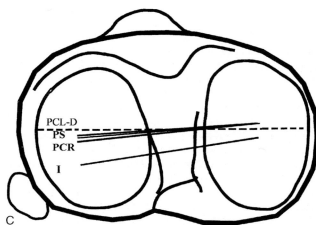

FIG. 5. Posterior femoral translation (PFT) of the lateral condyle **(A)** and medial condyle **(B)** under muscle loads. PCL-D, posterior cruciate ligament–deficient; PCR, PCL-retaining; PS, PCL-substituting; TKA, total knee arthroplasty. **C:** Schematic comparison of the translations of the lateral and medial femoral condyles at 30 degrees flexion in the intact knee (I) and after PCR TKA, PCL-D TKA, and PS TKA under a simulated co-contraction of the quadriceps and hamstrings (64).

TKA. Several possible causes may individually or in combination reduce the efficacy of the PCL. A loose flexion gap may result in a slack ligament (67). In the case of a tight flexion gap, one recommendation has been to recess the PCL (68). Unfortunately, there is currently no reliable method of accurately evaluating the correct tension, and the surgeon may thus release more than is needed. This again results in a loose flexion gap

with a partially incompetent PCL, which could explain the abnormal kinematics seen by some observers when the PCL is recessed (66). The PCL, after partial release, is less stiff than the intact PCL. However, the benefits of a PCL release when indicated have been established (68). Another explanation for the reduced PCL force is that the articular geometry of the femoral and tibial prosthetic components is different from that of the normal knee. Most prostheses are of the "curve on curve" (dished) design, and this is bound to change the kinematics and the forces limiting translation about the knee; therefore, this too could result in reducing the effect of the PCL.

Posterior Cruciate Ligament Substitution

An alternative to PCL retention is the PCL-substituting TKA. This prosthetic design allows for excision of the PCL, replacing it with a spine on the tibial polyethylene insert that engages with a cam built into the femoral component. The kinematics of this type of TKA have been studied using techniques similar to those used in the investigation of the PCL-retention procedure. Video fluoroscopy studies (62,63) have shown that the kinematics of this style of prosthesis mimic that of the native knee, although it begins with a tibiofemoral contact position more posterior than in the normal knee (63). These studies reported that the PCL-substituting TKA was better than the PCL-retaining TKA in restoring rollback. On the other hand, others (66) have shown that the posterior cruciate–substituting TKA does not restore rollback to the same extent as a PCL-retaining TKA.

Using a robotic device, we (64) were able to compare the cruciate-retaining and -substituting TKA directly under controlled conditions. We found that they both partially restored rollback with no statistically significant difference between them. However, the PCL-retaining TKA commenced rollback slightly earlier (60 degrees) than the PCL-substituting TKA (75 degrees) (Fig. 5). Thus, femoral rollback can occur in both the PCL-retaining and PCL-substituting TKA. Nonetheless, neither type of component fully restored intact knee kinematics.

The cam-spine mechanism is essential to rollback. Our study (64) showed that the contact forces between the cam and spine rise dramatically at flexion angles beyond 75 degrees, consistent with their engagement. Removing this mechanism resulted in markedly reduced rollback and altered kinematics. In the absence of a functioning PCL, the cam-spine mechanism is an essential substitute for rollback to occur. Furthermore, we found that the translations of the lateral and medial femoral condyles remained steady after cam-spine engagement, independent of the muscle loads applied. Thus, to improve rollback (and, hence, flexion), the mechanics of this engagement may need to be manipulated. Alterations to the geometry of the component or size and position of the cam-spine mechanism may affect the stability of the TKA, however, so that improvement in knee flexion may be limited by instability of the knee.

Using a two-dimensional computer model, Delp et al. (69) demonstrated that the position of the polyethylene spine on the tibial plateau is an important factor influencing the timing of the cam-spine engagement. The range of posterior translation of the femur at high flexion of the knee could be manipulated by varying the location of the tibial spine on the tibial plateau. A more anterior positioning of the tibial component results in less rollback and earlier impingement with subsequent loss of flexion. A

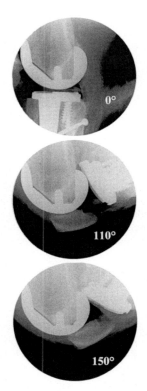

FIG. 6. Small femoral component size causes posterior bone and soft tissue impingement at high flexion.

posterior positioning of the component causes early cam-spine engagement and thus increases the extent of posterior femoral translation. Placing the spine more posteriorly, however, may result in exaggerated rollback and cause the femoral condyles to "roll off" the back of the tibial plateau, which leads to dislocation. Different surgical techniques as well as geometrical designs of the components could produce different timing of cam-spine engagement and improve flexion.

Given the kinematic similarities between PCL-retaining and PCL-substituting designs, it is not surprising that no definite clinical differences have been reported. Isokinetic strength testing and gait analysis, proprioception, and stair climbing have generally been found to be fairly similar (70–72). Interestingly, however, one paper (73) found a difference in the flexion range during a knee bend in association with a reduced femoral rollback. The authors found that the range of motion of patients with PCL-retention TKA (for which they measured less rollback) was significantly lower than that in patients with cruciate-substituting TKA under weightbearing conditions. This association confirms the importance of rollback to flexion. Tanzer et al. (74) compared cruciate-retaining and posterior-substituting TKA and found no significant difference in flexion between the two groups preoperatively or at any point postoperatively. They emphasized that meticulous balancing of the flexion and extension gaps has the greatest influence on the patient's motion. Based on the literature comparing posterior-substituting and cruciate-retaining TKA designs, neither can be recommended over the other in regard to optimizing range of motion.

Component Sizing

The size of the components is also important because it affects the tension of the PCL in cruciate-retaining TKA designs and affects the flexion gap in both designs. A component that is too small may result in a reduced posterior condyle offset, as discussed earlier, and cause impingement in flexion (Fig. 6). The loose flexion gap that may follow femoral component downsizing may also contribute to reduced flexion in association with midflexion instability and failure of the TKA. Furthermore, a loose flexion gap will result in a loose PCL, which, in a PCL-retaining TKA, may lead to reduced rollback and reduced flexion. On the other hand, a femoral component that is too large may result in a tight flexion gap that may restrict flexion. It may also cause "overstuffing" of the patellofemoral joint, and this, too, may result in unsatisfactory clinical outcome due to reduced flexion. Thus, accurate sizing of the components is important to obtain satisfactory range of motion after TKA.

A dilemma arises when the femur is between two sizes. Selecting the larger size may result in a tight flexion gap and an overstuffed patellofemoral joint. However, downsizing also has potential problems related to flexion gap instability as a result of the lower posterior femoral offset. Most surgeons recommend using the smaller size when choosing between two sizes. The problem of a loose flexion gap can be overcome by recutting the distal femur and by using a thicker polyethylene insert, despite the disadvantage of the resultant joint line elevation.

Component Positioning

The relative position of the tibial component on the cut tibial surface may also affect rollback, particularly under muscle loads. The more posterior the component is placed, the greater the capacity for posterior femoral translation, which would have a beneficial effect on flexion (Fig. 7). Computer analysis revealed that posterior displacement by 5 mm improved flexion by 5 degrees, whereas anterior displacement by 5 mm reduced flexion by 10 degrees (61). The posterior tibial border is usually the limiting factor, however, particularly in the posterolateral corner after it is aligned in rotation. Posterior overhang should

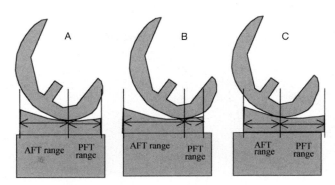

FIG. 7. Maximum ranges of posterior femoral translation (PFT) and anterior femoral translation (AFT) of the knee after total knee arthroplasty. **A:** Total knee arthroplasty with current surgical technique. **B:** Anteriorly positioned tibial component. **C:** Posteriorly positioned tibial component.

be avoided when positioning the component; otherwise, the posterior segment may impinge during flexion.

Positioning of the femoral component has also been shown to influence flexion. Walker and Garg (61) demonstrated that anterior displacement by 2.5 mm improved flexion by 15 degrees, whereas posterior displacement decreased flexion by 10 degrees. This effect is believed to be due to the reduction in PCL tension. The anteroposterior position of the femoral component can be altered in total knee systems that allow for an offset stem. This additional degree of freedom is vital in revision surgery but should also be recognized in primary surgery for a patient with deformity of the femur.

Improper rotation of the femoral component can also influence knee flexion. An internally rotated component can tighten the flexion gap on the medial side and result in a knee with less than optimal flexion. Malrotation of the components is a difficult diagnosis to make in the postoperative period but should be kept in mind as a potential cause for a stiff knee. One method, described by Berger et al. (75), is the use of computed tomography to access rotation of both the femoral and tibial components by using epicondylar axis and tibial tubercle. Using this technique the authors were able to show that these landmarks are reproducible on computed tomographic scan and can also be used intraoperatively to access for malrotation of the components (75).

Posterior Osteophytes

During TKA, it is important that the posterior femoral osteophytes be removed to improve flexion (Fig. 8). This is best done with an osteotome after the trial femoral component is removed. Failure to remove the posterior femoral osteophyte may result in early tibial impingement and thus reduce flexion. Similarly, careful attention must be paid to the tibial side. In particular, posterior overhang of the tibial component should be avoided, as it, too, may result in early impingement on the posterior distal femoral cortex. If present, osteophytes should be carefully removed. Removal of all

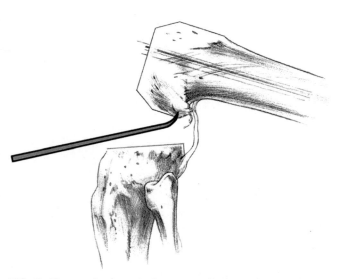

FIG. 8. Removal of posterior osteophytes using a curved osteotome.

the posterior osteophytes may also help in achieving full extension of the knee, as they cause tenting of the posterior capsule. Hence, adequate exposure of the proximal tibia is imperative.

Tibial Slope

The normal tibia has a natural posterior slope of approximately 10 degrees (76,77). Many TKA prostheses are designed so that the tibia is cut with a posterior slope (usually between 3 degrees and 10 degrees), the extent of which depending on the design. As the knee flexes, the femur articulates with a more posterior part of the tibial plateau or component. Failure to appreciate the posterior tibial slope may result in a tight flexion space, which, as discussed earlier, limits flexion (Fig. 2). It has also been shown that posterior tibial slope helps alleviate some of the stress on the PCL. Failure to restore the posterior tibial slope may result in a tight flexion space with a tight PCL. If a flexion gap is found to be tight, then the tibial slope should be checked and increased if necessary. Conversely, an excessive posterior slope may result in flexion gap laxity, which may lead to flexion instability and failure of the TKA.

Walker and Garg (61) have shown in a three-dimensional computer model that tibial slope is the most important surgical variable in optimizing flexion. Their model demonstrated that posterior tilt of the component by 10 degrees improved flexion by 30 degrees. Anterior tilt had the opposite effect due to the fact that this increased the tension of the PCL. Singerman (78) confirmed this finding in a cadaveric study that showed that increasing posterior tibial slope decreased the strain measured in the PCL. The increased strain was most notable at 100 degrees of flexion.

It is important to note, however, that posterior slope varies among patients. Some patients may have little or no posterior slope (and even an anterior slope), particularly after a high tibial osteotomy. In these patients, the PCL and other soft tissues may have adapted to this environment, and the standard posterior tibial slope cut may not be appropriate. The tibial cut may need to be modified to a lower posterior slope (but the tibia should not be cut with an anterior slope). This is particularly important in PCL-retaining TKA.

In a posterior-substituting TKA, however, the posterior slope may lead to anterior impingement of the spine on the femoral housing in extension. This could result in wear, because the knee joint itself needs to hyperextend at the prosthesis to achieve full clinical extension. Many posterior-substituting TKA designs do not allow more than 7 degrees of hyperextension at the prosthesis. The surgeon must therefore be careful not to cut the tibia in excessive posterior slope in a posterior-substituting TKA. Newer designs have advanced this by avoiding a closed femoral box.

Patellofemoral Joint

The patellofemoral joint has been one of the common reasons for failure and revision after TKA (79). As the source of many problems in TKA, it has given rise to controversy in treatment, particularly regarding whether or not to resurface the patella. Successful management of the patellofemoral joint is essential to the success of the TKA, because complications associated with the patellofemoral joint can cause reduced range of flexion. Overstuffing of the joint can be produced by using too large a femoral component. Use of a patellar bone

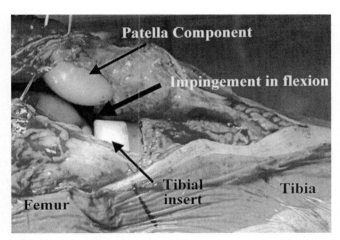

FIG. 9. Impingement of patella component with anterior edge of the tibial polyethylene component.

prosthesis composite that is thicker than the native patella can also cause this and result in reduced flexion. It has been demonstrated in cadavers that increasing patellar thickness significantly increases patellofemoral compressive forces when the knee is flexed more than 70 degrees (80). This creates problems both in terms of wear and in prevention of full flexion. To maintain patella composite height constant, the original patellar thickness must be measured, and a resection the depth of the intended prosthesis must be made. The patellar depth is then measured again to make sure that the resection is adequate and the new composite bone-prosthesis thickness is similar to the native patellar thickness.

The method of resurfacing has not been shown to affect range of motion. Results for three groups—patients treated with either a polyethylene component, a metal-backed component, or patellar débridement without resurfacing—were reviewed in a multicenter study. The authors (81) could not detect any difference with regard to range of motion, flexion or extension deficit, extension lag, walking distance, or ability to climb stairs.

Another problem related to the patellofemoral joint is elevation of the joint line by excessive distal femoral resection, which results in patella baja. A consequence of this is that, as the knee flexes, the patella may impinge on the anterior polyethylene insert (Fig. 9). The problem may be overcome by restoring the appropriate joint line through augmentation of the distal femoral surface, either with bone allograft or autograft (if sufficiently available) or with metallic augments. If this cannot be done, then the central anterior part of the tibial insert can be shaved off with a scalpel blade to allow more room for the patella. Some prostheses already have a concave surface on the central anterior aspect of the polyethylene insert for this reason, especially the thicker inserts that may be needed in cases in which the joint line has been elevated. It is thus important to observe the relative positions of the patella and tibial insert during flexion of the knee before the arthrotomy is closed.

Wound Closure

The position of the knee in flexion or extension during closure has been considered to be another factor that can affect the ulti-

mate range of motion of a knee. Emerson et al. (82,83) have reported that knees closed in 90 to 110 degrees of flexion have more flexion at 1-year follow-up. This finding was observed in both primary and revision TKA knees. Knees closed in flexion had a statistically significant difference in motion: 118 degrees compared to 113 degrees. All layers were closed in either full extension or flexion after the tourniquet was deflated. Another study (84), however, failed to show any benefit of capsular closure in flexion in relation to early postoperative rehabilitation at 3 months.

Intraoperative flexion against gravity after capsular closure appears to mimic the postoperative flexion the patient retains. Lee et al. (85) showed that 97% of knees had postoperative flexion within ±10 degrees of their intraoperative flexion, whereas only 55% of knees had a postoperative flexion within ±10 degrees of their preoperative flexion. Flexion against gravity at the conclusion of the surgery appears to be the best predictor of final motion and should be recorded to serve as the goal for the physical therapists.

Rehabilitation

Postoperative factors have been examined closely to determine their effect on the ultimate range of motion after TKA. CPM was first introduced by Salter et al. (86) but was made popular for postoperative use after TKA by Coutts et al. (87) in the early 1980s. Since that time, numerous articles have looked at CPM as a means of optimizing flexion, although the modality has potential complications. In addition, controversy exists regarding the possible benefit of decreasing narcotic requirements and thromboembolic events with the use of this device. Studies have shown that increased blood loss and wound complications occur if CPM is started in the recovery room. Johnson (88) showed that flexion beyond 40 degrees decreased the transcutaneous oxygen tension at the edges of the wound for the first 3 days after surgery. As the knee flexes, tension in the wound and surrounding soft tissues increases, which results in large increases in hydrostatic pressures and leads to reduced blood flow in the region. This would thus cause reduction in the transcutaneous oxygen tension and adversely affect wound healing. Delayed wound healing, prolonged drainage, and wound necrosis may be a consequence of this phenomenon; therefore, CPM should be used with caution.

Several prospective, clinical trials fail to show an advantage of CPM over physiotherapy alone in optimizing range of motion (89–92). MacDonald et al. (90) looked at three groups of patients assigned to either no CPM, CPM from 0 to 50 degrees, or CPM from 70 to 110 degrees. There were no statistical differences among any of the treatment groups regarding range of motion at any point during the postoperative period. This report also failed to show any differences in analgesic requirement, length of stay, or Knee Society scores. Pope et al. (92) reported similar results. At 1 week, the group placed on the CPM device with motion from 0 to 70 degrees showed significant increases compared with the non-CPM group in the amount of flexion (78 degrees vs. 56 degrees) and total range of motion (69 degrees vs. 50 degrees). At 1-year follow-up, however, there was no difference in mean flexion, overall range of motion, or fixed flexion deformity. This study stated that those treated with CPM had both a higher analgesic requirement and increased drainage postoperatively.

Similar flexion gains have been achieved using the drop-and-dangle protocol (93). On the first postoperative day, patients were positioned at the side of the bed and the foot was placed on the floor. Patients then moved their bodies forward with the foot firmly planted on the floor until 90 degrees of knee flexion was achieved, remaining in this position for 20 minutes twice a day. Patients in the drop-and-dangle group were discharged from the hospital 1 day earlier, had less drainage, and had a better extension range at 6 months.

Even though several studies (94–96) have failed to show a benefit in achieving greater postoperative flexion, CPM appears to decrease the need for knee manipulation under anesthesia. Ververeli et al. (96) reported a 10% rate of need for manipulation in the non-CPM group enrolled in a prospective study of 103 patients (52 non-CPM, 51 CPM). Knee manipulation was undertaken in patients with less than 50 degrees of flexion after the tenth postoperative day. There is uncertainty, however, regarding whether the motion gained with a manipulation under anesthesia will be retained at longer follow-up. Fox and Poss (97) reported that patients who underwent manipulation 2 weeks postoperatively improved their initial motion from a mean of 71 degrees to 108 degrees. At 1 week, however, the mean flexion was reduced to 88 degrees, and at 1 year, the motion was no different than in the nonmanipulated group. Esler et al. (98) reported on a prospective series in which 14% of the patients failed to increase their flexion beyond 80 degrees with routine physiotherapy. The patients who underwent manipulation improved and retained a 33-degree gain in motion. Even patients who underwent manipulation 4 to 5 months after their initial surgery showed sustained gains in their motion. Approximately one-third of the patients with restricted motion declined manipulation under anesthesia and did not show significant improvement in the flexion in their knees despite continued physiotherapy.

CONCLUSION

Flexion after TKA is dependent on several important variables that include preoperative flexion, surgical technique, component design, and rehabilitation. Even though the patient's final postoperative flexion depends heavily on the preoperative flexion, the surgeon still has a significant influence in optimizing the patient's motion. The mechanical limitations to motion must be recognized and addressed intraoperatively to allow the patient to maximize the motion allowed with a given implant. It is essential to balance the flexion-extension gap, restore tibial slope, remove posterior osteophytes, and avoid overstuffing the components. In addition, balancing of the soft tissues is necessary with special attention to the PCL. With investigation of both the motion of the native knee and the limitations of contemporary total knee designs, newer implants can be created that allow for improved flexion.

REFERENCES

1. Duffy G, Trausdale R, Stuart M. Total knee arthroplasty in patients 55 years old or younger. 10- to 17-year results. *Clin Orthop* 1998; 356:22–27.
2. Gill G, Joshi A. Long-term results of cemented, posterior cruciate ligament–retaining total knee arthroplasty in osteoarthritis. *Am J Knee Surg* 2000;14(4):209–214.
3. Gill G, Joshi A. Long-term results of retention of the posterior cruciate ligament in total knee replacement in rheumatoid arthritis. *J Bone Joint Surg Br* 2001;83(4):510–512.
4. Meding J, Ritter M, Faris P. Total knee arthroplasty with 4.4 mm of tibial polyethylene: 10-year followup. *Clin Orthop* 2001;388:112–117.
5. Pavone V, Boettner F, Fickert S, et al. Total condylar knee arthroplasty: a long-term followup. *Clin Orthop* 2001;388:18–25.
6. Robertsson O, Scott G, Freeman M. Ten-year survival of the cemented Freeman-Samuelson primary knee arthroplasty. Data from the Swedish Knee Arthroplasty Register and the Royal London Hospital. *J Bone Joint Surg Br* 2000;82:506–507.
7. Schai P, Thornhill T, Scott R. Total knee arthroplasty with the PFC system-results at a minimum of ten years and survivorship analysis. *J Bone Joint Surg Am* 1998;80:850–858.
8. Schai PA, Scott RD, Thornhill TS. Total knee arthroplasty with posterior cruciate retention in patients with rheumatoid arthritis. *Clin Orthop* 1999;367:96–106.
9. Laubenthal K, Smidt G, Kettlekamp D. A quantitative analysis of knee motion during activities of daily living. *Phys Ther* 1972;52:34.
10. Mulholland S, Wyss U. Activities of daily living in non-Western cultures: range of motion requirements for hip and knee joint implants. *Int J Rehab Res* 2001;24:191.
11. Hefzy MKB, Cooke TD, al-Baddah AM, et al. Knee kinematics in-vivo of kneeling in deep flexion examined by bi-planar radiographs. *Biomed Sci Instrum* 1997;33:453–458.
12. Rowe P, Myles C, Walker C, et al. Knee joint kinematics in gait and other functional activities measured using flexible electrogoniometry: how much knee motion is sufficient for normal daily life? *Gait Posture* 2000;12:143–155.
13. Kim J-M. Moon MS. Squatting following total knee arthroplasty. *Clin Orthop* 1995;313:177–186.
14. Aglietti P, Buzzi R, Gaudenzi A. Patellofemoral functional results and complications with the posterior stabilized total condylar knee prosthesis. *J Arthoplasty* 1988;3:17–25.
15. Dennis D, Clayton M, O'Donnell S, et al. Posterior cruciate condylar total knee arthroplasty: average 11-year followup evaluation. *Clin Orthop* 1992;281:168–176.
16. Emmerson K, Moran C, Pinder I. Survivorship analysis of the kinematic stabilizer total knee replacement: a 10- to 14-year followup. *J Bone Joint Surg Br* 1996;78:441–445.
17. Goldberg V, Figgie M, Figgie H, et al. Use of a total condylar knee prosthesis for treatment of osteoarthritis and rheumatoid arthritis: long-term results. *J Bone Joint Surg Br* 1988;70:802–811.
18. Insall J, Binazzi R, Soudry M, et al. Total knee arthroplasty. *Clin Orthop* 1985;192:13–22.
19. Insall J, Hood R, Flawn L, et al. The total condylar knee prosthesis in gonarthrosis. *J Bone Joint Surg Am* 1983;65(5):619–628.
20. Lee J, Keating E, Ritter M, et al. Review of the all-polyethylene tibial component in total knee arthroplasty: a minimum seven-year follow-up period. *Clin Orthop* 1990;260:87–92.
21. Malkani A, Rand J, Bryan R, et al. Total knee arthroplasty with the kinematic condylar prosthesis: a ten-year follow-up study. *J Bone Joint Surg Br* 1995;77:423–431.
22. Ranawat C, Flynn WJ, Saddler S, et al. Long-term results of the total condylar knee arthroplasty: a 15-year survivorship study. *Clin Orthop* 1993;286:94–102.
23. Ranawat C, Luessenhop C, Rodriguez J. The press-fit condylar modular total knee system: four-to-six-year results with a posterior-cruciate-substituting design. *J Bone Joint Surg Br* 1997;79:342–348.
24. Rand J. Comparison of metal-backed and all-polyethylene tibial components in cruciate condylar total knee arthroplasty. *J Arthoplasty* 1993;8:307–313.
25. Rosenberg A, Barden R, Galante J. Cemented and ingrowth fixation of the Miller-Galante prosthesis: clinical and roentgenographic comparison after three- to-six-year follow-up studies. *Clin Orthop* 1990;260:71–79.
26. Ritter M, Campbell E. Effect of range of motion on the success of a total knee arthoplasty. *J Arthoplasty* 1987;2:95–97.
27. Insall J, Scott W, Ranawat C. The total condylar knee prosthesis. A report of two hundred and twenty cases. *J Bone Joint Surg Br* 1979;61:173.
28. Insall J, Dorr L, Scott R, et al. Rationale of the Knee Society clinical rating system. *Clin Orthop* 1989;248:13–14.

29. Anouchi Y, McShane M, Kelly F, et al. Range of motion in total knee replacement. *Clin Orthop* 1996;331:87–92.

30. Harvey I, Barry K, Kirby S, et al. Factors affecting the range of movement of total knee arthroplasty. *J Bone Joint Surg Br* 1993;75:950–955.

31. Kawamura H, Bourne R. Factors affecting range of flexion after total knee arthroplasty. *J Orthop Sci* 2001;6:248–252.

32. Lizaur A, Marco L, Cebrian R. Preoperative factors influencing the range of movement after total knee arthroplasty for severe osteoarthritis. *J Bone Joint Surg Br* 1997;79:626–629.

33. Parlsley B, Engh G, Dwyer K. Preoperative flexion. Does it influence postoperative flexion after posterior-cruciate-retaining total knee arthroplasty? *Clin Orthop* 1992;275:204–210.

34. Ritter M, Stringer E. Predictive range of motion after total knee replacement. *Clin Orthop* 1979;143:115–119.

35. Schurman D, Matityahu A, Goodman S, et al. Prediction of postoperative knee flexion in Insall-Burstein II total knee arthroplasty. *Clin Orthop* 1998;353:175–184.

36. Schurman D, Parker J, Ornstein D. Total condylar knee replacement. A study of factors influencing range of motion as late as two years after arthroplasty. *J Bone Joint Surg Br* 1985;67:1006–1014.

37. Tew M, Forster I, Wallace W. Effect of total knee arthroplasty on maximal flexion. *Clin Orthop* 1989;247:168–174.

38. Iwaki H, Pinskerova V, Freeman MAR. Tibiofemoral movement 1: the shapes and relative movements of the femur and tibia in the unloaded cadaver knee. *J Bone Joint Surg Br* 2000;82(8):1189–1193.

39. Andriacchi T, Stanwyck T, Galante J. Knee biomechanics and total knee replacement. *J Arthroplasty* 1986;1:211–219.

40. Nakagawa S, Kadoya Y, Todo S, et al. Tibiofemoral movement 3: full flexion in the living knee studied by MRI. *J Bone Joint Surg Br* 2000;82(8):1199–1200.

41. Li G, Zayontz S, DeFrate L, et al. Kinematics of the knee at high flexion angles: an in vitro investigation. Unpublished data.

42. Covey D, Sapega A. Injuries of the posterior cruciate ligament. *J Bone Joint Surg Am* 1993;75:1376–1387.

43. Fanelli G, Giannotti B, Edson C. The posterior cruciate ligament arthroscopic evaluation and treatment. *Arthroscopy* 1994;10:673–688.

44. Girgis F, Marshall J, Al Monajem A. The cruciate ligaments of the knee joint: anatomical, functional and experimental analysis. *Clin Orthop* 1975;106:216–231.

45. Moyer R, Marchetto P. Injuries of the posterior cruciate ligament. *Clin Sports Med* 1993;12:307–315.

46. Harner C, Xerogeanes J, Livesay G, et al. The human posterior cruciate ligament complex: an interdisciplinary study. *Am J Sports Med* 1995;23:736–745.

47. Butler DL, Noyes FR, Grood ES. Ligamentous restraints to anterior-posterior drawer in the human knee: a biomechanical study. *J Bone Joint Surg Am* 1980;62(2):259–270.

48. Fox RJ, Harner CD, Sakane M, et al. Determination of the in-situ forces in the human posterior cruciate ligament using robotic technology. *Am J Sports Med* 1998;26:395–401.

49. Gollehon DL, Torzilli PA, Warren RF. The role of the posterolateral and cruciate ligaments in the stability of the human knee: a biomechanical study. *J Bone Joint Surg Am* 1987;69(2):233–242.

50. Markolf K, Slauterbeck J, Armstrong K, et al. A biomechanical study of replacement of the posterior cruciate ligament with a graft. *J Bone Joint Surg Am* 1997;79:381–387.

51. Noyes FR, Stowers SF, Grood ES, et al. Posterior subluxation of the medial and lateral tibiofemoral compartments. *Am J Sports Med* 1993;21(3):407–414.

52. Harner CD, Janaushek MA, Anamori A, et al. Biomechanical analysis of a double-bundle posterior cruciate ligament reconstruction. *Am J Sports Med* 2000;28(2):144–151.

53. Li G, Gill T, DeFrate L, et al. Biomechanical consequences of PCL deficiency—an in-vitro experimental study. *J Orthop Res* 2002;20(4):887–892.

54. Andriacchi T, Galante J. Retention of the posterior cruciate in total knee arthroplasty. *J Arthroplasty* 1988;3[Suppl]:S13–S19.

55. Keating E, Faris P, Meding J, et al. Comparison of the midvastus muscle-splitting approach with the median parapatellar approach in total knee arthroplasty. *J Arthroplasty* 1999;14:29–32.

56. Matsueda M, Gustilo R. Subvastus and medial parapatellar approaches in total knee arthroplasty. *Clin Orthop* 2000;371:161–168.

57. Parentis M, Rumi M, Deol G, et al. A comparison of the vastus splitting and median parapatellar approaches in total knee arthroplasty. *Clin Orthop* 1999;367:107–116.

58. Walker P, Sathasivam S. Design forms of total knee replacement. *Proc Inst Mech Eng* 2000;214(H):101–119.

59. Maloney W, Schurman D. The effects of implant design on range of motion after total knee arthroplasty laxity after ACL reconstructive surgery. *Clin Orthop* 1992;278:147–152.

60. Most F, Li G, Zayontz S, et al. Kinematics of intact, fixed and mobile bearing TKAs during passive flexion. *Trans ORS* 2002;48:945.

61. Walker P, Garg A. Range of motion in total knee arthroplasty: a computer analysis. *Clin Orthop* 1991;262:227–235.

62. Dennis D, Komistek R, Colwell C, et al. In-vivo anteroposterior femorotibial translation of total knee arthroplasty: a multicenter analysis. *Clin Orthop* 1998;356:47–57.

63. Dennis D, Komistek R, Hoff W, et al. In-vivo knee kinematics derived using an inverse perspective technique. *Clin Orthop* 1996;331:107–117.

64. Li G, Zayontz S, Most E, et al. Cruciate-retaining and cruciate-substituting total knee arthroplasty—an in-vitro comparison of the kinematics under muscle loads. *J Arthroplasty* 2001;16[Suppl]:150–156.

65. Li G, Zayontz S, Most E, et al. The posterior cruciate ligament after total knee arthroplasty—a quantitative in-vitro investigation using robotic technology. *J Bone Joint Surg Am* 2002; (*in press*).

66. Banks SA, Markovich GD, Hodge WA. In vivo kinematics of cruciate-retaining and -substituting knee arthroplasties. *J Arthroplasty* 1997;12:297–304.

67. Pagnano MW, Hanssen AD, Lewallen DG, et al. Flexion instability after primary posterior cruciate retaining total knee arthroplasty. *Clin Orthop* 1998;356:39–46.

68. Worland R, Jessup D, Johnson J. Posterior cruciate recession in total knee arthroplasty. *J Arthroplasty* 1997;12(1):70–73.

69. Delp SL, Kocmond JH, Stern SH. Tradeoffs between motion and stability in posterior substituting knee arthroplasty design. *J Biomech* 1995;28:1155–1166.

70. Becker M, Insall J, Faris P. Bilateral total knee arthroplasty. One cruciate retaining and one cruciate substituting. *Clin Orthop* 1991;271:122–124.

71. Bolanos A, Colizza W, McCan P, et al. A comparison of isokinetic stretch testing and gait analysis in patients with posterior cruciate-retaining and substituting knee arthroplasties. *J Arthroplasty* 1998;13:906–915.

72. Shoji H, Wolf A, Packard S, et al. Cruciate retained and excised total knee arthroplasty. A comparative study in patients with bilateral total knee arthroplasty. *Clin Orthop* 1994;305:218.

73. Dennis D, Komistek R, Stiehl J, et al. Range of motion after total knee arthroplasty—the effect of implant design and weight-bearing conditions. *J Arthroplasty* 1998;13(7):748–752.

74. Tanzer M, Barnet S, Smith K. Posterior stabilized versus cruciate retaining total knee arthroplasty: balancing the gap. Proceedings of American Academy of Orthopaedic Surgeons; 2001; San Francisco.

75. Berger RA, Crossett LS, Jacobs JJ, et al. Malrotation causing patellofemoral complications after total knee arthroplasty. *Clin Orthop* 1998;356:144–153.

76. Insall JN. Anatomy of the knee. In: Insall JN, ed. *Surgery of the knee*. New York: Churchill Livingstone, 1984:1–20.

77. Li G, Rudy TW, Allen C, et al. Effect of combined axial compressive and anterior tibial loads on in-situ forces in the anterior tibial ligament: a porcine study. *J Orthop Res* 1998;16:122–127.

78. Singerman R, Dean J, Pagan H, et al. Decreased posterior tibial slope increases strain in the posterior cruciate ligament following total knee arthroplasty. *J Arthroplasty* 1996;11(1):99–103.

79. Rand J. Patellofemoral joint in total knee arthroplasty. *J Bone Joint Surg Br* 1994;76:612–620.

80. Star M, Kaufman K, Irby S, et al. The effects of patellar thickness on patellofemoral forces after resurfacing. *Clin Orthop* 1996;322:279–284.

81. Braakman M, Verburg A, Bronsema G, et al. The outcome of three methods of patellar resurfacing in total knee arthroplasty. *Int Orthop* 1995;19:7–11.

82. Emerson RJ, Ayers C, Head W, et al. Surgical closing in primary total knee arthroplasties: flexion versus extension. *Clin Orthop* 1996;331:74–80.

83. Emerson RJ, Ayers C, Head W, et al. Surgical closing in total knee arthroplasty: a series followup. *Clin Orthop* 1999;368:176–181.

84. Masri B, Laskin R, Windsor R, et al. Knee closure in total knee arthroplasty. *Clin Orthop* 1996;331:81–86.
85. Lee D, Kim D, Scott R, et al. Intraoperative flexion against gravity as an indication of ultimate range of motion in individual cases after total knee arthroplasty. *J Arthoplasty* 1998;13:500–503.
86. Salter R, Simmonds D, Malcolm B, et al. The biological effect of continuous passive motion on the healing of full-thickness defects in articular cartilage. *J Bone Joint Surg Am* 1980;62:1232–1251.
87. Coutts R, Borden L, Bryan R, et al. The effect of continuous passive motion on total knee rehabilitation. *Orthop Trans* 1983;7:535–536.
88. Johnson D. The effect of continuous passive motion on wound-healing and joint mobility after knee arthroplasty. *J Bone Joint Surg Br* 1990;72:421–426.
89. Chen B, Zimmerman J, Soulen L, et al. Continuous passive motion after total knee arthroplasty: a prospective study. *Am J Phys Med Rehabil* 2000;79:421–426.
90. MacDonald S, Bourne R, Rorabek C, et al. Prospective randomized clinical trial of continuous passive motion after total knee arthroplasty. *Clin Orthop* 2000;360:30–35.
91. Maloney W, Schurman D, Hangen D, et al. The influence of continuous passive motion on outcome in total knee arthroplasty. *Clin Orthop* 1990;256:162–168.
92. Pope R, Corcoran S, McCaul K, et al. Continuous passive motion after primary total knee arthroplasty. *J Bone Joint Surg Br* 1997;79:914–917.
93. Kumar P, McPherson E, Dorr L, et al. Rehabilitation after total knee arthroplasty. *Clin Orthop* 1996;331:93–101.
94. McInnes J, et al. A controlled evaluation of continuous passive motion in patients undergoing total knee arthroplasty. *JAMA* 1992;268:1423–1428.
95. Romness D, Rand J. The role of continuous passive motion following total knee arthroplasty. *Clin Orthop* 1988;226:34–37.
96. Ververeli P, Sutton D, Hearn S, et al. Continuous passive motion after total knee arthroplasty. *Clin Orthop* 1995;321:208–215.
97. Fox J, Poss R. The role of manipulation following total knee replacement. *J Bone Joint Surg Br* 1981;63:357–362.
98. Esler C, Lock K, Harper W, et al. Manipulation of total knee replacements: is the flexion gained retained? *J Bone Joint Surg Br* 1999;81:27–29.

CHAPTER 87

Patellofemoral Problems in Total Knee Arthroplasty

Richard A. Berger, Craig J. Della Valle, and Harry E. Rubash

Patellofemoral complications are the most common postoperative problem associated with the current design of total knee prostheses and are a major cause of revision surgery (1–9). Patellofemoral complications affect 5% to 6% of all total knee replacements done in the United States. Although there is evidence that patellofemoral complications have diminished somewhat over the past decade (10), they are still a common reason for pain and dysfunction after total knee arthroplasty. In some series, up to 50% of the revisions performed were for a problem related to the patellofemoral articulation (6).

This chapter addresses patellofemoral complications from two perspectives. First, they are considered as they relate to primary total knee arthroplasty, to enable the surgeon to optimize patellofemoral tracking and minimize complications. The various aspects of primary total knee arthroplasty that affect the patellofemoral joint are covered so that these common complications can be avoided. In the second half of this chapter, the diagnosis and management of patellofemoral complications after total knee arthroplasties are addressed.

PATELLOFEMORAL JOINT IN PRIMARY TOTAL KNEE ARTHROPLASTY

Patellofemoral complications are the most common complications in total knee arthroplasty that can be avoided. Patellar tilt is a common radiographic finding and can range from minimal to dramatic. When patellar tilt is associated with a metal-backed patellar component, this can lead to eccentric wear and delamination with the possibility of eventual scoring of the femoral component, which necessitates complete revision surgery (Fig. 1). As the problems of the patellofemoral joint progress, subluxation and frank dislocation can occur. Patellar maltracking leads to shear forces over time that can result in either debonding of the patellar prosthesis from the native patella or shearing off of the prosthesis from the fixation lugs (Fig. 2). These shear forces on the patella over time can also lead to patella fragmentation or fracture.

Mythical Problem: The Tight Lateral Retinaculum

It has been the conventional wisdom that patellofemoral maltracking is secondary to a tight lateral retinaculum and, therefore, that the solution to this problem is a lateral retinacular release. Once a lateral retinacular release is performed, however, patellar tracking usually does not improve substantially. A few well-placed towel clips, however, can lead to the false conclusion that the patella is tracking appropriately. In these cases it is often found postoperatively that the patella is not tracking well, and with time patellofemoral maltracking and failure occur.

This gets back to the mythical problem of a tight lateral retinaculum. In most total knee arthroplasties with patellofemoral maltracking, the retinaculum is not the sole problem; it is really only a symptom indicating that, in some way, the patellofemoral articulation has been altered.

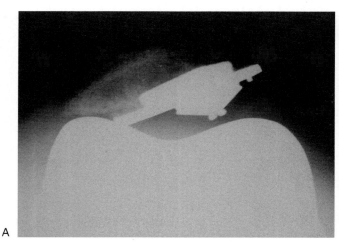
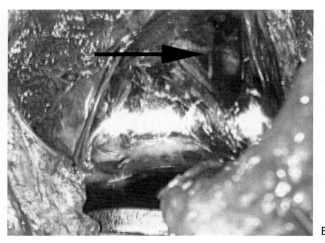

FIG. 1. Patellar tilt associated with a metal-backed patella. **A:** Radiograph. **B:** Intraoperative view of the femoral component that has been scored by the metal-backed patella (*arrow*) and requires revision.

Occasionally, such as in a knee with a valgus deformity, real lateral retinacular tightness is identified either preoperatively (Fig. 3) or intraoperatively after the arthrotomy has been performed. In these cases, the solution is a lateral retinacular release, which allows the patella to track in a more anatomic position in the trochlear groove. The majority of knees that require total knee arthroplasty are associated with a varus deformity, however, and in the majority of these cases, the patella tracks quite well before arthroplasty. Thus, if we recreate the patellar trochlear relationship that we started with, appropriate patellar tracking will result. If we alter that relationship, however, we end up with poor tracking that is manifest as lateral patellar tracking, subluxation, or frank dislocation. Thus, a tight lateral retinaculum is rarely the problem; it is only a symptom that intraoperatively the patellar trochlear relationship has been altered.

The problem of patellofemoral maltracking and the high rate of patellofemoral complications are a product of our surgical training. We have been taught to spend a great deal of time con-

centrating on balancing the flexion and extension gaps while obtaining balanced varus-valgus stability. Thus, patellar arthroplasty has, until recently, really been an afterthought. Normally, we take two towel clips, run a saw against the patella, apply a patellar button, and then wonder why the patella is not tracking the way it should. In general, the surgeon needs to spend more time reconstructing the patellofemoral joint and assessing how the patellofemoral joint is affected by multiple parameters.

Resection of the Patellofemoral Joint

As with the tibiofemoral articulation, the surgeon should take care in resecting the patellofemoral joint. In general, the patella should be restored millimeter for millimeter with polyethylene (11–13). Thus, the amount of bone resected should precisely equal the thickness of the patellar component to be implanted so that the final thickness of the patella-prosthesis composite is

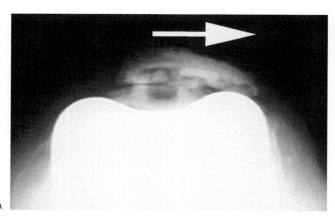
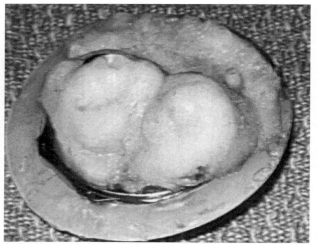

FIG. 2. A: Patellar maltracking has led to failure of the cemented patellar component secondary to shear forces (*arrow*). **B:** Failed metal-backed patellar component that has debonded from the surrounding cement mantle.

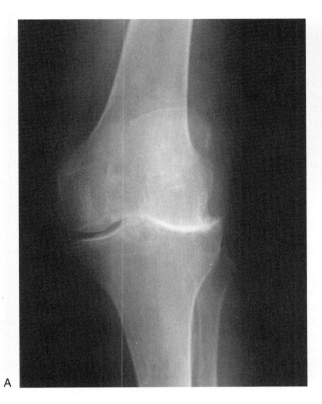

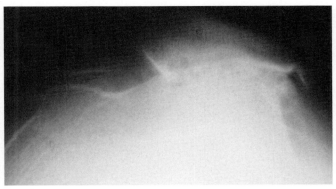

FIG. 3. Preoperative anteroposterior (**A**) and patellar view (**B**) of a knee with a valgus deformity with lateral patellar tracking noted preoperatively.

equivalent to the thickness of the native patella (Fig. 4). This is accomplished by first measuring the thickness of the native patella and then cutting it in the coronal plane, removing an amount of patellar bone that is equivalent to the thickness of the component to be inserted. The amount of bone resected is typically between 8 and 10 mm, which should correspond to the thickness of the patella component used. In general, at least 12 mm of patella should be left after resection.

It is important to resect the patella parallel to the coronal plane so that the patellar prosthesis is not tilted on the native patella. This can be accomplished by resecting some of the synovium around the patella so that the patellar tendon is exposed and cutting parallel to it. Booth et al. (14) have described the patellar nose as also a useful landmark for resecting the patella. Whatever landmark is chosen, it is important to resect the patella parallel to its anterior surface in the coronal plane and to remove an appropriate amount of bone that is equivalent to the thickness of the patellar component to be implanted. A useful rule of thumb is that the thickness of the final patella-prosthesis composite should be on the order of 21 to 23 mm for smaller

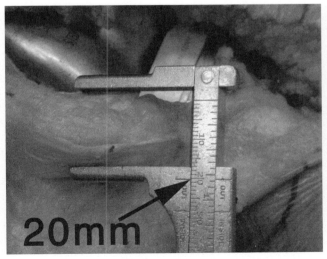

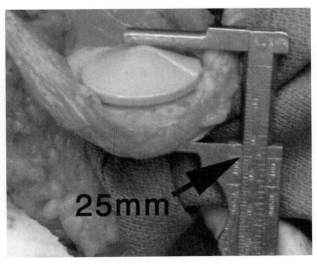

FIG. 4. **A:** Measurement of patellar thickness before resurfacing; the thickness is 20 mm. **B:** After resurfacing, with the trial component in place, the thickness is 25 mm. If additional bone is not resected, overstuffing of the patellofemoral joint will occur.

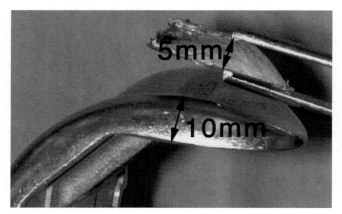

FIG. 5. The thickness of the anterior flange of the femoral component is 10 mm, whereas the bone resected from the anterior femur is only 5 mm in thickness. This can lead to overstuffing of the patellofemoral joint.

patients and 24 to 26 mm for larger patients. Thought and care should be taken when the combined thickness of the native patella and the patellar prosthesis is outside this range. Whether a patellar clamp, a patellar reamer, or a plain saw is used, it is important to adhere to these principles.

The consequences of not restoring the patellofemoral joint are significant (15–18). If patellar resection is excessive, so that the final construct of prosthesis plus native patella is significantly less than the native thickness, the quadriceps musculature is put at a substantial mechanical disadvantage, as the patella contributes approximately 30% to the extensor mechanism's moment arm (19,20). In addition, it is important to note that small differences in the final height of the patella are quite important. For example, if the patella before arthroplasty measures 25 mm and the final thickness of the resected patella plus the patellar implant is only 20 mm, the overall reduction in patellar thickness is 20%. Therefore, in this particular situation, 5 mm corresponds to a 20% reduction in patellar thickness, which will substantially affect quadriceps function (19).

Overstuffing the patellofemoral joint, although it improves quadriceps function, increases the resultant patellofemoral force and lateralizes the Q-angle force; this results in a tightened lateral retinaculum and lateral maltracking (21). As the patellofemoral joint is overstuffed with either too thick a patella or an oversized femoral component, the lateral retinaculum is stretched (22). The result is lateral patellar tracking, subluxation, and potentially dislocation (16). In addition to a tight lateral retinaculum secondary to overstuffing of the patellofemoral joint, other patellofemoral problems occur, many of which are associated with an increased Q angle, which further raises the resultant force that tends to pull the patella laterally (17,21,23).

The patellofemoral joint can also be overstuffed by failure to resect enough anterior femur (17). Most femoral components are 10 mm thick anteriorly, and in some patients, particularly women, the anterior trochlea that has been resected is not as thick as the component that replaces it (Fig. 5). In addition, the fear of notching the anterior femur has led many surgeons not to resect as much trochlea anteriorly as is being replaced by the component. This further leads to overstuffing of the patellofemoral joint. These problems can be avoided by carefully measuring the amount of bone resected from the trochlear groove and by ensuring that cutting guides are positioned appropriately.

Oversizing of the femoral component can also cause overstuffing of the patellofemoral joint (10,17). This is because, in flexion, the anteroposterior dimension of the femur contributes to the patellofemoral joint (Fig. 6). This problem is more commonly seen with posterior stabilized than with cruciate-retaining total knee arthroplasties, secondary to the tendency to upsize the femoral component, which makes it larger than the native anteroposterior diameter of the femur. This also tightens the retinaculum and makes it more likely that patellofemoral tracking problems will occur.

Many modern femoral components now have a deepened trochlear groove anteriorly, which prevents overstuffing of the joint (Fig. 7) (24,25). It is important to remember, however, that this should be thought of as adjunctive treatment for the patellofemoral joint, and care still must be taken to not overstuff it.

Femoral Component

Femoral component design, size, rotation, and placement all play an important role in patellofemoral tracking (23,24,26,27). The trochlear groove, being part of the femoral component, is related to placement and rotation of the femoral component itself. With the advent of the measured resection technique (28) in total knee arthroplasty, the initial thought was to remove equal amounts of bone from the medial and lateral posterior condyles (Fig. 8). However, when equal amounts of posterior condyle are resected in combination with a nonanatomic tibial cut (removing more lateral tibial bone than medial tibial bone), the femoral component is internally rotated on the tibia, which increases the Q angle of the knee and leads to patellar maltracking (24,26,29). To avoid this problem, in the majority of knees, more bone needs to be resected from the posterior medial femoral condyle than from the posterolateral femoral condyle (Fig. 9). In many modern total knee systems, the surgical protocols recommend cutting the femoral component with some external

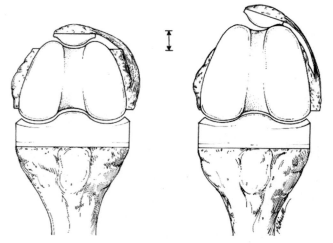

FIG. 6. Use of a larger femoral component **(right)** leads to overstuffing of the patellofemoral joint and creates the potential for patellar maltracking. (From Krackow KA. *The technique of total knee arthroplasty.* St. Louis, MO: Mosby, 1990:215, Fig. 6-25, with permission.)

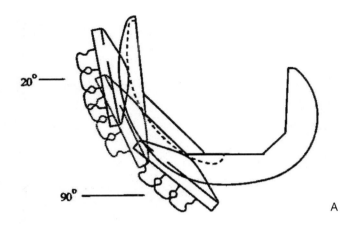

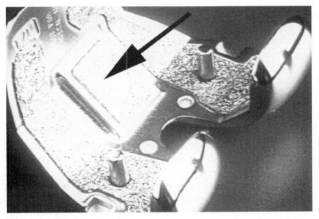

FIG. 7. A, B: Femoral component with a deepened trochlear groove (*arrow*).

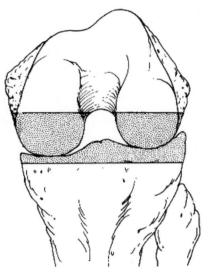

FIG. 8. Resection of equal amounts of bone from the posterior femoral condyles leads to internal rotation of the femoral component and poor patellar tracking. (From Krackow KA. *The technique of total knee arthroplasty.* St. Louis, MO: Mosby, 1990:131, with permission.)

In most varus knees, using either the epicondylar axis or the posterior condyles as a reference point for femoral component rotation works reasonably well. This is not true in valgus knees, however. Most valgus knees have hypoplasia of the posterior condyle that is present distally as well as posteriorly. Therefore, in the valgus knee, referencing the posterior condyles results in substantial internal rotation of the femoral component. This

rotation relative to the posterior condyles to optimize patellar tracking. Although external femoral rotation relative to the posterior condyles is helpful, a more accurate method of rotating the femoral component is to align the component parallel to the surgical epicondylar axis (Fig. 10).

The epicondylar axis can be found by identifying the lateral prominence of the lateral epicondyle and the medial sulcus of the medial epicondyle (Fig. 10) (30,31). If the medial sulcus is difficult to identify, the entire medial condyle is easy to palpate and is in essence a large prominence. If the center of that large prominence is then identified, that also corresponds to the sulcus of the medial epicondyle (15). The medial sulcus is the insertion point of the deep medial collateral ligament, and overlying this is the fan-like insertion of the superficial medial collateral ligament. These landmarks can be seen and felt intraoperatively in the majority of cases and routinely used to confirm appropriate femoral bone resection and component rotation.

Most surgeons and most instrumentation systems, however, still use the posterior femoral condyles as a reference point for femoral component alignment. Therefore, it is important to know the relationship between the posterior femoral condyles and the epicondylar axis. This has been shown to be approximately 3 degrees of external rotation, and thus many instrumentation systems rotate the femoral cutting block in 3 degrees of external rotation relative to the posterior femoral condyles (Fig. 11).

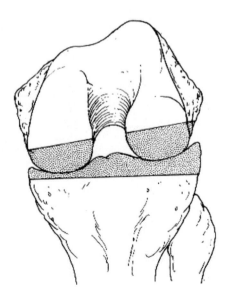

FIG. 9. Appropriate resection of bone from the posterior femoral condyles to avoid internal rotation of the femoral component. The cut is parallel to the epicondylar axis, with more bone being removed form the posteromedial than from the posterolateral condyle. (From Krackow KA. *The technique of total knee arthroplasty.* St. Louis, MO: Mosby, 1990:131, with permission.)

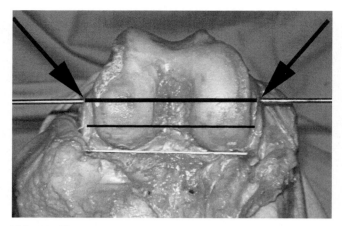

FIG. 10. The epicondylar axis has been marked by pins placed in the center of the medial and lateral epicondyles (*arrows*). The femoral cut is then made parallel to this line (*lower line*). Note that more bone will be resected from the medial than from the lateral condyle.

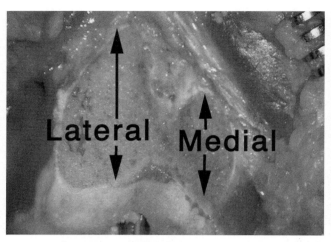

FIG. 12. View of the cut anterior surface of the distal femur (right knee). The exposed bone is substantially longer on the lateral side than on the medial side, which indicates appropriate external rotation of the femoral cuts.

leads to extremely poor patellofemoral tracking and is probably the principal reason that many valgus knees have poor patellofemoral tracking compared to varus knees. In the valgus knee, even though the lateral retinaculum is sometimes tight, correcting the axial deformity and properly aligning the components decreases the Q angle and improves patellar tracking; therefore, a lateral release is rarely required.

A useful intraoperative sign to ensure that appropriate femoral cuts have been made is the anterior trochlear groove. In the normal femur, the lateral side of the trochlear groove is more prominent than the medial side. Therefore, when the anterior surface of the trochlear groove is cut, more bone should be removed from the lateral than from the medial side of the trochlear groove. When viewed from above, the exposed bone on the medial side should be much shorter in length than the exposed bone on the lateral side (Fig. 12). This is often referred to as the "boot sign," with the toe on the medial side and the heel and shank on the lateral side. If the exposed bone on the medial side is equal or longer in length than on the lateral side, then the femoral component is internally rotated and the epicondylar axis should be identified and rotation reassessed and corrected.

In addition to the epicondylar axis and the posterior femoral condyles, a third landmark, which was described by Whiteside and Arima (32), is also useful. The Whiteside line, which is the

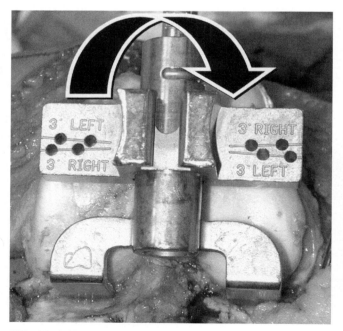

FIG. 11. Initial femoral guide for the NexGen total knee system as seen on a left knee. The guide orients the cutting block for the femoral component in 3 degrees of external rotation relative to the posterior condyles (*arrow*). Although this guide is accurate in the majority of knees, appropriate external rotation should always be confirmed using either the epicondylar axis or the Whiteside line.

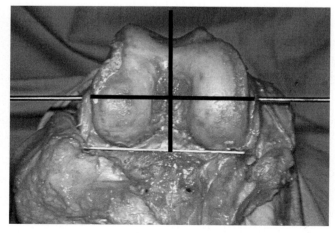

FIG. 13. Whiteside line is drawn in the deepest part of the trochlear recess and is perpendicular to the epicondylar axis, which has been marked with pins in the center of the medial and lateral epicondyles.

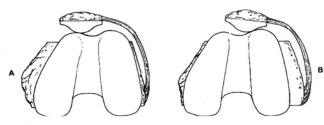

FIG. 14. Lateral placement of the femoral component **(A)** optimizes patellar tracking compared with medial placement **(B)**. (From Krackow KA. *The technique of total knee arthroplasty.* St. Louis, MO: Mosby, 1990:139, Fig. 5-12, with permission.)

deepest part of the trochlear recess, should be perpendicular to the epicondylar axis and is a useful final check to ensure that the femoral cutting block is oriented appropriately (Fig. 13).

In addition to rotation of the femoral component, mediolateral placement of the femoral component can also affect patellofemoral tracking (24). A component that is placed too far medially moves the entire trochlear groove medially, which results in relative lateral tracking of the patella (Fig. 14). Although, on most femurs, the mediolateral dimension of the component comes close to covering the exposed femur, oftentimes there are a few millimeters of uncovered femur. Therefore, the femur should be placed as close to the lateral edge of the exposed bone as possible. This helps in patellofemoral tracking by lateralizing the trochlear groove.

It is important, however, not to lateralize the femoral component so that the trochlear groove of the femoral component overhangs the bone anteriorly. This tends to tent the retinaculum and results in a tightening of the lateral retinaculum with associated pain and poor patellar tracking.

Tibial Component in Primary Total Knee Arthroplasty

Just as femoral component rotation is extremely important in patellofemoral tracking, so is tibial component rotation. Internally rotating the tibial component increases the Q angle and therefore increases the resultant force, which tends to dislocate the patella laterally. Externally rotating the tibial component decreases the Q angle, which reduces the resultant force that tends to dislocate the component laterally and results in improved patellar tracking (16). It must be stated, however, that excessive external rotation of the tibial component can lead to in-toeing, with subsequent problems such as tripping and cosmetic deformity.

It has been suggested that the proper rotational orientation of the tibial component is alignment with the center of the medial one-third of the tibial tubercle. However, this is a difficult landmark to assess. A better landmark is to use the tip of the tibial tubercle. Berger et al. (29) have described a technique to align the rotation of the tibial component. A pin is placed in the tibial tubercle at the tip and aimed towards the posterior cruciate ligament. This determines the orientation of the tibia. Then, the component is placed 18 degrees internal to the tip of the tibial tubercle (this is 3 minutes on a clock face). This point then corresponds roughly with the center of the medial one-third; however, it is a much more reproducible mark (Fig. 15). An

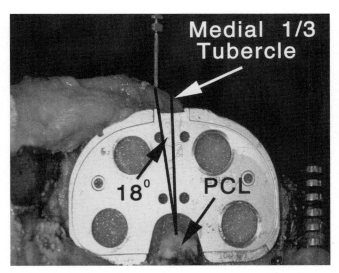

FIG. 15. Guidelines for obtaining appropriate external rotation of the tibial component. A pin is placed in the tibial tubercle at the tip and aimed toward the posterior cruciate ligament (PCL). This determines the orientation of the tibia. The component is then placed 18 degrees internal to the tip of the tibial tubercle (3 minutes on a clock face). This point corresponds roughly with the center of the medial one-third of the tibial tubercle.

alternative method to check proper rotation of the tibial component is to align the anterior edge of the component with the anterior edge of the native tibia (15).

Appropriate rotation of the tibial component is complicated by the asymmetric nature of the proximal tibia. With most symmetric tibial components, when they are placed on the tibia such that posterolaterally the tibial component is flush with the bone, some posteromedial bone will remain uncovered. This represents the proper tibial component rotation (Fig. 16). If, however, the component is too large and the surgeon tries to obtain perfect tibial coverage, internal rotation of the tibial component occurs

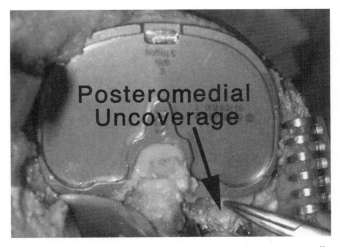

FIG. 16. When the tibial component has been externally rotated appropriately, the posteromedial portion of the proximal tibia is uncovered.

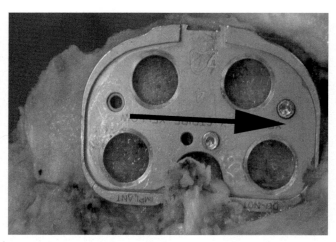

FIG. 17. View of the tibial trial appropriately positioned on a right knee. The component is placed as far lateral as is possible (*arrow*) to optimize patellar tracking, leaving medial bone uncovered. It is important to clear away adequate soft tissue to visualize the lateral border of the tibia and to place a retractor in this space to keep the patella retracted laterally.

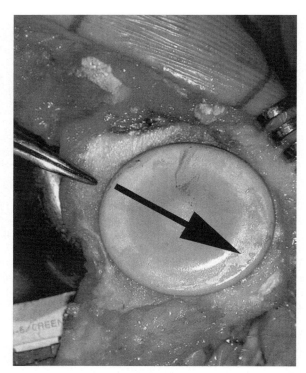

FIG. 18. The patellar button is placed medially on the native patella to optimize patellar tracking (*arrow*).

due to the attempt to cover the exposed posteromedial bone. It should be noted that this is also true with asymmetric tibial components, as they too usually do not fully cover the tibia if placed in an appropriate amount of external rotation. Therefore, the rotation of the tibial component should be determined independent of tibial coverage.

In addition, mediolateral tibial component placement can also affect the patellofemoral articulation and patellofemoral tracking. In addition, lateral placement of the tibial tray decreases the Q angle and improves patellofemoral tracking. Therefore, it is recommended that the tibial tray be placed as far lateral as possible; it is thus important to clear away enough soft tissue around the lateral edge of the tibia for it to be appropriately visualized (Fig. 17). As the majority of arthritic knees have a varus deformity, the small amount of proximal tibia that is uncovered on the medial side of the knee can then be removed, which aids in obtaining appropriate ligamentous balance by effectively lengthening the medial collateral ligament.

Patellar Component

In addition to recreating appropriate patellar thickness, mediolateral patellar component placement also plays a role in patellofemoral tracking. Most patellae are oblong with a larger medial-to-lateral distance than superior-inferior distance. Therefore, the patellar button usually can be placed either medially or laterally on the patella. Placing the patellar button medially on the native patella results in a decreased Q angle, whereas placing it laterally results in an increased Q angle (Fig. 18). Therefore, medial positioning helps patellofemoral tracking (25,33). In addition, it has been shown by Hofmann (33) that the normal center of the patella lies approximately 3 mm medial to the center of the underlying bone, and thus the center of the patellar button should be placed at least 3 mm medial to the center of the remaining bone. Further work by Miller et al. (23) found that patellar kinematics were improved with placement of

the patellar component 3.75 mm medial to the geometric center of the patella. Any remaining bone on the lateral side of the native patella should be removed as this bone can overgrow, causing patellofemoral impingement and pain. In addition, this small amount of bone tends to tent the retinaculum on the lateral side, tightening it with resultant poor patellofemoral tracking.

Conclusion

Multiple factors affect the patellofemoral joint in primary total knee arthroplasty. Avoidance of overstuffing the patellofemoral joint by replacing the anterior trochlear groove and the patella one for one with prosthesis for bone avoids overstuffing of the joint. Properly sizing the femoral component is also important. Overstuffing the joint with the normal Q angle of the knee results in tightening of the lateral retinaculum and the resultant force tends to dislocate the patella laterally.

Lateral placement of the femoral component on the femur as well as lateral placement of the tibial component on the tibia also tends to decrease the Q angle, as does medialization of the patellar component on the native patella. However, by far the most important contribution to patellofemoral tracking is femoral and tibial component rotation. Internal rotation of the femoral or tibial component results in poor patellofemoral tracking, whereas slight external rotation of the femoral and tibial components optimizes patellofemoral tracking (34). The femoral component should be rotated parallel to the epicondylar axis and the tibial component should be rotated 18 degrees from the tip of the tibial tubercle.

After all of the components are in place, a trial reduction should be performed to assess patellofemoral tracking. This assessment

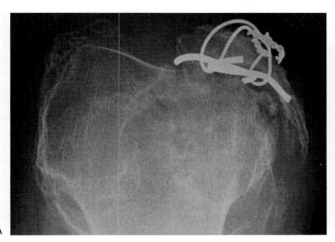
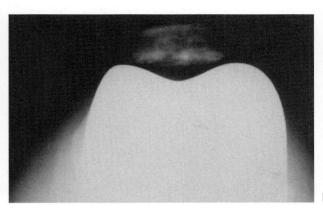

A   B

FIG. 19. A: Preoperative patellar view of a knee with severe lateral maltracking. The procedure was performed without a retinacular release but with special attention to appropriate component position. **B:** Postoperative patellar view.

should be done without towel clips in the retinaculum using the "no thumb" technique. If there is any concern about patellofemoral tracking, the tourniquet can be released, as this can affect patellofemoral tracking by binding of the quadriceps musculature. If the patella is still not tracking properly, attention should be directed to the components to determine if their rotation and position are optimal. A lateral retinacular release should be performed only if the lateral retinaculum was tight to begin with. If the lateral retinaculum was not tight preoperatively, then the surgeon affected the trochlear patellar relationship and therefore must determine which component or components have been malpositioned, malrotated, or improperly sized. The retinaculum should be released only if the retinaculum was a problem to begin with, and the problem that was created intraoperatively should be identified and corrected. With today's modern total knee systems, the most common problem is internal rotation of the femoral or tibial components. In conclusion, with attention to detail, alignment, rotation, and position, even the most complex patellofemoral joint can be handled and can track well postoperatively (Fig. 19).

REVISION TOTAL KNEE ARTHROPLASTY FOR PATELLAR MALTRACKING

As has been discussed earlier, it is important to strive to avoid patellofemoral complications by proper component rotation and alignment with attention to soft tissue balance. Patellofemoral complications sometimes do occur after total knee arthroplasty, however; the following section addresses the diagnosis and treatment of these problems.

Once patellofemoral problems occur, it is important to identify and address the underlying cause. Although it is appealing to believe that a simple lateral release will correct a subluxing or dislocating patella, if the underlying cause of the subluxation or dislocation is not identified, a lateral release merely provides a transient solution. Lateral releases with or without medial reefing should be considered only when the lateral retinaculum was tight preoperatively and was not released. The most commonly identified cause of patellar maltracking is internal rotation of the femoral or tibial component or both.

Assessment of Patellofemoral Maltracking

When patellofemoral problems are assessed, it is important to obtain a complete set of radiographs that includes a Merchant or skyline view. A long mechanical axis view should also be obtained to assess axial alignment. Although patellofemoral problems can result from axial malalignment, the problem is often improper rotation of the tibial or femoral component or both.

Berger et al. (29) have described a technique to allow for assessing component rotation preoperatively using noninvasive computed tomographic (CT) scanning methods. With this technique, the femoral component can be evaluated using a single cut through the epicondylar axis. The epicondylar axis is drawn from the lateral prominence to the medial sulcus and a second

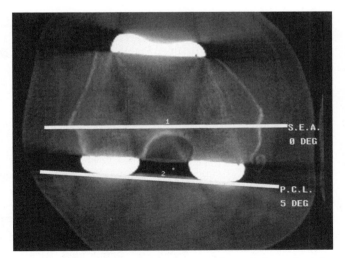

FIG. 20. Computed tomographic scan through the epicondylar axis of a right knee. The epicondylar axis (*upper line*) is compared with the position of the posterior condyles of the femoral component (*lower line*) to determine femoral component rotation. The component pictured is internally rotated 5 degrees. P.C.L., posterior condylar line; S.E.A., surgical epicondylar axis.

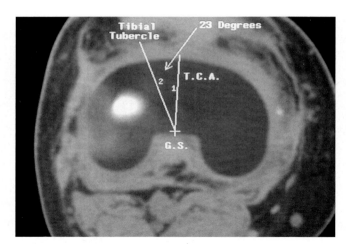

FIG. 21. Computed tomographic scan to determine tibial component rotation. A line is drawn from the tip of the tibial tubercle to the geometric center of the tibia and is compared to a line marking the anteroposterior axis of the tibial component. Appropriate rotation is 18 degrees. The component shown is internally rotated 5 degrees. G.S., geometric center; T.C.A., tibial component axis.

line is drawn in reference to the posterior condyles. The difference between these two angles is the femoral component rotation (Fig. 20). The femoral component should be parallel to the epicondylar axis, and any internal rotation may result in patellofemoral problems.

Tibial component rotation can also be assessed using this method. Three cuts through the tibia are obtained: one through the tibial tubercle, one through the proximal tibial plateau, and one through the tibial component. These three cuts are then superimposed. The geometric center of the tibial plateau is

found, and this point is connected to the tip of the tibial tubercle. This defines the orientation of the tibial tubercle. A second line is made in the anteroposterior axis of the tibial component. The difference between these two lines defines tibial component rotation (Fig. 21). Through previous studies, we have determined that appropriate component rotation using this method should be 18 degrees (29). If the tibial component rotation is more than 18 degrees, the tibial component is internally rotated and patellofemoral problems are likely.

We have shown in a study of 20 well-functioning total knee arthroplasties and 30 total knee arthroplasties with patellofemoral maltracking that the severity of patellofemoral problems in an otherwise well-aligned, well-balanced knee is related to the amount of overall internal rotation of the femoral component plus the tibial component (Fig. 22) (29). More severe complications were associated with greater amounts of combined internal rotation of the femoral or the tibial component or both. Subsequent authors have confirmed the accuracy of CT scanning for identifying femoral and tibial component rotation (35). If the overall problem is noted on the chart, then the amount of malrotation can be surmised. That is to say, with minor patellofemoral problems, only a mild amount of malrotation is likely to be present. With more serious patellofemoral problems, however, significant malrotation of both components is suspected.

Using CT, the amount and location of component malrotation can be easily assessed. If the problem lies with only one component, then an isolated component revision can be contemplated. If the problem is isolated tibial component internal rotation, an alternative to revising the tibial component is to have a custom externally rotated polyethylene liner made. This can be specially ordered from the manufacturer and has been successfully used in our experience to correct patellofemoral maltracking in the face of isolated internal rotation of the tibial component.

In addition to preoperative CT scans, an intraoperative assessment of component rotation can be made. When femoral

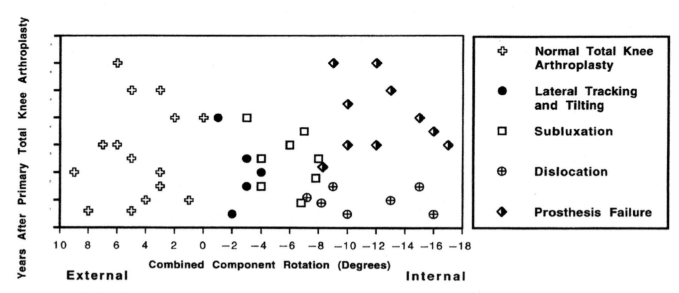

FIG. 22. Graphic representation of the results of combined femoral and tibial rotation on patellar tracking after total knee arthroplasty. With greater amounts of combined internal rotation, patellar maltracking and the risk of ultimate patellar failure increase with time. (From Berger RA, Crossett LS, Jacobs JJ, et al. Malrotation causing patellofemoral complications after total knee arthroplasty. *Clin Orthop* 1998;356:144–153, Fig. 7, with permission.)

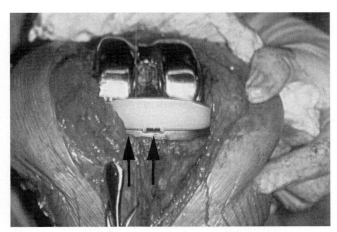

FIG. 23. Intraoperative assessment of tibial component rotation in a right knee. The center of the tibial component (*right arrow*) lies medial to the medial third of the tibial tubercle (*left arrow*) and, thus, is internally rotated. The tibial tubercle has a towel clamp placed around it, and the center of the tubercle is marked with an elevator.

component rotation is assessed, the epicondylar axis can be easily identified using the lateral prominence and the medial sulcus. Tibial component rotation can be assessed intraoperatively by noting where the center of the tibial component is located relative to the tip of the tubercle (Fig. 23). Although intraoperative assessment is important, it is strongly recommended that CT scans be used, as often anatomic variations,

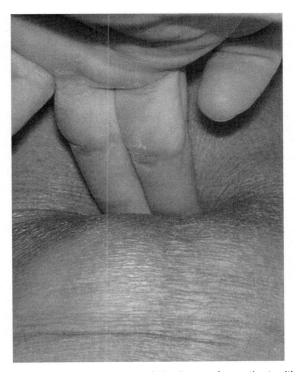

FIG. 24. Clinical photograph of the knee of a patient with a quadriceps tendon rupture after a total knee arthroplasty. There is a palpable defect proximal to the patella.

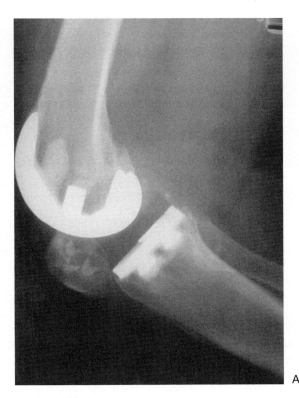

A

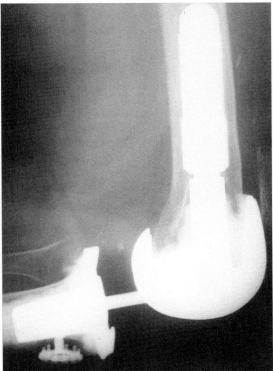

B

FIG. 25. A: Lateral radiograph of a quadriceps tendon rupture. The patella is seen to lie distal to its normal position. **B:** Lateral radiograph of a patellar tendon rupture showing the patella far proximal to its normal position. Note the hardware in the region of the tibial tubercle, which indicates that a portion of or the entire patellar tendon was damaged at the time of the revision surgery, and an attempt was made to repair the tendon using a soft tissue washer.

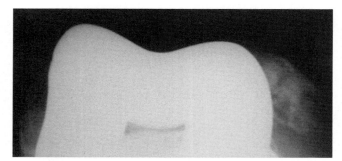

FIG. 26. Skyline or Merchant view of the right knee showing dislocation of the patella from the trochlea in a patient with a quadriceps tendon rupture.

which initially lead to abnormal rotation of the components, will still be present and can fool the revision surgeon, particularly if exposure is difficult.

Extensor Mechanism Disruption

Other extensor mechanism problems exist that may or may not be related to tibiofemoral component rotation. One of the more devastating complications after total knee arthroplasty is extensor mechanism disruption, which has been reported to occur in as many as 2.5% of cases (36). Although normally an

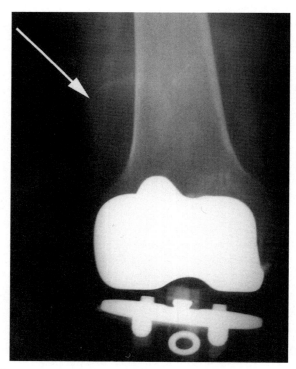

FIG. 27. Anteroposterior view of the right knee in a patient with a patellar tendon rupture. The "rising moon" sign is seen with the patella far proximal to its normal position. Note the metallic hardware present in the region of the tibial tubercle, indicative of an attempt to repair a partially or entirely detached patellar tendon at the time of the primary knee arthroplasty with a soft tissue washer.

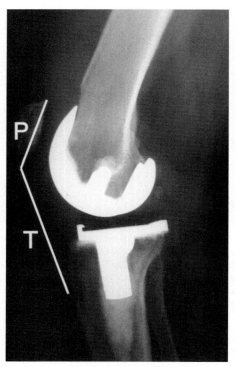

FIG. 28. Lateral radiograph of the knee of a patient with a patellar tendon disruption. The Insall ratio is determined by dividing the length of the patellar tendon (T) by the length of the patella (P). The normal value is 1, with values greater than 1.2 indicative of a patellar tendon disruption.

acute quadriceps rupture can be easily repaired primarily (8), a much more difficult situation develops with chronic quadriceps or patellar tendon ruptures (37).

Extensor mechanism disruptions manifest clinically as loss of active extension. When the quadriceps tendon is disrupted, a defect is often palpable proximal to the patella (Fig. 24). Radiographs often confirm the diagnosis of an extensor mechanism disruption, with the patella seen in a far more proximal or distal position than normal (Fig. 25), and a skyline or Merchant view shows that the patella is not present in the trochlear groove (Fig. 26). The "rising moon" sign, in which the patella is seen riding above the level of the top of the femoral component on the anteroposterior projection (Fig. 27), has been described for patellar tendon ruptures. On the lateral radiograph, the Insall-Salvati ratio can be used to assess the integrity of the patellar tendon (Fig. 28) (38). This is the ratio between the length of the patellar tendon (as measured from the insertion on the tibial tubercle to the insertion on the base of the patella) divided by the length of the patella. The normal ratio is approximately 1.2; values above this indicate patellar tendon disruption.

Patellar tendon ruptures can be divided into two broad categories: acute and chronic. Although the acute patellar tendon rupture can be addressed by primary repair with or without augmentation from a semitendinosus graft, chronic ruptures are more difficult to treat. Treatment of this catastrophic complication using primary direct repair or xenograft was associated with failure in 11 of 17 cases in one series (37). Alternative surgical techniques for management include reconstruction with autogenous semitendinosus tendon (36), medial gastrocnemius muscle transposition flap (39), or extensor mechanism allograft (40–43).

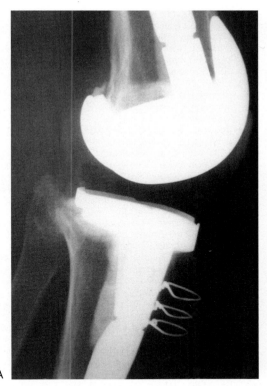
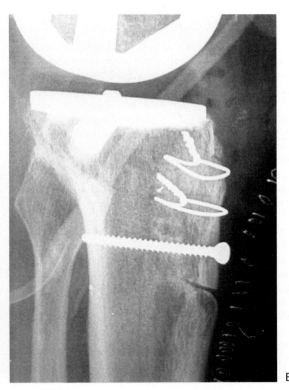

A
B

FIG. 29. Fixation methods for the tibial bone block of an extensor mechanism allograft. **A:** Six-month postoperative lateral radiograph showing a healed junction between the tibial bone block and the native tibia. The bone block was held in place using three wires. **B:** Immediately postoperative lateral radiograph after an extensor mechanism allograft in which adjunctive fixation was achieved using a bicortical screw.

Emerson et al. reported initial optimistic results in a group of 13 knees treated with a complete allograft extensor mechanism reconstruction, including the tibial tubercle, patellar tendon, patella, and quadriceps tendon for patellar tendon ruptures that occurred during or after total knee arthroplasty (40). They found reliable osseous union at the junction of the distal allograft bone plug (at the inferior portion of the allograft patellar tendon) and the host tibial tubercle, and no patient had an extensor lag of more than 20 degrees. A subsequent follow-up of the same group, however, found that three of the nine remaining patients had unacceptable extensor lags of 20 to 40 degrees (41). Using the original technique as described by Emerson, in which the graft was tensioned to allow for 60 degrees of flexion "without excessive tightness," our group previously reported poor results, with seven out of seven reconstructions having failed clinically at a mean of 39 months (42).

Better results were reported by Nazarian and Booth (43) in a series of 40 patients when the surgical technique was modified to include suturing the quadriceps anastomoses in full extension under maximal tension. Using this technique, we have found that the rate of recurrent extensor lag is greatly decreased, and we currently use an extensor mechanism allograft for patients with chronic extensor mechanism disruptions, severe patella baja, and patellar fragmentation, and for patients who have previously had a patellectomy with poor extensor mechanism function.

Our present surgical technique includes the use of fresh frozen allografts and tensioning of the graft in full extension. The patellar tendon insertion and tibial bone block are placed into a tight-fitting trough in the native tibia with fixation using multiple wires around the allograft; a bicortical screw is used if additional fixation is needed (Fig. 29). The native extensor tissue is

oversewn with the allograft using heavy nonabsorbable suture, and the patella is not resurfaced (Fig. 30). An alternative is reconstruction with a fresh frozen Achilles tendon allograft with an os calcis bone block using similar surgical technique and principles (44). Postoperative management includes the use of a brace locked in extension for 6 to 8 weeks followed by gentle active flexion exercises. Active extension is allowed at approximately 10 weeks postoperatively, and in our experience, flexion slowly improves over the subsequent 3 to 6 months. It is imperative that appropriate tibiofemoral component alignment and rotation be assessed both preoperatively and intraoperatively to prevent recurrence of extensor mechanism dysfunction, and in our experience, component revision is often necessary.

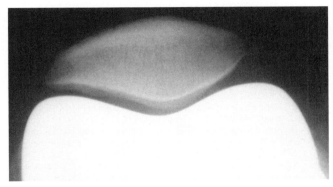

FIG. 30. Merchant view after an extensor mechanism allograft. The patella is not resurfaced and is seen tracking centrally.

Conclusion

Once patellofemoral problems occur and become clinically significant, it is important to identify and address the underlying cause of the malfunctioning patella; a simple lateral release alone merely results in a transient solution. Multiple factors may contribute to patellofemoral problems in the failed total knee arthroplasty. The most common cause of patellar maltracking, however, is internal rotation of the femoral or tibial component or both. Preoperatively, CT scans can assess and quantify this malrotation. Intraoperatively, the rotation of the femoral component can be assessed using the epicondylar axis and the tibial component's rotation can be assessed using the tibial tubercle. The offending component or components must be changed.

After all of the revision components are in place, a trial reduction should be performed to assess patellofemoral tracking. This assessment should be done without towel clips in the retinaculum using the "no thumb" technique. Subsequent alterations in the components can be performed until the patella tracks properly. When these techniques are used and attention is given to detail, alignment, rotation, and position, even the most complex patellofemoral joint problem can be handled, and the patella can track well postoperatively.

REFERENCES

1. Aglietti P, Buzzi R, Bassi PB. Arthroscopic partial meniscectomy in the anterior cruciate deficient knee. *Am J Sports Med* 1988; 16(6):597.
2. Aglietti P, Buzzi R, Gaudenzi A. Patellofemoral functional results and complications with the posterior stabilized total condylar knee prosthesis. *J Arthroplasty* 1988;3(1):17.
3. Brick GW, Scott RD. The patellofemoral component of total knee arthroplasty. *Clin Orthop* 1988;231:163.
4. Bryan RS, Rand JA. Revision total knee arthroplasty. *Clin Orthop* 1982;170:116.
5. Clayton ML, Thirupathi R. Patellar complications after total condylar arthroplasty. *Clin Orthop* 1982;170:152.
6. Doolittle KH 2nd, Turner RH. Patellofemoral problems following total knee arthroplasty. *Orthop Rev* 1988;17(7):696.
7. Insall JN, Binazzi R, Soudry M, et al. Total knee arthroplasty. *Clin Orthop* 1985;192:13.
8. Lynch AF, Rorabeck CH, Bourne RB. Extensor mechanism complications following total knee arthroplasty. *J Arthroplasty* 1987;2(2):135.
9. Webster DA, Murray DG. Complications of variable axis total knee arthroplasty. *Clin Orthop* 1985;193:160.
10. Kelly MA. Patellofemoral complications following total knee arthroplasty. *Instr Course Lect* 2001;50:403.
11. Hsu HC, Luo ZP, Rand JA, et al. Influence of patellar thickness on patellar tracking and patellofemoral contact characteristics after total knee arthroplasty. *J Arthroplasty* 1996;11(1):69.
12. Marmor L. Technique for patellar resurfacing in total knee arthroplasty. *Clin Orthop* 1988;230:166.
13. Oishi CS, Kaufman KR, Irby SE, et al. Effects of patellar thickness on compression and shear forces in total knee arthroplasty. *Clin Orthop* 1996;331:283.
14. Booth RE Jr, Bowen R, Nazarian DG, et al. The patellar nose: an anatomic guide for patellar resurfacing. Presented at: Knee Society Combined Specialty Day Meeting; 2000; Orlando.
15. Insall J, Easly ME. Surgical technique and instrumentation in total knee arthroplasty. In: Insall J, Scott WN, eds. *Surgery of the knee.* New York: Churchill Livingstone, 2001:1553.
16. Merkow RL, Soudry M, Insall JN. Patellar dislocation following total knee replacement. *J Bone Joint Surg Am* 1985;67(9):1321.
17. Rand JA. The patellofemoral joint in total knee arthroplasty. *J Bone Joint Surg Am* 1994;76(4):612.
18. Reuben JD, McDonald CL, Woodard PL, et al. Effect of patella thickness on patella strain following total knee arthroplasty. *J Arthroplasty* 1991;6(3):251.
19. Kaufer H. Patellar biomechanics. *Clin Orthop* 1979;144:51.
20. Wendt PP, Johnson RP. A study of quadriceps excursion, torque, and the effect of patellectomy on cadaver knees. *J Bone Joint Surg Am* 1985;67(5):726.
21. Huberti HH, Hayes WC. Patellofemoral contact pressures. The influence of q-angle and tendofemoral contact. *J Bone Joint Surg Am* 1984;66(5):715.
22. Briard JL, Hungerford DS. Patellofemoral instability in total knee arthroplasty. *J Arthroplasty* 1989;4[Suppl]:S87.
23. Miller MC, Zhang AX, Petrella AJ, et al. The effect of component placement on knee kinetics after arthroplasty with an unconstrained prosthesis. *J Orthop Res* 2001;19(4):614.
24. Rhoads DD, Noble PC, Reuben JD, et al. The effect of femoral component position on the kinematics of total knee arthroplasty. *Clin Orthop* 1993;286:122.
25. Yoshii I, Whiteside LA, Anouchi YS. The effect of patellar button placement and femoral component design on patellar tracking in total knee arthroplasty. *Clin Orthop* 1992;275:211.
26. Anouchi YS, Whiteside LA, Kaiser AD, et al. The effects of axial rotational alignment of the femoral component on knee stability and patellar tracking in total knee arthroplasty demonstrated on autopsy specimens. *Clin Orthop* 1993;287:170.
27. Miller MC, Berger RA, Petrella AJ, et al. Optimizing femoral component rotation in total knee arthroplasty. *Clin Orthop* 2001;392:38.
28. Hungerford DS, Krackow KA. Total joint arthroplasty of the knee. *Clin Orthop* 1985;192:23.
29. Berger RA, Crossett LS, Jacobs JJ, et al. Malrotation causing patellofemoral complications after total knee arthroplasty. *Clin Orthop* 1998;356:144.
30. Berger RA, Rubash HE, Seel MJ, et al. Determining the rotational alignment of the femoral component in total knee arthroplasty using the epicondylar axis. *Clin Orthop* 1993;286:40.
31. Poilvache PL, Insall JN, Scuderi GR, et al. Rotational landmarks and sizing of the distal femur in total knee arthroplasty. *Clin Orthop* 1996;331:35.
32. Whiteside LA, Arima J. The anteroposterior axis for femoral rotational alignment in valgus total knee arthroplasty. *Clin Orthop* 1995;321:168.
33. Hofmann AA, Tkach TK, Evanich CJ, et al. Patellar component medialization in total knee arthroplasty. *J Arthroplasty* 1997;12(2):155.
34. Berger RA, Rubash HE. Rotational instability and malrotation after total knee arthroplasty. *Orthop Clin North Am* 2001;32(4):639.
35. Jazrawi LM, Birdzell L, Kummer FJ, et al. The accuracy of computed tomography for determining femoral and tibial total knee arthroplasty component rotation. *J Arthroplasty* 2000;15(6):761.
36. Cadambi A, Engh GA. Use of a semitendinosus tendon autogenous graft for rupture of the patellar ligament after total knee arthroplasty. A report of seven cases. *J Bone Joint Surg Am* 1992;74(7):974.
37. Rand JA, Morrey BF, Bryan RS. Patellar tendon rupture after total knee arthroplasty. *Clin Orthop* 1989;244:233.
38. Insall J, Salvati E. Patella position in the normal knee joint. *Radiology* 1971;101(1):101.
39. Jaureguito JW, Dubois CM, Smith SR, et al. Medial gastrocnemius transposition flap for the treatment of disruption of the extensor mechanism after total knee arthroplasty. *J Bone Joint Surg Am* 1997;79(6):866.
40. Emerson RH Jr, Head WC, Malinin TI. Reconstruction of patellar tendon rupture after total knee arthroplasty with an extensor mechanism allograft. *Clin Orthop* 1990;260:154.
41. Emerson RH Jr, Head WC, Malinin TI. Extensor mechanism reconstruction with an allograft after total knee arthroplasty. *Clin Orthop* 1994;303:79.
42. Leopold SS, Greidanus N, Paprosky WG, et al. High rate of failure of allograft reconstruction of the extensor mechanism after total knee arthroplasty. *J Bone Joint Surg Am* 1999;81(11):1574.
43. Nazarian DG, Booth RE Jr. Extensor mechanism allografts in total knee arthroplasty. *Clin Orthop* 1999;367:123.
44. Sinha RK, Crossett LS, Rubash HE. Extensor mechanism disruption after total knee arthroplasty. In: Insall J, Scott WN, eds. *Surgery of the knee.* New York: Churchill Livingstone, 2001.

CHAPTER 88

Asian Knee

Shinro Takai, Masashi Kobayashi, and Nobuyuki Yoshino

The skeleton of the Asian is generally smaller than that of the Westerner. Bone morphology of the knee joint has been analyzed using cadaveric joints and measurements on radiographic and computed tomographic images. Body size is often expressed in terms of height and body weight. It is known that the size of the knee joint is correlated not with body weight but with height. Because the shape of the skull of Asians is evidently different from that of Westerners, the morphology of the bones making up the knee joint is also expected to be different for the two populations. Therefore, this chapter describes in detail the characteristics of the normal and osteoarthritic knee in Japanese individuals.

NORMAL KNEE

Miyasaka et al. (1) examined the bone morphology of the knee joint in the Japanese population. Their study included 500 knee joints that demonstrated no osteoarthritic changes on radiographic images and were considered normal clinically in individuals without any complaints related to knee joints; subjects were selected from among people who visited Keio University in Tokyo for other purposes.

The width of the femur at the articular level and the width of the tibia at the articular level were measured and digitized from the frontal radiographic image; the length of medial femoral condyle in anteroposterior view, the depth of the medial femoral condyle in the proximal-distal direction, and the length of the medial tibial condyle in the anteroposterior direction were measured and digitized from the lateral radiographic image (Fig. 1). The values were corrected for the radiographic magnification, which was set at 10%.

Values Measured for Various Regions

Results of measurement in 500 cases (500 joints) were as follows: maximum of 80.5 mm and minimum of 53.4 mm (mean, 68.4 mm) for the width of the femur at the articular level; 83.4 mm ~ 55.4 mm (mean, 71.6 mm) for the width of the tibia at the articular level; 69.2 mm ~ 44.1 mm (mean, 57.3 mm) for the length of the medial femoral condyle in the anteroposterior direction; 44.5 mm ~ 29.3 mm (mean, 36.7 mm) for the depth of the medial femoral condyle in the proximal-distal direction; and 54.6 mm ~ 33.4 mm (mean, 43.5 mm) for the length of the medial tibial condyle in the anteroposterior direction. When the correlation of values measured for various dimensions was examined, the coefficient of correlation with the width of the femur at the articular level was 0.99 for the width of the tibia at the articular level (Fig. 2), 0.70 for the length of the medial femoral condyle in the anteroposterior direction (Fig. 3), 0.77 for the depth of the medial femoral condyle in the proximal-distal direction (Fig. 4), and 0.92 for the length of the medial tibial condyle in the anteroposterior direction (Fig. 5).

Seedhom et al. (2) and Mensch et al. (3) have taken measurements on the knees of European and American subjects, using cadaveric knees and scout radiographic films.

According to these reports (2–4), a high positive correlation is found between the measured values for the width of the femur at the articular level and the values for the other dimensions, which is consistent with the results of Miyasaka et al. (1). However, the measured values for various dimensions of the knee joint are significantly greater for Western individuals than for Japanese individuals (Table 1). This is considered to be due to differences in the heights of the subjects. To compare the two groups in more detail, the width of the tibia at the articular level, the length of the medial femoral condyle in the

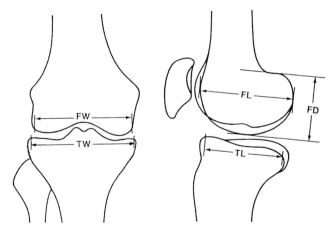

FIG. 1. Measured dimensions in the normal knee. FD, depth of the medial femoral condyle in the proximal-distal direction; FL, length of the medial femoral condyle in the anteroposterior direction; FW, width of the femur at the articular level; TL, length of the medial tibial condyle in the anteroposterior direction; TW, width of the tibia at the articular level.

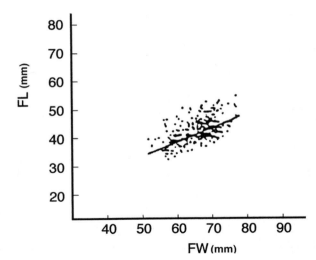

FIG. 3. Correlation between the width of the femur (FW) and the anteroposterior length of the femoral condyle (FL) in normal knees.

anteroposterior direction, and the length of the medial tibial condyle in the anteroposterior direction—dimensions for which the values were almost the same in the reports of Mensch et al. (3) and Miyasaka et al. (1)—were extracted and the ratios were calculated. The values obtained by dividing the length of the medial femoral condyle in the anteroposterior direction by the width of the tibia at the articular level (d) and the length of the medial tibial condyle in the anteroposterior direction by the width of the tibia (e) were $d = 0.86$ and $e = 0.65$ in the Western subjects versus $d = 0.80$ and $e = 0.61$ in the Japanese subjects. In other words, the knees of Japanese subjects are not only smaller than those of Western subjects but their length is relatively shorter than their width. This may suggest that the width of the knees of Japanese individuals tends to be relatively larger.

Correlation with Height and Body Weight

When the coefficient of correlation between height and the measured values for various dimensions was examined (1), the coefficient of correlation was found to be 0.67 for the width of the femur at the articular level, 0.67 for the width of the tibia at the articular level, 0.66 for the length of the medial femoral condyle in the anteroposterior direction, 0.27 for the depth of the medial femoral condyle in the proximal-distal direction, and 0.24 for the length of the medial tibial condyle in the anteroposterior direction. When the coefficient of correlation between body weight and values for various dimensions was examined (1), the coefficient of correlation was found to be 0.08 for the width of the femur at the articular level, 0.07 for the width of the

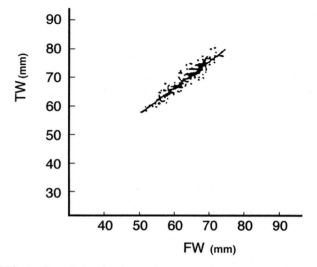

FIG. 2. Correlation between the width of the femur (FW) and the width of the tibia (TW) in normal knees.

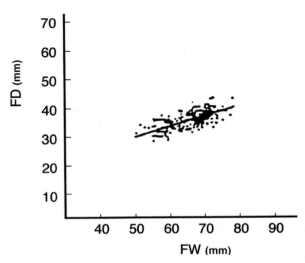

FIG. 4. Correlation between the width of the femur (FW) and the depth of the medial femoral condyle in the proximal-distal direction (FD) in normal knees.

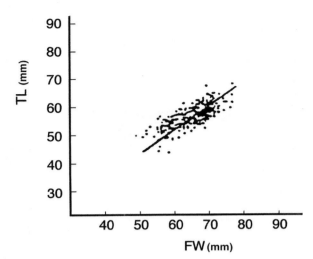

FIG. 5. Correlation between the width of the femur (FW) and the length of the medial tibial condyle in the anteroposterior direction (TL) in normal knees.

tibia at the articular level, 0.01 for the length of the medial femoral condyle in the anteroposterior direction, 0.003 for the depth of the medial femoral condyle in the proximal-distal direction, and 0.001 for the length of the medial tibial condyle in the anteroposterior direction.

With regard to the relation between height and body weight on the one hand and measured values for various dimensions on the other, measurements for the femur and tibia, which constitute the knee joint, showed a relatively high correlation with height but a very low correlation with body weight of less than 0.1. In estimating the size of the knee joint, therefore, the height rather than the body weight may serve as a better indicator.

Differences between the Sexes

The anthropometric values for the knee joint were measured for various dimensions, and values for males and females were compared by Miyasaka et al. (1). To evaluate potential differences between males and females in the same height group, 80 cases in which the height was between 155 cm and 160 cm (for which a large number of cases were available, including 34 males and 46 females) were extracted for analysis. The values measured were significantly larger in males than in females for

TABLE 1. *Differences in knee dimensions between Japanese and Western subjects*

	Western (mm)	Japanese (mm)
FL	65.2	57.3
FW	75.1	68.4
TL	49.8	43.5
TW	76.1	71.6

FL, length of medial femoral condyle in anteroposterior direction; FW, width of femur at articular level; TL, length of medial tibial condyle in anteroposterior direction; TW, width of tibia at articular level.

all dimensions. To clarify differences in morphology between the sexes, the ratios between the values for various dimensions were computed. The values obtained by dividing the length of the medial femoral condyle in the anteroposterior direction by the width of the femur at the articular level (*a*) and the depth of the medial femoral condyle in the proximal-distal direction by the width of the femur (*b*) were $a = 0.87 \pm 0.03$ and $b = 0.56 \pm 0.03$ for females versus $a = 0.81 \pm 0.04$ and $b = 0.52 \pm 0.03$ in males. The values obtained by dividing the length of medial tibial condyle in the anteroposterior direction by the width of the tibia at the articular level (*c*) were $c = 0.61 \pm 0.05$ in females versus $c = 0.59 \pm 0.04$ in males.

When the differences between the sexes were evaluated, the measured values for various dimensions were significantly larger in males than in females, even in individuals of the same height. Morphologically, the knees of males tended to be wider than those of females.

OSTEOARTHRITIC KNEE

In Japan, the population of people older than 65 years was 7,390,000 in 1970 and accounted for 7.1% of the total population. In 2000, the population older than 65 years was 21,870,000 and accounted for 17.2% of the total population. Thus, the percentage of elderly in the population has risen rapidly in the past 30 years. On the other hand, a tendency now exists for families to have fewer children, and the population older than 65 years exceeds the population aged 0 to 14 years. Therefore, the number of elderly as well as the proportion of the aged are expected to increase further. The population older than 65 years will reach 33,340,000 or 26.9% in 2020. The increase in the number of the elderly 20 years from now is equivalent to the present population of Tokyo.

In Japan, too, osteoarthritis of the knee joint develops preferentially in the elderly. The number of patients with osteoarthritic knees will increase dramatically. Total knee replacement is also expected to be indicated more frequently. We have reported that there is a difference in the shape of the knee between Japanese and Westerners with normal knees. However, no comparison has been made between these two populations with regard to the osteoarthritic knee. Many of the total knee prostheses are designed in the United States or Europe. We find during surgery that the total knee prosthesis does not always fit the shape of the osteoarthritic knee in Japanese patients.

At our hospital, 562 osteoarthritic knees rated as stage 1 or higher according to the osteoarthritic knee classification of Kellgren et al. (5) were selected randomly and analyzed radiologically. Quantifying the shape of bones that constitute the osteoarthritic knee is difficult because the knee is deformed. Thus a standard line as illustrated in Fig. 6 was drawn. The femoral lateral axis is a line connecting the midpoint of the distal femoral shaft with the center of the knee on the lateral radiographic image of the femur. Because the patellofemoral joint can be severely deformed in the osteoarthritic knee, the distance from the femoral axis to the anterior surface of the femur was measured. The distance from the femoral axis to the point farthest backward on the femoral condyle was also measured. The femoral frontal axis is a line connecting the midpoint of the distal femoral shaft with the center of the knee. The mediolateral width of the femoral condyle was measured 8 mm from the

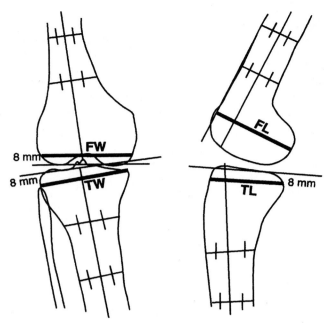

FIG. 6. Measured dimensions in osteoarthritic knees. FL, distance from the anterior surface of the femur to the point farthest backward on the femoral condyle; FW, width of the femur measured 8 mm from the articular surface; TL, anteroposterior length of the tibia measured at a posterior slope of 7 degrees to the tibial lateral axis; TW, width of the tibia measured 8 mm from the articular surface.

articular surface at an angle of 7 degrees from the femoral frontal axis. The mediolateral width of the tibia was measured 8 mm from the articular surface at an angle of 90 degrees to the tibial frontal axis. The anteroposterior length of the tibia was measured along a 7-degree posterior slope to the tibial lateral axis. The femoral frontal width was 68.1 ± 6.1 mm, whereas the tibial

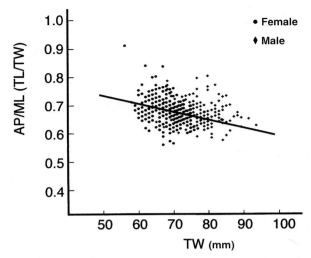

FIG. 8. Correlation between the tibial condyle width (TW) and the ratio of the anteroposterior length to the mediolateral width of the tibia (TL/TW or AP/ML) in osteoarthritic knees.

frontal width was 71.4 ± 6.6 mm. The femoral frontal width was statistically correlated with the tibial frontal width.

The distance from the femoral axis to the anterior flange of the femoral component ranged from 10.5 mm ~ 14.5 mm and averaged 12.9 ± 2.0 mm. The femoral component with a stem is often used for revision of total knee replacement. At present in Japan, however, many of the products used for revision of total knee arthroplasty are those imported from Europe or the United States. The distance from the central axis of the stem to the anterior surface of the femur is 15 mm at a minimum. When the anterior flange of the femoral component is to be placed along the anterior surface, the stem comes in contact with the posterior cortex, which precludes placement of the femoral component. When the stem is placed in line with the femoral axis, the anterior flange of the femoral component does not contact the anterior surface of the femoral condyle, and bone on the anterior surface of the femoral condyle is lost because of the large diameter of the stem. In designing a femoral component with a stem for revision, therefore, the diameter of the stem should be smaller and the stem should be positioned approximately 2 mm forward compared with the stems now commercially available in Japan. The supracondylar nail is very useful in the treatment of fracture of the femur after total knee arthroplasty. A wide opening of the intercondylar notch of the femoral component in the anterior and posterior directions is needed for the supracondylar nail in Japan.

The anteroposterior/mediolateral (AP/ML) ratio of the femur was obtained by dividing the anteroposterior length of the femoral condyle by the mediolateral width of the femoral condyle. The mean value of the AP/ML ratio was 0.74 ± 0.07. A statistically significant high negative correlation was found between femoral condyle width and AP/ML ratio (Fig. 7). As shown by the inclination of the regression line in Fig. 7, the larger the mediolateral width of the femur, the smaller the AP/ML ratio.

The AP/ML ratio of the tibia was obtained by dividing the anteroposterior length of the tibia by the mediolateral width of the tibia. The mean value of the AP/ML ratio was 0.68 ± 0.04. A sta-

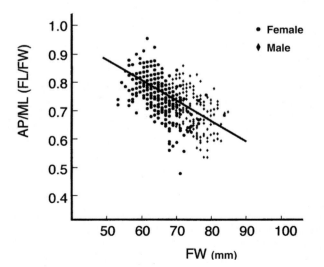

FIG. 7. Correlation between the femoral condyle width (FW) and the ratio of the anteroposterior length to the mediolateral width of the femur (FL/FW or AP/ML) in osteoarthritic knees.

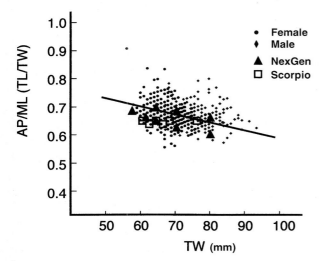

FIG. 9. Size variations in the tibial components of different sizes of two total knee prostheses and correlation between the tibial condyle width (TW) and the ratio of the anteroposterior length to the mediolateral width of the tibia (TL/TW or AP/ML) in osteoarthritic knees.

tistically significant high negative correlation was found between tibial width and AP/ML ratio (Fig. 8). As shown by the inclination of the regression line in Fig. 8, the larger the mediolateral width of the tibia, the smaller the AP/ML ratio. Generally, males are taller and have a larger mediolateral tibial width than females. Therefore, it may be concluded that the AP/ML ratio of the tibia is relatively smaller in males than in females.

The size variation of some tibial components used in Japan was examined (Fig. 9). The AP/ML ratio in these components was within the range of 0.6 ~ 0.7. It was found that the relation between the mediolateral width of the tibial component and the AP/ML ratio in the NexGen prosthesis was very close to that of the Japanese population in terms of the inclination of the regression line. Generally, the anteroposterior length of the lateral tibial condyle is smaller than that of the medial tibial condyle. Therefore, the tibial component in the NexGen prosthesis is symmetric, so the lateral portion of the tibial component may overhang and impinge on the popliteus tendon in some cases. In the case of the Scorpio prosthesis, small components have good bone coverage, but large ones do not necessarily fit Japanese patients because the anterior and posterior diameters are large. Although the size variation of the total knee prostheses commercially distributed in Japan is partially appropriate, the larger

components do not fit Japanese patients. The reason is that the difference in the AP/ML ratio compared to that in the Japanese population is pronounced in the larger sizes.

Finally, the mode of living in Japan requires deep knee flexion, typically of more than 135 degrees. Many elderly people stress the importance of this deep knee flexion for carrying out traditional activities. As Nakagawa et al. (6) have shown using magnetic resonance imaging, in deep knee flexion the tibia is rotated internally and the lateral femoral condyle is dislocated partially from the lateral tibial condyle. For such motion to occur with the prostheses now available, use of a mobile bearing on the tibial tray should be considered. Additional basic studies are required; however, if the goal of achieving deep knee flexion of more than 135 degrees with total knee arthroplasty is to be reliably attained.

SUMMARY

The geometry of the Asian knee has recently been evaluated because the Asian population undergoing total knee replacement is increasing. Most knee prostheses used in Asian countries are imported from Europe and the United States and do not necessarily fit the Asian population because of differences in the anterior and posterior diameters of the knee. Bone morphology of the knee joint of Japanese individuals was characterized in both normal and osteoarthritic knees. A statistically significant negative correlation was demonstrated between the width of the tibial condyle and the ratio of anteroposterior length to mediolateral width. That is, the Japanese knee is not only smaller than that of Westerners but also the length in the anteroposterior direction is shorter than the width in the mediolateral direction. This suggests that the relative width of the knee of Japanese individuals tends to be larger.

REFERENCES

1. Miyasaka T, Fujikawa K, Takeda T, et al. Measurement of the knee joint of Japanese [in Japanese with English abstract]. *J Tokyo Knee Soc* 1992;11:1–5.
2. Seedhom BB, et al. A technique for the study of geometry and contact in normal and artificial knee joints. *Wear* 1972;20:189–199.
3. Mensch JS, Amstutz HC. Knee morphology as a guide to knee replacement. *Clin Orthop Relat Res* 1975;112:231–241.
4. Seedhom BB, Longton EB, Wright V, et al. Dimensions of the knee. *Ann Rheum Dis* 1972;31:54–58.
5. Kellgren JH, et al. Radiological assessment of osteoarthritis. *Ann Rheum Dis* 1957;16:494–502.
6. Nakagawa S, Kadoya Y, Todo S, et al. Tibiofemoral movement 3: full flexion in the living knee studied by MRI. *J Bone Joint Surg Br* 2000;82:1199–1200.

CHAPTER 89

Total Knee Arthroplasty after Failed High Tibial Osteotomy

Nobuyuki Yoshino and Shinro Takai

ASIAN VERSUS WESTERN APPROACH TO OSTEOARTHRITIS

The Asian lifestyle requires deeper knee flexion than the Western lifestyle, such as in Japanese sitting, praying while sitting, and sitting on the floor with legs crossed. Therefore, many Japanese patients with arthritic knees want to preserve their range of knee motion, and some patients refuse to undergo total knee arthroplasty (TKA) because they will not be able to engage in Japanese-style sitting after TKA, even if TKA provides relief of knee pain. For this reason, high tibial osteotomy (HTO) is likely to be selected for treatment of medial unicompartmental osteoarthritis (OA) and medial and patellofemoral OA of the knee in Japan. To the authors' knowledge, more than 5,000 HTOs are performed in Japan yearly, whereas about 35,000 TKAs are performed. In Canada and the United States, the rates of HTO have decreased dramatically, whereas the rates of TKA have increased steadily (1). The results of HTO tend to deteriorate with time (2–6); therefore, many patients who have a failed HTO subsequently require TKA. The incidence of TKA after HTO will increase among elderly patients as the average life span increases. Thus, the effect of previous HTO on the results of subsequent TKA is of importance. More than 20 studies have been published in English concerning TKA after failed HTO (7–28); however, consensus has not been reached. There is still a great deal of debate as to whether or not TKA after HTO gives results equivalent to those of primary TKA.

SURGICAL OPTIONS FOR MEDIAL UNICOMPARTMENTAL OSTEOARTHRITIS

The management of medial unicompartmental OA of the knee remains a matter of controversy. Surgical options include arthroscopic débridement, arthrodesis, HTO, unicompartmental knee arthroplasty (UKA), and TKA. The patient's age, weight, occupation, activity level, and comorbid conditions are important considerations in the initial choice of treatment. There have been conflicting reports recommending the selection of HTO instead of TKA (28), TKA instead of HTO (27), UKA instead of HTO (29–31), and UKA instead of TKA (32–34).

The current widespread and successful adoption of TKA has simplified the management of most patients with OA. Reports from different institutions have shown stable long-term results for TKA with more than 90% survivorship at 10 years or longer in elderly patients (35–38). Even in patients 55 years old or younger, some authors have reported good long-term results similar to those in elderly patients (39–41). Concerns about potential problems such as aseptic loosening, however, and the need for multiple revisions have discouraged the widespread use of TKA for younger patients.

For young, active patients with medial unicompartmental OA, HTO may be preferable because this procedure can preserve the patient's own bone stock, maintain proprioception and knee motion, permit a high activity level, and provide sufficient relief of pain so that the need for TKA is at least delayed, if not precluded.

For elderly, less active patients, UKA is an attractive procedure with advantages over TKA, such as preservation of proprioception, bone stock, anterior and posterior cruciate ligaments, and the patellofemoral joint and opposite compartment to maintain normal knee kinematics with a functional range of motion. UKA with a modern condylar prosthesis design provides favorable long-term results for elderly patients (42–44). However, there is an increased risk of requiring conversion to TKA after 10 years for patients under the age of 65 (45). Furthermore, the results of revision TKA after failed UKA are controversial (46,47). Therefore, UKA is regarded as a viable option in the treatment of unicompartmental OA if proper patient selection and precise placement are assured.

The potential problems after primary TKA or UKA for young, active patients suggest that HTO should be the first choice for young patients from the perspective of long-term management.

RESULTS OF HIGH TIBIAL OSTEOTOMY

HTO was first introduced by Jackson (48) and popularized by Coventry (49). This procedure has been reported, in general, to have a satisfactory short-term result in 80% to 90% of patients. The results tend to deteriorate with time, however, and only approximately 60% maintain the earlier satisfactory results with longer follow-up (3,4,6). Several studies have identified risk factors associated with poor long-term results of HTO. Age, degree of medial compartment OA, preoperative alignment, correction and maintenance of alignment, ligamentous instability, lateral thrust, body weight, and preoperative arc of knee motion have been shown to influence HTO survival (2,3).

Several options exist to revise a failed HTO. If arthritic change is still limited to the medial unicompartment, re-osteotomy, UKA, or TKA may be selected. If arthritic changes have progressed to bi- or tricompartmental disease, TKA is the only choice. Therefore, many patients who have had a failed HTO subsequently require TKA.

The reasons for revision TKA include progression of OA to panarthritis, recurrence of varus deformity, and delayed union. In a study by the authors (14), the main reason for revision arthroplasty in patients who needed TKA within 3 years of the original surgery was pain due to the recurrence of varus deformity. The main reason for revision arthroplasty in patients who needed TKA more than 3 years after the original procedure was pain or hydrarthrosis due to the progression of OA to bicompartmental or tricompartmental changes. Therefore, revision TKA within 3 years might be precluded or delayed if proper alignment is obtained after HTO. Odenbring et al. reported that the revision rate was 54 in 170 in undercorrected knees and 8 in 144 in normalized or overcorrected knees, and estimated that, given 10 years, their osteotomy would have outlived contemporary arthroplasties (23). With refinement of the technique of HTO (50), early-revision TKA in undercorrected knees or cases of nonunion would be avoidable; however, revision TKA in well-aligned knees due to the deterioration of OA with time would be inevitable.

RESULTS OF REVISION TOTAL KNEE ARTHROPLASTY AFTER FAILED HIGH TIBIAL OSTEOTOMY

The results of TKA after HTO compared to the results of TKA in other circumstances is under debate. Several authors (7,9,11,13,14,16,24,28) reported results comparable to those for primary TKA. In contrast, several other studies (10,12,15, 20,25,27) found results inferior to those for primary TKA. Winsor et al. (25) reported results inferior to those for primary TKA and similar to those for revision TKA. Jackson et al. (19), Cameron and Park (15), and Gill et al. (17) compared the results of TKA after HTO with those of TKA after UKA. Jackson et al. (19) showed that TKA after HTO is associated with more complications than TKA after UKA, although Gill et al. (17) and Cameron et al. (15) reported superior results for TKA after HTO compared to TKA after UKA.

The reasons for these conflicting results are thought to involve many factors, such as selection of the control group, indication for HTO, age at surgery, degree of correction, type of prosthesis used, and scoring system employed. In previously reported studies, factors found to have potentially adverse effects on TKA after HTO include multiple surgical incisions, flexion contracture, peroneal nerve palsy after HTO, reflex sympathetic dystrophy after HTO, collateral ligament laxity, multiple previous surgeries, patella infera, soft tissue scarring, nonunion, retained hardware from HTO, truncated lateral tibial metaphysis, and overcorrected valgus deformity. The trend for more recent articles to show outcomes comparable to those of primary TKA may indicate a clearer understanding of such revision surgery and the lowering of complications in sophisticated HTO procedures (7,9,11,13, 14,16). The success of TKA after HTO depends on controlled bone resection, sometimes with bone grafting or metal augmentation; correct component alignment; proper soft tissue balancing, sometimes with reconstruction; restoration of a normal joint line; and accurate rotational alignment.

TECHNICAL FACTORS DURING REVISION TOTAL KNEE ARTHROPLASTY AFTER FAILED HIGH TIBIAL OSTEOTOMY

Conversion of the failed HTO to TKA presents technical challenges that are not generally encountered in primary TKA.

Skin Incision and Approach

The first technical difficulty in revision TKA after failed HTO is the decision regarding placement of the skin incision when a previous skin incision other than a median incision is encountered. The skin incision should optimally be median longitudinal regardless of the previous HTO incision.

The second technical difficulty is the eversion of the patella, and this difficulty is described in all the literature dealing with revision TKA after failed HTO. Crossing wedge osteotomies done proximal to the tibial tubercle lower the joint line and increase scarring in and around the patellar tendon (6,25,27). In one study (14), a tendency was seen for the patellar tendon to become shorter, the shorter the interval between HTO and TKA. The reason for this tendency was

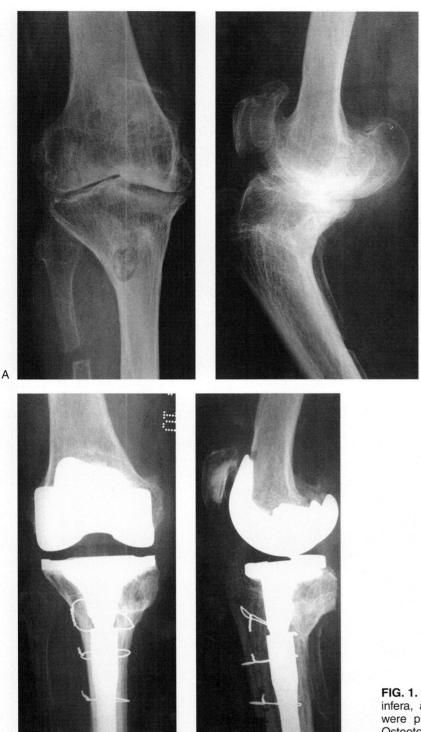

FIG. 1. A, B: Shift of the tibial shaft axis, patella infera, and posterior inclination of the tibial plateau were present before total knee arthroplasty. **C, D:** Osteotomy and transfer of the tibial tubercle were required for approach. Tibial component was set without re-osteotomy.

assumed to be that two major operations affecting the patellar tendon within a short interval accelerated the scarring. To obtain good exposure, various procedures, such as quadriceps snips, V-Y quadricepsplasty, early lateral retinacular release, femoral peel, tibial tubercle osteotomy, and a lateral approach, may be necessary (Fig. 1).

Loss of Bone Stock

Bony deformities present after HTO may reduce the amount of bone to be resected during TKA. The bone stock of the lateral side decreases in accordance with the amount of bone dissected in HTO to correct the anguler deformity. In overcorrected val-

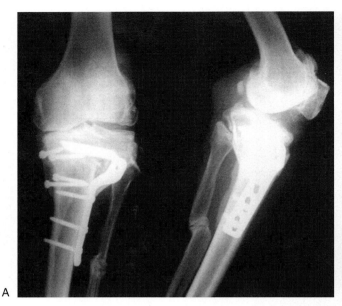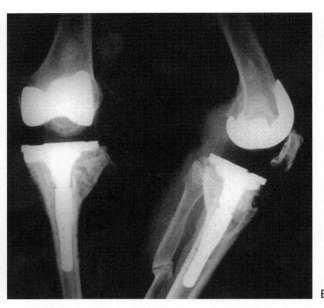

FIG. 2. A: Bone defect of the medial side due to recurrence of varus deformity, blade plate and screws, and anterior inclination of the tibial plateau were present before total knee arthroplasty. **B:** Wedge augmentation was required for bone defect.

gus knees, it is not uncommon to find that only a minimum amount of bone can be resected from the lateral tibial plateau (18,22,25,27). This leads to the elevation of the joint line on the lateral side. In the knee with recurrent varus deformity (Fig. 2), on the other hand, it is also not uncommon to find that a large bone defect must be created at the medial condyle to obtain proper alignment because the height of the lateral tibial plateau was reduced by HTO. This may necessitate the use of a very thick prosthesis to restore the joint line. Resecting enough bone to eliminate a defect would result in significant tibial bone loss

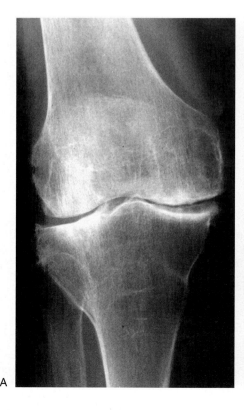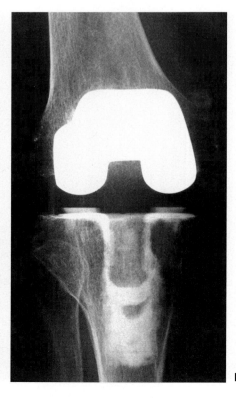

FIG. 3. A: Shift of tibial shaft axis was present before total knee arthroplasty. **B:** The lateral edge of the tibial component did not cover the cortical shell but was on the surface of cancellous bone.

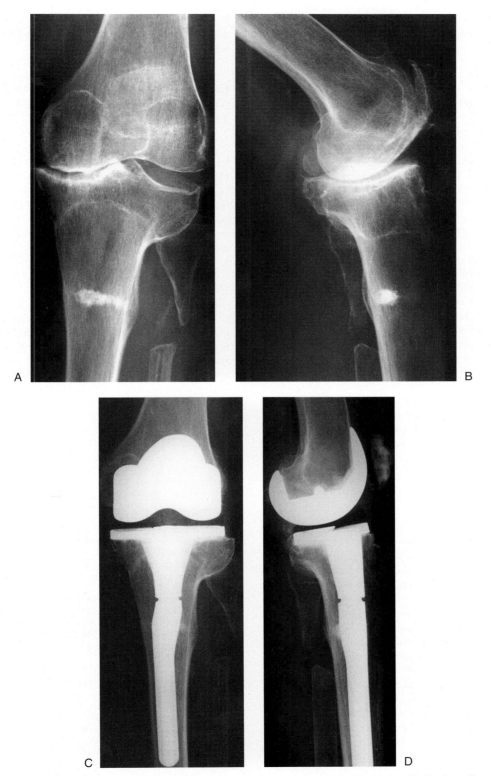

FIG. 4. A, B: Shift of tibial shaft axis was present before total knee arthroplasty. **C, D:** An offset long-stemmed component was used successfully.

and should be avoided. As these patients are relatively young, any maneuvers to conserve bone stock are critical. New techniques of HTO such as hemicallotasis may alleviate this problem (51).

Rotation and Inclination of the Tibial Plateau

Rotational deformity may occur after HTO because the bone can slip easily into internal or external rotation when the wedge osteotomy site is closed (18,21,25,27). In dome osteotomy, this deformity occurs less frequently. External rotation of the distal fragment increases the Q angle and sometimes requires compensation by medialization of the tibial tubercle during TKA to prevent patellofemoral instability. This deformity is difficult to evaluate intraoperatively; therefore, precise preoperative evaluation using computed tomography of the lower leg should be performed.

Change in the posterior inclination of tibial plateau (10,14,24) may also require careful preoperative planning to resect the tibial plateau (Figs. 1 and 2). Overlooking this deformity may result in overresection of the proximal tibia. In severe cases, re-osteotomy to reverse the overcorrected extraarticular deformity might be required before performing TKA (26), as in TKA for malunited extraarticular fracture around the knee (52). With regard to re-osteotomy, Cameron and Welsh (26) made several technical recommendations: The re-osteotomy should be dome type rather than wedge type to avoid further shortening of the leg; a fibular osteotomy should be performed to obtain adequate correction, as lateral scarring will make undercorrection more likely without it; a plate should be used to maintain position; and the tibial component should be equipped with a stem long enough to cross the re-osteotomy site.

Shift of Tibial Shaft Axis

HTO, even if it was performed by closing wedge osteotomy or dome osteotomy, alters the relative position of the tibial plateau in relation to the tibial medullary canal (7,14,16,21, 25,26,27). This shift of the tibial medullary canal is greater in knees undergoing dome osteotomy than in those undergoing closing wedge osteotomy (10). The axis of the tibial medullary canal shifts to the medial or anteromedial side, and a stemmed tibial component may therefore impinge on the lateral cortex even when it is centered on the tibial plateau (Fig. 1). If the center of the tibial component is placed on the tibial shaft axis, the lateral edge of the component will not cover the cortical shell but will be on the surface of cancellous bone (Fig. 3). This medial shifting of the tibial component may produce unbalanced stress to the proximal tibia and may lead to subsidence or loosening of the component. Use of the recently developed offset tibial stem may sometimes resolve this problem (Fig. 4).

Ligament Balancing

Ligamentous imbalance is not uncommon in knees with failed HTO and is especially prevalent in overcorrected valgus knees. Krackow and Holtgrewe (22) described a complex reconstruction that includes the reconstruction of the posterior cruciate ligament and advancement of the medial collateral ligament.

Hofmann and Kane recommended the resection of the posterior cruciate ligament and use of a more congruent insert on the tibial side (18).

COMPLICATIONS OF TOTAL KNEE ARTHROPLASTY AFTER FAILED HIGH TIBIAL OSTEOTOMY

Many patellofemoral complications of TKA after failed HTO have been reported in the literature, including skin necrosis (15,19), patellar subluxation (7,15), patellar avascular necrosis (15), and rupture of the patellar tendon (15). The rate of infection has been found by some authors (19,25) to be higher in patients undergoing TKA after HTO than in patients undergoing primary TKA. However, many other studies focusing on TKA after HTO report no difference.

CONCLUSION

TKA after failed HTO is technically demanding. The success of TKA after HTO depends on precise preoperative planning to identify preoperative deformities; controlled bone resection, sometimes with bone grafting or metal augmentation; correct component alignment; proper soft tissue balancing, sometimes with reconstruction; restoration of the normal joint line; and accurate rotational alignment.

REFERENCES

1. Wright J, Heck D, Hawker G, et al. Rates of tibial osteotomy in Canada and the United States. *Clin Orthop* 1995;319:266–275.
2. Majima T, Yasuda K, Katsuragi R, et al. Progression of joint arthrosis 10 to 15 years after high tibial osteotomy. *Clin Orthop* 2000;381:177–184.
3. Naudie DN, Bourne RB, Rorabeck CH, et al. Survivorship of the high tibial valgus osteotomy. A 10- to 15-year followup study. *Clin Orthop* 1999;367:18–27.
4. Rinonapoli E, Mancini GB, Corvalia A, et al. Tibial osteotomy for varus gonarthrosis. A 10- to 21-year followup study. *Clin Orthop* 1998;353:185–193.
5. Hernigou P, Medevielle D, Debeyre J, et al. Proximal tibial osteotomy for osteoarthritis with varus deformity. A ten to thirteen year follow up study. *J Bone Joint Surg Am* 1987;69:332–354.
6. Insall JN, Joseph DM, Muska C. High tibial osteotomy for varus gonarthrosis. A long term follow-up study. *J Bone Joint Surg Am* 1984;66:1040–1048.
7. Haddad FS, Bentley G. Total knee arthroplasty after high tibial osteotomy. A medium-term review. *J Arthroplasty* 2000;15:597–603.
8. Walther M, Konig A, Kirschner S, et al. Results of posterior cruciate-retaining unconstrained total knee arthroplasty after proximal tibial osteotomy for osteoarthritis. A prospective cohort study. *Arch Orthop Trauma Surg* 2000;120:166–170.
9. Meding JB, Keating EM, Ritter MA, et al. Total knee arthroplasty after high tibial osteotomy. *Clin Orthop* 2000;375:175–184.
10. Noda T, Yasuda S, Nagano K, et al. Clinico-radiological study of total knee arthroplasty after high tibial osteotomy. *J Orthop Sci* 2000;5:25–36.
11. Toksvig-Larsen S, Magyar G, Önsen I, et al. Fixation of the tibial component of total knee arthroplasty after high tibial osteotomy. *J Bone Joint Surg Br* 1998;80:295–297.
12. Nizard RS, Gardinne L, Witvoet J. Total knee replacement after failed tibial osteotomy. *J Arthroplasty* 1998;13:847–853.
13. Bergenudd H, Sahlström A, Sanzèn L. Total knee arthroplasty after

failed proximal tibial valgus osteotomy. *J Arthroplasty* 1997;12:635–638.

14. Takai S, Yoshino N, Hirasawa Y. Revision total knee arthroplasty after failed high tibial osteotomy. *Bull Hosp Joint Dis* 1997;56:245–250.

15. Cameron HU, Park YS. Total knee replacement following high tibial osteotomy and unicompartmental knee. *Orthopedics* 1996;19:807–808.

16. Marcacci M, Iacono F, Zaffagnini S, et al. Total knee arthroplasty after proximal tibial osteotomy. *Chir Organi Mov* 1995;80:353–359.

17. Gill T, Schemitsch EM, Brick GW, et al. Revision total knee arthroplasty after failed unicompartmental knee arthroplasty or high tibial osteotomy. *Clin Orthop* 1995;321:10–18.

18. Hofmann AA, Kane KR. Total knee arthroplasty after high tibial osteotomy. *Orthopedics* 1994;17:887–890.

19. Jackson M, Sarabgi PP, Newman JH. Revision total knee arthroplasty. Comparison of outcome following primary proximal tibial osteotomy or unicompartmental arthroplasty. *J Arthroplasty* 1994;9:539–542.

20. Mont MA, Antonaides S, Krackow KA, et al. Total knee arthroplasty after failed high tibial osteotomy. A comparison with a matched group. *Clin Orthop* 1994;299:125–130.

21. Mont MA, Alexander N, Krackow KA, et al. Total knee arthroplasty after failed high tibial osteotomy. *Orthop Clin North Am* 1994;25:515–525.

22. Krackow KA, Holtgrewe JL. Experience with a new technique for managing severely overcorrected valgus high tibial osteotomy at total knee arthroplasty. *Clin Orthop* 1990;258:213–224.

23. Odenbring S, Egund N, Lindstrend A, et al. Revision after osteotomy for gonarthrosis. A 10-19-year follow-up of 314 cases. *Acta Orthop Scand* 1990;61:128–130.

24. Amendola A, Roraback CH, Bourne RB, et al. Total knee arthroplasty following high tibial osteotomy for osteoarthritis. *J Arthroplasty* 1989;4:S11–S17.

25. Winsor RE, Insall JN, Vince KG. Technical consideration of total knee arthroplasty after failed proximal tibial osteotomy. *J Bone Joint Surg Am* 1988;70:547–555.

26. Cameron HU, Welsh RP. Potential complication of total knee replacement following tibial osteotomy. *Orthop Rev* 1988;17:39–43.

27. Katz MM, Hungerford DS, Krackow KA, et al. Results of total knee arthroplasty after failed proximal tibial osteotomy for osteoarthritis. *J Bone Joint Surg Am* 1987;69:225–233.

28. Staeheli JW, Cass JR, Morrey BF. Condylar knee arthroplasty after failed proximal tibial osteotomy. *J Bone Joint Surg Am* 1987;69:28–31.

29. Weale AE, Newman JH. Unicompartmental arthroplasty and high tibial osteotomy for osteoarthritis of the knee. *Clin Orthop* 1994;302:134–137.

30. Broughton WP, Newman JH, Baily RAJ. Unicompartmental replacement and high tibial osteotomy for osteoarthritis of the knee—a comparative study after 5-10 years follow-up. *J Bone Joint Surg Br* 1986;68:447–452.

31. Karpman RR, Volz RG. Osteotomy versus unicompartmental prosthetic replacement in the treatment of unicompartmental arthritis of the knee. *Orthopedics* 1982;5:989–991.

32. Laurencin CT, Zelicof SB, Scott RD, et al. Unicompartmental versus total knee arthroplasty in the same patient. *Clin Orthop* 1991;273:151–156.

33. Cobb AG, Kozinn SC, Scott RD. Unicondylar or total knee replacement: patient preference. *J Bone Joint Surg Br* 1990;72:166–170.

34. Cameron HU, Jung YB. A comparison of unicompartmental versus total knee replacement with total knee replacement. *Orthop Rev* 1988;17:983–988.

35. van Loon CJM, Wisse MA, de Waal Malefijit MC, et al. The kinematic total knee arthroplasty. A 10- to 15-year follow-up and survival analysis. *Arch Orthop Trauma Surg* 2000;120:48–52.

36. Font-Rodriguez DE, Scuderi GR, Insall JN. Survivorship of cemented total knee arthroplasty. *Clin Orthop* 1997;345:79–86.

37. Schai PA, Thornhill TS, Scott RD. Total knee arthroplasty with the PFC system. Results at a minimum ten years and survival analysis. *J Bone Joint Surg Am* 1997;79:575–582.

38. Malkani AL, Rand JA, Bryan RS, et al. Total knee arthroplasty with the kinematic condylar prosthesis. A ten-year follow-up study. *J Bone Joint Surg Am* 1995;77:423–431.

39. Duffy GP, Trousdale RT, Stuart MJ. Total knee arthroplasty in patients 55 years old or younger. *Clin Orthop* 1998;356:22–27.

40. Diduch DR, Insall JN, Scott WN, et al. Total knee replacement in young, active patients. *J Bone Joint Surg Br* 1998;80:850–858.

41. Gill GS, Chan KC, Mills DM. 5- to 18-years follow-up study of cemented total knee arthroplasty for patients 55 years old or younger. *J Arthroplasty* 1997;12:49–54.

42. Squire MW, Callaghan JJ, Goetz DD, et al. Unicompartmental knee replacement. A minimum 15 year follow up study. *Clin Orthop* 1999;367:61–72.

43. Berger RA, Nedeff DD, Barden RM, et al. Unicompartmental knee arthroplasty. Clinical experience at 6- to 10 year followup. *Clin Orthop* 1999;367:50–60.

44. Bert JM. 10-year survivorship of metal-backed, unicompartmental arthroplasty. *J Arthroplasty* 1998;13:901–905.

45. Knutson K, Lewold S, Robertson O, et al. The Swedish knee arthroplasty register: a nation-wide study of 30,003 knees 1976–1992. *Acta Orthop Scand* 1994;65:375–386.

46. Lewold S, Robertsson O, Knutson K, et al. Revision of unicompartmental knee arthroplasty. Outcome in 1135 cases from the Swedish knee arthroplasty study. *Acta Orthop Scand* 1998;69:469–474.

47. Levine WN, Ozuna RM, Scott RD, et al. Conversion of failed modern unicompartmental arthroplasty to total knee arthroplasty. *J Arthroplasty* 1996;11:797–801.

48. Jackson JP. Osteotomy for osteoarthritis of the knee. Proceedings of the British Orthopaedic Association. *J Bone Joint Surg Br* 1958;40:826.

49. Coventry MB. Osteotomy about the knee for degenerative and rheumatoid arthritis: indications, operative technique, and results. *J Bone Joint Surg Am* 1973;55:23–48.

50. Billings A, Scott DF, Camargo MP, et al. High tibial osteotomy with a calibrated osteotomy guide, rigid internal fixation, and early motion. *J Bone Joint Surg Am* 2000;82:70–79.

51. Magyar G, Tosvig-Larsen S, Lindstrand A. Open wedge tibial osteotomy by callus distraction in gonarthrosis. Operative technique and early results in 36 patients. *Acta Orthop Scand* 1998;69:147–151.

52. Wolff AM, Hungerford DS, Pepe CL. The effect of extraarticular varus and valgus deformity on the total knee arthroplasty. *Clin Orthop* 1991;271:35–51.

CHAPTER 90

Total Knee Replacement in Special Situations

Bennett S. Burns and Paul F. Lachiewicz

Although the majority of total knee arthroplasties are performed for primary osteoarthritis, there are rheumatologic, hematologic, metabolic, endocrine, and neurologic disorders that cause sufficient knee joint involvement to require surgical intervention. Although total knee arthroplasty has proven to be an effective treatment for most conditions that result in the loss of knee joint cartilage, the surgeon treating these patients with unusual conditions must be cognizant of specific features that may affect clinical decision making and treatment. These may involve the patients' ability to tolerate the surgery, may alter technical aspects of the procedure itself, or may affect the longevity of the prosthesis. This chapter reviews several of the most common conditions with which the knee surgeon must be familiar.

PAGET DISEASE

Paget disease of the bone is characterized by an increased rate of bone turnover. The incidence is from 2% to 4% of the population over the age of 40 (1–3). Symptomatic Paget disease is less common, however, affecting 10% or fewer of patients with the disorder. Back pain is the most common presenting symptom, followed by pain in the hip or knee. Although involvement of the hip joint is much more common than that of the knee, 10% to 12% of patients with knee disease develop symptomatic arthritis of the knee. Radiographs initially show diffuse osteopenia due to increased resorption, which later progresses to a mixed or sclerotic picture. Varus and anterior bowing of an enlarged distal femur is often seen (Fig. 1). Serum alkaline phosphatase levels are elevated in active disease due to the increased turnover of bone and serve as a marker of disease activity (4). Treatment with diphosphonates often relieves the

bone pain associated with the disease and should be used to assist in differentiating pain from arthritic joint involvement and pain from the underlying bone disorder. The presence of night pain and rest pain should alert the surgeon to the possibility of nonarthritic pain, either from untreated disease or from malignant degeneration (5).

In the rare knee that requires a total knee arthroplasty, several technical considerations should be anticipated. Most patients are in the sclerotic, or "burned out," phase of disease when presenting for arthroplasty, but clinical evaluation to rule out high-output cardiac failure should still be performed, especially in patients with polyostotic disease. The concerns about increased vascularity and increased perioperative bleeding with total knee arthroplasty are less important than when considering operative intervention for pathologic fractures or performing total hip arthroplasty. Gabel et al. reported a series of 16 total knee arthroplasties performed on patients with Paget disease. There was an average blood loss of 481 mL, but there was no significant difference between patients treated preoperatively with diphosphonates, calcitonin, or fluoride and those with no such treatment. Problems encountered during the knee arthroplasty included difficulty achieving satisfactory alignment, often due to increased femoral varus and anteversion (4). The use of intramedullary femoral guides may result in flexed or varus cuts of the distal femur and such guides should probably be used only in conjunction with extramedullary cutting guides. Anterior tibial bowing may also be present. Performance of the standard proximal tibial resection using an extramedullary guide may result in excessive bone removal anteriorly, with possible compromise of the extensor mechanism. Making a 10-degree posterior tilted cut and using a flat tibial component may avoid this. Medial bone loss and cysts may result in a fixed varus

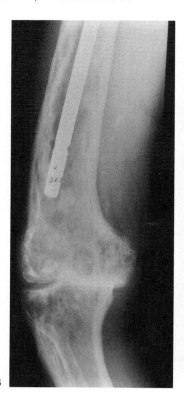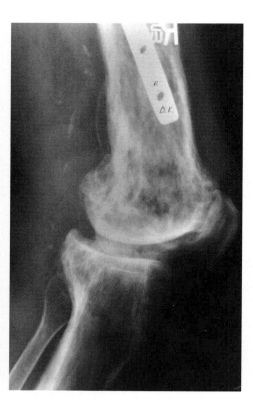

A,B

FIG. 1. A, B: Preoperative radiographs of patient with Paget disease about the knee.

deformity and tight medial structures. In this series, the authors achieved less than 5 degrees of valgus alignment in 10 of 16 knees. This was attributed to the deformities of the tibia and femur that shift the mechanical axis in both the sagittal and coronal planes. Because of this, use of extramedullary align-

ment guides for both the femoral and tibial resections were recommended. Full-length hip-knee-ankle radiographs, in both planes, may assist in preoperative planning. Anterior bowing of the tibia may require hyperextension of the prosthesis to keep the mechanical axis from falling behind the knee. Two patients

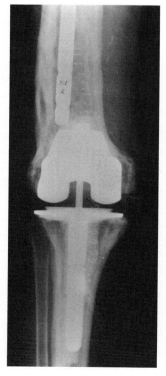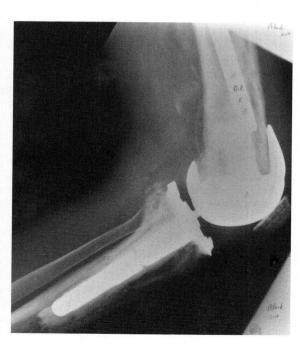

A,B

FIG. 2. A, B: Postoperative radiographs after total knee arthroplasty in patient with Paget disease.

in this series later sustained pathologic fractures through Pagetic bone (4). Because of the poor quality of this bone, cementing of all components and use of longer stems to prevent periprosthetic fracture is recommended. A posterior stabilized or, occasionally, constrained condylar prosthesis usually is required because of the preoperative knee deformity (Fig. 2). In the first report of seven arthroplasties in patients with Paget disease, the clinical results were similar to those obtained in patients with primary osteoarthritis. It was suggested that pagetic involvement of the knee should not preclude total knee arthroplasty (3).

POLIO

Although the incidence of poliomyelitis in the United States has been drastically reduced due to vaccination programs, the knee surgeon may occasionally evaluate a patient who suffers the sequelae of this disease. Due to weakness of the lower extremity, especially the extensor mechanism, the "screw home" or mechanical locking of the knee is often accentuated in these patients. As these patients back-knee to achieve mechanical stability in the stance phase of gait, joint mechanics are altered, which increases the frequency of osteoarthritis and progressive recurvatum. Other deformities of the knee associated with poliomyelitis include external rotation of the tibia and valgus instability. Initially, bracing with a drop-locked, hinged knee-ankle-foot orthosis may provide symptomatic relief and postpone the need for arthroplasty. If total knee arthroplasty is considered, the degree of recurvatum and extensor strength should be carefully assessed, as these will affect intraoperative balancing and overall patient satisfaction with the outcome.

Recurvatum may be corrected by resecting less of the femur or building up the femoral component to reduce the extension gap to take advantage of the cam effect of the collateral ligaments and the geometry of the femoral component. This may generate 5 to 10 degrees of flexion contracture. Patients with extensor weakness should be advised preoperatively that postoperative bracing may be required if the ability to hyperextend is lost. Alternatively, patients with known quadriceps weakness may be intentionally left with 5 to 10 degrees of recurvatum to allow them to continue to back-knee. However, this may increase the risk of component loosening and instability due to progressive recurvatum (6). The use of a long-leg brace with an extension stop has been proposed as a means of preventing loosening, but its efficacy remains unproven. In one small series of total knee arthroplasties in patients with a history of polio, the authors did not report increased loosening in patients who were not braced postoperatively (7).

Cemented posterior stabilized or constrained condylar total knee components, possibly with stem extensions, should be used to provide immediate stability and decrease the risk of early component loosening and instability. In one study, nine knees in nine patients with poliomyelitis and knee arthritis (mean age, 68 years) had cemented total knee arthroplasty. At a mean follow-up of 6.8 years, three of the nine knees required revision, one for late infection and two for recurrent instability (one posterior subluxation and one recurvatum). Three knees developed recurrent recurvatum, and bracing was unsuccessful in all cases (7). Patients should be warned that, even though the arthroplasty may provide stability and pain relief, their function may still continue to decline.

PARKINSONISM

Parkinson's disease is a progressive neurologic condition in which the basal ganglia, and specifically the substantia nigra, undergo progressive degeneration. This is usually an idiopathic disorder but may be secondary to a toxic insult. The latter type has been seen after recreational use of "designer drugs" and tends to be more severe and less responsive to therapy (8). Patients lose motor coordination, have muscle tremors, and may experience varying degrees of mental impairment. The mainstays of medical treatment include dopamine and dopaminergic agonists. Traditional teaching held that Parkinson's disease was a contraindication to total knee arthroplasty. There are scant reported data to support this, however. One study reported failures in three patients due to hamstring rigidity (9). Two studies, however, support the use of total knee arthroplasty in carefully selected patients (10,11). Patients considered for total knee arthroplasty should usually be ambulatory preoperatively and should have the physical and mental capacity to follow postoperative instructions. A more prolonged postoperative rehabilitation should be expected. Unfortunately, a continued decline in ambulation and overall function is associated with Parkinson's disease. One study recommended the use of semiconstrained implants in these patients, due to decreased muscle coordination. This impaired coordination, leading to more frequent falls, also places these patients at higher risk for periprosthetic fractures (12). Significant improvement in function may be achieved, however, and pain relief persists.

NEUROPATHIC ARTHRITIS

Neuropathic arthritis or Charcot arthropathy represents a form of joint destruction usually characterized by an insensate joint or impaired proprioception. It may accompany a number of disorders affecting the peripheral nervous system, including diabetes mellitus, tertiary syphilis (tabes dorsalis), and congenital indifference to pain. It is theorized to occur due to microtrauma to a joint that lacks protective sensation. The affected joint appears swollen and unstable but is usually painless relative to the degree of destruction. Approximately one-half of neuropathic joints, however, may be painful. Often inflammation is present, and the warm fragmented joint may be confused with an infected joint. Radiographs usually show destructive changes on both sides of the joint, and if the patient is left untreated, progressive angular deformity is common (Fig. 3) (13). The time course of the process is variable. Current research is assessing whether medical management, such as use of bisphosphonates, may alter the course of disease (14). Preoperatively, the patient should have a complete medical and neurologic evaluation to search for a treatable cause of the neuropathic joint. Serologic testing for syphilis, glucose tolerance testing, and complete blood count with indices to assess for vitamin B_{12} or thiamine deficiency should be obtained. Despite extensive testing, the cause of many cases remains unknown (15,16).

Traditionally neuropathic arthritis of the knee was considered an absolute contraindication for any surgical intervention, and bracing was recommended to treat the deformity and instability. Knee arthrodesis was initially recommended but generally abandoned due to mixed clinical results (17). As the disease process has become better understood, however, total knee arthro-

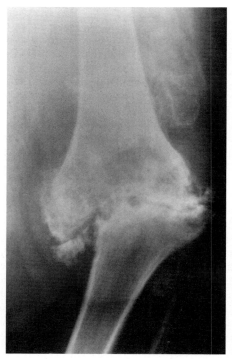

FIG. 3. Preoperative bone deficiency in patient with Charcot arthropathy.

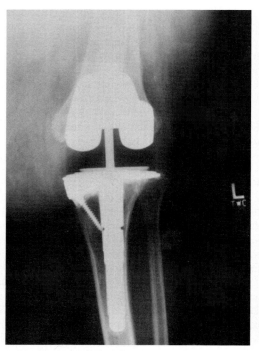

FIG. 4. Postoperative radiograph showing joint alignment restoration with wedges and bone cement in patient with Charcot arthropathy.

plasty has been reconsidered to treat the pain and disability of end-stage neuropathic arthritis. There are distinct stages of neuropathic arthritis. If the process is in the phase of coalescence and reconstruction, surgical reconstruction may be a viable option. Neuropathic arthritis presents a particular challenge to the knee surgeon. Not only is bone stock compromised, but the collateral ligaments are often deficient, which makes ligament balancing and stability difficult to obtain without the use of posterior stabilized or constrained condylar components (15,18). Finally, the bone quality is poor, and there is a higher risk of periprosthetic fracture (12).

There are relatively few reports of the results of total knee arthroplasty for neuropathic arthritis. In one series, nine arthroplasties were performed in seven patients with neuropathic arthritis. At an average of 3 years postoperatively, eight knees were graded as excellent, and one was good. It was concluded that total knee arthroplasty was a reasonable treatment for these patients. There are serious technical intraoperative challenges, however, including bone loss that may require augmented prostheses (wedges, blocks, etc.) or bone grafting, and care must be taken to restore ligament balance (15). Although another center reported a 50% failure rate at 5 years, due to loosening and instability, seven of the eight condylar prostheses had a satisfactory result (19). Another series compared modern prostheses to earlier designs. In 24 total knee arthroplasties in 18 patients with neuropathic arthritis, they reported 58% satisfactory results. When older designs (polycentric, geometric, and single-axis hinge prostheses) were compared to condylar prostheses, all of the former were found to fail, whereas 14 of 17 (82%) knees given condylar prostheses were satisfactory at 4 years' average follow-up (16). In still another series involving only five joints

in three patients with tabes dorsalis, the authors recommended the use of long-stemmed prostheses to redistribute stresses away from involved bone and felt that the presence of ataxia was a "critical" negative factor in outcome (18). Although the numbers were too small to draw a definite conclusion, the recommendations are biomechanically sound, and the use of cemented posterior stabilized or constrained condylar components with stem extensions is recommended (Fig. 4).

HEMOPHILIA

Disorders of hemostasis may arise from deficiencies anywhere in the clotting cascade, from platelet function through clot dissolution and resorption. The vascular phase of hemostasis involves local vessel constriction due either to local trauma or to sympathetic release in response to stress or hypovolemia. Exposed tissue factors promote platelet aggregation and activate both the intrinsic and extrinsic pathways. The most common pathologies resulting in musculoskeletal complications are defects in the intrinsic pathway, namely defects in factor VII (classic hemophilia or hemophilia A) and factor IX (Christmas disease or hemophilia B).

Hemophilia most often involves the joints as a result of recurrent bleeds into the joints. The knee is the most common site of both hemarthrosis and arthropathy, which occur as many as four times more frequently here than in the hip. The synovium initially becomes inflamed and subsequently contracts. Aggressive prophylactic treatment of hemarthrosis is recommended to decrease the risk of arthropathy (Fig. 5) (20). If the patient develops an inhibitor, however, this can become difficult. Synovectomy, either

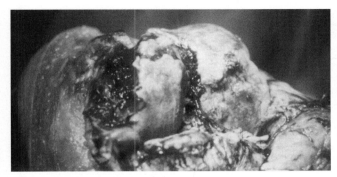

FIG. 5. Distal femur in patient with hemophilic synovitis.

open, arthroscopic or with radioactive isotopes, may slow the progression of synovitis to joint destruction (21). Radiographs typically reveal squaring of the patella (Jordan sign), enlargement of the intercondylar notch, and enlarged femoral condyles, which result in femoral-tibial mismatch (22).

The incidence of human immunodeficiency virus 1 (HIV-1) infection ranges from 33% to 92% in patients with hemophilia A, and from 14% to 52% in patients with hemophilia B (23). The patient's immune status and anticipated longevity should be considered preoperatively, although continued advances are being made in the medical treatment and survival of patients with acquired immune deficiency syndrome. Synovectomy and total knee arthroplasty should be performed at centers with experience in managing hemophilia and major surgery. If nonprosthetic management fails, modern techniques with total knee arthroplasty may offer significant relief of pain and improve function. Factor VIII and inhibitor levels should be assessed preoperatively, and factor levels should be 100% of

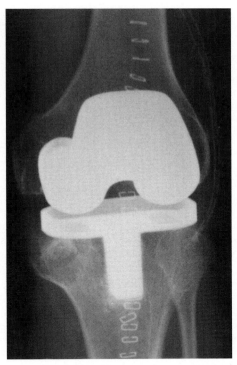

FIG. 7. Postoperative radiograph showing bone graft in cysts in patient with hemophilic arthropathy.

normal before surgery. Factor levels should be maintained at higher than 75% of normal for the first 5 days postoperatively, higher than 50% for days 6 through 10, and higher than 25% for days 11 through 15. Each unit of factor infused per kilogram of body weight should result in a 2% increase in factor levels (24). Patients with inhibitors are resistant to conventional therapy. The severity of an inhibitor is defined in Bethesda units of inhibitor activity per milliliter of plasma. Inhibitor levels higher than 20 Bethesda units were previously considered a contraindication to surgery. However, techniques that overwhelm the inhibitor with high doses of factor may allow surgery to be performed safely. The cost of this treatment is extremely high.

Additional preoperative evaluation includes complete blood count with differential and platelet count, serum albumin level, and, if HIV positive, the CD4 lymphocyte count. Functional assessment preoperatively should include the femoral nerve, as it may occasionally be compromised by an iliacus hematoma (25). Based on one study of elective orthopedic procedures in hemophilia, a CD4 level of less than 200×10^9 per L is generally considered a contraindication to surgery, whereas levels higher than 400×10^9 per L with and albumin level higher than 25 g per L are associated with a minimally increased risk of infection (26).

When total knee arthroplasty is indicated for severe pain and disability, several technical considerations should be addressed. Joint contractures are the rule, and all three planes are involved. Flexion contracture (often severe), valgus, and external rotation are the most common (Fig. 6). Reconstruction of multiple deformities usually requires the use of posterior stabilized components. Cementing of all components is recommended to obtain immediate fixation (Fig. 7) (27,28).

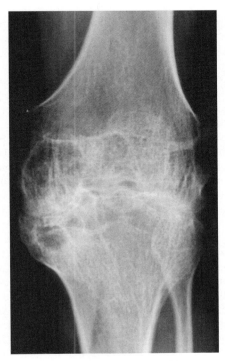

FIG. 6. Hemophilic arthropathy. Note cysts.

TABLE 1. *Results of total knee arthroplasty in patients with hemophilia*

Study	No. knees	No. patients	Follow-up (yr)	Good/excellent results (%)	Increased ROM (degrees)	Infection (%)
Goldberg et al. (29)	13	10	2–6	31	13	8
McCollough et al. (70)	10	8	0.3–4.5	—	0	10
Karthaus et al. (33)	11	8	2–8	82	20	0
Kjaersgaard-Andersen et al. (28)	13	9	1–6	100	13	0
Lachiewicz et al. (27)	24	14	2–9	88	23	8
Unger et al. (32)	26	15	1–9	50	28	0

ROM, range of motion.

Most of the long-term complications of total knee arthroplasty in hemophilia are deep infections, often secondary to HIV infection. In one study of 24 total knee arthroplasties, 21 knees (81%) had an excellent or good result at a median follow-up of 3.6 years with use of total condylar or posterior stabilized prostheses. There were two late infections requiring implant removal (27). Another series of 13 knees in ten patients followed 2 to 6 years reported only 31% good and excellent results, with a 31% revision rate, including two (8%) deep infections (29). Still another study followed 23 arthroplasties in 15 knees a mean of 7.5 years. They reported only four good and excellent results, and seven patients died during the study, all from complications of HIV (30). In another study of 19 knees, there were six failures at a mean follow-up of 9.5 years. Two knees required additional surgery for patellar resurfacing, two required revision of a loose tibial component, and one knee with a deep infection required prosthesis removal and arthrodesis (31).

Several authors have addressed the rate of infectious complications in HIV-positive hemophilia patients undergoing total knee arthroplasty. Most have examined a small number of HIV-positive patients who were a subset of their total study population (28,30). One study of 13 knee arthroplasties in nine patients reported no major complications related to the procedure, and 100% good and excellent results. Two knees developed hematomas, however, two in one patient had prolonged drainage, and 44% of the patients died during the observation period (28). Another study reported 88% good and excellent results with 26 total knee arthroplasties in 15 patients followed for an average of 6.4 years. The investigators reported no deaths, infections, or revisions, but two knees in one patient developed recurrent hemarthrosis, and 13 knees (50%) required manipulation (32) (Table 1).

DIABETES MELLITUS

Diabetes mellitus is a systemic disorder affecting 2% to 4% of the population in the United States (34). Although it may involve almost any organ system, most pathology arises from its effect on the vascular system, especially small vessels, with resultant ischemia.

Primary joint involvement may be more frequent than in the nondiabetic population (35). Most of the concern regarding patients evaluated for total knee arthroplasty, however, centers on the impact of the disease on wound healing, the risk of infection, and the patient's ability to tolerate the stress of surgery. The extent of systemic impairment correlates with duration of disease and adequacy of control of blood glucose level. The preoperative evaluation of cardiac and renal function is crucial, as silent ischemia and impaired renal function may be present without clinical symptoms. As many as 50% of patients with adult-onset diabetes eventually die of coronary artery disease (36). Bone healing and strength have been shown in experimental models to be adversely affected in hyperglycemia. Diabetic patients also have an increased susceptibility to both deep and superficial infections after surgery, possibly due to impaired phagocytosis (37,38).

In a study of 59 cemented total knee arthroplasties in 40 diabetic patients, there was an overall infection rate of 7% despite prophylactic administration of antibiotics, and a wound complication rate of 12%. The rate of deep infection in diabetic patients was statistically higher than in nondiabetic patients. There were two deaths due to myocardial infarction. The overall rate of revision was 10% at a mean follow-up of 4.3 years. Bone cement admixed with an antibiotic was recommended for fixation of the components in these patients (39).

PSORIASIS

Psoriasis is a skin disorder affecting 1% to 2% of the population. Skin manifestations include scaly patches that are localized preferentially on the extensor surfaces of the limbs but that may occur anywhere on the body. Chronic inflammatory arthritis affects fewer than 10% of patients, so most commonly patients present with osteoarthritis and concurrent psoriasis. Psoriatic skin lesions are known to show higher bacterial counts than healthy skin (40). An additional consideration is the possibility of a flare of disease due to the stress of surgery, termed the Koebner phenomenon (41). Patients may also be taking corticosteroids for the disorder, which increases concerns about perioperative infection. Only two reports address the results of total knee arthroplasty in patients with psoriasis. One study of 27 arthroplasties in 18 patients reported 29% poor results, including a rate of deep infection of 17% at 4 years postoperatively. This study included patients with active psoriasis and osteoarthritis as well as patients with inflammatory arthritis and psoriasis. The group with inflammatory arthritis, however, included a number of patients with rheumatoid arthritis (42). The only other study of psoriasis and total knee arthroplasty involved 50 knees in 34 patients followed for an average of 4.5 years. The authors reported only one deep infection at 25 weeks, with all patients receiving perioperative antibiotics. This study concluded that psoriatic arthritis conferred no increased risk of infection with total knee arthroplasty (43).

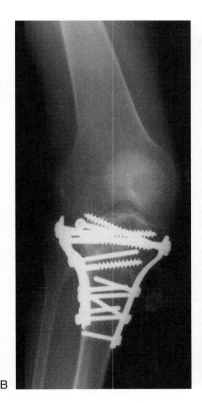
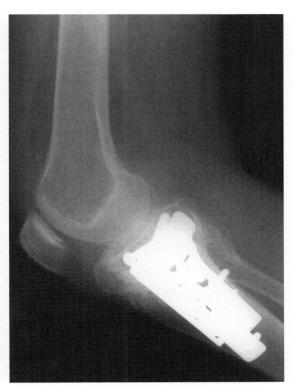

A,B

FIG. 8. A, B: Posttraumatic arthritis with valgus deformity.

Although routine perioperative skin preparation and systemic prophylactic antibiotics should be adequate in reducing the incidence of infection in these patients (43), it seems wise to optimize treatment of the local disease before undertaking an elective procedure. For this reason, and to allow early treatment of flares, dermatologic consultation is recommended preoperatively.

POSTTRAUMATIC ARTHRITIS

Posttraumatic gonarthrosis poses a unique set of circumstances for total knee replacement. Patients tend to be younger, more active, predominantly male, and, if employed, more likely to have a physically demanding job. The contralateral knee is likely to be normal. These patients probably have a longer life expectancy than the usual patient with osteoarthritis and are more likely to have recently enjoyed full pain-free function of the involved knee. Many have had fractures with additional complicating factors of bone or ligament deficiency, compromised skin, or osteomyelitis—either from pin tracts or open fractures. For these reasons, patient expectations and the demands placed on the posttraumatic knee reconstruction tend to be higher than those in the primary arthritic population, and the surgery may be more technically demanding.

Previous skin incisions, scars, and burn injuries must be assessed to determine whether healing of total knee arthroplasty incisions may be compromised. Many patients have had surgery on the distal femur and proximal tibia, and these incisions may jeopardize healing of common total knee incisions. Comorbidities, such as smoking, also impair healing and should be minimized. The more time that has passed since a previous incision was made, the lower the risk of compromise. Incisions should be as far apart as possible, and if they must intersect, a right angle

is preferable to an acute angle. A good rule of thumb is that, if the skin bridge between two incisions is longer than the length of the incision, circulation should be sufficient for healing (44). All flaps should be developed below the deep fascia, as the plexus feeding the skin and adipose tissue lies above this (45). Most of the deep perforators arise medially, so one should use the most lateral incision that can be made without compromising exposure (44). If there is doubt about the ability of an incision to heal, tissue expanders, planned flap coverage, or a sham incision before arthroplasty may be used to avoid flap necrosis, a potentially devastating complication.

Due to the possibility of prior ligament injury or deficiency, posterior stabilized and constrained condylar prostheses should be available. The preoperative assessment of collateral ligament instability in the setting of bone loss may not be completely reliable. After correction of joint alignment, ligament stability may be restored, which allows the use of less constrained designs. Wedges, blocks, or bone grafts should be considered for the augmentation of periarticular bone loss. Preoperative templating from full-length films can determine whether intramedullary or extramedullary alignment guides should be used. When the deformity or bone loss is localized near the joint, or when a stemmed prosthesis is planned, use of intramedullary guides is attractive. When there is a malunion away from the joint in either the tibia or femur, however, use of extramedullary guides gives a more accurate mechanical axis.

Patients with posttraumatic arthritis may also have hardware that must be removed to perform a knee arthroplasty (Fig. 8). Screw holes or incomplete union may create stress risers predisposing to fracture. In this situation, prophylactic nail insertion may prevent periprosthetic fracture (46), or alternatively, a longer stem extension may be used (Fig. 9). When a malunion exceeds 5 degrees in the coronal plane or 10 degrees in the sagittal plane,

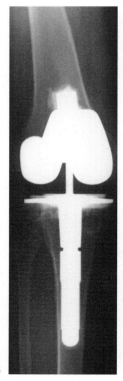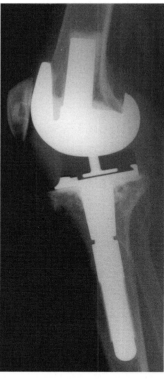

A,B

FIG. 9. A, B: Postoperative radiograph showing long-stemmed constrained implant in patient with posttraumatic arthritis.

consideration must be given to correcting the malunion acutely, either with an osteotomy and long-stemmed prosthesis, or an osteotomy alone over an intramedullary nail. Retrograde nails should be used in the femur and antegrade in the tibia to allow ease of retrieval at time of arthroplasty (47). There are anecdotal reports of patients obtaining several years of pain-free ambulation from the realignment alone. As a rule, varus and femoral deformity may be corrected by intraarticular bone resection, as lateral instability is better tolerated than medial, and the closer a deformity is to the knee, the greater its impact on joint mechanics (48).

The few series in the literature emphasize the high complication rate and poorer outcomes in total knee arthroplasties in patients with posttraumatic arthritis. One study of 31 total knee arthroplasties performed in 30 patients an average of 13 years after trauma reported 71% good or excellent postoperative results at 46 months. However, 57% of patients experienced significant complications (49). Similar results were obtained in another series of 40 total knee arthroplasties in 40 patients with posttraumatic arthritis who were followed an average of 4.3 years. These investigators reported 79% good and excellent results but an 8% rate of deep infection rate requiring revision (50). Another study compared ten knees replaced for work-related posttraumatic arthritis with ten knees in age- and sex-matched controls. Patients were evaluated with the Hospital for Special Surgery knee scoring system. Despite similar alignment and radiographic appearance of the knee, patients in the posttraumatic group scored significantly worse (64.1 vs. 91.9) (51).

Arthroplasty in the posttraumatic knee may be substantially more difficult to perform technically than the usual primary total knee arthroplasty. Complications are increased, and revision for loosening or wear may be required during the patient's lifetime. Patient factors are equally important to the outcome, and early intervention in the form of vocational retraining to deskwork, if possible, is recommended. Trauma, especially vehicular trauma, is not a random event, and care must be taken in patient selection for arthroplasty to decrease the risk of early failure.

ARTHROPLASTY AFTER HIGH TIBIAL OSTEOTOMY

Despite the enviable long-term success enjoyed with total knee replacements, in younger patients or those with high activity demands (such as manual laborers), proximal tibial osteotomy is an option that has been traditionally considered.

The goal of the procedure is to realign the weightbearing (mechanical) axis of the limb so that it passes through the less involved compartment. Normally the medial compartment bears 60% of the force whereas the lateral bears 40%. As medial- or lateral-sided arthritis progresses, the mechanical axis shifts, which increases the load on the affected compartment and accelerates the degenerative process. Secondary laxity of the collateral ligaments may add a static (opening) or dynamic (thrust) component to the problem. In varus or medial gonarthrosis, a proximal valgus-producing osteotomy of the tibia is the procedure of choice. Conversely, in valgus or lateral gonarthrosis, a varus-producing distal femoral osteotomy is preferred (52).

As the results of osteotomy for arthritis tend to deteriorate over time (53–57) and the operation is done in a younger population, a number of patients eventually require conversion to total knee arthroplasty. Planning for a knee arthroplasty should therefore begin at the time of osteotomy. Longitudinal incisions should be sufficiently short and posterior to allow maintenance of a viable skin bridge between the osteotomy incision and any future arthroplasty incision. Transverse incisions also provide good exposure, however, and have not been associated with increased wound complications after later arthroplasty (52,57).

Choice of fixation is a more theoretical concern. Distraction osteogenesis with fixators may preserve more bone stock, but the possibility that later pin tract infection and chronic osteomyelitis will increase the risk of infection at later total knee arthroplasty should be considered. One series of 95 knee arthroplasties in 82 patients with prior tibial osteotomies reported one deep infection, which occurred 1 month after arthroplasty (58). Proximal tibial osteotomy is contraindicated in patients with more than 10 degrees of varus. As angular correction increases, however, even within these limits consideration should be given to performing a dome rather than a wedge osteotomy to minimize changes in position of the patella and joint line. These considerations are less important in distal femoral osteotomies (53).

There are several technical difficulties in the conversion of a previous proximal tibial osteotomy to a total knee arthroplasty. Problems may include patella infera and difficulty with exposure (59–61). The need for a vastus snip or tibial tubercle osteotomy to adequately expose the joint should be considered. Retained hardware may usually be removed through standard exposures (Fig. 10), but this may not always be necessary (57,62). Sclerotic bone at the osteotomy may impinge on central pegs. Metal or cement augmentation can replace smaller defects of the proximal tibia. Larger defects may require bone grafting, however, either from femoral

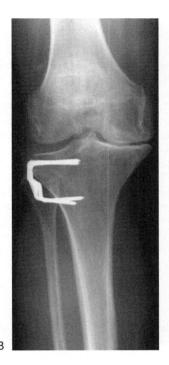
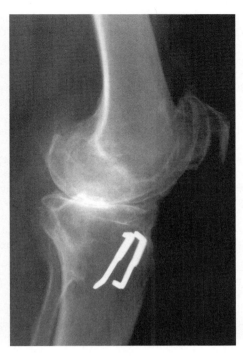

A,B

FIG. 10. A, B: Knee after proximal tibial osteotomy.

cuts or from allograft femoral head. The tibial template and hole for the stem should be placed as medially as possible without over-hang. Offset tibial stems may need to be considered in patients with overcorrections and should be available if stemmed prosthesis or bone grafting is anticipated. Posterior slope may be decreased, which requires minimal anterior bone resection, and the tibial tubercle is a less reliable guide for rotation than in routine primary

total knee arthroplasty (57). One study of 21 knees followed for 2.9 years comparing patients with a previous proximal tibial osteotomy and a matched control group without osteotomy reported only 81% satisfactory results in the patients with a prior osteotomy versus 100% in patients without a prior osteotomy (63). A study of 45 knees in 41 patients, who were followed for an average of 55 months, reported only 80% good or excellent results after osteot-

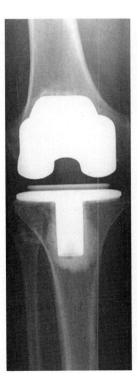
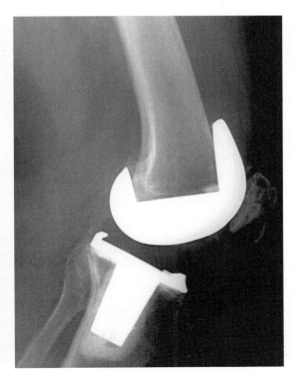

A,B

FIG. 11. A, B: Total knee arthroplasty with hardware removal and use of standard implants in a patient with previous tibial osteotomy.

omy. These findings were similar to those of a group who had a revision knee arthroplasty (62). Two other studies, however, reported no significant difference in outcome between patients with total knee arthroplasties and previous proximal tibial osteotomies, and those with routine primary total knee arthroplasties. The first report compared 42 total knee arthroplasties in 39 patients with failed proximal tibial osteotomies and 41 primary total knee arthroplasties in 39 patients. At an average follow-up of 37 months, investigators reported an average of 14 degrees greater range of motion in the control group but otherwise similar results in the two groups (59). Another study of 35 condylar resurfacing arthroplasties in 35 patients followed a minimum of 2 years reported 89% good and excellent results. These compared favorably with results in historic controls undergoing primary total knee arthroplasty (61) (Fig. 11).

ARTHROPLASTY AFTER FUSION

Conversion of the surgically fused knee to total knee arthroplasty is supported by only a few scattered case reports. This is due in large part to the difficulty encountered in restoring an effective extensor mechanism. Extensor mechanism deficiency has usually been considered an absolute contraindication to total knee arthroplasty and an indication for arthrodesis. If conversion to total knee arthroplasty is to be considered, the surgeon should have reasonable assurance that the quadriceps mechanism is intact (the ability to perform a straight leg raise is necessary, but not sufficient). Lack of extensor function requires locking in hyperextension during the stance phase of gait, which leads to increased stress on the prosthesis and failure due to loosening and wear (64). The frequency of falls is also increased (65).

Decreased bone stock is expected, and care must be taken to restore the joint line to as near anatomic as possible to avoid patellar complications. The collateral and cruciate ligaments will most likely be contracted or absent, so the use of constrained, stemmed prostheses should be anticipated. Exposure is often difficult due to contracture of the tissues, so that extensile approaches, quadriceps snip, or tubercle osteotomy is required to allow sufficient exposure of the joint (44). There are only two reported series of total knee arthroplasty after knee arthrodesis. One study reported 59% good and excellent results, but a 53% complication rate, in 17 patients followed for 1 to 10 years (66). The second study reported on 37 knees in 35 patients followed for an average of 90 months. There was a satisfactory outcome in only 29% and a 57% complication rate, including a 14% rate of infection (67). Both studies concluded that success was possible, but that patients should be counseled regarding the very high rate of serious complications.

RECURVATUM

One of the guiding principles of total knee arthroplasty is the restoration of proper knee alignment. The mechanical axis in the coronal plane should pass from the center of the femoral head, through the center of the knee joint to the center of the ankle. The mechanical axis should also be centered in the sagittal plane. Severe recurvatum of the knee has traditionally been considered a contraindication to total knee arthroplasty. However, it is difficult to find studies to support this (68).

In planning total knee arthroplasty in a patient with painful gonarthrosis and recurvatum, attempts should be made to determine the cause of the deformity. Ankle equinus and quadriceps weakness may cause recurvatum at the knee and should be addressed before attempting total knee arthroplasty. Posttraumatic malunion of the proximal tibia can also lead to unilateral recurvatum. If a correctable cause is found it should be remedied either preoperatively or at the time of surgery to decrease the risk of recurrent deformity or loosening. As previously discussed with reference to treatment of polio-related deformities, recurvatum deformity may be corrected using the cam effect of the shape of the femoral condyles. Resecting less bone from the distal femur or building up the distal femur with blocks or graft decreases the extension gap, which limits the knee's ability to hyperextend. Krackow and Weiss have also suggested transposing the collateral ligaments posteriorly on the femur to achieve the same effect (69). This carries with it the risk of disruption of the transposed ligaments from their new locations with loss of varus-valgus stability.

If the deformity is the result of anterior tibial bowing, increasing the angle of the tibial cut and using a flatter tray prevents excessive anterior bone resection and possible compromise of the extensor mechanism.

CONCLUSION

Although total knee arthroplasty may be attempted in the medical conditions discussed previously, adequate preoperative evaluation of the patient's medical condition and type of deformity is crucial to the outcome. Even more than with hip arthroplasty, the outcome of total knee arthroplasty is dependent on alignment and soft tissue balance for successful outcome. There can be no substitute for adequate preoperative planning. Techniques and implants needed to achieve stability must be anticipated and readily available. With strict attention to the overall care of the patient and adherence to the principles of knee arthroplasty, improvement in patient function, pain relief, and quality of life may be achieved.

REFERENCES

1. McDonald DJ, Sim FH. Total hip arthroplasty in Paget's disease. A follow-up note. *J Bone Joint Surg Am* 1987;69:766–772.
2. Merkow RL, Pellicci PM, Hely DP, et al. Total hip replacement for Paget's disease of the hip. *J Bone Joint Surg Am* 1984;66:752–758.
3. Broberg MA, Cass JR. Total knee arthroplasty in Paget's disease of the knee. *J Arthroplasty* 1986;1:139–142.
4. Gabel GT, Rand JA, Sim FH. Total knee arthroplasty for osteoarthrosis in patients who have Paget's disease of bone at the knee. *J Bone Joint Surg Am* 1991;73(5):739–744.
5. Hadjipavlou A, Lander P, Srolovitz H, et al. Malignant transformation in Paget disease of bone. *Cancer* 1992;70(12):2802–2808.
6. Moran MC. Functional loss after total knee arthroplasty for poliomyelitis. *Clin Orthop* 1996;323:243–246.
7. Patterson BM, Insall JN. Surgical management of gonarthrosis in patients with poliomyelitis. *J Arthroplasty* 1992;7[Suppl]:419–426.
8. Langston JW, Ballard P, Tetrud JW, et al. Chronic parkinsonism in humans due to a product of meperidine-analog synthesis. *Science* 1983;219(4587):979–980.
9. Oni OO, MacKenney RP. Total knee replacement in patients with Parkinson's disease. *J Bone Joint Surg Br* 1985;67:424–425.
10. Vince KG, Insall JM, Bannerman CE. Total knee arthroplasty in the patient with Parkinson's disease. *J Bone Joint Surg Br* 1989;71:51.
11. Duffy GP, Trousdale RT. Total knee arthroplasty in patients with Parkinson's disease. *J Arthroplasty* 1996;11(8):899–904.
12. Engh GA, Ammeen DJ. Periprosthetic fractures adjacent to total knee implants. *J Bone Joint Surg Am* 1997;79(7):1100–1113.
13. Gupta R. A short history of neuropathic arthropathy. *Clin Orthop* 1993;296:43–49.
14. Selby PL, Young MJ, Boulton AJ. Bisphosphonates: a new treatment for diabetic Charcot neuroarthropathy? *Diabet Med* 1994;11(1):28–31.
15. Soudry M, Binazzi R, Johanson NA, et al. Total knee arthroplasty

in Charcot and Charcot-like joints. *Clin Orthop* 1986;208:199–204.

16. Doherty WP, Rand JA, Bryan RS. Total knee arthroplasty in neuropathic arthropathy. In: *Proceedings of the Knee Society.* Park Ridge, IL: The Knee Society, 279–285.

17. Drennan DB, Fahey JJ, Maylahn DJ. Important factors in achieving arthrodesis of the Charcot knee. *J Bone Joint Surg Am* 1971; 53:1180.

18. Yoshino S, Fujimori J, Kajino A, et al. Total knee arthroplasty in Charcot's joint. *J Arthroplasty* 1993;8(3):335–340.

19. Lachiewicz PF. Total joint replacement in special medical conditions. In: Callaghan JJ, Dennis DA, Paprosky WG, et al., eds. *Orthopaedic knowledge update—hip and knee reconstruction.* Chicago: American Academy of Orthopaedic Surgeons, 1995:79–86.

20. Ribbans WJ, Giangrande P, Beeton K. Conservative treatment of hemarthrosis for prevention of hemophilic synovitis. *Clin Orthop* 1997;343:19–24.

21. Wiedel JD. Arthroscopic synovectomy of the knee in hemophilia: a 10-to-15 year followup. *Clin Orthop* 1996;328:46–53.

22. Greene WB, Yankasakas BC, Guilford WB. Roentgenographic classifications of hemophilic arthropathy. *J Bone Joint Surg Am* 1989;71(2):237–244.

23. Stehr-Green JK, Evatt BL, Lawrence DN. Acquired immune deficiency syndrome associated with hemophilia in the United States. *Instr Course Lect* 1989;38:357–365.

24. Greene WB, DeGnore LT, White GC. Orthopaedic procedures and prognosis in hemophilic patients who are seropositive for human immunodeficiency virus. *J Bone Joint Surg Am* 1997;72:2–11.

25. Goodfellow J, Fearn CB, Matthews JM. Iliacus haematoma. A common complication of haemophilia. *J Bone Joint Surg Br* 1967;49: 748–756.

26. Ragni MV, Crossett LS, Herndon JH. Postoperative infection following orthopaedic surgery in human immunodeficiency virus-infected hemophiliacs with CD-4 counts ≤200/mm³. *J Arthroplasty* 1995;10(6):716–721.

27. Lachiewicz PF, Inglis AE, Insall JN, et al. Total knee arthroplasty in hemophilia. *J Bone Joint Surg Am* 1995;67:1361–1366.

28. Kjaersgaard-Andersen P, Christiansen SE, Ingerslev J, et al. Total knee arthroplasty in classic hemophilia. *Clin Orthop* 1990;256:137–146.

29. Goldberg VM, Heiple KG, Ratnoff OD, et al. Total knee arthroplasty in classic hemophilia. *J Bone Joint Surg Am* 1981;63:695–701.

30. Thomasson HC, Wilson FC, Lachiewicz PF, et al. Knee arthroplasty in hemophilic arthropathy. *Clin Orthop* 1999;360:169–173.

31. Figgie MP, Goldberg VM, Figgie HE III, et al. Total knee arthroplasty for the treatment of chronic hemophilic arthropathy. *Clin Orthop* 1989;248:98–107.

32. Unger AS, Kessler CM, Lewis RJ. Total knee arthroplasty in human immunodeficiency virus-infected hemophilics. *J. Arthroplasty* 1995;10(4):448–452.

33. Karthaus RP, Novakova IRO. Total knee replacement in hemophilic arthropathy. *J Bone Joint Surg Br* 1988;70:382–385.

34. Cahill GF. Disorders of carbohydrate metabolism. In: Wyngaarden JB, Smith LH, eds. *Cecil textbook of medicine.* Philadelphia: WB Saunders, 1982:1053–1071.

35. Pastan RS, Cohen AS. The rheumatologic manifestations of diabetes mellitus. *Med Clin North Am* 1978;62:829.

36. Fishman MC, et al. *Medicine.* Philadelphia: JB Lippincott, 1981:221–234.

37. Menon TJ, Thjellesen D, Wroblewski BM. Charnley low-friction arthroplasty in diabetic patients. *J Bone Joint Surg Br* 1983;65:580.

38. Wong RY, Lotke PAS, Ecker ML. Factors influencing wound healing after total knee arthroplasty. *Orthop Trans* 1986;10:497.

39. England SP, Stem SH, Insall JN, et al. Total knee arthroplasty in diabetes mellitus. *Clin Orthop* 1990;260:130–134.

40. Marples RR, Heaton CL, Kligman AM. *Staphylococcus aureus* in psoriasis. *Arch Dermatol* 1973;107:568.

41. Krueger GG, Christophers E, Draper RE. Psoriasis: clinical features and pathogenesis. In: Gerber LH, Espinoza LR, eds. *Psoriatic arthritis.* Orlando, FL: Grune and Stratton, 1985:147–165.

42. Stern SH, Insall JH, Windsor RE, et al. Total knee arthroplasty in patients with psoriasis. *Clin Orthop* 1989;248:108–111.

43. Beyer CA, Hanssen AD, Lewallen DG, et al. Primary total knee arthroplasty in patients with psoriasis. *J Bone Joint Surg Br* 1973;73(2):258–259.

44. Younger ASE, Duncan CP, Masri BA. Surgical exposures in revision total knee arthroplasty. *J Am Acad Orthop Surg* 1998;6(1):55–64.

45. Haertsch PA. The blood supply to the skin of the leg: a post mortem investigation. *Br J Plast Surg* 1981;34:470–477.

46. Reis MD. Prophylactic intramedullary femoral rod during total knee arthroplasty with simultaneous femoral plate removal. *J Arthroplasty* 1998;13(6):718–721.

47. Paley D, Herzenberg JE, Bor N. Fixator assisted nailing of femoral and tibial deformities. *Tech Orthop* 1997;12(4):260–275.

48. Wolff AM, Hungerford DS, Pepe CI. The effect of extraarticular varus and valgus deformity on total knee arthroplasty. *Clin Orthop* 1991;271:35–51.

49. Lonner JH, Pedlow FX, Siliski JM. Total knee arthroplasty for post-traumatic arthrosis. *J Arthroplasty* 1999;14(8):969–975.

50. Zelicof SB, Scuderi GR, Vince KG, et al. Total knee arthroplasty in post-traumatic arthritis. *Orthop Trans* 1988;12:547–548.

51. Brinker MR, Savory CG, Weeden SH, et al. The results of total knee arthroplasty in workers' compensation patients. *Bull Hosp Joint Dis* 1998;57(2):80–83.

52. Kelley MA. Nonprosthetic management of the arthritic knee. In: Callaghan JJ, Dennis DA, Paprosky WG, et al., eds. *Orthopaedic knowledge update—hip and knee reconstruction.* Chicago: American Academy of Orthopaedic Surgeons, 1995:245–249.

53. Coventry MB, Ilstrup DM, Wallrichs SL. Proximal tibial osteotomy: a critical long-term study of eighty-seven cases. *J Bone Joint Surg Am* 1993;75:196–201.

54. Hernigou P, Medevielle D, Debeyre J, et al. Proximal tibial osteotomy for osteoarthritis with varus deformity: a ten to thirteen year follow-up study. *J Bone Joint Surg Am* 1987;69:332–354.

55. Holden DL, James SL, Larson RL, et al. Proximal tibial osteotomy in patients who are fifty years old or less: a long-term follow up study. *J Bone Joint Surg Am* 1988;70(7):977–982.

56. Insall JN, Joseph DM, Msika C. High tibial osteotomy for varus gonarthrosis: a long-term follow up study. *J Bone Joint Surg Am* 1984;66:1040–1048.

57. Johnson BP, Dorr LD. Total knee arthroplasty after high tibial osteotomies. In: Lotke, PA, ed. *Master techniques in orthopaedic surgery, knee arthroplasty.* New York: Raven Press, 1995:177–192.

58. Meding JB, Keating M, Ritter MA, et al. Total knee arthroplasty after high tibial osteotomy. *Clin Orthop* 2000;375:75–184.

59. Annuniato A, Roraveck CH, Bourne RB, et al. Total knee arthroplasty following high tibial osteotomy for osteoarthritis. *J Arthroplasty* 1989;4[Suppl]:S11–S17.

60. Scuderi GR, Windsor RE, Insall JN. Observations on patellar height after proximal tibial osteotomy. *J Bone Joint Surg Am* 1989;71(2):245–248.

61. Staeheli JW, Cass JR, Morrey BF. Condylar total knee arthroplasty after failed proximal tibial osteotomy. *J Bone Joint Surg Am* 1987;69(1):28–31.

62. Windsor RE, Insall JN, Vince KG. Technical considerations of total knee arthroplasty after proximal tibial osteotomy. *J Bone Joint Surg Am* 1988;70:547–554.

63. Katz MM, Hungerford DS, Krackow KA, et al. Results of total knee arthroplasty after failed proximal tibial osteotomy for osteoarthritis. *J Bone Joint Surg Am* 1987;69(2):225–233.

64. VanKrieken FM, DenHeeten GJ, Pedersen DR, et al. Prediction of muscle and joint loads after segmental femur replacement for osteosarcoma. *Clin Orthop* 1985;198:273–283.

65. Lord SR, Clark RD. Simple physiologic and clinical tests for the accurate prediction of falling in older people. *Gerontology* 1996;42:199–203.

66. Cameron HU, Hu C. Results of total knee arthroplasty following takedown of formal knee fusion. *J Arthroplasty* 1996;11(6):732–737.

67. Naranja RJ Jr, Lotke PA, Pagnano MW, et al. Total knee arthroplasty in a previously ankylosed or arthrodesed knee. *Clin Orthop* 1996;331:234–237.

68. Laskin RS. Modular total knee-replacement arthroplasty. A review of eighty-nine patients. *J Bone Joint Surg Am* 1976;58(6):766–773.

69. Krackow KA, Weiss APC. Recurvatum deformity complicating performance of total knee arthroplasty. *J Bone Joint Surg Am* 1990;72(2):268–271.

70. McCollough NC, Enis JE, Lovitt J, et al. Synovectomy or total replacement of the knee in hemophilia. *J Bone Joint Surg Am* 1979;61:69.

CHAPTER 91

Bilateral Total Knee Arthroplasty

David G. Lewallen

Primary osteoarthritis of the knee, inflammatory arthritic conditions, and posttraumatic degenerative changes combine to make total knee arthroplasty a common orthopedic procedure required for management of recalcitrant knee symptoms. Because of the pathophysiology and natural history of the conditions most commonly producing destructive changes in the knee, a large percentage of patients experience with bilateral knee pain symptoms during their lifetime and a substantial subset have bilateral knee symptoms at the time of presentation for medical care. Gunther et al. have documented that in a large cohort of patients presenting with knee osteoarthritis for consideration of total knee arthroplasty, 87.4% have radiographic changes of osteoarthritis in the contralateral knee (1). In a study by Mont et al., 43% of those presenting for unilateral total knee arthroplasty eventually had the other knee replaced as well, with 44% having bilateral symptoms at the time of the first surgery (2). A common clinical scenario is the patient with severe symptoms in both knees and equivalent or nearly equivalent impairment produced by the arthritic changes present. When pain symptoms and limitations imposed by the symptoms justify consideration of total knee arthroplasty in both knees, patients and surgeons face a decision regarding timing of the two operative procedures. The first decision is whether to perform both total knee arthroplasties during the same anesthesia (one stage) or during two separate surgical procedures (two stage), separated by days, weeks, or months. If the two procedures are performed during one stage, an additional decision is required by the surgeon regarding whether to arrange for the surgery to be performed by two surgical teams simultaneously or whether to perform the two procedures in sequential fashion, one after the other, during the same, more prolonged period of anesthesia. The following factors deserve consideration in deciding on the timing of the second surgical procedure: clinical results, general medical risks and complication rates, expense and efficiency of the various options, and, finally, individual patient and surgeon preference.

CLINICAL RESULTS AFTER BILATERAL TOTAL KNEE ARTHROPLASTY

Total knee arthroplasty has emerged as one of the most successful operative procedures in orthopedics, with initial pain relief, functional improvement, and longer-term durability of the procedures sufficient to provide a major impact on the patient's quality of life (3). No major differences have been shown in the clinical outcome of total knee arthroplasty when performed in simultaneous bilateral fashion or as an isolated unilateral procedure (4–9). No data are available in the literature to show a significant impact on patient functional outcome, standardized knee scores, or long-term implant survivorship due to timing of surgery for the second knee in patients with bilateral disease (Table 1). In the absence of significant clinical differences with regard to function and outcome of the total knee arthroplasty, the decision on whether to perform bilateral simultaneous procedures or staged reconstructions therefore should rest on general medical considerations, risks of complications, and other factors such as expense and preference.

MEDICAL COMPLICATIONS AND RISKS

Overall complication rates in patients undergoing bilateral versus unilateral total knee arthroplasty are similar, which suggests that for the average patient there appears to be no increased risk posed by the larger bilateral surgery (10–12).

For the individual patient, however, the physiologic insult produced by bilateral total knee arthroplasties performed during the same anesthetic period is substantially greater than that produced by a unilateral total knee arthroplasty. Operative time is typically 1.5 to 2.0 times longer for those procedures done sequentially during the same period of anesthesia, depending on the degree of overlap between the two procedures (6). Bilateral simultaneous procedures subject patients to greater acute blood

TABLE 1. *Studies reviewing complications, outcomes, and costs in bilateral total knee replacement*

Study	No. patients and procedure	Findings
Cohen et al. (5)	86 Simultaneous sequential bilateral TKRs 100 Unilateral TKRs	Patients undergoing simultaneous bilateral TKR had no increased morbidity or compromise in postoperative function. No difference in complication rate, but greater blood loss and transfusion in bilateral procedures.
Jankiewicz et al. (4)	99 Simultaneous sequential bilateral TKRs 56 Staged bilateral TKRs	Complication rate similar for both groups. Simultaneous group had greater blood loss and transfusion, shorter hospitalization, less therapy, and decreased costs.
Lane et al. (7)	100 Simultaneous sequential bilateral TKRs 100 Unilateral TKRs	Greater postoperative confusion, cardiopulmonary complications, transfusion requirement, and rehabilitation stays in simultaneous group. No difference in length of hospital stay. Implicit financial advantage to simultaneous TKRs, but partially offset by rehabilitation need.
Liu and Chen (6)	64 Simultaneous sequential bilateral TKRs 24 Bilateral staged (7 d) TKRs	Complication rates similar for both groups. No difference in blood loss or functional scores. Simultaneous group had shorter operative time and hospitalization.
Morrey et al. (10)	290 Simultaneous sequential bilateral TKRs 228 Staggered, single hospitalization 234 Bilateral, separate hospitalizations 501 Unilateral TKRs	No difference in complication rates, incidence of reoperation, or mortality.
Ritter et al. (3,8)	93 Unilateral TKRs 65 Single-stage bilateral TKRs	Significant improvements from preoperative in quality-of-life measures; no significant differences between unilateral and bilateral TKRs.
Ritter et al., HCFA data (1985–1990) (3,8)	12,622 Simultaneous TKRs 4,354 Bilateral staged TKRs (6 wk) 4,524 Bilateral staged TKRs (3 mo) 9,829 Bilateral staged TKRs (6 mo) 31,401 Bilateral staged TKRs (1 yr)	Simultaneous group had double the ICU days of staged group (0.48 vs. 0.21). Length of stay and cost were less with simultaneous TKRs. Infections were similar in all groups. 30-d mortality highest in simultaneous group, but rates similar by 2 yr.
Soudry et al. (12)	56 Simultaneous sequential bilateral TKRs 18 Staged bilateral TKRs	Outcome rating similar for all groups. Complications similar except higher DVT and PE in staged group.
Williams-Russo et al. (26)	51 Simultaneous sequential bilateral TKRs	Forty-one percent had acute postoperative delirium. Predictive factors for delirium were age, gender, and preoperative EtOH use.
Worland et al. (9)	213 Simultaneous sequential bilateral TKRs 107 Matched unilateral TKRs	No difference in knee function scores. Lower complication rate in the bilateral series.

DVT, deep venous thrombosis; EtOH, ethanol; HCFA, Health Care Financing Administration; ICU, intensive care unit; PE, pulmonary embolism; TKR, total knee replacement.

loss and a higher potential for fluid shifts, with bleeding from both wounds and inflation and deflation of pneumatic tourniquets on both lower extremities (13,14). Bierbaum et al. documented increased allogenic blood transfusion in patients with bilateral total knee arthroplasty, and in this same study transfusion of allogenic blood was associated with increased risk of infection, fluid overload, and duration of hospitalization (15). It would appear that the increased blood loss observed when bilateral knee arthroplasties are performed during the same anesthetic period is due to more than simply twice the amount of surgery. Bould et al. have demonstrated that blood loss is greater by a mean of 323 mm during the second of two knee surgeries when the procedures are staged, and documented that clotting studies performed during the procedure show a prolongation of prothrombin time, activated partial thromboplastin time, and thrombin time after release of the first tourniquet, which potentially increases blood loss with the second knee surgery (13).

Thrombocytopenia occurs after total knee arthroplasty and is more pronounced after a bilateral procedure (16). Coagulation and fibrinolytic activation as measured by thromboelastography has been documented during bilateral sequential total knee arthroplasty after release of the first tourniquet and, even more so, the second tourniquet, and persists up to and beyond 2 hours postoperative (17). The significantly larger blood loss observed in patients undergoing bilateral knee arthroplasties compared to those undergoing a unilateral procedure has been documented by other authors as well (4,18). In one review, the average drop in hemoglobin for unilateral total knee arthroplasties was found to be 3.85 g per dL compared to 5.42 g per dL in the group of patients undergoing bilateral knee replacements during this same operative procedure (18). The effects of this greater blood loss may also be compounded by differences in physiologic response to the second of two total knee arthroplasties observed during bilateral knee replacements. Huang et al. (14) studied hemodynamic changes after release of the first and second tourniquets in a group of patients undergoing one-stage bilateral total knee replacements. Systolic and diastolic blood pressure decreased significantly after deflation of both the first and second tourniquets; however, the decrease was much more marked after second tourniquet deflation. The need for vasopressor drugs was greater after deflation of the second tourniquet in this same study.

Total knee arthroplasty also subjects all patients to varying levels of embolization of fat and marrow contents from the medullary canal of the tibia and femur. Release of this material into the right-sided circulation has been documented by catheter aspiration from the right atrium and noninvasively by transesophageal echo imaging, and can produce pulmonary and more widespread systemic effects culminating in the fat embolism syndrome (19–22). The response to this embolic material is highly variable among patients. Adverse clinical outcomes have been correlated with larger volumes of material, and performance of bilateral total knee arthroplasties during the same anesthetic period could be expected to subject patients to at least twice the amount of embolized fat and marrow debris. Clinically significant fat embolism syndrome has been reported in association with bilateral total knee arthroplasties (19,23). Dorr et al. studied 65 patients undergoing bilateral total knee arthroplasty; they found a 12% incidence of fat embolism syndrome diagnosed clinically and reported one death due to adult respiratory distress syndrome 1 week postoperatively (23). Fat embolism has been documented as a cause of death in the early postoperative period after total knee arthroplasty by Monto et al. (20). Sulek et al., in a study of total knee arthroplasty patients, used both transesophageal echocardiography and transcranial Doppler ultrasonography to document the release of echogenic material into the right-sided circulation in patients undergoing both unilateral and bilateral procedures (24). Cerebral emboli were detected in 60% of patients undergoing unilateral knee arthroplasty and 57% of the patients undergoing bilateral total knee arthroplasty; echogenic material was identified in the left atrium via a patent foraminal ovale in two patients, whereas in an additional six patients, left atrial echogenic material was present, with access presumably via pulmonary veins and opening of recruitable pulmonary vessels. In this study, emboli counts were significantly higher in patients undergoing bilateral total knee arthroplasty than in those undergoing unilateral arthroplasty, and all patients with echogenic material in the left atrium on transesophageal echocardiography were documented to have emboli on transcranial Doppler ultrasonography. Paradoxical embolization has the potential to cause catastrophic neurologic injury and has even been the cause of death during bilateral total knee arthroplasty (25). Clearly, these widespread and common effects of knee arthroplasty are well tolerated by the majority of patients; however, response to embolized fat and marrow contents can be catastrophic, particularly in the elderly, those with preexisting significant cardiopulmonary disease, and a subgroup of patients with potential right-to-left shunts at the cardiac level. Changes in technique that avoid instrumentation of the bone with rods or provide for overdrilling, venting, or flutes on rods can reduce but not eliminate these effects (22,23). Although these catastrophic outcomes are rare and the majority of patients appear to tolerate either unilateral or bilateral total knee arthroplasties well, it is possible that the fairly common perioperative confusion and delirium observed with these procedures, particularly in the elderly, are due in part to embolic effects. The overall incidence of acute delirium has been documented to be in the neighborhood of 41% of patients after bilateral knee replacement (26). The overall incidence of acute delirium has been documented to be significantly higher in bilateral total knee arthroplasty than in unilateral total knee arthroplasty in patients over the age of 80 (27). In their review of 65 bilateral total knee cases, Dorr et al. observed hallucination, confusion, lethargy, stupor, hemiparesis, and aphasia in the early postoperative period in addition to one death (23). An advantage of bilateral sequential arthroplasties over the simultaneous method is that observation of any hemodynamic instability during the first procedure allows the surgeon to abort the second procedure and thereby minimize the operative insult.

Several large reviews, however, suggest that bilateral procedures are very safe for most patients. Morrey et al., in a review of complications and mortality associated with bilateral and unilateral knee arthroplasties, documented an overall complication rate of 9.3% in 290 bilateral simultaneous total knee arthroplasties compared to 7% in 228 bilateral staged knee arthroplasties performed during the same hospitalization, and a complication rate of 12% in 234 procedures staged over longer time periods with two separate hospitalizations (10). The complication rate in this same series for 501 unilateral procedures was 11%. No statistically significant difference was observed in the mortality rate, and these authors concluded that no difference exists overall for large cohorts of patients between simultaneous bilateral total knee arthroplasties and staged procedures performed during two periods of anesthesia. Jankiewicz et al. (4) similarly demonstrated no difference in morbidity between 99 sequential procedures performed during the same anesthetic period and 56 staged bilateral knee arthroplasties, although blood loss was greater in the one-stage bilateral group. In a prospective review of 100 bilateral versus 100 unilateral total knee arthroplasties, fourfold higher rates of postoperative confusion were documented, threefold higher risk of cardiopulmonary complications, and greater transfusion requirements in the group undergoing simultaneous bilateral arthroplasties. These authors suggest that preexisting cardiac disease is a relative contraindication to simultaneous bilateral total knee arthroplasties. The more substantial physiologic insult posed by simultaneous bilateral procedures is substantiated by data collected by Ritter et al. (3,8) from 339,152 total knee arthroplasties performed between 1985 and 1990 as recorded in the Health Care Financing Administration database. Patients undergoing bilateral total knee arthroplasty required twice as many intensive care unit days and had over a threefold higher mortality rate at 30 days after surgery than those undergoing staged procedures 3 to 6 months apart (0.99% vs. 0.30%). Two studies have focused specifically on the safety and risk of medical complications of bilateral versus unilateral total knee arthroplasties in the elderly. Lynch et al. reviewed 98 consecutively treated patients age 80 or older who underwent bilateral simultaneous total knee arthroplasties and matched these patients with a retrospective group of patients undergoing unilateral total knee arthroplasty. Four patients in the bilateral simultaneous arthroplasty group died in the early postoperative period, whereas no deaths were observed in the unilateral arthroplasty group. A significantly higher incidence of cardiovascular and neurologic problems was noted in the bilateral arthroplasty group, and this study has led the senior author to abandon performance of bilateral total knee arthroplasties during the same anesthetic period in elderly patients and those with significant prior cardiovascular disease (27). Adili et al. reviewed a group of patients over 75 years of age and examined complications and functional outcomes based on whether the procedure was sequential bilateral knee arthroplasties or a unilateral knee arthroplasty procedure. Eighty-two patients in the bilateral group were matched with 82 unilateral knee arthroplasty patients. Cardiovascular complications were again found to be significantly greater in the bilateral group and were associated with preoperative cardiac risk factors. These authors recommend staged procedures for patients with cardiovascular disease who are elderly (28).

From these studies, it appears that the overall risk of medical complications is not significantly greater for the general population of knee arthroplasty patients when bilateral knee arthroplasty procedures are performed during the same anesthetic period than when procedures are unilateral or staged. It is clear, however, that the operative insult of bilateral procedures is greater, with increased blood loss, substantially greater hemodynamic effects, and significantly greater embolization of fat and marrow elements despite technical measures designed to reduce the amount of material released, and that in selected patient subgroups, bilateral procedures place the patient at greater risk of complications and potentially catastrophic and even fatal adverse effects. Specifically, elderly patients older than 75 or 80 years of age; those with significant medical comorbidity, particularly those with cardiovascular problems; and certainly those with known right-to-left shunts at the cardiac level should be managed with careful monitoring during surgery and should undergo unilateral staged procedures.

EXPENSE AND EFFICIENCY

A clear benefit is seen to bilateral one-staged total knee arthroplasties compared to staged procedures with regard to period of disability, efficient use of resources, and overall expense (7,29,30). In a study of hospital charges, Lane et al. demonstrated a difference of over $12,000 in favor of bilateral simultaneous procedures ($53,186 for bilateral simultaneous total knee arthroplasty versus $32,598 for each side for staged bilateral total knee arthroplasties). This cost differential is partly offset, however, by a much greater chance that the patient will require posthospital rehabilitative services or short-term residence in a rehabilitation facility. Eighty-nine percent of patients in the simultaneous bilateral total knee arthroplasty group required a rehabilitation stay versus 45% of patients in the unilateral total knee arthroplasty group (7). In a review of medical and financial aspects of same-day bilateral total knee arthroplasties, Kovacik et al. found that, even when the usage and financial charges for extended care facilities and home health care after discharge from the hospital were factored in, same-day bilateral total knee arthroplasties were significantly less costly than staged bilateral procedures, with no difference observed in complication rates compared to unilateral procedures (30).

Thus, when the issue is viewed from an economic perspective, and particularly when the inconvenience and economic impact of the period of disability experienced by the patient after surgery is factored in, performance of bilateral total knee arthroplasties during the same anesthesia followed by a single recovery period clearly provides the most efficient means of addressing significantly symptomatic bilateral knee arthritis requiring arthroplasty.

PATIENT AND SURGEON PREFERENCE

It is a very common and interesting observation that patients who have undergone total knee arthroplasty on both knees tend to prefer and recommend the sequence or timing of the procedures that they themselves experienced. Patients who have undergone bilateral knee arthroplasties during the same anesthetic period express satisfaction that they made that decision and underwent one period of convalescence, and are pleased they do not have to confront the prospect of a second surgery, the postoperative pain involved, and a second period of rehabilitation. Likewise, those patients who have undergone staged knee arthroplasties state that they have difficulty imagining having to convalesce or recover from two such procedures all at the same time and are for the most part pleased with the choice that they have made. Thus, clinical experience would suggest that, with either approach, barring perioperative complications that might affect the outcome of the procedure, the prospects for patient satisfaction are high.

Surgeon preference regarding sequence and timing of bilateral knee arthroplasties is multifactorial and is impacted by the availability of support services in the operating room that facilitate performing bilateral procedures during the same anesthesia. When the procedures are performed simultaneously, two operating surgeons are needed. When they are performed sequentially, it is still helpful to have additional support staff so that some overlap between the two procedures can occur for efficiency's sake. Reimbursement for both hospitals and surgeons varies greatly by payer for bilateral procedures performed in a single stage or in two separate stages during two separate hospitalizations. The economics of reimbursement may play a role in surgeon preference and decision making regarding bilateral knee arthroplasty procedures. Katz et al. have documented significant demographic variation in rates of knee replacement among Medicare patients across the United States (31). A significant regional variation is likely to be observed in patterns of performance of simultaneous bilateral total knee arthroplasties as well and can be expected to result from a complex interplay between patient preference; surgeon background training, experience, and preference; availability of hospital support services and practices; and specific economic incentives or disincentives for these procedures.

CONCLUSION

Bilateral total knee arthroplasty is frequently required for treatment of arthritic conditions involving the knees due to the frequent bilaterality of the disease processes affecting the knee and culminating in the need for arthroplasty procedures. Thus, decision making about the timing for bilateral knee arthroplasty procedures will continue to be a common dilemma faced by patients and surgeons. Available data suggest that patients who are elderly or who have major medical complications or problems, specifically cardiovascular disease or structural cardiac anomalies that subject them to potential right-to-left shunting at the cardiac level, are poor candidates for performance of bilateral total knee arthroplasties during the same operative procedure. For the average patient presenting for bilateral knee arthroplasty, bilateral simultaneous procedures during the same anesthetic period or staged procedures during the same anesthetic period are a reasonable choice. In these cases, simple measures to reduce the degree of physiologic insult imposed by the procedure seem reasonable. Careful monitoring and management of fluid status during the procedure are even more important than during a unilateral knee arthroplasty because of the greater blood loss and more significant fluid shifts that can be expected as a result of the procedure. Overdrilling of the medullary canal and use of fluted rather than solid rods for intramedullary guides during the course of knee arthroplasty should be routine but are of particular importance in patients undergoing bilateral procedures. Because of the increase in fat and marrow embolization produced by intramedullary instrumentation, use of extramedullary alignment guides, at least on the tibia, is a reasonable consideration in those undergoing bilateral knee arthroplasty during the same anesthesia. Fortunately, total knee arthroplasty remains one of the most effective and successful procedures in orthopedics. Whether the procedure is performed in a single stage or in two stages, the patient with severe arthritic changes in both knees who is facing total knee arthroplasty can rely on a very high probability of excellent results and reliable relief of symptoms, regardless of the timing chosen for the two arthroplasties.

REFERENCES

1. Gunther KP, Sturmer T, Sauerland S, et al. Prevalence of generalized osteoarthritis in patients with advanced hip and knee osteoarthritis. The Ulm Osteoarthritis study. *Ann Rheum Dis* 1998;57(12):717–723.
2. Mont MA, Mitzner DL, Jones LC, et al. History of the contralateral knee after primary knee arthroplasty for osteoarthritis. *Clin Orthop* 1995;321:145–150.
3. Ritter MA, Albohm MJ, Keating EM, et al. Comparative outcomes of total joint arthroplasty. *J Arthroplasty* 1995;10(6):737–741.
4. Jankiewicz JJ, Sculco TP, Ranawat CS, et al. One-stage versus 2-stage bilateral total knee arthroplasty. *Clin Orthop* 1994;309:94–101.
5. Cohen RG, Forrest CJ, Benjamin JB. Safety and efficacy of bilateral total knee arthroplasty. *J Arthroplasty* 1997;12(5):497–502.
6. Liu TK, Chen SH. Simultaneous bilateral total knee arthroplasty in a single procedure. *Int Orthop* 1998;22(6):390–393.
7. Lane GJ, Hozack WJ, Shah S, et al. Simultaneous bilateral versus unilateral total knee arthroplasty. Outcomes analysis. *Clin Orthop* 1997;345:106–112.
8. Ritter M, Mamlin LA, Melfi CA, et al. Outcome implications for the timing of bilateral total knee arthroplasties. *Clin Orthop* 1997;345:99–105.
9. Worland RL, Jessup DE, Clelland C. Simultaneous bilateral total knee replacement versus unilateral replacement. *Am J Orthop* 1996;25(4):292–295.
10. Morrey BF, Adams RA, Ilstrup DM, et al. Complications and mortality associated with bilateral or unilateral total knee arthroplasty. *J Bone Joint Surg Am* 1987;69:484–488.
11. Kolettis GT, Wixson RL, Peruzzi WT, et al. Safety of one-stage bilateral total knee arthroplasty. *Clin Orthop* 1994;309:102–109.
12. Soudry M, Binazzi R, Insall JN, et al. Successive bilateral total knee replacement. *J Bone Joint Surg Am* 1985;67:573–576.
13. Bould M, Freeman BJ, Pullyblank A, et al. Blood loss in sequential bilateral total knee arthroplasty. *J Arthroplasty* 1998;13(1):77–79.
14. Huang CH, Wang MJ, Chen TL, et al. Blood and central venous pressure responses after serial tourniquet deflation during bilateral total knee replacement. *J Formos Med Assoc* 1996;95(6):496–499.
15. Bierbaum BE, Callaghan JJ, Galante JO, et al. An analysis of blood management in patients having a total hip or knee arthroplasty. *J Bone Joint Surg Am* 1999;81(1):2–10.
16. Stern SH, Insall JN. Hematologic effects of total knee arthroplasty. A prospective evaluation. *Clin Orthop* 1993;286:10–14.
17. Hsu HW, Huang CH, Chang Y, et al. Perioperative alterations of the thromboelastography in patients receiving one-stage bilateral total knee arthroplasty. *Acta Anaesthesiol Sin* 1996;34(3):129–134.
18. Keating EM, Meding JB, Faris PM, et al. Predictors of transfusion risk in elective knee surgery. *Clin Orthop* 1998;357:50–59.
19. Lu CC, Chang YT, Hwang CC, et al. Fat embolism syndrome following bilateral total knee replacement with total condylar prosthesis—a case report. *Acta Anaesthesiol Sin* 1995;33(1):69–71.
20. Monto RR, Garcia J, Callaghan JJ. Fatal fat embolism following total condylar knee arthroplasty. *J Arthroplasty* 1990;5(4):291–299.
21. Ries MD, Rauscher LA, Hoskins S, et al. Intramedullary pressure and pulmonary function during total knee arthroplasty. *Clin Orthop* 1998;356:154–160.
22. Fahmy NR, Chandler HP, Danylchuk K, et al. Blood-gas and circulatory changes during total knee replacement. Role of the intramedullary alignment rod. *J Bone Joint Surg Am* 1990;72(1):19–26.
23. Dorr LD, Merkel C, Mellman MF, et al. Fat emboli in bilateral total knee arthroplasty. Predictive factors for neurologic manifestations. *Clin Orthop* 1989;248:112–128; discussion, 118–119.
24. Sulek CA, Davies LK, Enneking FK, et al. Cerebral microembolism diagnosed by transcranial Doppler during total knee arthroplasty: correlation with transesophageal echocardiography. *Anesthesiology* 1999;91(3):672–676.
25. Weiss SJ, Cheung AT, Stecker MM, et al. Fatal paradoxical cerebral embolization during bilateral knee arthroplasty. *Anesthesiology* 1996;84(3):721–723.
26. Williams-Russo P, Urquhart BL, et al. Postoperative delirium. Predictors and prognosis in elderly orthopedic patients. *J Am Geriatr Soc* 1992;40(8):759–767.
27. Lynch NM, Trousdale RT, Ilstrup DM. Complications after concomitant bilateral total knee arthroplasty in elderly patients. *Mayo Clin Proc* 1997;72(9):799–805.
28. Adili A, Bhandari M, Petrucelli D, et al. Sequential bilateral total knee arthroplasty under 1 anesthetic in patients ≥75 years old. *J Arthroplasty* 2001;16:271–278.
29. Reuben JD, Meyers SJ, Cox DD, et al. Cost comparison between bilateral simultaneous, staged, and unilateral total joint arthroplasty. *J Arthroplasty* 1998;13(2):172–179.
30. Kovacik MW, Singri P, Khanna S, et al. Medical and financial aspects of same-day bilateral total knee arthroplasties. *Biomed Sci Instrum* 1997;33:429–434.
31. Katz BP, Freund DA, Heck DA, et al. Demographic variation in the rate of knee replacement: a multi-year analysis. *Health Serv Res* 1996;31(2):125–140.

CHAPTER 92

Prevention of Deep Venous Thromboembolism after Total Knee Arthroplasty

Jay R. Lieberman and Janet Baker

Total knee arthroplasty is effective in relieving pain, increasing mobility, and improving the patient's quality of life. Patients undergoing both total hip and knee arthroplasty are at high risk for developing venous thromboembolic disease. Because total joint arthroplasty is usually an elective procedure performed in relatively healthy individuals, pulmonary embolism may be a devastating complication. The first manifestation of venous thromboembolic disease may be a fatal pulmonary embolism. Therefore, selection of an effective method of prophylaxis is an essential part of the care of patients undergoing this operation (1).

Despite the completion of a number of well-designed clinical trials that have assessed the efficacy and safety of a variety of different modalities for prophylaxis, the prevention of deep venous thrombosis (DVT) after major knee surgery remains problematic. The ideal method of prophylaxis is still to be determined. The selection of a prophylactic regimen is influenced not only by its ability to prevent DVT but also by the pressures of cost containment and decreased duration of hospital stay (2).

Total knee arthroplasty differs from total hip arthroplasty with regard to venous thromboembolism in a number of critical elements. First, the overall DVT rate is higher in patients undergoing total knee arthroplasty than in those undergoing total hip arthroplasty without prophylaxis. Second, it is more difficult to suppress venous thrombus formation in patients undergoing total knee arthroplasty than in those undergoing total hip arthroplasty despite the use of the same prophylactic regimens. There are lower rates of symptomatic pulmonary embolism after total knee arthroplasty, however. Finally, bleeding complications associated with total knee arthroplasty are of greater concern because of an increased risk of development of hematomas that require surgical intervention (1–3). In this chapter, we review the available data on DVT prophylaxis after total knee arthroplasty.

PATHOGENESIS

The triad of venous stasis, hypercoagulability, and endothelial injury is associated with thrombus formation and is present in the perioperative period in patients undergoing total knee arthroplasty. A large proportion of thrombi have been shown to begin intraoperatively. Venous stasis often occurs in these patients as a result of the use of a tourniquet on the thigh, knee flexion for a prolonged period of time, and reduced postoperative mobility (1–4). The trauma of the procedure itself can result in a sustained activation of tissue factor and other clotting factors, which then localize at the sites of vascular injury and areas of venous stasis. Postoperative reduction in antithrombin III levels and inhibition of the endogenous fibrinolytic system may allow for continued thrombus growth (1,4–6) (Fig. 1).

In a study of circulatory indices of thrombosis and fibrinolysis, Sharrock et al. noted minimal increases in fibrinopeptide A, thrombin-antithrombin complexes, and D-dimer during total knee arthroplasty as long as the tourniquet was inflated but significant increases in these indices immediately after deflation of the tourniquet (7). Maynard et al. assessed patients undergoing unilateral total knee arthroplasty for the development of DVT using serial contrast venography. Nineteen of 42 limbs (45%) had venographically documented DVT, and two limbs (5%) had

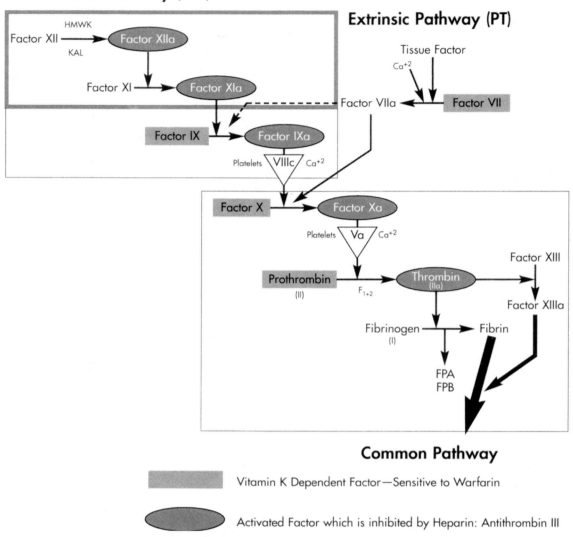

FIG. 1. Coagulation pathways. Both the intrinsic and extrinsic pathways converge, which leads to activation of factor X and the subsequent formation of thrombin. The prothrombin time (PT) measures the function of the extrinsic and common pathways. The partial thromboplastin time (PTT) measures the function of the intrinsic and common pathways. FPA, fibrinopeptide A; FPB, fibrinopeptide B; HMWK, high-molecular-weight kininogen; KAL, potassium. (Adapted from Stead RB. Regulation of hemostasis. In: Goldhaber SZ, ed. *Pulmonary embolism and deep venous thromboembolism*. Philadelphia: WB Sanders, 1985:32.)

popliteal thrombi within 24 hours after the operation. Nineteen of the 22 limbs that eventually showed a positive finding on venogram developed it within 24 hours after surgery (8). These results provide further evidence that the development of DVT occurs during the course of total knee arthroplasty and suggests that the main purpose of prophylaxis is limiting clot propagation rather than preventing clot formation.

EPIDEMIOLOGY

The prevalence of thromboembolic complications after total knee arthroplasty in the absence of prophylaxis is 40% to 80% for venographically verified postoperative DVT and 0.3% to 3.0% for pulmonary embolism (1–3). DVT usually develops locally in the areas of deep flow with frequent initiation at the valve cusp of the soleal veins or other veins in the calf. Most distal thrombi are small and clinically insignificant. Proximal venous thrombosis may also be nonocclusive and asymptomatic, but there is a strong association between proximal DVT and pulmonary embolism. Even nonocclusive, silent proximal thrombi may result in a symptomatic or fatal pulmonary embolism (4,9).

Thrombosis of the veins in the calf is generally an asymptomatic, self-limiting process that spontaneously resolves. Calf thrombi carry a low risk of embolization and chronic venous insufficiency. Extension of the distal thrombus may occur more

TABLE 1. *Risk factors for venous thromboembolic disease*

Clinical risk factors
  Advanced age
  Fractures of the pelvis, hip, femur, or tibia
  Paralysis or prolonged immobility
  Prior venous thromboembolic disease
    Surgery—operations involving the abdomen, pelvis,
      lower extremities, and abdomen
    Obesity
    Congestive heart failure
    Myocardial infarction
    Stroke
Hemostatic abnormalities (hypercoagulable states)
  Antithrombin III deficiency
  Protein C deficiency
  Protein S deficiency
  Dysfibrinogenemia
  Presence of lupus anticoagulant and antiphospholipid
    antibodies
  Myeloproliferative disorders
  Heparin-induced thrombocytopenia
  Disorders of plasminogen and plasminogen activation

frequently in patients who have had a total joint arthroplasty than in patients with other risk factors and seems to be associated with the size of the clot (4,9).

Oishi et al. used duplex ultrasonography to screen 273 consecutively treated patients who underwent total hip and knee arthroplasty to determine the prevalence and clinical course of distal DVT. In this group, 41 patients (15%) developed a distal vein thrombosis. The prevalence of deep venous thrombi was significantly higher after total knee arthroplasty (23%) than after total hip arthroplasty (9%). Follow-up duplex scans were performed at 7 and 14 days postoperatively on all patients with initially positive scan findings. Of these patients, 7 (17%) had evidence of proximal propagation by postoperative day 14 (9).

Factors associated with the development of venous thromboembolism include advanced age, prior venous thromboembolism, prolonged immobilization, varicose veins, obesity, and cardiac dysfunction (Table 1). These risk factors are often present in patients undergoing total knee arthroplasty. Even in the absence of these risk factors, however, all patients undergoing a total knee arthroplasty are at increased risk for development of DVT or pulmonary embolism. Prophylaxis is mandatory in these patients (3,4).

DEEP VEIN THROMBOSIS PROPHYLAXIS AFTER TOTAL KNEE ARTHROPLASTY

A variety of pharmacologic and mechanical approaches have been used to decrease the risk of venous thromboembolism after total knee arthroplasty. The pharmacologic approaches have included administration of warfarin sodium, low-molecular-weight heparins (LMWHs), standard heparin sodium, and aspirin. Mechanical approaches have included early mobilization, use of graded compression stockings, use of sequential intermittent pneumatic compression boots, and intermittent plantar compression. In addition, there are a number of new agents with significant clinical potential that are presently being analyzed.

Randomized clinical trials are the gold standard for assessing the efficacy of any therapeutic modality. Fortunately, there have been a number of well-designed clinical trials evaluating the efficacy of different prophylactic regimens. There are some caveats that must be noted when reviewing these studies. First, because symptomatic pulmonary emboli are relatively rare events, venographically documented asymptomatic DVT is used as a surrogate outcome measure. However, the clinical relevance of asymptomatic distal thrombi has not been established. Second, there are no large randomized trials evaluating the efficacy of these agents in limiting the formation of symptomatic DVT or pulmonary emboli after total knee arthroplasty that would provide more valuable information for the clinician. Third, the assessment of bleeding complications usually involves either relatively inaccurate measurements of blood loss or arbitrary criteria that have been established to define major blood loss. Finally, few studies have evaluated either wound drainage or wound appearance, both of which are important to surgeons.

Warfarin

Warfarin blocks the transformation of vitamin K in the liver and thereby inhibits production of vitamin K–dependent clotting factors II, VII, IX, and X (10). Warfarin has been shown to be a safe and effective prophylactic agent after total knee arthroplasty for the past 30 years (1,4,11). The major advantages of warfarin prophylaxis include oral administration and low cost. Prophylaxis with warfarin is usually initiated with a 5- or 10-mg dose either the evening before or the evening of the operation. In the past, subsequent doses were determined by measuring the prothrombin time (PT), and the target PT level for low-dose warfarin prophylaxis was 1.3 to 1.5. The anticoagulant effect associated with a particular PT level varies in different institutions, however, depending on the thromboplastin sensitivity. Presently, the international normalized ratio (INR) is used to determine anticoagulation levels because it incorporates a correction factor, the international sensitivity index, into the PT ratio to account for differences in thromboplastin reactivity. Therefore, the INR represents the PT ratio that would have been measured if the international reference thromboplastin had been used rather than a local reagent (1,10). The target INR is 2.0 (range, 1.8 to 2.5) to provide effective prophylaxis and to limit bleeding complications.

Since 1993, six randomized trials have been published comparing the efficacy of adjusted low-dose warfarin (INR = 2.0 to 3.0) and different LMWHs as prophylactic agents after total knee arthroplasty (11–16). In these trials, postoperative venography was used to determine the prevalence of clot formation. The results of these trials reveal a significantly higher risk of overall asymptomatic DVT formation when using warfarin than when using LMWHs (Table 2). Postoperative DVT prevalence rates with low-dose warfarin prophylaxis range from 38% to 55%. However, there was no significant difference between warfarin and LMWHs in symptomatic proximal clot formation or rates of symptomatic pulmonary embolism. The LMWHs were associated with increased bleeding complications. One study showed an increase in the incidence of major bleeds (13); in another study there was a significantly increased risk of hemorrhage at the operative site (17); and three studies found a significant increase in blood loss or transfusion requirements among patients receiving an LMWH (3,13,16,17).

The clinical significance of the thrombi that were noted in these studies is difficult to ascertain because almost all of these

TABLE 2. *Prophylaxis with warfarin versus low-molecular-weight heparin after total knee arthroplasty[a]*

Study	No. patients	Successful venography	DVT (%) Overall	DVT (%) Proximal	Pulmonary embolism (%)	Bleeding (%)
Hull et al. (13)						
Warfarin sodium	324	277	54.9	12.3	0.0	2.4
Logiparin (14)	317	258	45.0	7.8	0.0	4.4
RD heparin						
Warfarin sodium	147	147	41.0	10.0	0.0	NA
RD heparin (twice daily)	150	150	25.0	6.0	0.0	NA
Hamulyak et al. (15)						
Warfarin sodium	61	NA	37.7	9.8	0.0	1.3
Nadroparine	65	NA	24.6	7.7	0.0	2.6
Leclerc et al. (12)						
Warfarin sodium	334	211	51.7	10.4	0.9	1.8
Enoxaparin sodium	336	206	36.9	11.7	0.3	2.1
Heit et al. (16)						
Warfarin sodium	279	222	38.0	7.0	0.04	4.4
Ardeparin	277	232	27.0	6.0	0.0	7.9
Fitzgerald et al. (17)						
Warfarin sodium	176	122	45.0	11.0	0.6	3.4
Enoxaparin sodium	173	108	25.0	1.7	0.0	6.9

DVT, deep venous thrombosis; NA, not applicable.
[a]Randomized trials.

clots were asymptomatic. Postoperative venography may not be the appropriate surrogate measure to use when one is really concerned about the development of symptomatic venous thromboembolism and fatal pulmonary embolism. These asymptomatic clots may be associated with the development of chronic venous stasis disease but this has not been documented.

Low-dose warfarin prophylaxis has been used successfully at the University of California, Los Angeles, Medical Center for the past three decades. We reported the results of a series of 815 consecutively treated primary and revision total knee arthroplasty patients who received low-dose warfarin prophylaxis (11). The average time until the attainment of the target level of anticoagulation (PT ratio of 1.3 to 1.5) was 3 days. The average duration of warfarin prophylaxis was 12 days. Overall, three symptomatic pulmonary emboli occurred in 815 patients (0.3%; 95% confidence interval, 0.08% to 1.1%), and there were eight symptomatic DVTs (1%), all distal. Two patients (0.2%) died, but death was not secondary to a pulmonary emboli. Hematomas developed after surgery in 17 knees (2.5%); two of these patients required drainage of the knee (11). In another clinical trial of 257 total knee arthroplasty patients who received low-dose warfarin as prophylaxis for a mean duration of 9.8 days, the overall incidence of symptomatic venous thrombosis 90 days after surgery was only 0.8% (18). The results of these two studies demonstrate that low-dose warfarin prophylaxis is safe and effective in preventing symptomatic pulmonary embolism and symptomatic DVT after total knee arthroplasty.

A number of disadvantages are associated with warfarin prophylaxis, including the need for regular monitoring of the INR, a 1% to 5% prevalence of major bleeding, and a delayed onset of action that potentially leaves the patient unprotected during the period of greatest risk for the initiation of thrombosis (1,2,11–17). This delayed onset of action is of particular concern in total knee arthroplasty patients because most clots form during the course of the surgical procedure or in the early postoperative period (7,8). Therefore, the major goal of warfarin prophylaxis is to prevent proximal propagation of the clots. The low rates of pulmonary embolism associated with extended warfarin prophylaxis suggest that clinically silent, early thrombi may be prevented from propagating and causing a symptomatic pulmonary embolism.

Another drawback of warfarin prophylaxis is that it interacts with a large number of medications. In particular, the combination of warfarin with nonsteroidal antiinflammatory drugs has been shown to be associated with an increased risk of development of peptic ulcers (19). There are also a number of pharmacologic agents that could potentiate the effect of warfarin anticoagulation. Some of these agents are trimethoprim, phenytoin, cimetidine, and cefamandole. If patients are ingesting these drugs and warfarin at the same time, the INR must be closely monitored (2).

Heparin and Low-Molecular-Weight Heparins

Standard unfractionated heparin is a heterogeneous mixture of glycosaminoglycans. Heparin contains a unique pentasaccharide that binds antithrombin III with a high affinity. The interaction of heparin with antithrombin III accelerates the ability of heparin to inhibit the coagulation enzymes, thrombin, factor IX, and factor Xa. This anticoagulation effect requires the formation of a ternary complex by the binding of the heparin molecule with at least 18 saccharides to both thrombin and antithrombin III. Heparin molecules (i.e., LMWH) that contain fewer than 18 saccharide units are unable to bind to both thrombin and antithrombin simultaneously and are thus unable to induce thrombin inhibition (Fig. 2) (4,20).

Low-molecular-weight fractions of commercial heparin are generally prepared by either chemical or enzymatic depolymer-

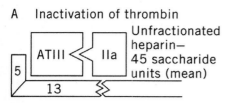

A Inactivation of thrombin

Unfractionated heparin— 45 saccharide units (mean)

- Inhibition of thrombin— binds to ATIII and to thrombin. Binding of heparin IIa is necessary for inhibition.

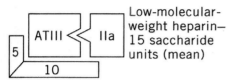

Low-molecular-weight heparin— 15 saccharide units (mean)

- No inhibition of thrombin— binds to ATIII but not to thrombin.

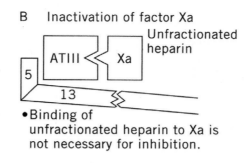

B Inactivation of factor Xa

Unfractionated heparin

- Binding of unfractionated heparin to Xa is not necessary for inhibition.

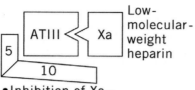

Low-molecular-weight heparin

- Inhibition of Xa— binds to ATIII.

FIG. 2. A: Inactivation of thrombin. Heparins must bind antithrombin III (ATIII) via the high-affinity pentasaccharide and thrombin through an additional 13-saccharide unit to inactivate thrombin. Low-molecular-weight heparins that do not contain 18-saccharide units bind to ATIII but not to thrombin. **B:** Inactivation of factor Xa. Heparins bind to ATIII via the high-affinity pentasaccharide to inactivate factor Xa. Both standard heparin and low-molecular-weight heparins can inactivate factor Xa. (From Hirsh J, Levine MN. Low molecular weight heparin. *Blood* 1992;79:2, with permission.)

ization of heparin. The LMWHs are relatively homogeneous in size, with molecular weights between 1,000 and 10,000 d (mean of approximately 4,500 d). The primary effect of LMWHs is the inhibition of factor Xa. Because a minimum chain length of 18 saccharides is required for ternary complex formation (heparin-antithrombin-thrombin), LMWH is able to inhibit factor Xa but not thrombin (4,20,21).

LMWHs induce less bleeding than standard heparin because inhibition of platelet function is reduced and there is also less microvascular permeability. LMWHs have a bioavailability of at least 90%, with substantially reduced binding to either plasma proteins, vascular endothelium, or other circulating cells. The prolonged half-life of LMWHs allows for once to twice per day dosing. In addition, these properties result in limited interindividual variation in antithrombotic effect. Dosages used for DVT prophylaxis do not increase the activated partial thromboplastin time, and therefore no laboratory monitoring is required (4,19,21). The LMWHs are metabolized in the kidney, and modifications in dosing are necessary in patients with elevated creatinine levels.

The LMWHs provide safe and effective prophylaxis after total knee arthroplasty. There have been a number of randomized clinical trials comparing the efficacy of the LMWHs with a placebo, unfractionated heparin, or warfarin for prevention of DVT after total knee arthroplasty. Leclerc et al. evaluated the LMWH enoxaparin sodium in a double-blind trial of 111 patients undergoing major knee surgery (80% with arthroplasty). The risk reduction in total DVT was 71% with the enoxaparin (*p* <.0001) compared to the placebo (22). Proximal vein thrombosis was documented in 19% (12 patients) of the control group and in none of the patients who received the LMWH (*p* <.001). There was no difference in bleeding in the two groups. Colwell et al. compared the LMWH enoxaparin with unfractionated heparin (5,000 U administered subcutaneously every 8 hours). The proximal and distal venous thrombosis rate was 24.6% (56 of 228) in the LMWH group and 34.2% (72 of 225) in the LMWH group. There was no difference in major bleeding episodes between the two groups (23). The use of adjusted-dose unfractionated heparin has never become popular in North

America because, in addition to causing concerns about bleeding, the regimen requires three subcutaneous injections per day and daily monitoring.

As stated previously, there have been several randomized trials comparing the efficacy of different LMWHs with warfarin. In general, the results of these studies demonstrate that LMWHs are more effective than warfarin in preventing DVT formation after total knee arthroplasty. When the results of six randomized trials assessing different LMWHs and warfarin are pooled together, the DVT rates are found to be 31.5% (388 of 1,231) and 46.2% (505 of 1,094) for the LMWHs and warfarin, respectively (3). In one study, there was a significantly lower prevalence of proximal clot formation in patients treated with enoxaparin than in those treated with warfarin (17). However, the low LMWHs appear to be associated with an increased risk of bleeding episodes compared with warfarin (11–16). There have been no randomized trials comparing the efficacy and safety of different LMWHs.

Aspirin

The role of aspirin as a prophylactic agent after total knee arthroplasty remains controversial. Aspirin irreversibly binds and inactivates cyclooxygenase in platelets. Aspirin use has been demonstrated to be associated with a relatively small reduction in risk of DVT after total knee arthroplasty compared with other agents such as warfarin, LMWH, or even compared with the use of intermittent pneumatic compression boots (3,24–26). Advantages of aspirin prophylaxis include oral administration, lack of need for laboratory monitoring, and excellent patient compliance.

Advocates of aspirin prophylaxis point to the results of the Pulmonary Embolism Prevention trial as demonstrating the efficacy of this agent in preventing symptomatic pulmonary embolism and DVT. Aspirin was effective in preventing symptomatic pulmonary embolism in hip fracture patients. The Pulmonary Embolism Prevention trial analyzed data for 17,444 patients who received either low-dose aspirin (160 mg) or placebo for

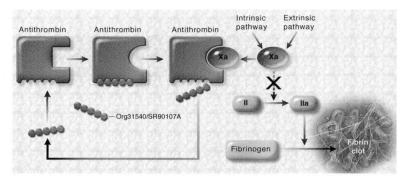

FIG. 3. The synthetic pentasaccharide fondaparinux sodium (Org31540/SR90107A) is an indirect inhibitor of activated factor X (denoted by *X*) and leads to interruption of the coagulation cascade by preventing the activation of thrombin. The synthetic pentasaccharide Org31540/SR90107A binds with high affinity to the pentasaccharide-binding site on antithrombin, producing an irreversible conformational change in antithrombin, which then binds to and inhibits activated factor Xa. The agent is then released and made available to bind to other antithrombin molecules. (From Turpie AG, Gallus AS, Hoek JA. A synthetic pentasaccharide for the prevention of deep-vein thrombosis after total hip replacement. *N Engl J Med* 2001;344:619–625, with permission.)

prophylaxis after hip fracture surgery or total hip or knee arthroplasty. Only 1,440 patients, however, were randomly assigned to receive to either aspirin (715 patients) or a placebo (725 patients) after total knee arthroplasty. Pulmonary embolism or DVT was confirmed in 23 patients (1.1%) randomly assigned to the aspirin group and 28 patients (1.4%) assigned to the placebo group. Twenty-seven percent of the patients also received other nonsteroidal antiinflammatory medications, and 35% received LMWH prophylaxis after total knee arthroplasty. There was no significant reduction in symptomatic clot formation in patients receiving aspirin (25). Clearly, more randomized trials comparing the efficacy of aspirin with LMWHs or warfarin are necessary to determine its true efficacy and its role as a prophylactic agent after total knee arthroplasty.

Fondaparinux Sodium

Fondaparinux sodium is a new agent that is an entirely synthetic pentasaccharide that is structurally related to the antithrombin binding site of heparin. The pentasaccharide selectively binds to antithrombin, causing it to rapidly inhibit factor Xa, which is a key enzyme in the coagulation pathway (Fig. 3). The agent is administered subcutaneously to patients 6 to 12 hours after the surgical procedure. Fondaparinux has been demonstrated to provide effective prophylaxis in patients undergoing total knee arthroplasty (35), hip fracture surgery (36), and total hip arthroplasty (37). This drug has now received the approval of the Food and Drug Administration.

In a double-blind randomized study, 1,049 patients undergoing elective knee surgery received either a once-daily 2.5-mg dose of the synthetic pentasaccharide fondaparinux or enoxaparin 30 mg twice daily. The group given fondaparinux had a significantly lower incidence of DVT than the group receiving enoxaparin (12.5% vs. 27.8%). There was a trend toward reduced proximal clot formation in those given fondaparinux with an overall risk reduction of 54.5% compared with enoxaparin ($p = .006$). Major bleeding was documented more frequently in the group receiving the synthetic pentasaccharide ($p = .006$). There was no significant difference in bleeding requiring reoperation. The reduction in DVT rates associated with the synthetic pentasaccharide was clearly quite impressive, particularly for total knee arthroplasty patients, but further study is required to determine its safety with regard to bleeding.

Mechanical Methods

Intermittent pulsatile compression boots and intermittent plantar compression (foot pump) are two mechanical methods that have been shown to be efficacious in limiting clot formation after total knee arthroplasty. Intermittent pulsatile compression boots prevent DVT formation by increasing the velocity of venous blood flow in the extremities, decreasing venous stasis, and enhancing endogenous fibrinolytic activity (27,28). Intermittent plantar compression of the foot simulates the hemodynamic effects that occur during normal walking, and this theoretically increases venous return (26,29). The appeal of both of these types of device is that they do not require any laboratory monitoring, there is no potential for bleeding, and they are generally well tolerated by patients. These mechanical methods of prophylaxis seem to be particularly well suited for patients undergoing total knee arthroplasty in view of concerns about the effects of bleeding and the influence of hematoma formation on postoperative range of motion (4).

The results of several randomized trials demonstrated that intermittent pneumatic compression provides effective prophylaxis in patients undergoing total knee arthroplasty (30–32). There have also been two small trials demonstrating the efficacy of the foot pump in preventing DVT after total knee arthroplasty (26,33). In all of these studies, there were significant reductions in both proximal and overall DVT rates with the use of these devices. The limitations of these mechanical devices are that the patient is receiving no prophylaxis when the device is not on, there are problems with compliance, and prophylaxis cannot be continued after hospital discharge. Large multicenter randomized trials comparing these mechanical methods to pharmacologic prophylaxis are necessary to clarify the role of these prophylactic agents.

Another potential mechanical method of prophylaxis is the use of a continuous passive motion machine after total knee arthroplasty. It has been hypothesized that the use of this device would not only maintain motion but would reduce clot formation by stimulating venous flow. In one prospective randomized study, patients who were assigned to receive treatment with a continuous passive motion device postoperatively did not experience a lower rate of thrombotic events than patients who were treated without the use of the passive motion machine (34).

New Agents on the Horizon

New antithrombotic preparations that appear to have promise as prophylactic agents are presently being tested. One agent that is presently under development is a direct oral thrombin inhibitor. Melagatran is a small molecule that provides potent, competitive, and direct inhibition of free and clot-bound thrombin. This molecule, however, must be administered parenterally. In contrast, ximelagatran is an oral prodrug that is converted to melagatran, the active metabolite. A randomized parallel dose-finding study of patients undergoing elective total knee arthroplasty was performed to determine the optimum dose of ximelagatran to use as prophylaxis against DVT. The conclusion of this study was that a fixed dose of 24 mg twice daily of unmonitored ximelagatran provides as safe and effective a prophylaxis as enoxaparin 30 mg administered subcutaneously twice daily (38). Another randomized trial comparing the efficacy of ximelagatran with that of warfarin demonstrated that ximelagatran was as safe and effective as warfarin. There was a trend toward lower overall DVT rates in the group given ximelagatran than in patients receiving warfarin prophylaxis ($p = .70$), but this difference was not statistically significant (39). This type of prophylaxis is obviously attractive to orthopedic surgeons because it is an oral agent that does not require any monitoring. However, further studies regarding the efficacy and safety of this drug are necessary for it to receive U.S. Food and Drug Administration approval.

The development of a new delivery system has made it possible to administer heparin or LMWH orally. To facilitate heparin absorption by the gut, synthetic amino acids such as sodium N-(8[2-hydroxybenzoy]amino)caprylate are used as delivery systems (40,41). Phase III trials are presently underway to assess the efficacy of this drug as a prophylactic agent for patients undergoing total hip and knee arthroplasty.

DURATION OF PROPHYLAXIS

Postoperative prophylaxis to prevent DVT formation has clearly become the standard of care after total knee and hip arthroplasty procedures. The optimal duration of treatment is not known, however. The duration of prophylaxis used by orthopedic surgeons varies considerably, although most studies recommend 7 to 14 days of therapy with either an LMWH or warfarin. In clinical practice, DVT prophylaxis is often administered only until the time of hospital discharge because of concerns about bleeding complications and patient compliance. Given the current trend toward shorter hospitalizations after total knee arthroplasty, numerous patients may receive an inadequate course of DVT prophylaxis. Previous studies have demonstrated that routine duplex ultrasonographic screening for asymptomatic DVT before hospital discharge is not effective (18,42). The question is how long patients should be given prophylaxis.

Several controlled, randomized clinical trials have directly compared extended out-of-hospital LMWH prophylaxis (at least 21 days of prophylaxis) to administration of a placebo after total hip arthroplasty and total knee arthroplasty. In most of these studies, the patients received LMWH prophylaxis during the period of hospitalization, which ranged from 4 to 15 days. At the time of hospital discharge, patients were randomly assigned to receive either extended-duration LMWH treatment or placebo for an additional 21 to 35 days (43–46). The results of these randomized trials have found that an extended regimen of LMWH prophylaxis is superior to a placebo in reducing the incidence of asymptomatic DVT events after total hip arthroplasty, but no similar benefit was noted in total knee arthroplasty patients (43–48). There have been no studies evaluating long-term prophylaxis with warfarin.

White et al. used a linked hospital discharge database provided by the state of California to identify cases diagnosed as having DVT or pulmonary embolism within 3 months of unilateral total hip or knee arthroplasty. There were 19,586 primary hip arthroplasties and 24,059 primary total knee arthroplasties. There was a low incidence of DVT or pulmonary embolism a few months after surgery of 2.8% (556 patients) after total hip arthroplasty and 2.1% (508 patients) after knee arthroplasty. The diagnosis of thromboembolism was made after hospital discharge in 76% and 47% of the total hip and knee arthroplasty patients, respectively (49). The median time to diagnosis was 17 days after total hip arthroplasty and 7 days after total knee arthroplasty. The results of these studies suggest that perhaps DVT prophylaxis regimens may have to be different for total hip and knee arthroplasty patients. This issue requires further study, but our recommendation at this time is to continue prophylaxis for at least 10 to 14 days after total knee arthroplasty.

PROPHYLAXIS IN THE HIGH-RISK PATIENT

It has been hypothesized that patients with a history of symptomatic pulmonary embolism or DVT are at an increased risk of developing symptomatic venous thromboembolic disease after total joint arthroplasty. In our evaluation of total knee arthroplasty patients, none of the patients with a prior history of symptomatic venous thromboembolic disease developed a symptomatic pulmonary embolism (11). These results suggest that these individuals may not require special prophylactic regimens, but these data must be confirmed by further studies of a larger patient population.

Despite the findings from our study, we believe that adjustments in prophylactic regimens should be considered in patients with a prior history of symptomatic venous thromboembolic disease. Consideration should be given to prolonging the duration of prophylaxis. In addition, prophylactic regimens that can be started preoperatively or have a rapid onset of action may be preferable. Therefore, if warfarin is the prophylactic regimen of choice, perhaps one should consider administering the drug the night before the procedure or in combination with an LMWH or some type of mechanical device to provide better protection for patients until the target INR is attained. Our general recommendation at this time for patients who have had a prior DVT or symptomatic pulmonary embolism is 1 month to 6 weeks of prophylaxis.

RECOMMENDATIONS

There is general agreement that patients undergoing total knee arthroplasty are at high risk of developing DVT and pulmonary embolism. Primary prophylaxis with an effective regimen is mandatory in these patients. Although none of the modalities for prophylaxis available today is ideal, there are some that safely protect patients against venous thromboembolic events. For patients undergoing total knee arthroplasty, the LMWHs, low-dose warfarin, fondaparinux, and pneumatic compression boots are effective in reducing the prevalence of pulmonary embolism and proximal clot formation. A number of randomized trials have demonstrated that LMWHs are more effective than warfarin in reducing asymptomatic clot formation, but these same agents may be associated with higher bleeding rates. There have been no significant differences noted in the rates of symptomatic pulmonary emboli in patients receiving these two agents. Mechanical devices have been shown to be effective, but there are concerns about poor compliance and limited duration of prophylaxis. Further studies are clearly necessary to determine the reduction in risk of clot formation when using devices such as pneumatic compression boots and intermittent plantar compression. The optimal duration of prophylaxis for patients undergoing hip or knee arthroplasty has not yet been determined. A number of recent studies have raised concerns about postdischarge thromboembolic events. Our present recommendation is to continue with DVT prophylaxis after total knee arthroplasty for 10 to 14 days. There are several new drugs that are being studied that also show promise as effective prophylactic agents.

REFERENCES

1. Lieberman JR, Geerts WH. Current concepts review. Prevention of venous thromboembolism after total hip and knee arthroplasty. *J Bone Joint Surg Am* 1994;76:1239–1249.
2. Lieberman JR. Warfarin prophylaxis after total knee arthroplasty. *Am J Knee Surg* 1999;12:49–53.
3. Geerts WH, Heit JA, Clagett GP, et al. Prevention of venous thromboembolism. *Chest* 2001;119[Suppl]:132S–175S.
4. Lieberman JR. Prevention of deep venous thromboembolism following primary and revision hip and knee arthroplasty. In: Bono JV, McCarthy JC, Thornhill TS, et al., eds. *Revision total hip arthroplasty.* New York: Springer-Verlag, 1999:401–417.
5. Francis CW, Ricotta JJ, Evarts CM, et al. Long-term clinical observations and venous functional abnormalities after asymptomatic venous thrombosis following total hip or knee arthroplasty. *Clin Orthop* 1988;232:271–278.
6. Stulberg BN, Francis CW, Pellegrini VD, et al. Antithrombin III/low-dose heparin in the prevention of deep-vein thrombosis after total knee arthroplasty: a preliminary report. *Clin Orthop* 1989;248:152–157.
7. Sharrock Ne, Go G, Sculco TP, Ranawat CS, et al. Changes in circulatory indices of thrombosis and fibrinolysis during total knee arthroplasty performed under tourniquet. *J Arthroplasty* 1995;10:523–528.
8. Maynard MJ, Sculco TP, Gehlman B. Progression and regression of deep vein thrombosis after total knee arthroplasty. *Clin Orthop* 1991;273:125–130.
9. Oishi CS, Grady-Benson JC, Otis SM, et al. The clinical course of distal deep venous thrombosis after total hip and total knee arthroplasty, as determined with duplex ultrasonography. *J Bone Joint Surg Am* 1994;76:1658–1663.
10. Fiore L, Deykin D. Anticoagulant therapy. In: Beutler E, ed. *Williams hematology.* New York: McGraw-Hill, 1995:1562–1583.
11. Lieberman JR, Sung R, Dorey F, et al. The efficacy of low dose warfarin prophylaxis after total knee arthroplasty. *J Arthroplasty* 1997;12:180.
12. Leclerc JR, Geerts WH, Desjardins L, et al. Prevention of venous thromboembolism after knee arthroplasty: a randomized, double-blind trial comparing enoxaparin with warfarin. *Ann Intern Med* 1996;124:619–626.
13. Hull R, Raskob G, Pineo G, et al. A comparison of subcutaneous low-molecular-weight heparin with warfarin sodium for prophylaxis against deep-vein thrombosis after hip or knee implantation. *N Engl J Med* 1993;329:1370–1376.
14. The RD Heparin Arthroplasty Group. RD heparin compared with warfarin for prevention of venous thromboembolic disease following total hip or total knee arthroplasty. *J Bone Joint Surg Am* 1994;76;1174–1185.
15. Hamulyak K, Lensing AWA, van der Meer J, et al. Subcutaneous low-molecular-weight heparin or oral anticoagulants for the prevention of deep-vein thrombosis in elective hip and knee replacement. *Thromb Haemost* 1995;74:1428–1431.
16. Heit JA, Berkowitz SD, Bona R, et al. Efficacy and safety of low molecular weight heparin (ardeparin sodium) compared to warfarin for the prevention of venous thromboembolism after total knee replacement surgery: a double-blind, dose-ranging study. *Thromb Haemost* 1997;77:32–38.
17. Fitzgerald RH Jr, Spiro TE, Trowbridge AA, et al. Enoxaparin Clinical Trial Group. Prevention of venous thromboembolic disease following primary total knee arthroplasty. A randomized multicenter, open-label, parallel-group comparison of enoxaparin and warfarin. *J Bone Joint Surg Am* 2001;83:900–906.
18. Robinson KS, Anderson DR, Gross M, et al. Ultrasonographic screening before hospital discharge for deep venous thrombosis after arthroplasty: the Post-Arthroplasty Study: a randomized, controlled trial. *Ann Intern Med* 1997:127:439–445.
19. Shorr RI, Ray WA, Daugherty J, et al. Concurrent use of nonsteroidal anti-inflammatory drugs and oral anticoagulants places elderly persons at high risk for hemorrhagic peptic ulcer disease. *Arch Intern Med* 1993;153:1665–1670.
20. Hirsh J, Warkentin TE, Shaughnesy SG, et al. Heparin and low molecular weight heparin: mechanism of action, pharmacokinetics, dosing, monitoring, efficacy and safety. *Chest* 2001;119[Suppl]:64S–94S.
21. Hirsh J, Levine MN. Low molecular weight heparin. *Blood* 1992;79:1–17.
22. Leclerc JR, Geerts WH, Desjardins L, et al. Prevention of deep vein thrombosis, double-blind trial comparing a low molecular weight heparin fragment (enoxaparin) to placebo. *Thromb Haemost* 1992;67:417–423.
23. Colwell CW Jr, Spiro TE, Trowbridge AA, et al. Efficacy and safety of enoxaparin versus unfractionated heparin for prevention of deep vein thrombosis after elective knee arthroplasty. *Clin Orthop* 1995;321:19–27.
24. Lotke PA, Palevsky H, Keenan AM, et al. Aspirin and warfarin for thromboembolic disease after total joint arthroplasty. *Clin Orthop* 1996;324:251–258.
25. Pulmonary Embolism Prevention (PEP) Trial Collaborative Group. Prevention of pulmonary embolism and deep vein thrombosis with low dose aspirin: Pulmonary Embolism Prevention (PEP) trial. *Lancet* 2000;355:1295–1302.
26. Westrich GH, Sculco TP. Prophylaxis against deep venous thrombosis after total knee arthroplasty: pneumatic plantar compression and aspirin compared with aspirin alone. *J Bone Joint Surg Am* 1996;78:826–834.
27. Allenby F, Boardman L, Pflug JJ, et al. Effects of external pneumatic intermittent compression of fibrinolysis in man. *Lancet* 1973;2:1412–1414.
28. Weitz J, Michelsen J, Gold K, et al. Effects of intermittent pneumatic calf compression on postoperative thrombin and plasmin activity. *Thromb Haemost* 1986;56:198–201.
29. Gardner AMN, Fox RH. The venous footpump: influence on tissue perfusion and prevention of venous thrombosis. *Ann Rheum Dis* 1992;51(10):1173–1178.
30. Hull R, Demore TJ, Hirsh J. Effectiveness of intermittent pulsatile elastic stockings for the prevention of calf and thigh vein thrombosis in patients undergoing elective knee surgery. *Thromb Res* 1979;16:37–45.
31. McKenna R, Galante J, Bachmann F, et al. Prevention of venous thromboembolism after total knee replacement by high-dose aspirin or intermittent calf and thigh compression. *BMJ* 1980;280:514–517.

32. Haas SB, Insall JN, Sucuderi GR, et al. Pneumatic sequential compression boots compared with aspirin prophylaxis of deep-vein thrombosis after total knee arthroplasty. *J Bone Joint Surg Am* 1990;72:27–31.

33. Wilson NF, Das SK, Kakkar VV, et al. Thrombo-embolic prophylaxis in total knee replacement: evaluation of the A-V impulse system. *J Bone Joint Surg Br* 1992;74:50–52.

34. Lynch AF, Bourne RB, Rorabech CH, et al. Deep vein thrombosis and continuous passive motion after total knee arthroplasty. *J Bone Joint Surg Am* 1988;70:11–14.

35. Bauer KA, Erickson BI, Lassen MR, et al. Fondaparinux compared with enoxaparin for the prevention of venous thromboembolism after elective major knee surgery. *N Engl J Med* 2001;345:1305–1310.

36. Lynch AF, Bourne RB, Rorabeck CH, et al. Deep-vein thrombosis and continuous passive motion after total knee arthroplasty. *J Bone Joint Surg Am* 1988;70:11–14.

37. Turpie AG, Gallus AS, Hoek JA. A synthetic pentasaccharide for the prevention of deep-vein thrombosis after total hip replacement. *N Engl J Med* 2001;344:619–635.

38. Hirt JA, Colwell CW, Francis CW, et al. Comparison of the oral direct thrombin inhibitor Ximelagatran with enoxaparin as prophylaxis against venous thromboembolism after total knee replacement. *Arch Intern Med* 2001;161:2215–2221.

39. Francis CW, Davidson BL, Berkowitz SD, et al. Randomized double-blind comparative study of H376/95, an oral direct thrombin inhibitor and warfarin to prevent venous thromboembolism after total knee arthroplasty. *Thromb Haemost* 2001;Suppl. Abstracts from the XVIII Congress of the International Society on Thrombosis and Haemostasis; July 6–12, 2001; Paris, France. CD-ROM.

40. Weitz JI, Hirsh J. New anticoagulant drugs. *Chest* 2001;119[Suppl]: 95S–107S.

41. Gonze MD, Manord JD, Leone-Bay A, et al. Orally administered heparin for preventing deep vein thrombosis. *Am J Surg* 1998;176: 176–178.

42. Ciccone WJ, Fox PS, Neumyer M, et al. Ultrasound surveillance for asymptomatic deep venous thrombosis after total joint replacement. *J Bone Joint Surg Am* 1998;80:1167–1174.

43. Planes A, Vochelle N, Darmon JY, et al. Risk of deep-venous thrombosis after hospital discharge in patients having undergone total hip replacement: double-blind randomized comparison of enoxaparin versus placebo. *Lancet* 1996;348:224–228.

44. Dahl OE, Andreassen G, Aspelin T, et al. Prolonged thromboprophylaxis following hip replacement surgery—results of a double-blind prospective, randomized placebo-controlled study with dalteparin (Fragmin). *Thromb Haemost* 1997;77:26–31.

45. Heit JA, Elliot CG, Trowbridge AA, et al. Ardeparin sodium for extended out-of-hospital prophylaxis against venous thromboembolism after total hip or knee replacement. *Ann Intern Med* 2000;132:853–861.

46. Comp PC, Spiro TE, Friedman RJ, et al. Prolonged enoxaparin therapy to prevent venous thromboembolism after primary hip or knee replacement. *J Bone Joint Surg Am* 2001;83:336–345.

47. Hull RD, Pineo GF, Stein PD, et al. Extended out-of-hospital low-molecular-weight heparin prophylaxis against deep venous thrombosis in patients after elective hip arthroplasty: a systematic review. *Ann Intern Med* 2001;135:858–869.

48. Eikelboom JW, Quinlan DJ, Douketis JD. Extended-duration prophylaxis against venous thromboembolism after total hip or knee replacement: a meta-analysis of the randomised trials. *Lancet* 2001;358:9–15.

49. White RH, Romano PS, Zhou H, et al. Incidence and time course of thromboembolic outcomes following total hip or knee arthroplasty. *Arch Intern Med* 1998;158:1525–1531.

CHAPTER 93

Blood Management

Geoffrey H. Westrich and Pamela M. Sanchez

Blood lost during orthopedic surgery is significant, especially from tissue dissection, exposure, and decortication of bone that, in itself, can produce a substantial amount of bleeding. On average, total knee arthroplasty patients lose 1,000 mL of blood in a primary cemented replacement and a minimum of 500 mL in a primary noncemented knee replacement (1,2). Consequently, blood management is essential in the knee arthroplasty patient to minimize the amount of blood loss and thus avoid the use of allogeneic transfusion.

Blood management should begin preoperatively; however, it can also be accomplished intraoperatively. The intraoperative reduction of blood lost can be managed through careful hemostasis, atraumatic technique, use of regional anesthesia, and reduction of surgical time. Cushner and Scott (3) report that the use of a cemented prosthesis, bone plugging of the intramedullary canal, and tourniquet deflation decrease the amount of blood lost intraoperatively.

Patients should be assessed preoperatively for their respective transfusion risks. Studies have demonstrated an inverse relationship between baseline hemoglobin levels and the need for postoperative blood transfusion. Specifically, patients with a baseline hemoglobin level higher than 10 g per dL but less than or equal to 13 g per dL have shown a higher probability of requiring postoperative blood transfusion than patients with a baseline hemoglobin level higher than 13 g per dL (4–8). This association supports the use of preoperative screening to identify anemic patients at risk for requiring transfusion. Specific indications for transfusion have been debated over the years; however, a general rule is to review the patient's overall health, mainly the rate of change in the hemoglobin level, including the absolute level, and the occurrence of cardiovascular symptoms such as shortness of breath, angina, hypertension, and dizziness (9).

There are two main forms of blood donation, allogeneic and autologous. Allogeneic blood donation is associated with increased risk of postoperative infection; thus, autologous blood donation has become routine practice in orthopedic surgery. Autologous blood donation can occur at different intervals preoperatively, intraoperatively, and postoperatively. In addition, the use of pharmacologic agents has been gaining popularity for their ability to increase red blood cell (RBC) mass, hemoglobin concentration, and hematocrit levels and thus decrease the requirement for postoperative allogeneic transfusion.

ALLOGENEIC BLOOD DONATION

The use of allogeneic blood donation, originally known as homologous blood donation, in orthopedic surgery cases consists of postoperative transfusion of packed RBCs (1 U = 200 to 300 mL) (9). The practice of allogeneic transfusion began during the early 1900s, and it was commonly used until the 1980s. During the 1980s, the blood-donor population decreased as a result of rising incidences of disease transmission; thus, the American Association of Blood Banks (AABB) established extensive criteria for allogeneic blood donors. These criteria include a hemoglobin level of 12.5 g per dL or higher, a minimum age of 18 years, a weight of more than 50 kg, and negative results on testing for hepatitis, syphilis, and human immunodeficiency virus (HIV) (10). According to AABB guidelines, nine tests are performed on each unit of donated blood: hepatitis B surface antigen, antibodies to the Hepatitis B core, antibodies to the hepatitis C virus, antibodies to HIV types 1 and 2, HIV type 1 p24 antigen, antibodies to human T-lymphotropic virus types 1 and 2, syphilis, nucleic acid amplification testing, and confirmatory testing (10). The risk of HIV trans-

TABLE 1. *Risks associated with allogeneic blood transfusion*

Risk	Frequency (per unit)
Disease transmission	
Human immunodeficiency virus infection	1:200,000–1:2,000,000
Hepatitis A	1:1,000,000
Hepatitis B	1:30,000–1:250,000
Hepatitis C	1:30,000–1:150,000
Transfusion reaction	
Acute lung injury	1:5,000
Acute hemolysis	1:250,000–1:1,000,000
Delayed hemolysis	1:1,000
Bacterial contamination	
Platelets	1:12,000
Red cells	1:500,000

Data from Goodnough LT, Brecher ME, Kanter MH, et al. Transfusion medicine. First of two parts—blood transfusion. *N Engl J Med* 1999;340:438–447; Fernandez MC, Gottlieb M, Menitove JE. Blood transfusion and postoperative infection in orthopedic patients. *Transfusion* 1992;32:318–322; and Wagner S. Transfusion-related bacterial sepsis. *Curr Opin Hematol* 1997;4:464–469.

mission through allogeneic transfusion has been reported to be as high as 1 in 200,000, whereas the risk of hepatitis C transmission has been reported to be as high as 1 in 30,000 (11) (Table 1).

In addition to the risk of disease transmission, allogeneic blood donation is associated with transfusion reactions such as febrile response, allergic or immune response, and hemolysis. Febrile responses consist of chills or severe pain, which can be caused by an antibody response against leukocytes in the donated blood (9,12). Immunologic incompatibilities result from the antigenic diversity that exists. Immune or allergic reactions produce symptoms such as chills, fever, and urticaria; these symptoms can occur immediately, afterward, or not at all. Immune reactions can also cause other more serious complications, for instance, hemolysis, acute lung injury, anaphylaxis, thrombocytopenic purpura, graft versus host disease, and immunodilation. A less common but more serious transfusion reaction is immediate hemolysis. Hemolysis, a potentially fatal complication, can be diagnosed with the presence of fever, chills, chest pain, circulatory collapse, hemoglobinuria, and coagulopathy (9,13). Septic shock as a result of bacterial contamination is another adverse transfusion reaction that can occur. Bacteria transmission can be linked to the donor, to contaminated blood collection equipment, or to bacterial entry after blood collection. The U.S. Food and Drug Administration reported rates of septic deaths related to platelet and red cell transfusion to be 1 in 12,000 U and 1 in 500,000 U, respectively (11).

Allogeneic transfusion is associated with a four- to tenfold higher risk of infection compared with autologous transfusion (14–17).

AUTOLOGOUS BLOOD DONATION

The donation of autologous blood can be accomplished through various methods: preoperative autologous blood dona-

tion (PAD), normovolemic hemodilution (NVHD), intraoperative blood salvage, or postoperative reinfusion. Although, PAD is the standard for many orthopedic surgeons, PAD is not cost effective relative to the use of allogeneic blood; consequently, the other techniques have received much more consideration. Nevertheless, each method has its advantages and disadvantages, as well as specific indications, which are outlined in the following sections.

Preoperative Autologous Donation

Preoperative autologous blood is best suited for elective orthopedic operations, especially when ample time exists before the surgery. Patients have their blood drawn at weekly intervals, with circumstantial donations at 3- to 5-day intervals (18,19). Preoperative autologous blood (whole blood) donation cannot occur within 72 hours of the surgery because the patient must be able to recover a sufficient amount of RBCs before surgery. Upon donation, whole blood is separated into its elements: RBCs, platelets, plasma, cryoprecipitate, and granulocytes. Each component can be transfused to different individuals, because each patient differs in specific deficiencies. To aid the RBC recovery process after PAD donation, iron supplements are prescribed to patients to be taken before and after donation. As indicated by the AABB, collected RBCs can be refrigerated for a maximum of 42 days or frozen for up to 10 years (10).

Patients who opt to donate blood must also meet standards set by the AABB; however, these standards are not as extensive as those established for allogeneic blood donors. Autologous blood donors are not limited by a minimum age or weight requirement; however, they must have a hemoglobin level higher than 11 g per dL (9,10). Certain contraindications to autologous blood donation, such as the presence of active infection or the existence of an uncontrolled cardiac disease, may be negative factors; however, this depends on the physician. Predonation nevertheless has been successful in the presence of these conditions (9,18).

Transfusion of autologous blood donated preoperatively has significant advantages over allogeneic blood transfusion. One of the main benefits is the decreased risk of disease transmission such as HIV infection and hepatitis A, B, and C. When the costs of treating the infectious diseases that can result from allogeneic blood transfusion are considered, PAD presents itself as a cost-effective option. Furthermore, PAD primes the bone marrow and commences the generation of reticulocytes before the stimulus initiated by surgical blood loss. PAD also decreases red cell mass and thus decreases the amount of RBCs lost during surgery.

Another benefit of PAD is its role as a complementary prophylaxis for deep venous thrombosis (DVT). Anders et al. reported PAD to have a significant effect on the reduction of DVT after total knee arthroplasty (20). Bae et al. (21) conducted a study comparing the DVT incidence in a group of patients who donated blood preoperatively and a group who did not donate blood before total hip arthroplasty. The patients who donated blood preoperatively experienced a statistically significantly lower rate of DVT (9.0% vs. 13.5%). In addition, a direct correlation was found between increasing preoperative hemoglobin levels and an increasing prevalence of DVT (Fig. 1) (21).

It is important to note, though, the disadvantages of autologous blood donation. First, there is room for human error, which can lead to serious mistakes such as the transfusion of incorrect autologous units or unwarranted autologous blood donation.

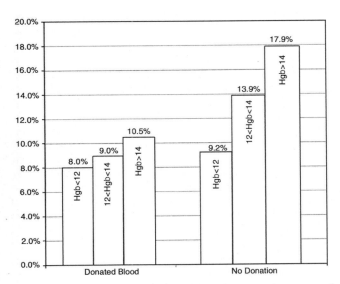

FIG. 1. Preoperative hemoglobin (Hgb) levels and incidence of deep venous thrombosis in patients who did and did not donate blood preoperatively. (From Bae H, Westrich GH, Sculco TP, et al. The effect of preoperative donation of autologous blood on deep-vein thrombosis after total hip arthroplasty. *J Bone Joint Surg Br* 2001;83:676–679, with permission.)

The risk of transfusing incorrect units has been estimated to be between 1 in 16,000 and 1 in 30,000 U (18,22–24).

Whereas cost effectiveness is an advantage of PAD, it is also a disadvantage due to the large amount of unused blood. The option of preoperative donation tends to be overused as a result of predeposition of excess blood or unwarranted predeposition of blood. It is important that guidelines be set for the amount of blood donated preoperatively to avoid waste and, most important, to avoid PAD-induced anemia and subsequently increased risk of the need for transfusion. Patients who donate blood preoperatively often do not experience an increase in erythropoietin levels or do not reach their baseline hematocrit levels before surgery; this is especially true for patients with initial hemoglobin levels lower than 13 g per dL. Hence, to avoid such circumstances, it has been recommended that primary unilateral total knee replacement patients donate between 1 and 2 U of autologous blood, knee revision patients donate at least 2 U, and bilateral knee replacement patients donate between 2 and 3 U of autologous blood (2,3,25).

Preoperative Hemodilution

Originally known for its success in prostate surgery (26), NVHD is gaining recognition for its effectiveness in orthopedic surgery. NVHD is a process, performed in the operating room, in which the concentration of erythrocytes is diluted and the hematocrit is decreased by 20% to 30% (9). After the induction of anesthesia, as many as 4 U of blood are removed, which can then be reinfused postoperatively.

The main benefit of NVHD is that the removal of blood at this time, when blood loss is minimal, decreases RBC mass and thus yields a lower RBC loss during surgery. Furthermore, the blood retrieved from NVHD is fresh and has a higher concentration of viable RBCs, platelets, and coagulation factors, none of which is present in processed units of autologous red blood cells (19,27). Another advantage of NVHD is its associated lower cost, relative to PAD (9).

NVHD is challenging to perform, however, in centers where the surgical volume is high and a rapid case turnover is necessary. For NVHD to be effective, a dedicated anesthesia team is needed, as well as careful monitoring and efficient protocol (27).

Ness et al. (26) reported that PAD and NVHD are equally effective in reducing the need for allogeneic blood transfusion in elective surgery.

Intraoperative Salvage

Intraoperative salvage, a form of autologous blood donation, is yet another alternative to allogeneic transfusion. Intraoperatively shed blood is recovered and is recycled throughout surgery for subsequent reinfusion, either as whole blood or as filtered, packed RBCs. The process of whole blood reinfusion involves suctioning blood from the wound, collecting this blood in a device, and then reinfusing the whole blood postoperatively. The shed blood collected in the device is treated with an anticoagulant such as heparin sodium, and after the shed blood is filtered, it is reinfused into the patient. The salvaged blood contains erythrocytes, platelets, fibrinogen, and clotting factors (9,28). Approximately 60% of the RBCs shed can be collected and subsequently reinfused (27). Reinfusion of unwashed shed blood has the advantages of technical ease and lower cost relative to reinfusion of filtered, packed RBCs.

Alternatively, there are devices (i.e., Haemonetics Cell Saver) that intraoperatively salvage blood, centrifuge, and subsequently wash the blood. The processed blood is then filtered and reinfused as packed RBCs. The retrieval of RBCs in this manner is said to preserve or increase the levels of 2,3-diphosphoglycerate, which is responsible for improving the ability of RBCs to deliver oxygen to tissues (29). This technique has been reported to have a 50% to 60% rate of RBC salvage (30). Devices such as the Cell Saver are cost effective when the expected blood loss is 1,000 mL or more (19) or when the expected blood loss is 20% or more of the patient's blood volume (10).

The disadvantages of devices like the Cell Saver are the associated high costs of the software used in retrieving the blood and the trained technician or physician required to supervise the procedure. This method is not as applicable in total knee replacement surgeries with tourniquet use, because patients must have a significant amount of blood loss to prime the system. Furthermore, this technique should not be used in patients with active infection or neoplasm.

Postoperative Salvage

Wound drainage fluid can also be collected in the early postoperative period and subsequently be reinfused. Blood lost in the early postoperative period is collected in a drainage tube at the surgical site and is then transfused into the patient. The blood transfused into the patient can be washed or unwashed; however, in most cases unprocessed blood is reinfused. The reinfusion of washed blood is associated with high costs; on the other hand, it is considered the safest method of reinfusion.

Reinfusing unwashed RBCs is gaining popularity in orthopedic cases (31); however, controversy exists regarding the quality of the blood. Many opponents of this technique believe that the wound drainage is contaminated with bone debris, fat particles, free hemoglobin, fibrin and fibrinogen degradation products, vasoactive agents, infection, or tumor (9,27,28,31). The presence of these superfluous particles can result in complications such as hyperthermia, hypotension, changes in vital signs, or increased levels of interleukins 1α, 1β, 6, and 8 (9,27,28,32).

To reduce the postoperative complication rate resulting from reinfusion of unwashed blood, it is recommended that the amount of blood be limited to 2 U and that it be transfused to the patient within 4 to 6 hours after the initiation of collection (9,10).

Although this technique has demonstrated a reduction in allogeneic blood transfusion requirements, the amount of RBCs lost in the early postoperative period is minimal compared to the total RBCs lost throughout patient hospitalization. Umlas et al. (33) reported that only 16% of the blood loss in unilateral knee arthroplasty patients occurs in the perioperative period.

PHARMACOLOGIC AGENTS

Erythropoietin and vasopressin are examples of pharmacologic agents whose objective is to decrease transfusion risks by decreasing the amount of surgical blood loss.

Recombinant Human Erythropoietin (Epoetin Alfa)

Erythropoietin is a natural glycoprotein secreted by the kidneys that stimulates RBC production. Recombinant human erythropoietin, epoetin alfa, is identical to the natural form of erythropoietin. Epoetin alfa has been approved by the U.S. Food and Drug Administration to treat anemia associated with renal failure (as well as acquired immunodeficiency syndrome and nonmyeloid malignant disease) (8), as it increases preoperative RBC mass, hemoglobin concentration, and hematocrit level. In addition, epoetin alfa is suitable for operations in which there is a significant, predicted blood loss, as in complex joint revision, bilateral joint arthroplasty, or spinal fusion surgeries.

Recombinant human erythropoietin is an effective blood management tool when used in conjunction with PAD or when used exclusively. Orthopedic patients are more prone to have an insufficient amount of RBCs; thus, a treatment for anemia minimizes their risk of requiring perioperative allogeneic transfusion. PAD patients tend to have lower postoperative hematocrit values; consequently, they are more likely to be transfused earlier and more frequently than non-PAD patients. Administration of epoetin alfa mitigates PAD-induced anemia by increasing RBC mass when blood donation immediately precedes the erythropoietin injection. When used along with PAD, erythropoietin injections produce a greater amount of donated blood. In a study performed by Goodnough et al. (34), patients who received erythropoietin donated an average of 5.4 U of blood preoperatively, whereas patients who received a saline injection donated an average of 4.1 U of blood preoperatively. Erythropoietin also reduces the need for allogeneic transfusion in those who cannot participate in PAD programs, such as Jehovah's Witnesses who refuse blood transfusions due to religious policy.

Epoetin alfa treatment has two variable categories: (a) subcutaneous versus intravenous administration, and (b) daily doses versus weekly doses. Subcutaneous injection is preferable because the drug has a longer circulating half-life than an intravenous dose (approximately four times as long). The weekly regimen is administered in doses of 300 to 600 U per kg, by intravenous or by subcutaneous injection, 3 weeks before surgery and on the day of surgery, for a total of four doses. The single-dose amount is widely disputed, but the standard is 600 U per kg. The daily regimen is also administered by intravenous or subcutaneous injection, in doses of 300 U per kg for 10 days preoperatively, on the day of surgery, and 4 days postoperatively, for a total of 14 to 15 doses. There has been no reported difference in the effectiveness of the daily and weekly regimens; however, a weekly regimen is more patient friendly, mainly because of the total number of doses administered. A weekly regimen has the potential for a maximum total dose of 2,400 U per kg, whereas a daily regimen has the potential for a maximum total dose of 4,500 U per kg; thus, the weekly regimen is the most cost-effective option because treatment costs are on a per-dose basis. Erythropoietin treatment is also supplemented by iron sulfate, which is taken throughout the treatment period.

Numerous studies have evaluated the efficacy of perioperative administration of epoetin alfa in patients undergoing elective surgery. Patients who received epoetin alfa experienced a 50% reduction in risk of requiring allogeneic transfusion compared with placebo-treated patients (4,6,7). There is recent work demonstrating the efficacy of erythropoietin in between stages of two-stage exchange for infected total hip and total knee arthroplasties.

Erythropoietin treatment is still under much investigation to evaluate its efficacy. In addition, epoetin alfa treatment may not be cost efficient. Hospitals have reported epoetin alfa costs to be higher than $200 per dose.

Vasopressin

Studies have shown that vasopressin is effective in reducing the amount of surgical blood loss; however, more research is needed before vasopressin can be recommended as a blood management tool.

CONCLUSION

Blood management is essential in knee surgery, especially due to the potential amount of blood loss and the risks of allogeneic transfusion. Patients are likely to be anemic after surgery; therefore, consideration of the blood management tools discussed should be part of the preoperative evaluation.

Allogeneic transfusion should be avoided if possible in elective orthopedic surgery. Consequently, this chapter has evaluated the various autologous blood donation mechanisms, as well as the pharmacologic agents that are used to treat anemia. With regard to autologous blood donation, preoperative blood donation is the most efficient option provided that strict guidelines are used with respect to the number of blood units collected. Collecting an excessive number of units places the patient at greater risk of needing postoperative transfusion. In addition, collection of an unwarranted number of units creates a surplus of blood that generally goes to waste.

Recombinant human erythropoietin, a pharmacologic agent, is also an effective and proactive measure in treating anemia. Although erythropoietin has been approved by the U.S. Food and Drug Administration to treat anemia associated with renal failure, it is still under investigation regarding its role in orthopedic surgery. In addition, this treatment is expensive.

REFERENCES

1. Pope RO, Corcoran S, McCaul K, et al. Continuous passive motion after primary total knee arthroplasty. Does it offer any benefits? *J Bone Joint Surg Br* 1997;79:914–917.

2. Yasher AA, Colwell CW. Postoperative management and rehabilitation. In: Lotke PA, Garino JP, eds. *Revision total knee arthroplasty.* Philadelphia: Lippincott–Raven Publishers, 1999:311–327.

3. Cushner FD, Scott WN. Evolution of blood transfusion management for a busy knee practice. *Orthopedics* 1999;22:S145–S147.

4. Canadian Orthopedic Perioperative Erythropoietin Study Group. Effectiveness of perioperative recombinant human erythropoietin in elective hip replacement. *Lancet* 1993;341:1227–1232.

5. Carson JL. Morbidity risk assessment in the surgically anemic patient. *Am J Surg* 1995;170:32S–36S.

6. Faris PM, Ritter MA, Abels RI. The effects of recombinant human erythropoietin on perioperative transfusion requirements in patients having a major orthopaedic operation. The American Erythropoietin Study Group. *J Bone Joint Surg Am* 1996;78:62–72.

7. Faris PM, Spence RK, Larholt KM, et al. The predictive power of baseline hemoglobin for transfusion risk in surgery patients. *Orthopedics* 1999;22:S135–S140.

8. Spence RK, Cernaianu AC, Carson J, et al. Transfusion and surgery. *Curr Probl Surg* 1993;30:1101–1180.

9. Lemos MJ, Healy WL. Blood transfusion in orthopaedic operations. *J Bone Joint Surg Am* 1996;78:1260–1270.

10. Walker RH. *American Association of Blood Banks technical manual,* 11th ed. Bethesda, MD: American Association of Blood Banks, 1993:1–29.

11. Goodnough LT, Brecher ME, Kanter MH, et al. Transfusion medicine. First of two parts—blood transfusion. *N Engl J Med* 1999;340:438–447.

12. Goodnough LT, Shuck JM. Risks, options, and informed consent for blood transfusion in elective surgery. *Am J Surg* 1990;159:602–609.

13. Pisciotto PT. Transfusion reactions. In: Pisciotto PT, ed. *Blood: transfusion therapy. A physician's handbook*, 3rd ed. Arlington, VA: American Association of Blood Banks, 1989:77–85.

14. Blumberg N, Triulzi DJ, Heal JM. Transfusion-induced immuno-modulation and its clinical consequences. *Transfus Med Rev* 1990;4:24–35.

15. Fernandez MC, Gottlieb M, Menitove JE. Blood transfusion and postoperative infection in orthopedic patients. *Transfusion* 1992;32:318–322.

16. Mezrow CK, Bergstein I, Tartter PI. Postoperative infections following autologous and homologous blood transfusions. *Transfusion* 1992;32:27–30.

17. Murphy P, Heal JM, Blumberg N. Infection or suspected infection after hip replacement surgery with autologous or homologous blood transfusions. *Transfusion* 1991;31:212–217.

18. Hatzidakis AM, Mendlick RM, McKillip T, et al. Preoperative autologous donation for total joint arthroplasty. An analysis of risk factors for allogenic transfusion. *J Bone Joint Surg Am* 2000;82:89–100.

19. Sculco TP. Global blood management in orthopaedic surgery. *Clin Orthop* 1998;357:43–49.

20. Anders MJ, Lifeso RM, Landis M, et al. Effect of preoperative donation of autologous blood on deep-vein thrombosis following total joint arthroplasty of the hip or knee. *J Bone Joint Surg Am* 1996;78:574–580.

21. Bae H, Westrich GH, Sculco TP, et al. The effect of preoperative donation of autologous blood on deep-vein thrombosis after total hip arthroplasty. *J Bone Joint Surg Br* 2001;83:676–679.

22. Linden JV, Kaplan HS. Transfusion errors: causes and effects. *Transfus Med Rev* 1994;8:169–183.

23. Linden JV, Paul B, Dressler KP. A report of 104 transfusion errors in New York State. *Transfusion* 1992;32:601–606.

24. Yomtovian R. Autologous transfusion complications. In: Popovsky MA, ed. *Transfusion reactions*. Bethesda, MD: American Association of Blood Banks, 1996:237–280.

25. Jankiewicz JJ, Sculco TP, Ranawat CS, et al. One-stage versus 2-stage bilateral total knee arthroplasty. *Clin Orthop* 1994;309:94–101.

26. Ness PM, Bourke DL, Walsh PC. A randomized trial of perioperative hemodilution versus transfusion of preoperatively deposited autologous blood in elective surgery. *Transfusion* 1992;32:226–230.

27. Sculco TP. Blood management in orthopedic surgery. *Am J Surg* 1995;170:60S–63S.

28. Keeling MM, Schmidt-Clay P, Kotcamp WW, et al. Autotransfusion in the postoperative orthopedic patient. *Clin Orthop* 1993;291:251–258.

29. Silva R, Moore EE, Bar-Or D, et al. The risk:benefit of autotransfusion—comparison to banked blood in a canine model. *J Trauma Injury Infect Crit Care* 1984;24:557–564.

30. McMurray MR, Birnbaum MA, Walter NE. Intraoperative autologous transfusion in primary and revision total hip arthroplasty. *J Arthroplasty* 1990;5:61–65.

31. Jensen CM, Pilegaard R, Hviid K, et al. Quality of reinfused drainage blood after total knee arthroplasty. *J Arthroplasty* 1999;14:312–318.

32. Goodnough LT, Verbrugge D, Marcus RE. The relationship between hematocrit, blood lost, and blood transfused in total knee replacement. Implications for postoperative blood salvage and reinfusion. *Am J Knee Surg* 1995;8:83–87.

33. Umlas J, Foster RR, Dalal SA, et al. Red cell loss following orthopedic surgery: the case against postoperative blood salvage. *Transfusion* 1994;34:402–406.

34. Goodnough LT, Rudnick S, Price TH, et al. Increased preoperative collection of autologous blood with recombinant human erythropoietin therapy. *N Engl J Med* 1989;321:1163–1168.

35. Wagner S. Transfusion-related bacterial sepsis. *Curr Opin Hematol* 1997;4:464–469.

CHAPTER 94

Clinical Pathways and Cost Efficiency for Total Knee Arthroplasty

William L. Healy, Paul D. Warren, and Richard Iorio

During the early 1990s, health care expenses in the United States increased to 14% of the gross domestic product. Health care economists and government officials studied this unprecedented rise in health care expenditures, and they told Americans the health care delivery system was inefficient and too much money was being spent on health care. The Clinton administration tried to reengineer the health care economy with broad legislation designed to develop a market-oriented health care system based on managed competition. Although the Clinton health plan failed in Congress, Americans endorsed the concept of market-oriented health care and health care reform. The agents of health care reform in this "era of economic accountability" (25) were managed care, Medicare reform, and managed Medicare.

Concurrent with the development of economic accountability in health care, public expectations for high-quality health care increased. Americans wanted better access to health care, technologic improvements in care, and lower costs for health care. This demand for high-quality, cost-effective care stimulated the development of clinical guidelines and critical pathways in medicine. This chapter discusses clinical pathways and cost efficiency in total knee arthroplasty.

ECONOMICS OF TOTAL KNEE ARTHROPLASTY

Total knee arthroplasty is among the most successful medical and surgical treatments developed during the twentieth century. Total knee arthroplasty successfully relieves pain, corrects deformity, and improves function for patients with painful, arthritic knees. More than 90% of patients with knee replacements are expected to have good to excellent results for 10 or more years. In 2000, 335,176 total knee arthroplasty procedures were performed in the United States (22). This number is likely to increase based on a 16.3% increase in the American population during the 1990s and the increased average age of the population documented by the 2000 census (3). Furthermore, the baby boom generation is moving into the "knee replacement years."

In addition to being popular and clinically successful, knee replacement operations are expensive. Total joint arthroplasty of the hip and knee is one of the largest expense categories for Medicare, and expenditures for total joint arthroplasty are increasing. During the 1990s, health care payers targeted total knee arthroplasty for cost control.

In general, hospital reimbursement for knee replacement operations is currently based on case-price payment. Medicare, which pays for two-thirds of the total knee arthroplasty operations in the United States, pays hospitals for these operations according to Diagnosis Related Group (DRG) 209 case payment. All expenses related to the hospital cost of the total knee arthroplasty operation must be deducted from the fixed amount of payment dollars. Profit or loss depends on whether expenses exceed payment. At present, hospital expenses are increasing due to labor shortages, new pharmaceuticals, new services, and inflation, but hospital payment for total knee arthroplasty operations is not increasing. The Centers for Medicare and Medicaid Services decreased hospital payment for total knee arthroplasty (DRG-209) by 1.8% to $9,057 on October 1, 2001 (22). Hospital payment for total knee arthroplasty by Medicare and other health care payers is not keeping pace with inflation.

To deliver total knee arthroplasty operations without losing money, hospitals developed cost-reduction programs. These cost-reduction programs were designed to reduce use of supplies and services required to deliver an operation or reduce the unit costs of supplies and services required to deliver the operation. Development of clinical pathways was one of the early cost-reduction programs designed to reduce the use of hospital resources for total knee arthroplasty. Several of the desired outcomes of clinical pathways for knee replacement were to reduce use of supplies, reduce hospital length of stay, and reduce hospital cost.

Another method of reducing hospital cost for total knee arthroplasty is to reduce the unit cost of supplies and services required for the operation. The largest single unit cost for total knee arthroplasty is the cost of the knee implants (1,12). Implant cost-reduction methods include vendor discounts, implant standardization, consignment negotiations, price caps, competitive bid purchasing, and single price/case price purchasing (14). Hospitals that controlled their cost for knee implants were able to control or reduce the overall hospital cost for total knee arthroplasty.

Cost efficiency for total knee arthroplasty is achieved when minimal hospital resources are used and low prices are paid for the supplies and services required to deliver high-quality knee replacement operations. Healy et al. studied hospital costs for total joint arthroplasty after early hospital cost-reduction programs were implemented. Eighty percent of hospital costs for total joint replacement operations are incurred during the first 48 hours of hospitalization in the operating room, recovery room, nursing units, and pharmacy. The largest direct cost in the operating room is the cost of the knee implant. This study suggests that control of the hospital cost for total knee arthroplasty should focus on the first 48 hours of hospitalization and on the cost of knee implants. This analysis further suggested that when length of stay is reduced to 6 days or fewer, incremental savings are difficult to achieve by further reducing length of stay (13). Stern et al. studied the hospital cost of total knee arthroplasty and reported that control of the hospital cost of total knee replacement surgery might be best achieved by controlling the direct cost of implants and supplies rather than by reducing hospital length of stay (28). At present, control of hospital cost for surgical procedures requires control of use and control of unit costs for the supplies and services required to deliver the operation.

CLINICAL PATHWAYS IN HEALTH CARE

A clinical pathway is an algorithm developed for a specific diagnosis or procedure that establishes a standardized, streamlined plan of care for designated patient populations from preadmission to postdischarge (9). The pathways may also include tracking mechanisms and outcome measures. Synonyms for clinical pathways include care maps, care continuum, algorithms, guidelines, practice parameters, and protocols (16). A clinical pathway is designed as a flow chart. The clinical pathway concept originated in methods used for guiding complex engineering and construction projects (23). The goals of clinical pathways include improvement in quality of care, enhanced interdisciplinary practice, standardization of care delivery, reduction of unnecessary variation in care, reduction of hospital length of stay, improved patient outcomes, increased patient satisfaction, and reduction of cost for care.

Clinical pathways were first used in health care in the 1980s to map the care of hospital inpatients, improve efficiency, and reduce the unit cost of care (17,27). At present, most health care organizations recognize the wisdom of pathway planning in an effort to minimize the use of resources, supplies, and time; reduce duplication and variation; and enhance overall efficiency in the care of patients.

Clinical pathways represent a method of quality improvement technique used in industry called *total quality management*. Clinical pathways are the application of total quality management principles to clinical care. There is a shared premise that quality improvement can be achieved through reduction in process variation (7,11).

For a clinical pathway process to be effective, it should be comprehensive, multidisciplinary, and based on evidence and consensus, and it should have administrative support. Individuals from each discipline and hospital department who encounter the particular patient group or participate in their care should be involved in developing, evaluating, and modifying the clinical pathway. The hospital administration should provide appropriate resources, including designated personnel and support for progressive information systems (18). The process of establishing a clinical pathway fosters better intra- and interdisciplinary communication (11). In 1995, 80% of health care organizations used clinical pathways as demonstrated in a national poll of 188 health care providers. Most of the remaining 20% planned to use pathways in the near future (16).

A segment of most clinical pathways focuses on education of the patient and his or her family regarding the disease or procedure in question. Patient education is achieved with monographs, brochures, videotapes, and interpersonal sessions such as one-on-one counseling, group classes, or seminars. Patients who attend preadmission classes and information seminars have been reported to have shorter hospital stays (8).

Patient and family satisfaction can be enhanced by clinical pathways, which create an opportunity to address specific and individual concerns. Tahan et al. suggest the use of separate patient and family pathway versions. The family version reinforces the important information in the patient's care, using a language understood by everyone, that is, it "does not exceed the fourth-grade level." A layperson-friendly version of the clinical pathway improves patient and family understanding of the care to be rendered (29).

From time to time, some physicians consider clinical pathways as intrusions into the practice and art of medicine that reduce patient care to the level of "cookbook medicine." Pathways and algorithms may threaten a physician's autonomy, ability to innovate, and ability to vary patient care to meet the specific needs of their patients. Physicians who evaluate clinical pathways with an open mind, however, frequently realize that patient care can be improved by a hospital and staff committed to the clinical pathway process.

Clinical pathways define the processes, time lines, and responsibilities associated with a patient's clinical needs from preadmission to postdischarge. In such a setting, everyone involved in treating the patient understands what is to be done, by whom, and when. Clinical pathways allow physicians to plan ahead and educate patients and families regarding reasonable expectations, which results in less patient worry and confusion. However, not all patients are candidates for clinical pathways. Physicians and hospitals need to recognize when a patient requires individualized care that varies from the clinical pathway. Variation allows patients in unique circumstances to deviate from the pathway. Later in the care episode, the patient can return to the care plan (19).

In an era of economic accountability in health care in general and orthopedic surgery in particular, orthopedic surgeons have compelling reasons to learn the basic principles of quality management and cost management. As a patient advocate, a surgeon must balance the role of physician and businessman. The primary goal for orthopedic surgeons in the new millennium should be to create and maintain quality in musculoskeletal care. A second but possibly equally important goal is to control the cost of care delivered.

A financial benefit of using clinical pathways is that they enable health care institutions to predict costs and thus accurately to bid to obtain managed care contracts. The adherence to a clinical pathway may also serve as a marketing tool to attract more managed care contracts (29). The adherence to clinical pathways demonstrates to managed care organizations the commitment of the hospital and various disciplines to achieve both cost-effective and high-quality patient care.

LAHEY CLINIC CLINICAL PATHWAY FOR TOTAL KNEE ARTHROPLASTY

The Lahey Clinic clinical pathway for total knee arthroplasty begins when an orthopedic surgeon and a patient decide to schedule a knee replacement operation. The pathway stresses education of both patients and families. The clinical pathway focuses on virtually all aspects of patient care, and it includes both an acute and a postacute plan of care (Figs. 1 and 2). Total knee arthroplasty patients at the Lahey Clinic are usually discharged to home on postoperative day 4 or to a postacute care facility on postoperative day 3. The pathway arranges for the involvement of appropriate consulting services, including social services for discharge planning, the primary care physician, the physical therapy department for total knee protocol and continuous passive motion monitoring, and phlebotomy services for routine laboratory studies. The pathway provides guidelines for the nursing staff for most nursing care concerns, including the use of antithrombotic measures such as thromboembolic disease stockings and Venodyne devices, surgical site examination, patient safety, nutrition, medication, and elimination issues. Variance from the pathway is documented.

Adherence to the clinical pathway for total knee arthroplasty at the Lahey Clinic has been associated with a reduction in length of hospital stay and a reduction in hospital costs. Between 1992 and 1995, use of the pathway was associated with a decrease in length of stay from 6.79 days to 4.16 days, and with a 19% reduction in hospital costs for total knee arthroplasty. No significant adverse short-term patient outcomes have been associated with the clinical pathway (15). Other studies confirm these results, reporting overall reductions in total hospital costs ranging from 11% to 19% (20,21). The overall average length of stay for all knee replacement operations at the Lahey Clinic in 2000 was 4 days.

Use of the clinical pathway for knee replacement at the Lahey Clinic was associated with a change in the disposition of patients from the acute care hospital. In 1992, 39.3% of patients were discharged to rehabilitation hospitals. In 1995, 99.1% of patients were discharged to rehabilitation hospitals. This practice of early discharge to rehabilitation hospitals or skilled nursing facilities enables patients to leave acute care hospitals earlier than if they were discharged to home. When patients were discharged to postacute care facilities, the acute care hospital collected the full case price payment and reduced the expenses for service. This practice

has been called *cost shifting* because the patients generate new costs at the postacute care facility. The practice of cost shifting has been discouraged by the Balanced Budget Act of 1997, which imposed financial penalties on hospitals when DRG-209 patients were discharged to postacute care facilities earlier than the average Centers for Medicare and Medicaid Services length of stay for DRG-209. In 2000, 24% of knee replacement patients were discharged from the acute care hospital to home and 76% were discharged to postacute care facilities. Managed care organizations have developed home care programs to avoid the use of rehabilitation facilities. It remains to be seen how effective these programs are, and their influence on the outcome of total knee arthroplasty needs to be measured.

CLINICAL PATHWAY OUTCOMES

Clinical pathway implementation can result in better, more cost-effective medical care. The use of clinical pathways is associated with reduced length of hospital stay for hip and knee replacement operations in several well-documented studies (8,21). After implementation of a clinical pathway for total knee arthroplasty, Mabrey et al. reported a 57% reduction in length of stay from 10.9 days in 1994 to 4.7 days in 1996 (20). Earlier ambulation after total joint arthroplasty has also been associated with clinical pathway implementation. Analysis showed that time to ambulation was the only significant contributor to reduction in length of stay in the clinical pathway group compared with a control group (8).

Clinical pathways have successfully addressed use, variation, and cost in health care. However, patient satisfaction has also been improved by the use of clinical pathways. With pathway implementation, patients believe that they have an increased level of participation in their care. Patient satisfaction is critical to achieve a quality outcome, and the patient's perception of involvement or participation enhances the patient's satisfaction, continued well-being, and health status (2,4,10,26).

The impact of clinical pathways on postoperative complications after total joint arthroplasty is not clear. Some studies have shown no difference in the prevalence of postoperative complications (24), whereas other studies of joint replacement clinical pathway patients suggest that fewer complications occur in clinical pathway patients (8). Mabrey et al. found that patients using a total knee arthroplasty clinical pathway were 4.6 times less likely to experience a complication than patients not using the pathway (20). Pearson et al. noted that reducing the length of hospital stay with a clinical pathway has not been associated with an increase in readmissions or complications within 6 months (24). Dowsey et al. reported a 4.3% readmission rate for knee replacement patients managed with a clinical pathway and a 13% readmission rate for knee replacement patients managed without a clinical pathway (8). They suggest that readmission and complication rates during a follow-up period of 3 months after discharge are lower in total joint arthroplasty patients following a clinical pathway (8).

LEGAL RAMIFICATIONS AND BENEFITS OF CLINICAL GUIDELINES AND PATHWAYS

The implementation of clinical pathways has created medical-legal concerns for some physicians. The concern involves

TOTAL KNEE ARTHROPLASTY

Lahey Clinic
DEPARTMENT OF ORTHOPAEDIC SURGERY

PATIENT: _____ LAHEY CLINIC # _____ SURGEON: _____

	Operative Decision for TKA 4–6 W	PREOP VISIT (completed by 1 week preop)	DAY OF SURGERY	PO DAY 1	PO DAY 2
CONSULTATIONS	•Orthopaedic Surgeon	•Social Service •Consult Primary Care M.D. •Physical Therapy		•S.S. •P.T. in A.M. •O.T. consult for ADLs if plan d/c to home	•P.T.
PROCEDURES & TESTS	•HADF	•Pre-Admission Testing •H & P •Begin Autologous Blood Donation/ Collection	**OPERATION – TKA** •TKA Standard Post-Op Orders (attached) •Autologous blood available	•CBC, PT, PTT, lytes, BUN, Cr in AM	•CBC, PT, PTT, lytes, BUN, Cr in AM

TREATMENTS			•VS q shift
			•Incentive spirometry
			•TED stockings bilaterally
			
			Assess:
			  •Pulses
			  •Neurosensory
			  •Presence of Homans sign
			  •Skin
			  •Bowel sounds
				•VS q shift
				•Incentive spirometry
				•TED stockings bilaterally
				•Continue assessments
				
				Exercises:
				  •Quad & Ham sets
				  •Supine AA to active hip/knee flexion
				  •AA→AROM with involved knee
				  •Dangle
				  •ROM BID
				  •Transfers/Ambulation
					•VS q shift
					•Incentive spirometry
					•TED stockings bilaterally
					•Continue assessments
					
					Exercises:
					  •Quad & Ham sets
					  •SLR
					  •Supine AA to active hip/knee flexion
					  •AA→AROM with involved knee
					  •Dangle
					  •ROM BID
					  •Transfers/Ambulation

ACTIVITIES			•Bedrest with CPM 20 out of 24 hours when ordered by surgeon •CPM 15 sec extension pause	•Transfer to bed/chair •Ambulate with walker •Sit in chair •Full WBAT •CPM when in bed as ordered by surgeon	•OOB B.I.D. with walker •Transfer training •Ambulate •RN to get pt. OOB to chair for meals •CPM when in bed as ordered by surgeon

MEDICATION			**Analgesia:**
			  •IM
			  •PO
			  •IV – PCA (per anesthesia)
			•IV antibiotics postop x 24 hours
			•Anticoagulation therapy
				Analgesia:
				  •IM
				  •PO
				  •IV – PCA (per anesthesia)
				•IV antibiotics
				•Anticoagulation therapy
					•Pain medication
					•Anticoagulation therapy

FIG. 1. Guidelines and clinical pathways for total knee arthroplasty patients. AA, active-assistive; ADL, activities of daily living; AROM, active range of motion; BUN, blood urea nitrogen; CBC, complete blood count; CPM, continuous passive motion; Cr, creatinine; DAT, diet as tolerated; d/c, discharge; D/C, discontinue, discharge; dsg, dressing; f/u, follow-up; HADF, hospital admission data form; H & P, history and physical; HL, heparin lock; INR, international normalized ratio; IPN, integrated progress note; MOM, milk of magnesia; OOB, out of bed; OT, occupational therapy; PCA, patient-controlled analgesia; PO, postoperative; pt., patient; PT, prothrombin time, physical therapy; PTT, partial thromboplastin time; ROM, range of motion; SLR, straight leg raise; S.S., social services; TED, thromboembolic disease; THR, total hip replacement; TKA, total knee arthroplasty; VS, vital signs; WBAT, weightbearing as tolerated. (From the Lahey Clinic, with permission.)

TKA

DISCHARGE RN:_____

PO DAY 3	PO DAY 4	PO DAY 5	OUTCOMES
•P.T.	•P.T.	*Discharge by 12 noon.*	
•PT/INR in AM	•PT/INR in AM	•PT/INR in AM	
•VS q shift •Continue assessments •Incentive spirometry •TED stockings bilaterally •Wound exam & Dsg change **Exercises:** •Quad & Ham sets •SLR •Supine AA to active hip/knee flexion •AA→AROM with involved knee •Dangle •ROM BID •Transfers/Ambulation	•VS q shift •Continue assessments •Incentive spirometry •TED stockings bilaterally •Wound exam & Dsg change **Exercises:** •Quad & Ham sets •SLR •Supine AA to active hip/knee flexion •AA→AROM with involved knee •Dangle •ROM BID •Transfers/Ambulation	•VS q shift •Continue assessments •Incentive spirometry •TED stockings bilaterally •Wound exam & Dsg change **Exercises:** •Quad & Ham sets •SLR •Supine AA to active hip/knee flexion •AA→AROM with involved knee •Dangle •ROM BID •Transfers/Ambulation	•Patient has TED stockings on bilaterally as ordered and understands importance. •Patient understands exercise program - (Quad & Ham sets) • ROM is a priority • Ambulation
•Ambulate with walker or crutches •OOB T.I.D. and P.R.N. •RN to get pt. OOB to chair for meals •CPM when in bed as ordered by surgeon	•Stairs with crutches if plan discharge home •Independent ambulation on level floor with crutches •Full review of exercises •RN to get pt. OOB to chair for meals •CPM when in bed as ordered by surgeon	•Full review of home exercise program and precautions •ROM goal for discharge home is >90 degrees flexion and <5 degrees extension •RN to get pt. OOB to chair for meals •CPM when in bed as ordered by surgeon	
•Pain medication • Anticoagulation therapy	•Pain medication • Anticoagulation therapy	•Pain medication • Anticoagulation therapy	•Patient receiving anticoagulation therapy as ordered. •Patient has a coumadin teaching booklet. •PT/INR f/u sent with patient if D/C to rehab.

Patient Stamp

DISCHARGE DATA

REASON FOR ADMISSION
☐ Primary TKA
☐ Revision TKA
☐ Fracture
☐ Complication of TKA

TYPE OF ADMISSION
☐ Elective
☐ Urgent
☐ Emergency
☐ Readmission within 4 weeks

Admission date_____ DC date____
Date of Surgery_____ LOS_____

Number of autologous blood units donated
☐ 0
☐ 1
☐ 2
☐ 3
☐ >3

Number of autologous units used
☐ 0
☐ 1
☐ 2
☐ 3
☐ >3

Number of homologous blood units used
☐ 0
☐ 1
☐ 2
☐ 3
☐ >3

Total # of visits by Physical Therapy
_____

Was knee arc of motion >90 degrees flexion and <5 degrees extension on discharge?
☐ YES
☐ NO

DISCHARGE DISPOSITION
☐ Home
☐ Home with services
☐ Post acute care facility

*Cut along dotted line

FIG. 1. *Continued.*

SAFETY			•Needs assessed •Fall Risk Safety Guide	•Assess q shift •Fall Risk Safety Guide
NUTRITION			•P.O. fluids as tolerated	•Clear liquid diet • IV to HL when tolerating p.o. fluids >500cc in 8 hours.
ELIMINATION			•Foley catheter to gravity PRN •MOM q.h.s. till bowel movement	•D/C Foley at 6:00 A.M.(if present) (Due to void by 14:00) •MOM q.h.s.until bowel movement
PATIENT EDUCATION	•Patient education •Admission process letter	•Teach patient the expected goals and activities	•Needs assessed	•Review of THR safety precautions •Patient given coumadin teaching booklet
DISCHARGE PLANNING		•Discharge plan reviewed with patient and/or caregiver		•Discharge plan reviewed with patient and/or caregiver
	ON TARGET ____ *VARIANCE ____ *Documentation in IPN required	ON TARGET ____ *VARIANCE ____ *Documentation in IPN required	ON TARGET ____ *VARIANCE ____ *Documentation in IPN required	ON TARGET ____ *VARIANCE ____ *Documentation in IPN required
SIGNATURES	_____ _____ _____ _____	_____ _____ _____ _____	_____ _____ _____ _____	_____ _____ _____ _____

Lahey Clinic guidelines and pathways are designed to assist clinicians by providing an analytical framework are not intended to replace a clinician's judgment or to establish a protocol for all patients with a particular more than one appropriate approach for a given medical condition.

FIG. 1. *Continued.*

adherence to and deviation from pathways, and the potential of a malpractice claim if an unexpected, unfavorable result occurs. However, these concerns may not be warranted. A clinical pathway is a guideline for care. Variation from the pathway to meet the specific and unique needs of a patient is expected. In the course of delivering care, a physician has the opportunity to document the reasons for a deviation from a pathway (5,19).

Clinical pathways, which are developed by a multidisciplinary care team and implemented as a clinical guideline, should minimize risk of malpractice litigation. Clinical pathways may be considered the standard of care in a medical community. As the law evolves to a national standard of care, however, clinical pathways should be reviewed annually and improved with new information obtained from a review of the literature (5). Each discipline represented in patient care should benefit from adherence to established protocols as well as from continuing review and process improvement (29).

Defensive medicine is frequently cited as one of the reasons for the rapidly increasing rate of health care expenditures. Defensive medicine is defined as "care that does not benefit the patient, and is provided solely to avoid malpractice claims" (6). It has been estimated that defensive medical costs, when computed as a percentage of physician and hospital malpractice insurance premiums, range from $5 billion to $15 billion per year (6). Efforts to reduce these costs would likely slow the rate of increase of health care system costs. Adherence to clinical pathways could be helpful in this endeavor. Clinical pathways serve as standards of care, reduce the uncertainty of treatment decisions, and free physicians from having to practice defensive medicine (11).

The inclusion of a disclaimer within the text of the clinical pathway documentation can be helpful in reducing the chances of malpractice claims. The objective of adding a disclaimer is to reduce the number of situations in which breach of warranty may occur. It allows practitioners the right to deviate as necessary from the rigidity of a pathway to meet the needs of individual patients (29). A disclaimer on each pathway lessens the risk of liability claims. Furthermore, if unique patient circumstances indicate the need for deviation from the standard of care, the reasons should be documented. This documentation should strengthen the doctor's position (5).

•Assess q shift •Fall Risk Safety Guide	•Fall Risk Safety Guide	•Fall Risk Safety Guide	•Fall Risk Safety Guide	•Patient understands fall risk safety.
•Advance to DAT if BS ⊕	•DAT	•DAT	•DAT	•Patient is tolerating diet as ordered.
•If no bowel movement — suppository or Fleets •MOM q.h.s. until bowel movement	•If no bowel movement — suppository or Fleets •MOM q.h.s. until bowel movement	•If no bowel movement — suppository or Fleets •MOM q.h.s. until bowel movement		•Patient has had a bowel movement prior to discharge.
•Review coumadin teaching	•Instruct in home exercise program if plan to d/c patient to home	•Review home exercise program if plan to d/c patient to home	•Review home exercise program if plan to d/c patient to home	•Patient understands importance of ROM.
•PT/INR f/u information •SS and PT to formalize / recommended discharge (Home vs. Rehab) •D/C summary for patients to rehab on eve of discharge. •Complete patient care referral forms			•Discharge	•Patient understands outpatient anticoagulation management
ON TARGET ____ *VARIANCE ____ *Documentation in IPN required	ON TARGET ____ *VARIANCE ____ *Documentation in IPN required	ON TARGET ____ *VARIANCE ____ *Documentation in IPN required	ON TARGET ____ *VARIANCE ____ *Documentation in IPN required	
_____ _____ _____ _____ _____	_____ _____ _____ _____ _____	_____ _____ _____ _____ _____	_____ _____ _____ _____ _____	

for the diagnosis and treatment of specific medical problems. They may be used for patient education and assist in planning future care. They condition. In many circumstances, individual patients will not fit the clinical conditions contemplated by a guideline. Usually there is

FIG. 1. *Continued.*

The state of Minnesota has passed legislation requiring hospitals to implement clinical pathways (11). It has been suggested that the statutory adoption by states of clinical guidelines for inpatient hospital care can be cited as affirmative defenses in physician and hospital malpractice suits. Adherence to these clinical pathways is believed to demonstrate that physicians and hospitals have met the requisite standard of care. Adherence to the specified clinical practice guideline could be raised only by the defense. If a physician had felt the need to deviate from the guidelines, he or she would not introduce the guidelines as an affirmative defense. Adherence to clinical practice guidelines over a 5-year period could reduce defensive medicine costs by 25%. Costello et al. suggested that, if physicians and hospitals had a clear indication of the standards by which their cases would be judged, they would be more willing to accept certain limitations imposed by guidelines (6).

Education of both patients and families, which is associated with patient satisfaction, has clear benefits and likely minimizes the risk of malpractice claims. Satisfaction during the course of the patient and family encounter is affected by many factors.

Several factors under the influence of health care practitioners that can be affected by the implementation of clinical pathways are using a proactive approach to the identification of patient needs and foreseeable problems and ensuring patient and family awareness of the initiation of clear and appropriate efforts at resolution of any such problems. Patient and family acknowledgment and understanding of the proposed pathway allow them to make educated and well-informed decisions about the rendered care. This involvement makes the patient and family more satisfied and minimizes the risk of malpractice claims (5).

CONCLUSION

Implementation of clinical pathways for knee replacement operations enhances the quality of patient care while reducing resource use and cost. The benefits of clinical pathways include optimization of resources, time, and personnel for the treatment; increased patient satisfaction; standardization of the care process for medical and nonmedical personnel; and potential medical-legal benefits for physicians and hospitals.

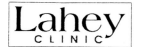

Total Knee Arthroplasty
Recommended Post-Acute Plan of Care
February 12, 2002

Patient: _____ Date of Surgery: _____

	PO DAY 4	PO DAY 5	PO DAY 6	PO DAY 7
ACTIVITIES	**PT** • Ambulate—WBAT Review Lahey Clinic's TKA exercises • Progress to crutches Stairs with crutches when able • Transfer Independence **OT** • ADLs • Out of bed for meals	**PT** • Ambulate—WBAT Review Lahey Clinic's TKA exercises • Progress to crutches Stairs with crutches when able • Transfer Independence **OT** • ADLs • Out of bed for meals	**PT** • Ambulate—WBAT Review Lahey Clinic's TKA exercises • Progress to crutches Stairs with crutches when able • Transfer Independence **OT** • ADLs • Out of bed for meals	**PT** • Ambulate—WBAT Review Lahey Clinic's TKA exercises • Progress to crutches Stairs with crutches when able • Transfer Independence **OT** • ADLs • Out of bed for meals
TREATMENTS	• Wound check & dressing change • TED stockings bilaterally • Heel roll on affected side to maximize extension • Exercises: Supine AA to A • Hip / knee flexion • SLR • AA to AROM with involved knee • ROM goal: >90° flexion <5° extension	• Wound check & dressing change • TED stockings bilaterally • Heel roll on affected side to maximize extension • Should have 80° flexion • Exercises	• Wound check & dressing change • TED stockings bilaterally • Heel roll on affected side to maximize extension • Exercises	• Wound check & dressing change • TED stockings bilaterally • Heel roll on affected side to maximize extension • Exercises **MUST** have 90° flexion prior to discharge; **If not, call MD**
TESTS	PT / INR	PT / INR		PT / INR
MEDICATION	• Anticoagulation therapy • Any other ordered medications	• Anticoagulation therapy • Any other ordered medications	• Anticoagulation therapy • Any other ordered medications	• Anticoagulation therapy • Any other ordered medications
SAFETY	Needs Assessed	Needs Assessed	Needs Assessed	Needs Assessed
NUTRITION	Diet as Ordered	Diet as Ordered	Diet as Ordered	Diet as Ordered
PATIENT TEACHING	• Needs assessed • Review Total Knee Precautions: 1. Avoid low chairs 2. Avoid slippery surfaces which may cause the knee to give way 3. Avoid twisting the knee for 6–8 weeks 4. Avoid sitting longer than 45 minutes at a time	• Needs assessed • Review Total Knee Precautions	• Needs assessed • Review Total Knee Precautions	• Needs assessed • Review Total Knee Precautions

FIG. 2. Postacute plan of care for total knee arthroplasty patients. AA, active-assistive; ADL, activities of daily living; D/C, discontinue; DVT, deep venous thrombosis; INR, international normalized ratio; OT, occupational therapy; PO, postoperative; PT, prothrombin time, physical therapy; R/O, rule out; ROM, range of motion; SLR, straight leg raise; TED, thromboembolic disease; TKA, total knee arthroplasty; WBAT, weightbearing as tolerated. (From the Lahey Clinic, with permission.)

Date of Discharge from Hospital: _____   Date of Arrival to Post-Acute Care Facility: _____

PO DAY 8	PO DAY 9	PO DAY 10	PO DAY 11
PT • Ambulate—WBAT Review Lahey Clinic's TKA exercises • Progress to crutches Stairs with crutches when able • Transfer Independence **OT** • ADLs • Out of bed for meals	**PT** • Ambulate—WBAT Review Lahey Clinic's TKA exercises • Progress to crutches Stairs with crutches when able • Transfer Independence **OT** • ADLs • Out of bed for meals	**PT** • Ambulate—WBAT Review Lahey Clinic's TKA exercises • Progress to crutches Stairs with crutches when able • Transfer Independence **OT** • ADLs • Out of bed for meals	**PT** • Ambulate—WBAT Review Lahey Clinic's TKA exercises • Progress to crutches Stairs with crutches when able • Transfer Independence **OT** • ADLs • Out of bed for meals
• Wound check & dressing change • TED stockings bilaterally • Exercises	• Wound check & dressing change • TED stockings bilaterally • Exercises	• Wound check & dressing change • TED stockings bilaterally • Exercises ROM Goal: 100° flexion 0–5° extension **Call MD if not achieved**	• Wound check & dressing change • TED stockings bilaterally • Exercises
	PT / INR		**PT / INR**
• Anticoagulation therapy • Any other ordered medications	• Anticoagulation therapy • Any other ordered medications	• Anticoagulation therapy • Any other ordered medications	• Anticoagulation therapy • Any other ordered medications
Needs Assessed	Needs Assessed	Needs Assessed	Needs Assessed
Diet as Ordered	Diet as Ordered	Diet as Ordered	Diet as Ordered
• Needs assessed • Review Total Knee Precautions	• Needs assessed • Review Total Knee Precautions	• Needs assessed • Review Total Knee Precautions	• Needs assessed • Review Total Knee Precautions

FIG. 2. *Continued.*

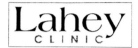

Total Knee Arthroplasty
Recommended Post-Acute Plan of Care
February 12, 2002

Patient: _____ Date of Surgery: _____ Date of Discharge from Hospital: _____

	PO DAY 12	PO DAY 13

ACTIVITIES	**PT**
	• Ambulate – WBAT
	  Review Lahey Clinic's TKA exercises
	• Progress to crutches
	  Stairs with crutches when able
	• Transfer Independence
	
	OT
	• ADLs
	• Out of bed for meals
		PT
		• Ambulate – WBAT
		  Review Lahey Clinic's TKA exercises
		• Progress to crutches
		  Stairs with crutches when able
		• Transfer Independence
		
		OT
		• ADLs
		• Out of bed for meals

TREATMENTS	• Wound check & dressing change • TED stockings bilaterally • Exercises	• Wound check & dressing change • TED stockings bilaterally • Exercises
TESTS		PT / INR
MEDICATION	• Anticoagulation therapy • Any other ordered medications	• Anticoagulation therapy • Any other ordered medications
SAFETY	Needs Assessed	Needs Assessed
NUTRITION	Diet as Ordered	Diet as Ordered
PATIENT TEACHING	• Needs assessed • Review Total Knee Precautions	• Needs assessed • Review Total Knee Precautions

FIG. 2. *Continued.*

Date of Arrival to Post-Acute Care Facility: _____

PO DAY 14	* OUTCOMES AT DISCHARGE TO HOME

PT
• Ambulate — WBAT
  Review Lahey Clinic's TKA exercises
• Progress to crutches
  Stairs with crutches when able
• Transfer Independence
 	
OT
• ADLs
• Out of bed for meals
	• Assist to single assist device (cane) as
	  tolerated — after 2 – 4 weeks
	• Safe ambulation on level, slopes and stairs
	  according to weight bearing orders
	• Able to do Lahey Clinic's TKA exercises
	  independently
	• Home safe for ADL

• Wound check & dressing change
• TED stockings bilaterally
• Exercises
 	
• **ROM goal:**
  100° + flexion
  0–5° extension
	• Staple removal and steri-strips applied to
	  wound POD# 10–14
	• Clinically evaluate to R/O DVT
	• POD# 10–14
	  D/C Coumadin
	  Start Ecotrin 325 mg 1 PO BID until
	  6 weeks postop
	• TED stockings bilaterally for 6 weeks

• Anticoagulation therapy
• Any other ordered medications
	• If patient is discharged before POD# 14,
	  they must remain on Lahey Clinic's
	  anticoagulation protocol through
	  POD# 14

Needs Assessed	Home Safety
Diet as Ordered	Arrangements for nutrition in place
• Needs assessed • Review Total Knee Precautions	Patient understands Lahey Clinic Total Knee Precautions

FIG. 2. *Continued.*

REFERENCES

1. *Am Acad Orthop Surg Bull* January 1996;44(1).
2. Blegen MA, Reiter RC, Goode CJ, et al. Outcome of hospital-based managed care: a multivariate analysis of cost and quality. *Obstet Gynecol* 1995;86(5):809–814.
3. Census gain largest ever. *Boston Globe* April 3, 2001:A4.
4. Brody DS, Miller SM, Lerman CE, et al. Patient perception of involvement in medical care: relationships to illness attitudes and outcomes. *J Gen Intern Med* 1989;4:506–511.
5. Brugh LA. Automated clinical pathways in the patient record: legal implications. *Nurs Case Manag* 1998;3(3):131–137.
6. Costello M, Murphy KM. Clinical guidelines: a defense in medical malpractice suits. *Physician Exec* 1995;21(8):10–12.
7. Deming WE. *Out of the crisis.* Washington: W. Edwards Deming Institute, 1986:cp 2.
8. Dowsey MM, Kilgour ML, Santamaria NM, et al. Clinical pathways in hip and knee arthroplasty: a prospective randomized controlled study. *Med J Aust* 1999;170:59–62.
9. Graybeal KB, Gheen M, McKenna B. Clinical pathway development: the Overlake Model. *Nurs Manage* 1993;24(4):42–45.
10. Greenfield S, Kaplan S, Ware JE. Expanding patient involvement in care: effects on patient outcomes. *Ann Intern Med* 1985;102:520–528.
11. Hardt R, Musfeldt C. MD-directed critical pathways: it's time. *Hospitals* 1992;66:56.
12. Healy WL, Finn D. The hospital cost and the cost of the implant for total knee arthroplasty. *J Bone Joint Surg Am* 1994;76:801–806.
13. Healy WL, Iorio Richard, Richards JA, et al. Opportunities for control of hospital costs for total joint arthroplasty after initial cost containment. *J Arthroplasty* 1998;13(5):504–507.
14. Healy WL, Iorio R, Lemos M, et al. Single price/case price purchasing in orthopaedic surgery: experience at Lahey Clinic. *J Bone Joint Surg Am* 2000;82(5):607–612.
15. Healy WL, Iorio R, Ko J, et al. Impact of cost reduction programs on short-term outcome and hospital cost of total knee arthroplasty. *J Bone Joint Surg Am* 2002;84-A(3):348–353.
16. Howe JG, Lambert B. Critical pathways in total hip arthroplasty. In: Callaghan JJ, Rosenberg AG, Rubash HE, eds. *The Adult Hip.* Philadelphia: Lippincott–Raven Publishers, 1998: 865–870.
17. Isozaki LF, Fahndrick J. Clinical pathways—a perioperative application. *AORN J* 1998;67:376, 379–386, 389–392.
18. Krampf L. Physician-led teams develop critical pathways. *OR Manager* 1995;11:28–30.
19. Lowe C. Care pathways: have they a place in "the new National Health Service"? *J Nurs Manag* 1998;6:303–306.

20. Mabrey JD, Toohey JS, Armstrong DA, et al. Clinical pathway management of total knee arthroplasty. *Clin Orthop Relat Res* 1997;345:125–133.

21. Macario A, Horne M, Goodman S, et al. The effect of a perioperative clinical pathway for knee replacement surgery on hospital costs. *Anesth Analg* 1998;86:978–984.

22. Mendenhall S. *Orthop Network News* 2001;12:19.

23. Patterson P. ORs streamline patient care, control resource utilization. *OR Manager* 1994;10:1–7.

24. Pearson S, Moraw I, Maddern GJ. Clinical pathway management of total knee arthroplasty: a retrospective comparative study. *Aust N Z J Surg* 2000;70:351–354.

25. Relman AS. Assessment and accountability. *N Engl J Med* 1988;319(18):1220–1222.

26. Rost K. The influence of patient participation on satisfaction and compliance. *Diabetes Educ* 1989;15(2):139–143.

27. Sommers LS, Schurman DJ, Jamison JQ, et al. Clinician-directed hospital cost management for total hip arthroplasty patients. *Clin Orthop Relat Res* 1990;258:168–175.

28. Stern SH, Singer LB, Weissman SE. Analysis of hospital cost in total knee arthroplasty: does length of stay matter? *Clin Orthop* 1995;321:36.

29. Tahan HA. The multidisciplinary mandate of clinical pathways enhancement. *Nurs Case Manag* 1998;3(1):46–51.

CHAPTER 95

Preoperative Medical Evaluation

Anthony B. Fiorillo and Francis X. Solano, Jr.

This chapter acquaints the reader with an approach to the patient undergoing knee replacement, describes strategies for preoperative assessment, and discusses the management of common medical conditions in the perioperative period.

The preoperative assessment of patients undergoing knee replacement follows the basic principles of preoperative assessment of patients undergoing anesthesia and noncardiac surgery. Inherent in this population are comorbid conditions that may increase their surgical risk. The goal of preoperative assessment is to identify the patient's known and occult medical conditions, optimize medical care, and intervene with therapy to improve the surgical outcome. An added benefit is the chance for the assessing physician to share with the patient the risk and benefit of surgery given his or her comorbid conditions.

The most important tools of preoperative assessment are the history and physical examination. History can predict fitness in 96% of general surgical patients (1). The findings of the history and physical examination direct the physician in efficient use of preoperative laboratory tests and diagnostic studies. The elderly orthopedic population presents a challenge in that a patient's history may not adequately predict risk due to the functional limitations of the joint disease. This is especially true with regard to cardiac and pulmonary assessment.

LABORATORY TESTING

There have been many studies addressing the utility of routine laboratory testing for surgical patients (1–4). The laboratory findings add a new diagnosis in 0.7% of patients (1). Twenty percent of patients show abnormal results on screening studies. For 40%, studies are ordered for a recognizable indication. It is important to realize that, statistically, 5% of patients on a given test fall outside the reference range (5). On a standard 20-item chemistry panel, 64% of patients in a healthy population will have at least one abnormal finding.

The next important question is, How do these abnormal results influence surgical risk? In many studies that have looked at this issue, the answer is a resounding, "Very little!" The chance of finding a significant laboratory abnormality that will affect the surgical outcome is much lower than 1%. Most clinicians are now using selective testing in their approach to preoperative assessment of patients (3).

The complete blood count is important in orthopedic patients, because many of these patients have been on nonsteroidal antiinflammatory agents, which can result in iron deficiency anemia owing to indolent gastrointestinal bleeding. Patients with inflammatory arthritides can have anemia of chronic disease. Both situations can cause severe anemia (hemoglobin level less than 8 g per dL) that impacts surgical risk. Knee replacement and knee revision arthroplasty can be associated with significant blood loss, so it is important to have a baseline value. Studies on the preoperative value of the white blood cell count have demonstrated an abnormality rate in the range of 0.0% to 9.5%. Severe abnormalities are uncommon (less than 0.7%). In orthopedic patients who have rheumatoid arthritis (RA), leukopenia may be found (but infrequently) with Felty syndrome in the setting of splenomegaly. Leukopenia resulting from the use of drugs such as methotrexate sodium, gold, and nonsteroidal antiinflammatory agents can also be seen, but this is uncommon. Leukocytosis caused by steroid use is also possible, but it is uncommon in patients on low-dose corticosteroids (less than the equivalent of 7.5 mg prednisone every day) for inflammatory arthritis. Abnormal platelet counts are seen in 0.0% to 11.8% of patients. Severe abnormalities con-

TABLE 1. *Preoperative testing schedule*

Preoperative condition	HCT	PT	PTT	Na, K	Creat, BUN	Glucose	Radiography	EKG	Urine pregnancy test	T/SS
Procedure with blood loss	X									X
Procedure without blood loss										
40–49 yr								X[a]		
50–64 yr								X		
65 yr and older					X			X		
Cardiovascular disease										
Hypertension										
Mild										
Moderate to severe							X	X		
Congestive heart failure	X						X	X		
Ischemic heart disease	X							X		
Vascular disease										
Carotid disease								X		
Abdominal aorta disease								X		
Peripheral vascular disease								X		
Pulmonary disease							X	X		
Hepatic disease	X	X								
Renal disease	X			X	X					
Suspected pregnancy									X	
Diabetes				X	X	X		X		
Use of diuretics				X	X					
Use of digoxin				X	X			X		
Use of steroids				X		X				
Use of carbamazepine (Tegretol)				X						
Use of warfarin sodium (Coumadin)		X								
Use of heparin sodium			X							

BUN, blood urea nitrogen; Creat, creatinine; EKG, electrocardiogram; HCT, hematocrit; PT, prothrombin time; PTT, partial thromboplastin time; T/SS, type and screen units of red blood cells.

[a] Men.

tributing to an increased risk of bleeding are uncommon. In the postoperative period, patients who have undergone knee arthroplasty occasionally have thrombocytopenia caused by consumptive coagulopathy, and they require platelet transfusion. It is therefore reasonable to obtain a baseline platelet count.

Chemistry studies to assess renal function, hepatic enzyme abnormalities, serum glucose levels, and electrolyte abnormalities also are of limited usefulness as screens for asymptomatic disease. Renal function, however, can be adversely affected in older patients, in those who have congestive heart failure (CHF), and in those who are taking nonsteroidal antiinflammatory agents. Therefore, it is important to assess renal function in patients such as these who will undergo knee replacement. Liver enzyme abnormalities in orthopedic patients are also uncommon, but hepatitis secondary to acute viral disease and alcohol use can have adverse effects on morbidity and mortality. Therefore, the history should identify patients with these risk processes. Although the prevalence of type 2 diabetes can approach 5% in the adult population, identifying it preoperatively has not been shown to benefit the surgical outcome. Suggestions of wound healing difficulties in patients with poorly controlled diabetes have been supported by *in vitro* studies (6), but the impact in orthopedic patients undergoing joint replacement has not been investigated. Abnormalities in leukocyte phagocytosis and antibody response to Gram-positive organisms may be impaired when serum glucose level exceeds 250 mg per dL. This degree of poor control may also predispose the patient to

postoperative sepsis due to Gram-negative organisms (7). Coronary artery disease is four times more prevalent in patients with established diabetes than in age-matched controls, and it may account for an increase in perioperative ischemia and myocardial infarctions (MIs) (8).

Coagulation studies are not helpful in identifying asymptomatic patients who will have bleeding problems. Clearly, the history and physical examination are most important in assessing hemostasis. Determination of bleeding time is of little utility in predicting postoperative hemorrhage. In the orthopedic population, patients may have been taking aspirin or nonsteroidal antiinflammatory agents, which affects bleeding time.

Urinalysis is not very helpful in identifying patients at risk for infectious complications. It is difficult to demonstrate that treating a patient for asymptomatic bacteriuria will diminish the risk of knee infection. Asymptomatic bacteriuria can be found in 25% to 50% of elderly patients, and, in general, treatment does not lead to lasting cures. It is advisable to treat asymptomatic bacteriuria preoperatively, however, because many patients will undergo urologic instrumentation in the perioperative period, with postoperative catheter placement or intermittent catheterization.

Chest radiographic abnormalities are very common in patients over 60 years of age (3,9), but the influence of a preoperatively identified abnormality on the outcome of knee surgery is small (10). Although chronic obstructive lung disease changes and abnormalities consistent with heart failure may influence management decisions, the history and physical examination

TABLE 2. *Preoperative assessment classification*

ASA status	Examples of preoperative patients
Class 1: No disease	Healthy 25-yr-old
Class 2: Mild to moderate systemic disease	65-yr-old with well-controlled DM type 2
Class 3: Severe systemic disease	70-yr-old with CHF and rest angina
Class 4: Life-threatening systemic disease	30-yr-old with DM type 1 in ketoacidosis
Class 5: Morbidly ill	70-yr-old with angina and mesenteric ischemia
E is added to each class if surgery is an emergency.	

ASA, American Society of Anesthesiology; DM, diabetes mellitus; CHF, congestive heart failure.
Adapted from Dripps RD. New classification of physical status. *Anesthesiology* 1963;24:111.

remain more important in assessing pulmonary or cardiac risk than the radiograph.

The abnormal preoperative electrocardiogram (EKG) probably deserves the most attention. Up to 52.7% of patients may have an abnormality on routine EKG. Goldman (11) has demonstrated the poor predictive value of ST-segment and T-wave changes in predicting cardiac events. Detection of a silent MI based on EKG is a rare event (0.3%), but detection of an MI may have some validity in risk stratification. Patients with recent MI appear to be at highest risk for perioperative MI. Bifascicular block rarely progresses to complete heart block during surgery and is not an indication for temporary pacemaker placement.

There are other reasons to perform preoperative laboratory testing. Often, the institution in which surgery is being performed has baseline requirements that are mandated by the hospital or by the medical or anesthesia staff. Medicolegal issues, and the fear of omission, are a major reason for testing. Presently, the standards of care promoted by textbooks, physician organizations, and the current literature on laboratory testing include a selective testing approach (Table 1).

In summary, laboratory testing should be selective rather than routine in patients undergoing surgery. It is difficult to find significant abnormalities that will influence management decisions regarding surgery.

CLASSIFICATION OF RISK

The American Society of Anesthesiology has adopted Dripps's stratification system (Table 2) to predict perioperative mortality (Table 3). This system was originally designed to classify patients for a research protocol, but it was found to have predictive value for clinical outcomes.

Because there is some subjectivity in the American Society of Anesthesiology scale, other authors have sought more objective criteria for surgical risk stratification. Goldman et al. (12) and Detsky et al. (13) used multivariate analysis to stratify risk. The index of Goldman et al. was based on data collected on 1,001 consecutively treated patients admitted to their institution for a variety of nonthoracic surgeries (Table 4). They developed a multivariate point sys-

TABLE 3. *American Society of Anesthesiology status and deaths per 10,000 patients*

Class	Deaths from anesthesia	Postoperative deaths
1	1	6
2	1	47
3	29	440
4	75	2,345
5	155	5,980

Adapted from Marx GF, Mateo CV, Orkin LR. Computer analysis of postanesthetic deaths. *Anesthesiology* 1973;39:54.

tem that has been validated at other institutions as a predictor of cardiac complication after nonthoracic surgery (Table 5).

Detsky et al. (13) modified the risk index by looking at the timing of MI, current or previous pulmonary edema, Canadian Cardiovascular Society angina classification, and institution-specific complication rates for types of surgical procedures (Table 6). Using the criteria of Detsky et al., a specific cardiac risk can be assigned to the individual by plotting the summed points on a nomogram. The exact calculation is not as important as the recognition that criteria have been established and validated to allow the clinician to preoperatively estimate cardiac risk. There are limitations to applying multivariate analysis for predicting risk in a patient; many additional factors influence outcome.

The variables (or clinical parameters) of these indices offer the clinician a structure for assessment. This information can be offered to the patient, anesthesiologist, and surgeon to maximize the success of surgery. Following are some specific risk categories of patients undergoing knee replacement.

Cardiovascular Disorders

The patient undergoing knee replacement often has limited functional capacity because of age or arthritis, which makes cardiovascular fitness assessment difficult.

TABLE 4. *Goldman multifactorial risk index*

Factor	Points
Age older than 70 yr	5
Myocardial infarction within 6 mo	10
S_3 gallop or JVD	11
Significant aortic stenosis	3
Rhythm other than sinus or PACs on EKG	7
Greater than 5 PVCs per min	7
Poor medical status (PO_2 >60, PCO_2 >50, K^+ <3.0, HCO_3 <20, BUN >50, Creat >3.0 mg%, abnormal SGOT, or bedridden)	3
Abdominal, intrathoracic, or aortic surgery	3
Emergency surgery	4
Total	53

BUN, blood urea nitrogen; Creat, creatinine; EKG, electrocardiogram; JVD, jugular venous distention; PAC, premature atrial contraction; PVC, premature ventricular contraction; SGOT, serum glutamic-oxaloacetic transaminase.
Adapted from Goldman L, Caldera DL, Nussbaum SR, et al. Multifactorial index of cardiac risk in noncardiac surgical procedures. *N Engl J Med* 1977;297:845.

TABLE 5. *Goldman cardiac risk index*

Class	Points	No or minor risk (%)	Life-threatening complications (%)	Cardiac death complications (%)
I (n = 537)	0–5	532 (99)	4 (0.7)	1 (0.2)
II (n = 316)	6–12	295 (93)	16 (5)	5 (2)
III (n = 130)	13–25	112 (86)	15 (11)	3 (2)
IV (n = 18)	>26	4 (22)	4 (22)	10 (56)

Adapted from Goldman L, Caldera DL, Nussbaum SR, et al. Multifactorial index of cardiac risk in noncardiac surgical procedures. *N Engl J Med* 1977;297:845.

Stable angina has been shown not to be a risk factor for noncardiac surgery by several authors (12,13). Patients with unstable angina or angina at a low level of activity should be considered at high risk, and cardiovascular evaluation should be performed before proceeding. Recent coronary artery bypass grafting does not appear to increase risk.

Noninvasive pharmacologic stress tests using dipyridamole (Persantine) (14,15), adenosine thallium (16,17), or dobutamine hydrochloride echocardiography (18,19) have been helpful in assessing patients undergoing vascular or noncardiac surgery. Dipyridamole increases intracoronary adenosine, which leads to vasodilatation of the coronary circulation. This creates intracoronary steals in areas of fixed coronary obstruction, which results in a relative decrease in perfusion that can be detected with thallium, and more recently on echocardiography, as segmental wall motion abnormalities. These techniques have limitations, particularly in determining whom to screen and then what to do with the information obtained (14,17). All of the modalities available have good sensitivity and specificity for detection of coronary disease, but they do not give an ischemic threshold.

TABLE 6. *Detsky et al. modified multifactorial index*

Status	Points
Coronary artery disease	
MI within 6 mo	10
MI >6 mo earlier	5
CSS angina class 3	10
CSS angina class 4	20
Unstable angina within 3 mo	10
Alveolar pulmonary edema	
Within 6 mo	10
Ever	5
Valvular disease	
Suspected hemodynamically significant aortic stenosis	20
EKG	
Nonsinus or sinus rhythm, with frequent PACs on preoperative test	5
More than 5 PVCs on EKG	5
Poor medical status	5
Age >70 yr	5
Emergency operation	10
Total maximum points	125

CSS, carotid sinus stimulation; EKG, electrocardiogram; MI, myocardial infarction; PAC, premature atrial contraction; PVC, premature ventricular contraction.
Adapted from Detsky AS, Abrams HB, McLaughlin JR, et al. Predicting cardiac complications in patients undergoing non-cardiac surgery. *J Gen Intern Med* 1986;1:212.

Eagle et al. (16) validated a clinical index used in conjunction with pharmacologic stress testing. Patients were classified into low-, intermediate-, and high-risk groups based on the presence of five risk factors: age over 70, angina, prior MI, prior CHF, and diabetes mellitus. Risk factor number correlated with postoperative cardiac events. Among patients with no risk factor, 1 patient out of 29 had a cardiac event. Among patients with more than two risk factors, 50% had an event. Evaluating according to these factors put patients into risk categories correctly 71% of the time. If a patient anticipating knee surgery has risk factors for coronary events, as identified by Eagle and functional capacity is unassessable because of arthritis or age, it is advisable to perform pharmacologic stress testing.

It has been shown that there is a correlation between the degree of abnormality on thallium imaging and risk (14,19). An abnormal thallium test result with fixed defects, or an abnormal test result with reversible ischemia in one coronary territory, is not an indication for catheterization or revascularization. These patients can be treated medically and have an acceptable cardiac risk. Patients with global ischemia or with two or more significant areas of myocardium at risk should be studied with coronary arteriography before proceeding with knee replacement. As in all risk assessments, the risk of knee surgery and revascularization (angioplasty, vascular stent, atherectomy, or coronary artery bypass grafts) must be weighed against the benefit of the knee surgery itself (15,20).

Recent Myocardial Infarction

Unstable angina and a recent MI (less than 6 months previously) remain the strongest predictors of perioperative myocardial ischemia. Thus it is customary to wait until 6 months after an MI before proceeding with nonthoracic surgery. This practice is based on the work of Tahran et al. (21) in the early 1970s, and it was validated by Goldman et al. (12) during their classic preoperative study in 1977 and then by Steen et al. (22). Tahran et al. (21) studied 38,877 patients who had undergone anesthesia and found 422 with prior infarction. Of these 422, 37% had another infarction if they had surgery within 3 months of the prior infarction, 16% if the surgery was within 3 to 6 months, and 5% if the surgery was after 6 months. Tahran obtained statistically similar results again 6 years later. Rao et al. (23) used invasive hemodynamic monitoring in patients with recent MI and demonstrated a 5.7% risk of MI when surgery followed the prior MI by 3 months or less and a 2.3% risk when the surgery was within 3 to 6 months of the prior MI.

Because of increased knowledge about MI, improved hemodynamic monitoring, and availability of a larger array of cardiac medications, some have questioned the convention of waiting 6 months. Others have suggested that the location of the ischemic event has a bearing on perioperative risk; for example, an uncomplicated inferior wall MI is less risky than an anterior or lateral wall MI. Mortality from a perioperative MI remains high (50%) in some series (22). Only 50% of patients have typical chest pain and many have atypical symptoms, such as arrhythmia, confusion, hypotension, or CHF, which makes the diagnosis more challenging. Thus, although the risk of perioperative MI less than 6 months from a prior MI is probably lower than originally estimated, given the consequence of a perioperative MI, it is advisable to postpone surgery for 6 months, during which time the patient's internist or cardiologist can assess further myocardial risk and optimize medical care.

Preexisting Congestive Heart Failure

CHF can be the consequence of many forms of cardiac disease (myocardial ischemia, aortic or mitral valvular disease, arrhythmias) and noncardiac disease (hypertension, anemia, hemochromatosis). The underlying disease and cardiac function should be optimally managed before surgery. Patients who have a history of CHF have a 6% risk of recurrent CHF and a 5% mortality (12). Those patients with an S_3 gallop, jugular venous distention, or rales have a 20% mortality rate. It is important to identify the cause and to reverse the CHF, if possible. Echocardiography to assess left ventricular function and the presence of significant valvular disease can be helpful preoperatively. Patients with severe impairment of left ventricular function (ejection fraction less than 25%) are at increased risk for CHF and death. These patients should be monitored with a Swan-Ganz catheter and arterial lines. If available, transesophageal echocardiography can be used to facilitate management of fluid balance as well.

Valvular Disease

Patients with significant aortic stenosis and mitral stenosis are at greatest risk for perioperative morbidity, because these lesions tend to cause a fixed cardiac output, which in turn makes them intolerant of increased preload (excessive intravenous fluids intraoperatively) or decreased afterload (vasodilation with spinal or epidural anesthesia). Perioperative CHF, dysrhythmias, and death occur as a consequence. Patients with mitral stenosis, in particular, can have significant problems with tachyarrhythmias, which can compromise ventricular filling and lead to CHF. Because many anesthetic agents are afterload-reducing agents, regurgitant valves such as in mitral insufficiency and aortic insufficiency do well if cardiac output is preserved. These patients should receive prophylaxis for subacute bacterial endocarditis, particularly if the genitourinary tract will be manipulated in the perioperative period.

Patients with *mechanical valves* who receive warfarin sodium (Coumadin) should discontinue use 3 to 5 days in advance of surgery, and treatment should be converted to heparin sodium. Generally, the heparin can be stopped 4 to 6 hours before surgery and can be resumed within 24 hours of knee replacement. These patients should also receive subacute bacterial endocarditis prophylaxis.

Patients with *atrial fibrillation* but controlled ventricular rates generally pose no special problems. It is reasonable, however, to be concerned about the cause of the atrial fibrillation and its impact on risk. Warfarin is widely used in the treatment of atrial fibrillation to prevent stroke, and its use must be managed at the time of surgery (Table 7). In patients with only atrial fibrillation, it is generally appropriate to stop warfarin treatment 3 to 5 days in advance of surgery and to resume it on the evening of surgery. Patients who have had embolic strokes, like those who have had valve replacement, should be converted to heparin preoperatively.

Patients who have significant ventricular arrhythmias are maintained on their usual medication. If they have ectopy with normal left ventricular function and no hemodynamic compromise, their arrhythmias are not treated. Patients with implantable defibrillators should be assessed by a cardiologist so that their defibrillators can be turned off during the surgical procedure to avoid spontaneous activation by operating room equipment.

Perioperative Cardiac Therapy

The physician's ability to identify patients at risk for perioperative cardiac complication has improved significantly over the last 20 years. For those patients with recent unstable angina or MI, surgery should be postponed for 6 months and their cardiac risks stabilized. Low-risk patients with no cardiac risk factors or physical findings of left ventricular dysfunction need no further workup and should proceed with surgery. Similarly, patients with risk factors who are by history asymptomatic are also at low risk for perioperative events. Those symptomatic patients with risk factors, particularly diabetes mellitus, should be considered for cardiac testing. Before testing, the assessing physician must weigh the benefit of delaying surgery against the risk of cardiac intervention.

Until recently, limited clinical evidence has existed to support initiating new therapies to reduce the incidence of perioperative cardiac complications. These therapies fall into three categories: preoperative revascularization, perioperative medical therapy, and perioperative monitoring. Other than in the observational study of Rao et al. (23), perioperative monitoring has not been shown to reduce the incidence of perioperative events. No randomized trials have been done prospectively assessing perioperative and intraoperative monitoring in nonvascular surgery. Medical therapies that have been evaluated include use of β-blockers, calcium channel blockers, nitrates, and α-adrenergic agonists. Administration of β-blockers has been shown in two prospective blinded studies to reduce perioperative ischemia. Mangano et al. (24) administered atenolol 50 mg intravenously or orally 2 days before surgery and 7 days postoperatively in 200 high-risk patients undergoing nonvascular surgery. The group given atenolol had a significant reduction in perioperative ischemia and higher event-free survival at 6 months. Poldermans et al. (25) studied the use of bisoprolol fumarate in elective vascular surgery in patients who had many risk factors and evidence of inducible myocardial ischemia by dobutamine echocardiography. Use of bisoprolol resulted in a 91% reduction in perioperative MI or cardiac death compared with placebo.

The use of α_2-adrenergic agonists, calcium channel antagonists, and nitrates has been studied in patients at high risk for coronary disease or with known cardiac disease and has not been shown to reduce perioperative ischemia, MI, or cardiac death.

TABLE 7. *Stopping and restarting medication in the perioperative period*

Medication	Recommendation	Comment
Insulin	Half dose of NPH or lente, sliding scale	i.v. fluid D5W ~2 mL/kg/h (see text)
Oral hypoglycemic	Discontinue 1–2 d preop	Chlorpropamide long acting, stop 3 d preop
L-thyroxine	Give equal dose p.o. or i.v. day of surgery	Long-acting hormone
Propylthiouracil	Continue through morning of surgery, check level (see text)	If NPO is prolonged, administer i.v. β-blocker labetalol hydrochloride 10 mg q15min, propranolol hydrochloride 1–2 mg q1h
Estrogens		
Oral contraceptives	Stop 3 wk preop	Increased risk of thrombosis
Replacement therapy	Stop equine 1 wk preop	Transdermal may decrease thrombogenic risk
	Stop estradiol 3 wk preop	Equine estrogen 0.625 mg qd = transdermal estradiol q3d
Cardiac		
Digoxin	Continue	Check level
Antiarrhythmic agents		
Quinidine sulfate	For SVT, hold day of surgery, substitute i.v. verapamil hydrochloride	For VT, may substitute lidocaine
Procainamide hydrochloride	For SVT, hold day of surgery, i.v. available	
Amiodarone hydrochloride	Hold	T$_{1/2}$ 30–60 d, hold and resume when p.o.
Nitrates	Continue	Change from p.o. to transdermal equivalents?
Calcium channel blockers	Continue	Anesthetic complication
Diuretics	Consider discontinuing	Check K$^+$ level, assess fluid status
β-blockers	Continue	May substitute i.v. propranolol, metoprolol tartrate, or labetalol
Pulmonary	Continue all medications	If on theophylline, check level (see text)
Antihypertensives		
Diuretics	See above	
β-blockers	See above	
Calcium channel blockers	Continue	Anesthetic complication
ACE inhibitors	Continue	Check K$^+$ level, i.v. enalaprilat available
Central-acting agents	Continue, associated with withdrawal	Methyldopa, reserpine, are long-acting, clonidine withdrawal increases BP and tachycardia
Peripheral-acting agents	Continue	Prazosin hydrochloride, hydralazine hydrochloride
Perioperative urgencies	i.v. labetalol 10 mg q10min, methyldopa 250 mg q4h, nifedipine 10 mg s.l. (see text)	
Neurologics/psychotropics		
Monoamine oxidase inhibitors	May be continued with caution	Recent studies of chronic users show low complication rate; caution with narcotics
Antidepressants		
Tricyclics	Hold day of surgery	Resume postop
SSRIs	Hold day of surgery	Resume postop
Phenytoin	Continue through morning of surgery, check level	Resume postop p.o. or through NG tube; i.v. available, but has potential for cardiac toxicity
Anticoagulation with warfarin sodium		
Prosthetic mitral valve	Stop warfarin 3 d before surgery, begin i.v. heparin sodium with a PTT goal of 50–70 sec; start warfarin postop, evening of surgery	Resume heparin 6–12 h postop until INR 2.5–3.5
Prosthetic aortic valve	Stop warfarin 3 d before surgery, begin i.v. heparin with a PTT goal of 50–70 sec; start warfarin postop, evening of surgery	No heparin necessary postop
Nonvalvular atrial fibrillation	Stop warfarin 3 d before surgery; start warfarin postop, evening of surgery	No preop heparin necessary

ACE, angiotensin-converting enzyme; BP, blood pressure; D5W, 5% dextrose in water; INR, international normalized ratio; NPH, neutral protamine Hagedorn; NPO, nothing by mouth; PTT, partial thromboplastin time; SSRI, selective serotonin reuptake inhibitor; SVT, supraventricular tachycardia; T$_{1/2}$, half-life; VT, ventricular tachycardia.

Modified from Cygan R, Waitzkin H. Stopping and restarting medications in the perioperative period. *J Geriatr Med* 1987;2: 270; Guarnieri KM, Mekeon BP. *Perioperative medicine.* New York: McGraw-Hill, 1994:479.

Revascularization

In Washington State, a retrospective study was done on hospital records of patients who had undergone surgery from 1987 to 1993. The authors compared patients who had noncardiac surgery with known coronary artery disease and had recently undergone percutaneous angioplasty with similar patients who had not undergone angioplasty. Patients who underwent revascularization by percutaneous transluminal coronary angioplasty (PTCA) longer than 90 days before surgery had a lower incidence of perioperative cardiac complications. Undergoing the procedure fewer than 90 days earlier did not confer a benefit (26). There are no data regarding the now-common use of vascular stents with PTCA in reducing perioperative cardiac events. As with PTCA, only retrospective data are available on the coronary artery bypass graft procedure to support a positive benefit (reduced cardiac death and incident of MI) in noncardiac surgery.

Given these findings, in the absence of contraindications the use of preoperative β-blocker therapy should be considered in all patients at high risk for coronary events who are undergoing knee replacement. The β-blockers should be started 3 to 7 days before surgery to achieve a resting heart rate of 60 beats per minute. Atenolol 50 mg a day or metoprolol tartate 25 to 50 mg twice a day is recommended. Either one should be continued up to 7 days after surgery or indefinitely if hypertension is a preexisting condition.

Pulmonary Disorders

Pulmonary complications after surgery remain a leading cause of surgical morbidity (27). Unlike with cardiac evaluation, there are no proven pulmonary risk stratification indices. A history and physical examination with review of daily activity and medications offer the best method of evaluation for risk of pulmonary complications.

Thoracic and upper abdominal procedures pose the highest risk and ophthalmologic procedures the lowest. The total knee replacement procedure results in small changes in vital capacity and functional residual capacity due to positioning on the operative table. Epidural or spinal anesthesia is often recommended in patients with underlying lung disease, yet the literature is mixed in demonstrating lower complication rates. This has little impact on the morbidity of the procedure. After knee replacement an ileus can occur, which decreases diaphragmatic excursion and forced vital capacity, and results in atelectasis. Aspiration pneumonia, pulmonary edema from intravenous fluids, and pulmonary embolism are the major problems seen postoperatively (28).

Patients with morbid obesity or skeletal or neuromuscular disorders may have restrictive lung disease with increased risk of postoperative atelectasis. Those with primary restrictive lung disease, that is, pulmonary fibrosis, do well because respiratory drive is preserved.

Chronic obstructive airway disease and asthma are the most common respiratory diseases encountered by medical consultants. In patients with poorly controlled reversible airway disease or an acute exacerbation, elective surgery should be postponed. Aggressive management with inhaled steroids, oral steroids, inhaled β-agonists, and inhaled ipratropium bromide will decrease postoperative pulmonary complications. There are few data on the preoperative benefit of individual drugs. All maintenance medications should be continued through the perioperative period.

There is no clear-cut level of forced expiratory volume in 1 second (FEV_1) or other spirometric measurements to predict complications. Some authors have suggested that an FEV_1 of 1.2 to 2.0 L is predictive of risk (27,29,30). A more useful predictor of pulmonary risk is the maximum voluntary minute ventilation, which is a measure of respiratory drive. Patients who have values below 50% of predicted are at risk for pulmonary complications. Of interest is the fact that there have been no studies to define a lower limit of FEV_1 at which surgery should not be performed. Williams and Brenowitz (31) studied 16 patients with severe chronic obstructive pulmonary disease and found a 19% incidence of major pulmonary complications. For arterial blood gases, PCO_2 is a better predictor of risk than PO_2. Patients with PCO_2 above 45 mm Hg are at risk for increased pulmonary complications.

In summary, a patient's functional capacity is assessed through a history and physical examination. If the patient is not limited in routine daily activity, and if no pulmonary disease exists, no further evaluation is necessary. In patients who have preexisting airway disease, smoking should be stopped, bronchodilators (oral theophylline, β₂-agonist, and anticholinergic inhalers), and inhaled corticosteroids should be used on a continuous basis pre- and postoperatively. Antibiotics should be used if there is evidence of bacterial infection of the airway (i.e., abnormal chest radiograph or a change in sputum). Pre- and postoperative respiratory therapy, instruction in the use of incentive spirometry, coughing, and deep breathing exercises should be implemented (32). Early ambulation after surgery should also be encouraged.

Hypertension

Little has been published on hypertension as it relates to preoperative assessment and surgical risk, even though there are probably 55 million people who have hypertension in the United States. In most of these studies, the patients had mild hypertension. The standard has been that, in patients with diastolic pressure above 110 mm Hg or systolic hypertension above 200 mm Hg, surgery should be postponed until the blood pressure is adequately controlled. This was based on data from studies performed in the 1950s, 1960s, and early 1970s, on poor autoregulation of the central nervous system and renal blood flow, on the risk of myocardial ischemia, and on arrhythmias. Since those early days, it is difficult to find patients with this severe degree of hypertension who have undergone surgical treatment (33). In patients with mild to moderate hypertension, there appears to be no significant perioperative risk. Any reported morbidity has resulted from exacerbation of underlying hypertension (34).

Interestingly enough, ability to control blood pressure preoperatively does not predict the degree of perioperative difficulties. Twenty-five percent of patients develop an exaggeration of blood pressure independent of their preoperative blood pressure (35). Wide swings in intraoperative blood pressure in patients with uncontrolled hypertension account for the morbidity and mortality. There are three periods during which hypertensive episodes are seen: at induction of anesthesia (associated with hemodynamic instability and myocardial ischemia), in the immediately postoperative period (usually secondary to pain or hypoxia), and between days 3 and 5 (when worsening postoperative hypertension is associated with mobilization of third-space fluid; these patients respond to diuretic therapy).

Patients with hypertension often have concomitant risk factors for surgery such as ischemic heart disease, renal disease, CHF, cerebrovascular disease, or prior MI. When these factors are also considered, the risk can be more accurately assessed.

Patients should be given their hypertension medications preoperatively and the medications should be resumed as soon as possible postoperatively (Table 7). If patients are unable to take their medications orally, many agents can be given intravenously, but the substituted intravenous agent should be of the same class as the oral medication, if possible. It is important to avoid abrupt withdrawal of some antihypertensive agents, which can lead to rebound hypertension [e.g., central-acting agents such as clonidine (36) and β-blockers (35)]. Most antihypertensive agents have beneficial effects on the hemodynamic instability that occurs with anesthesia. Only the withdrawal of diuretics is recommended before the surgery, but this remains controversial (Table 7). Use of diuretics reduces plasma volume further in hypertensive patients already depleted in volume. This volume reduction, along with the direct effect of these agents on renal distal tubular secretion of potassium, results in intravascular and cellular potassium depletion. Hypokalemia tends to potentiate the effects of muscle relaxants; it increases the probability of cardiac atrial and ventricular arrhythmias, and it increases the risk of a paralytic ileus. Many clinicians stop diuretic administration a few days before surgery to decrease the risk of hypovolemia or hypokalemia or both. All patients taking diuretics should have preoperative laboratory evaluation with correction of hypokalemia, potassium levels higher than 4.0 mEq per L, and intravascular volume abnormalities.

Fortunately, monoamine oxidase inhibitors are rarely used in the management of hypertension today, but they should be avoided before surgery to prevent accelerated hypertension and hyperpyrexia. Aggressive attempts to lower blood pressure within 48 hours of surgery can have detrimental effects on hemodynamic stability and should be avoided.

Diabetes Mellitus

Evaluation

Diabetes mellitus affects approximately 5% of the population. Type 1 diabetes (insulin-dependent diabetes) is a state of insulin deficiency associated with ketoacidosis; it is commonly seen in the young but can present as late as the third decade of life. Type 2 diabetes entails a relative resistance to endogenous insulin and is not associated with ketoacidosis. The latter type is more common in the adult patient presenting for arthroplasty, who is usually older and overweight. Type 2 diabetes is managed by diet, oral hypoglycemic agents, insulin, or combinations of the three. Complications in the form of end-organ damage are normal for both types (Table 8).

Several studies in the 1970s (12) and 1980s (13) suggested that diabetes itself is not an independent risk factor for perioperative morbidity and mortality, but cardiac, renal, vascular, and neurologic abnormalities are predictors of complications.

The clinician's approach to these patients is to assess the end-organ damage. A physical examination is done with special

TABLE 8. *Complications of diabetes*

Organ system	Impact
Coronary arteries	Angina, myocardial infarction, silent ischemia
Vascular disease	Coronary artery disease, peripheral artery insufficiency, carotid disease, stroke
Kidneys	Proteinuria, decreased glomerular filtration, acidosis, hyperkalemia, prolongation of drug metabolism with decreased renal clearance
Peripheral neuropathy	Decreased nociception with increased risk of infection; impact on rehabilitation postoperatively
Autonomic neuropathy	Orthostatic hypotension, perioperative swings in blood pressure, delayed gastric emptying, urinary retention with increased risk of infection

attention to the existence of retinopathy (which often indicates the presence of nephropathy), the presence of vascular bruits and diminished pulses (suggestive of vascular disease), and an orthostatic blood pressure change of greater than 15 mm Hg without pulse increase or the presence of peripheral neuropathy (which implies the existence of autonomic neuropathy).

A preoperative EKG is a requirement for all diabetic patients. The finding of a loss of R-R variation on a resting EKG may indicate autonomic neuropathy. The presence of Q waves may identify an old transmural MI. Many times the patient may be unaware of previous myocardial ischemia. The incidence of silent ischemia is higher in the diabetic population than in the general population. Disappointingly, current screening tests and exercise and pharmacologic stress tests have poor predictive value for silent ischemia. The clinician should be aware of this and have a high index of suspicion and a low threshold for obtaining an EKG on postoperative days 1 through 5.

Renal function assessment should include a physical examination, with note of the volume status of the patient, and laboratory tests for serum electrolytes, blood urea nitrogen, and creatinine. A urinalysis for protein is also essential. Knowledge of the presence of renal dysfunction is necessary when choosing perioperative medications such as antibiotics or radiocontrast dyes. Because asymptomatic bacteriuria is common, a urine culture should be performed before arthroplasty.

The presence of autonomic neuropathy may complicate the postoperative course due to blood pressure and pulse variations. Diabetic patients may also have profound hypoglycemia without symptoms. Postoperative nausea with gastroparesis is frequent in diabetic patients and is successfully treated with intravenous metoclopramide, 10 to 30 mg every 6 to 8 hours. It is a good first-line medication, for it has an antiemetic effect as well as improving gastric emptying.

Glucose Management

The goal of glucose management in the perioperative period is to minimize fluctuations in glucose levels to avoid disruption of the metabolic state and return the patient to stable levels as soon as possible. This goal of a stable glycemic level is not always easy to achieve, even in those patients with excellent preoperative control. On the surgical day the carbohydrate intake of the patient is limited (decreases glucose levels) and muscle activity is at a minimum (increases glucose levels), and the stress of surgery imparts a state of insulin resistance with increased production of glucagon, epinephrine and norepinephrine, and other glycemic endocrine modulators. This resistant state is most severe in the first 24 hours postsurgery but resistance remains relatively elevated for 5 days postoperatively.

A numeric goal for optimal glucose level in the perioperative period can only be inferred from the clinical literature and *in vitro* studies of phagocytosis and fibroblast cellular metabolism. There are no studies available documenting a difference in infection rates or wound healing based on levels of glycemic control in any joint replacement surgery. Recognizing this paucity of data and extrapolating from other forms of surgery (37), one can say that glycemic levels in the perioperative period should be optimal at 120 mg to 200 mg per dL.

For patients with type 2 diabetes who are using diet modification and oral agents, medication should be withheld the day of surgery; if the medication is longer-acting chlorpropamide, it should be withheld the day before surgery. The blood glucose level should be checked the morning of surgery, or preoperatively, and then every 4 to 6 hours intra- and postoperatively. Human synthetic regular insulin can be administered on a sliding scale for any blood glucose levels over 250 mg per dL (Table 7). Intravenous solutions of 5% dextrose should be administered to avoid starvation ketosis. On the morning after surgery, an 1,800-calorie American Diabetes Association diet can be started, along with the oral hypoglycemic agent if the patient is taking food well.

Patients with type 2 diabetes taking insulin can be managed in a fashion similar to that outlined earlier. Whether to administer a long-acting insulin on the morning of surgery is a clinical judgment and should be individualized. The dosage of 0.5 U per kg of long-acting insulin [less than 40 U of neutral protamine Hagedorn (NPH) or lente insulin] per 24 hours can be selected as a cutoff point.

If the patient takes less than this amount, the long-acting insulin can be withheld on the morning of surgery and short-acting insulin used every 4 to 6 hours as needed. If the patient takes more than 0.5 U per kg per 24 hours, then one-third to one-half the usual dose is given on the morning of surgery, and any glucose elevations are treated on a sliding scale. It is important to remember that the insulin resistance of the patient with type 2 diabetes imparts the need for a larger dose of regular insulin per glucose increment than for patients with type 1 diabetes. Also, the commonly used Humulin 70/30 is a combination insulin (70% NPH and 30% regular), so if insulin is given on the morning of surgery, one-third the usual amount of insulin is given in the form of NPH.

Many insulin-management protocols for patients with type 1 diabetes have been suggested. European clinicians used intraoperative infusion of a premixed insulin–10% dextrose solution or a variable continuous insulin infusion (38). Practice in the United States, however, has favored a reduced dose of long-acting insulins given subcutaneously, with frequent monitoring and administration of short-acting insulin as needed. There are no comparative studies of these regimens evaluating glycemic control and perioperative complications in orthopedic surgery.

Good control of blood glucose level should begin weeks before surgery. The patient with type 1 diabetes, with the guidance of the physician, should strive to attain a stable blood glucose level (100 to 200 mg per dL) for at least 7 days before the operation. Adherence to the appropriate diet with control of glucose should replete hepatic glycogen stores, reducing the risk of intraoperative hypoglycemia. Because of insulin deficiency, patients with type 1 diabetes are at risk for perioperative hyperglycemia and ketoacidosis.

The patient with well-controlled type 1 diabetes can be treated with a half-dose of the morning NPH or lente insulin and frequent serum glucose monitoring (every 4 hours). Treatment on a sliding scale with short-acting insulin should be used throughout the first 24 postoperative hours. The following morning, the patient should be returned to the standard insulin dose only if able to consume a full American Diabetes Association diet.

For patients with type 1 diabetes who demonstrate a wide variation in preoperative glucose levels or a history of poor control (i.e., brittle diabetes), an insulin drip is most appropriate. The NPH or lente insulin should be reduced to 80% of the patient's standard dose the night before surgery to avoid morning hypoglycemia. When the patient arrives at the preoperative area, blood glucose level should be measured and an intravenous 5% or 10% dextrose solution begun at 100 mL per hour. Administration of dextrose avoids potential starvation ketosis. Through a separate line, an insulin infusion can be instituted by mixing 100 U of regular insulin in 500 mL of normal saline (1 U per 5 mL). The infusion is started at 2 U per hour (10 mL per hour). The blood glucose level must be monitored hourly and the infusion increased or decreased by 5 mL to maintain a blood glucose level between 150 and 240 mg per dL.

The continuous infusion can be maintained for the first 24 postoperative hours. The morning after surgery, two-thirds of the patient's usual morning insulin should be administered subcutaneously, and the insulin infusion can be stopped 3 hours later. Coverage with a sliding scale of regular insulin is then appropriate.

For patients with type 1 diabetes managed on a continuous ambulatory subcutaneous infusion, such as with an insulin pump, the pump may be stopped at midnight before the surgery, an intravenous 5% dextrose solution can be started, and the insulin drip can be used as described.

New insulins have been developed during the last decade and have not been evaluated for use in the perioperative period. Readers may encounter them during their practice and may wish to consult an endocrinologist regarding their use.

Lispro insulin (Humalog) is a synthetic insulin equal in potency to regular insulin, but it reaches a peak serum level 30 to 90 minutes after administration. This insulin is well suited for postprandial blood glucose control.

Glargine insulin (Lantus) is a synthetic insulin that is injected once a day. Subcutaneous injection results in a relatively constant concentration-time profile over 24 hours with no pronounced peak. It is commonly administered at 10 p.m., which results in a steady basal insulin level. This is an ideal insulin for type 1 diabetes to achieve optimal control.

Cerebral Vascular Disease

Patients who have asymptomatic carotid stenosis have a 1% to 2% risk of stroke after anesthesia. Patients with previous but now stable cerebral vascular disease (i.e., the last event was more than 1 year before surgery) are at low risk (less than 1%) for perioperative events. The approach in cases of an asymptomatic carotid bruit with significant stenosis (more than 70% occlusion on Doppler ultrasonography) is a controversial area in preoperative management (39,40). Data suggest that patients with asymptomatic carotid disease should undergo surgical treatment if the stenosis is greater than 75% (39,40). This refutes the consensus from many studies in the 1970s and 1980s that medical therapy is preferable. The prior recommendations were based on risk-benefit analysis. Because the annual risk of stroke from asymptomatic carotid stenosis (more than 50% occlusion by Doppler ultrasonography) is 1% to 2%, morbidity from medical therapy was lower than morbidity associated with carotid endarterectomy (CEA), in which complication rates varied from 2% to 21% (41,42). As surgical skills and postoperative care improve, the benefit may outweigh the risk and CEA may be considered.

Most of the studies of prophylactic CEA have been done on patients undergoing cardiac and vascular surgeries, and the results are mixed. There have been no studies done on prophylactic CEA preceding total knee arthroplasty. Thus, given our current knowledge and the small risk of stroke in the asymptomatic patient, it appears to be acceptable to proceed with knee surgery before addressing the asymptomatic carotid stenosis.

Patients who have had recent transient ischemic attacks are at increased risk for stroke, particularly within 6 weeks of the event (43); most strokes occur within the first year after a transient ischemic attack. These symptomatic patients should be thoroughly investigated for the cause of the transient ischemic attack before any surgery is performed. If the patient has hemodynamically significant carotid stenosis (more than 75% occlusion), a CEA should be performed before elective knee surgery (44). If the stenosis is noncritical (less than 70% occlusion), CEA may not be necessary, and elective total knee arthroplasty can be scheduled. It seems prudent, however, to wait at least 4 to 6 weeks after the event (45), based on the timing used to schedule a CEA after a stroke or transient ischemic attack.

Rheumatoid Arthritis

Patients with RA commonly are candidates for total joint replacement as well as other surgeries. RA is associated with anatomic and physiologic changes that must be evaluated before general anesthesia, including cervical spine disease, anemia, and pleural and pulmonary involvement.

Studies have shown that 30% to 40% of RA patients admitted to the hospital have radiographic evidence of cervical spine subluxation (46), which commonly involves the first and second cervical vertebrae. Between 2% and 5% have demonstrable long-tract findings (47). Subluxation of a diseased atlantoaxial joint during endotracheal intubation may compromise the respiratory center of the medulla. Taking a careful history for symptoms of pain in the C1-C2 nerve root during routine daily activity is necessary. Dynamic flexion and extension radiographs can identify this problem. If there is any question, a computed tomographic scan of the upper cervical spine is obtained. Furthermore, a small subset of these patients (2% to 3% of adults with RA) may have involvement of the temporal mandibular joint, which makes intubation difficult (46).

Lung disease in RA patients has many manifestations. Pleuritis, interstitial fibrosis, and pleura-based nodules can result in restrictive lung disease manifested by exertional dyspnea. In addition, the interstitial fibrosis may inhibit alveolar-capillary gas exchange, lowering resting PaO_2. A history of exertional dyspnea or rales should be evaluated by a chest radiograph and spirometry, with or without carbon monoxide diffusion capacity. Although intervention to modify the pulmonary disease uncovered by this assessment is unlikely to reverse existing disease, it is important to have this baseline information to help in the assessment of postoperative hypoxemia and dyspnea.

Heart disease in RA patients may include pericarditis, myocarditis, noninfective vegetation on the valves, conduction defects, and, rarely, coronary arteritis. A history, physical examination, and EKG are sufficient screening for RA patients, following the guidelines set down previously. If a murmur exists, antibiotic prophylaxis is necessary. Anemia of chronic inflammatory disease is often found in this patient population, and preoperatively a complete blood count should always be obtained.

The use of corticosteroids is common in this patient population and should be managed as outlined later.

Ankylosing spondylitis involves the cervical and thoracic spine and results in a restrictive lung disease. This can increase the risk of postoperative pulmonary complications. Rigidity of the cervical spine makes intubation difficult.

Similarly, patients with *juvenile rheumatoid arthritis* may also have extensive ankylosis of the cervical spine, which makes hyperextension for visualization of the vocal cord difficult for the anesthesiologist.

Gout commonly flares in the postoperative patient with a history of gouty arthropathy. Management is complicated by the fact that these patients are commonly on anticoagulants, which contraindicates the use of nonsteroidal antiinflammatory drugs. Colchicine is the drug of choice but its use is limited by the occurrence of gastrointestinal distress. Colchicine 0.6 mg, intravenously or by mouth, can be given every hour until pain is relieved or diarrhea occurs (but without exceeding six doses over 24 hours).

Long-Term Glucocorticoid Use

Many of the comorbid conditions (e.g., asthma, chronic obstructive pulmonary disease, RA, and inflammatory bowel disease) in patients who present for total knee arthroplasty require long-term glucocorticoid therapy. Some patients may have been taking steroids for nonchronic conditions (e.g., dermatitis) within the 12 months preceding surgery. Theoretically, these patients may have hypothalamic-pituitary-adrenal axis suppression and are at risk for adrenal insufficiency intra- and postoperatively. Anecdotal reports in the 1950s, 1960s, and 1970s documented adrenal insufficiency in the long-term steroid user during the perioperative period, sometimes with fatal outcomes. Consensus is difficult because the studies were heterogeneous in design, with small numbers of patients, different steroid preparations, and different durations of use. They often had poorly defined end points. The symptoms of adrenal insufficiency can be very subtle, including anorexia, low-grade fever, mild to moderate hypotension, malaise, myalgias, and arthralgias. These symptoms may be overlooked because of their common occurrence in the postoperative period.

Two tests are available to assess adrenal reserve: synthetic adrenocorticotropic hormone (ACTH; Cortrosyn) stimulation, and metapyrone sulfate challenge. The ACTH stimulation test is the simplest to perform and has been validated by Jasani et al. (48) for prediction of adrenal response in surgery. The test can be done at any time of day and rarely causes side effects. A baseline serum cortisol level is determined, followed by intravenous

TABLE 9. *Steroid equivalents*

Steroids	Glucocorticoid potency	Equivalent dose (mg)
Short acting		
Cortisol (hydrocortisone)	1	20
Cortisone	0.8	25
Prednisone	4	5
Prednisolone	4	5
Methylprednisolone	5	4
Intermediate acting		
Triamcinolone	5	4
Long acting		
Dexamethasone	30	0.75
Betamethasone	25	0.60

administration of 250 μg of synthetic ACTH. Thirty-minute and 60-minute cortisol levels are obtained. A positive adrenal response from a baseline serum cortisol level of 6 to 25 μg per dL is a rise of more than 7 μg per dL from baseline or to more than 20 μg per dL at 60 minutes.

The following issues remain controversial: How much glucocorticoid steroid is needed for suppression? What is the minimum duration of steroid use to demonstrate suppression, and, once steroids are stopped, how long are the adrenal glands suppressed?

Graber et al. (49), in 1965, tried to answer these questions when they studied the hypothalamic-pituitary-adrenal axis response after cessation of steroids. They discovered that the equivalent of 7.5 mg of prednisone (Table 9) given daily for 7 days or more was sufficient for suppression of this axis. They found that the hypothalamic output of corticotropin-releasing hormone returned first, followed by pituitary secretion of ACTH, and finally adrenal production of cortisol. Adrenal response became appropriate 9 months, on average, after cessation of steroids. Based on these data, some clinicians conservatively recommend administration of stress steroids for up to 1 year after a patient stops taking steroids in any patient who has received the equivalent of 7.5 mg of prednisone daily for 5 days. Because there is wide variation in individual responses to these steroids, this approach has led to excessive use of steroids. Thus, when time permits in the preoperative period, it is prudent to perform the ACTH stimulation test.

The literature is filled with regimens of steroid coverage and taper, but no comparative studies have been done. The following protocol, based on physiologic adrenal response, is widely used. A functional adrenal gland produces the equivalent of 250 to 300 mg of cortisol in 24 hours when challenged. The goal of replacement is to equal this output with equivalent exogenous steroid (Table 9). A suggested regimen is 100 mg of intravenous hydrocortisone 30 to 60 minutes before the procedure, followed by 100 mg intravenously every 8 hours for two more doses. Patients who are not taking steroids long term or who use less than physiologic doses (less than 7.5 mg per day of prednisone) do not need a tapering regimen. Patients taking steroids above this dose over the long term should receive 50 mg intravenous hydrocortisone every 8 hours for three doses on postoperative day 1 and 25 mg every 8 hours for three doses on postoperative day 2. On the third postoperative day, the patients are returned to the standard daily dose. Monitoring of fluid volume (input and output), blood pressure, glucose, and electrolytes is necessary. Some clinicians favor the use of a histamine (H_2) antagonist to avoid the theoretical possibility of steroid/stress-induced gastric ulcers.

Obesity

Because excessive weight results in damage to lower extremity joints or acceleration of underlying arthritis, obesity is a common comorbid condition in adults undergoing total knee arthroplasty. One must be aware of the related medical problems of obesity and anticipate potential perioperative problems. Anecdotal consensus is that obesity imparts an increase in complications in the perioperative period (e.g., increased atelectasis, wound dehiscence, higher rate of wound infection), yet there are very few studies to document these beliefs.

Obesity imparts perioperative risk by its association with other medical conditions. It is associated with hypertension, hyperlipidemia, atherosclerotic vascular disease, left ventricular hypertrophy, changes in pulmonary function, diabetes mellitus, cholelithiasis, and gout. The clinician's responsibility is to recognize these associations and assess the patient accordingly.

Changes in pulmonary dynamics have the greatest potential impact on outcome during and after surgery. Obesity can result in increased minute ventilation, decreased compliance of the chest wall, and an increase in the energy expenditure of breathing (all to maintain a normal Po_2 and a reduced Pco_2). Abnormalities can occur in spirometric measurements, with a decrease in expiratory reserve volume and functional residual capacity. Respiratory rate increases to maintain minute ventilation. Shallow breathing is common, and it produces overventilation of the upper and underventilation of the lower lung fields. Perfusion is unchanged, so that ventilation-perfusion mismatches are common.

Preoperative assessment should include a careful history, physical examination, and laboratory testing to screen for the comorbidities of obesity. Special attention should be paid to respiratory symptoms, functional abilities in day-to-day life, and sleep disturbance. A chest radiograph, EKG, and complete blood count are appropriate in all morbidly obese patients (more than 100% above ideal body weight), regardless of symptoms.

It would be reasonable to expect a higher incidence of postoperative atelectasis and pneumonia given these functional changes. Yet in a study of consecutively treated cholecystectomy patients, no difference was found in the incidence of atelectasis (50). Other studies in abdominal surgery showed no difference in postoperative pneumonia between obese and nonobese patients (28). In addition, a larger gastric volume and the frequent presence of a hiatal hernia theoretically makes postoperative aspiration more likely. The amount of data in the orthopedic literature documenting these complication rates is scant.

Thyroid Disease

Because total knee arthroplasty is almost exclusively an elective procedure, surgery should be delayed until evaluation and treatment are begun for the hypothyroid or hyperthyroid state.

A hypothyroid condition, both treated and untreated, is common in the population undergoing knee replacement. Hypothyroidism is seen in patients with Hashimoto thyroiditis or hypofunctional goiter, and in those who had previous thyroid surgery or iodine-131 radiation therapy. Patients maintained on L-thyroxine are at low risk for complications, even in the presence of mild under- or overreplacement. The preoperative assessment of these patients should include evaluation of thyroid status. On physical examination, the reflexes can be most helpful (i.e., hyperreflexia in hyperthyroidism and a delayed return of the reflex response in hypothyroidism). If there is any question about the patient's thyroid status, or no laboratory assessment has been done within 1 year of proposed surgery, then a highly sensitive thyroid-stimulating hormone (TSH) study should be done. A TSH level of under 0.5 µU per dL suggests a hyperthyroid state, whereas a TSH level of over 5.0 µU per dL indicates a hypothyroid condition.

In the rare instance when knee replacement cannot be delayed in the profoundly hypothyroid patient, 300 to 500 µg of intravenous L-thyroxine along with 100 mg intravenous hydrocortisone should be administered preoperatively. This should be followed with 100 mg hydrocortisone, intravenously or by mouth, daily for 1 week. Postoperatively, 25 or 50 µg of L-thyroxine should be given by mouth daily (Table 7).

Hyperthyroid patients maintained in a euthyroid state using propylthiouracil or methimazole are at no greater risk for surgery than those without the disorder. The medication can be administered by mouth or via the nasogastric tube perioperatively. A TSH test should be performed preoperatively. Surgery should be delayed for the thyrotoxic patient. If surgery is urgent, the severely hyperthyroid patient should receive 1 g oral propylthiouracil and 300 mg intravenous hydrocortisone followed by 5 drops of saturated solution of potassium iodine (50 mg of iodide per drop) orally three times a day, or 1 g sodium iodine intravenously three times a day. Propranolol hydrochloride is given 1 mg per minute intravenously or 20 to 40 mg orally every 6 hours to manage the tachycardia and hypertension associated with thyrotoxicosis. Intravenous esmolol hydrochloride or labetalol hydrochloride may be substituted.

CONCLUSION

A patient presenting for total knee arthroplasty commonly has numerous comorbid conditions that can impact the immediate surgical success and long-term recovery of the patient. Although a consultant should not be asked to clear a patient for surgery and general anesthesia, he or she can be asked to preoperatively assess the patient. The objective is to identify treatable comorbid conditions, to identify comorbid conditions that are not reversible and may adversely impact the surgical outcome, and to identify occult conditions that can be corrected. Thus, patients are evaluated so that they may be in an optimal medical condition to undergo the proposed surgery.

REFERENCES

1. Turnbull JM, Buck C. The value of preoperative screening investigations in otherwise healthy individuals. *Arch Intern Med* 1987;147:1101–1105.
2. Kaplan EB, Sheiner LB, Boeckman AJ, et al. The usefulness of preoperative laboratory screening. *JAMA* 1985;23:3576–3581.
3. Macpherson DS. Preoperative laboratory testing: should any tests be routine before surgery? *Med Clin North Am* 1993:77(2):289–308.
4. Sander DP, McKinney FW, Harris WH. Clinical evaluation and cost effectiveness of preoperative laboratory assessment on patients undergoing total hip arthroplasty. *Orthopedics* 1989;12(11):1449–1453.
5. Galen RS, Gambino SR. *Beyond normality: the predictive value and efficiency of medical diagnosis.* New York: John Wiley and Sons, 1975.
6. McMurry J. Wound healing with diabetes mellitus. *Surg Clin North Am* 1984;64:769–778.
7. Nolan CM, Beaty HN, et al. Further characterization of the impaired bactericidal function of granulocytes in patients with poorly controlled diabetes. *Diabetes* 1978;27:889–894.
8. Hollenberg M, Mangan DT, et al. Predictors of postoperative myocardial ischemia in patients undergoing noncardiac surgery. The Study of Perioperative Ischemia Research Group. *JAMA* 1992;268(2):205–209.
9. Tae T, Mushlin A. The utility of routine chest radiographs. *Ann Intern Med* 1986;104:663–670.
10. Rucker L, Frye EB, et al. Usefulness of screening chest roentgenograms in preoperative patients *JAMA* 1983;250:3209–3211.
11. Goldman L. Cardiac risks and complications of noncardiac surgery *Ann Intern Med* 1983;98:504–513.
12. Goldman L, Caldera DL, Nussbaum SR, et al. Multifactorial index of cardiac risk in noncardiac surgical procedures. *N Engl J Med* 1977;297:845–850.
13. Detsky AS, Abrams HB, McLaughlin JR, et al. Predicting cardiac complications in patients undergoing non-cardiac surgery. *J Gen Intern Med* 1986;1:211–219.
14. Lette J, Waters D, Lapointe J, et al. Usefulness of the severity and extent of reversible perfusion defects during thallium-dipyridamole imaging for cardiac risk assessment before noncardiac surgery. *Am J Cardiol* 1989;64:276–281.
15. Mangano DT, Goldman L. Current concepts: preoperative assessment of patients with known or suspected coronary disease. *N Engl J Med* 1995;333:1750–1756.
16. Eagle KA, Coley CM, Newell JB, et al. Combining clinical and thallium data optimizes preoperative assessment of cardiac risk before major vascular surgery. *Ann Intern Med* 1989;110:859–866.
17. Seeger JM, Rosenthal GR, Self SB, et al. Does routine stress thallium cardiac scanning reduce postoperative cardiac complications? *Ann Surg* 1994;219:654–663.
18. Lane RT, Sawada SG, Segar DS, et al. Dobutamine stress echocardiography for assessment of cardiac risk before noncardiac surgery. *Am J Cardiol* 1991;68:976–977.
19. London MJ, Tubau JF, Wong MG, et al. The natural history of segmental wall motion abnormalities in patients undergoing noncardiac surgery. *Anesthesiology* 1990;73:644–655.
20. Zeldin RA. Assessing cardiac risk in patients undergoing noncardiac surgical procedures. *Can J Surg* 1984;27:402–404.
21. Tahran S, Moffitt EA, Taylor WF, et al. Myocardial infarction after general anesthesia. *JAMA* 1972;220:1451–1454.
22. Steen PA, Tinker JH, Tarhan S. Myocardial re-infarction after anesthesia and surgery. *JAMA* 1978;239:2566–2570.
23. Rao TL, Jacobs KH, El Etr AA. Reinfarction following anesthesia in patients with myocardial infarction. *Anesthesiology* 1983;59:499–505.
24. Mangano DT, Layug EL, Wallace A, et al. Effect of atenolol on mortality and cardiovascular morbidity after non-cardiac surgery. *N Engl J Med* 1996;335:1713–1720.
25. Poldermans D, Boersma E, Bax JJ, et al. The effect of bisoprolol on perioperative mortality and myocardial infarction in high-risk patient under going vascular surgery. *N Engl J Med* 1999;341:1789–1794.
26. Posner KL, Van Norman GA, Chan V. Adverse cardiac outcomes after non-cardiac surgery in patients with prior percutaneous transluminal coronary angioplasty. *Anesth Analg* 1999;89:553–560.
27. Tisi GM. Preoperative evaluation of pulmonary function. *Am Rev Respir Dis* 1979;119:293–310.
28. Presley AP, Alexander-Williams J. Postoperative chest infection. *Br J Surg* 1974;61:448.
29. Celli BR. What is the value of preoperative pulmonary function testing. *Med Clin North Am* 1993;77:309–325.
30. Gass GD, Olsen GN. Preoperative pulmonary function testing to predict postoperative morbidity and mortality. *Chest* 1986;89:127–135.
31. Williams CD, Brenowitz JB. Prohibitive lung function and major surgical procedures. *Am J Surg* 1976;132:763–766.
32. Ford GT, Guenter CA. Toward prevention of postoperative pulmonary complications. *Am Rev Respir Dis* 1984;130:4–5.
33. Prys-Roberts C. Hypertension and anesthesia. Fifty years on. *Anesthesiology* 1979;50:281.

34. Goldman L, Caldera DL. Risks of general anesthesia and elective operation in the hypertensive patient. *Anesthesiology* 1979;50:285–292.

35. Goldman L. Noncardiac surgery in patients receiving propranolol: case reports and a recommended approach. *Arch Intern Med* 1981;141:193.

36. Brodsky JB, Bravo JJ. Acute postoperative clonidine withdrawal syndrome. *Anesthesiology* 1976;44:519.

37. Golden SH, Peart-Vigilance C, Kao WH, et al. Perioperative glycemic control and the risk of infectious complications in a cohort of adults with diabetes. *Diabetes Care* 1999;22(9):1408–1414.

38. Alberti KG, Thomas DJB. The management of diabetes during surgery. *Br J Anaesth* 1979;51:693–708.

39. Executive Committee for the Asymptomatic Carotid Atherosclerosis Study. Endarterectomy for asymptomatic carotid artery stenosis. *JAMA* 1995;273:1421–1428.

40. Moore WS, Barnet HJM, Beebe HG, et al. Guidelines for carotid endarterectomy. *Stroke* 1995;26:188–201.

41. Nunn DB. Carotid endarterectomy in patients with territorial transient ischemic attacks. *J Vasc Surg* 1988;8:447–452.

42. Toole JF, Yuson CP, Janeway R, et al. Transient ischemic attacks: a prospective study of 225 patients. *Neurology* 1988;18:746–753.

43. Whisnant JP, Sandok BA, Sundt TM. Carotid endarterectomy for unilateral carotid system transient cerebral ischemia. *Mayo Clin Proc* 1983;56:171–175.

44. North American Symptomatic Carotid Endarterectomy trial collaborators. Beneficial effects of carotid endarterectomy in symptomatic patients with high grade stenosis. *N Engl J Med* 1991;325:445–453.

45. Harrison MJG, Marshall J. The finding of thrombus at carotid endarterectomy and its relationship to the timing of surgery. *Br J Surg* 1977;64:511–512.

46. Sledge CB. Introduction to surgical management. In: Kelly W, ed. *Textbook of rheumatology.* Philadelphia: WB Saunders, 1985:1745.

47. Tsahakis PJ, et al. Surgical care of the patient with rheumatoid arthritis. In: Kelly W, ed. *Textbook of rheumatology.* Philadelphia: WB Saunders, 1985:1823.

48. Jasani MK, Freeman PA, Boyle JA, et al. Studies of the rise in plasma 11-hydroxycorticosteroid (11-OHCS) in corticosteroid-treated patients with rheumatoid arthritis during surgery: correlations with the functional integrity of the hypothalmo-pituitary-adrenal axis. *QJM* 1968;37:407.

49. Graber AL, Ney RI, Nicholson WE, et al. Natural history of pituitary adrenal recovery following long-term suppression with corticosteroids. *J Clin Endocrinol Metab* 1965;25:11.

50. Poe Rh, Kally MC, Dass T, et al. Can postoperative pulmonary complications after elective cholecystectomy be predicted? *Am J Med Sci* 1988;295:29–34.

Management of the Stiff Knee

Thomas P. Sculco

Restriction of knee motion is a challenging dilemma for the surgeon both in the initial knee replacement surgery and should motion be compromised after knee arthroplasty. In addition to pain relief and improved ambulatory ability, patients expect to achieve improved knee flexion. However, periarticular fibrosis with knee stiffness in the primary knee with degenerative arthritis is predictive of postoperative motion in knee replacement. Although numerous factors may contribute to failure to achieve a mobile total knee replacement, poor motion preoperatively is the most correlative (1). Therefore, it is important to inform the patient of the more limited expectations of knee motion if there is severe restriction of flexion preoperatively. Surgical management in knees with significant limitation of motion requires more extensive soft tissue surgery and often a slower recovery. There is also an increased risk for postoperative complication, with a greater chance of knee swelling, hematoma, and reformation of periarticular scar. This chapter deals with the surgical management and postoperative rehabilitation of the patient with a stiff knee undergoing knee replacement. The complication of knee stiffness after arthroplasty and the treatment algorithm for this difficult problem are also addressed.

STIFF KNEE PREOPERATIVELY

Severe loss of motion in the arthritic knee may occur in a number of pathologic conditions. Patients with prior infection in the knee joint will often present with marked knee joint stiffness. The intraarticular global nature of the infection leads to the development of both intraarticular and periarticular fibrosis in addition to the destruction of the joint surfaces. Patients with hemophilia and the ankylosing type of rheumatoid or inflammatory arthritis often demonstrate severe knee stiffness. In addition, this limitation of motion is usually associated with severe

deformity, most commonly with valgus and external rotation. Trauma to the knee joint with intraarticular fracture of the femoral condyles or tibia plateau will also lead to severe knee joint fibrosis and knee stiffness (Fig. 1). In all of these conditions, prior surgical procedures usually have been performed (e.g., synovectomy, internal fixation, débridement) and this further increases scar formation and loss of motion. The extensive nature of these procedures themselves may promote extensive scar formation in the joint and in its surrounding soft tissues. Postoperative rehabilitation after these initial procedures can be difficult and painful, resulting in further loss of motion.

Patients with infected total knee arthroplasty often develop significant loss of motion even if methylmethacrylate or implant spacers are used. The knee is often stiff in extension, and, if delay in reimplantation extends beyond 8 to 12 weeks, the probability of motion beyond 90 degrees is unlikely.

Limitation of motion may be quantified into (a) severe, with a resultant arc of less than 30 to 45 degrees, (b) moderate, with an arc of 45 to 70 degrees, or (c) mild, with motion possible from 70 to 90 degrees. In the moderate and mild cases, knee replacement can usually be performed with extensive soft tissue releases about the joint and aggressive excision of scar and fibrotic tissue. The extent of these soft tissue releases is determined by the degree of knee stiffness. In the severely limited cases, radical subperiosteal soft tissue release will be necessary with resection of scar in a more global fashion. Often the entire distal femur and proximal tibia will be devoid of soft tissue and additional procedures may be necessary to elongate the contracted extensor mechanism.

In evaluation of the stiff knee preoperatively it is important to document if the knee is contracted in extension or flexion. Knees that have severe limitation of motion and are stiff in extension are the most difficult to mobilize. There are a number of reasons for this but the main problem in these knees is that the entire extensor

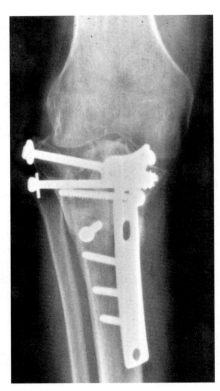

FIG. 1. Posttraumatic knee with severe articular damage and marked stiffness.

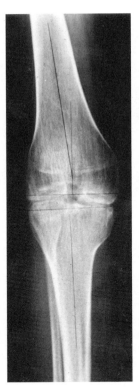

FIG. 2. Radiograph of a prior septic arthritis of the knee joint with fibrous ankylosis.

mechanism is shortened and almost always lengthening of the extensor mechanism will be necessary to achieve satisfactory knee flexion. If the knee is stiff in flexion, management is much easier. In these patients, the extensor mechanism is generally not as contracted because the knee has been in the flexed position. The extensor mechanism is not as shortened in these patients because the knee has contracted in the flexed position. Generally, release and elevation of subperiosteal periarticular scar will allow mobilization of the knee, and quadricepsplasty and tibial tubercle osteotomy are not necessary.

SURGICAL MANAGEMENT OF THE STIFF KNEE

In the most severe cases of knee stiffness, when there is complete absence of knee motion, it is important to determine if there is a fibrous or bony ankylosis. This can be identified on plain radiographs of the knee; if a joint line is still perceptible, the ankylosis is fibrous (Fig. 2). If there are bony trabeculations extending across the knee joint between the femur and tibia, identification of the joint may be more complex at the time of knee replacement, and ultimate motion in these knees tends to be less.

Whenever feasible, as part of the surgical approach, previous incisions should be used. If the knee joint destruction is the result of trauma and internal fixation has been used, removal of these screws or plates is performed at the time of the arthroplasty. If there is a history of infection or a suspicion exists of infection around the hardware, a two-stage procedure should be performed with removal of the plate as a separate procedure.

The approach to the knee joint is similar to a standard knee replacement. Once through the subcutaneous tissue, the interval between the quadriceps tendon and the vastus medialis is identified. In knees with little motion, there may be little subcutaneous tissue, and the skin may be adherent to the underlying scar. In these patients, care must be taken not to devascular the skin edges by excessive retraction and extensive undermining of the skin. Two to 3 mm of tendon is left on the vastus medialis muscle as the joint is entered to allow for a tendinous closure at the end of the procedure.

In the most severe cases of joint stiffness, the patella may be ankylosed to the knee joint and it may be necessary to osteotomize it and reflect it laterally. Wide soft tissue releases are performed subperiosteally starting on the medial and lateral surfaces of the femur and tibia. It is important to be extensive with this elevation of the adherent fibrotic soft tissue, and this is best done with a scalpel or cautery. The underlying bone is often osteoporotic, and the aggressive use of periosteal elevators and osteotomes may damage the underlying bony surfaces. In the most severe cases, the entire distal femur (Fig. 3) and proximal tibia will be skeletized to allow flexion of the knee. If there is a fibrous ankylosis, the knee should be flexed gently, and the joint line can usually be identified. Sharp dissection continues in the intraarticular area, and cruciate ligaments are removed if still present.

Posterior release of soft tissues from the posterior aspect of the tibia and femur is necessary, particularly if the knee is stiff and fixed in flexion (Fig. 4). The tibia can be mobilized anteriorly and, using electrocautery, the adherent posterior capsule, gastrocnemius, and medial and lateral hamstrings can be released from the posterior tibia. In severe flexion deformity,

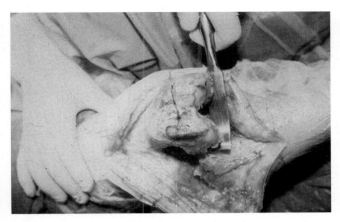

FIG. 3. Femoral skeletization procedure for severe knee stiffness.

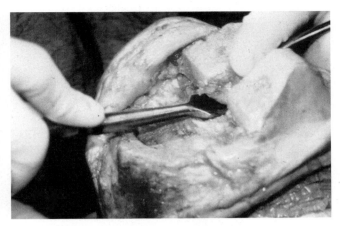

FIG. 5. Subperiosteal posterior release in intercondylar notch for stiff knee in flexion.

femoral release should also be performed. Sharp dissection will generally be necessary in the intercondylar area of the femur. Using a periosteal elevator the soft tissues can then be released in a proximal direction from the back of the femur (Fig. 5).

The knee is gradually flexed to a greater degree, and the patella is everted laterally. In severely contracted knees, mobilization of the adherent soft tissues of the knee must be radical before attempting to evert the patella. A lateral release may be necessary to allow eversion of the patella. A fixation pin should be inserted into the patellar tendon if it appears to be at risk as the knee is flexed. This generally prevents avulsion of the patellar tendon. It is important not to force the knee into flexion, as often the bone is osteoporotic and fracture may occur as well as avulsion of the patellar tendon. Continued subperiosteal soft tissue releases should be performed by palpating the tight structures as the knee is flexed. If patella eversion is not possible, the patella may be subluxed laterally and held away from the joint by the use of an angled Hohmann retractor.

If after release of the periarticular soft tissues knee flexion is still limited because of a tight quadriceps tendon, a "lateral snip" of the tendon may be performed. With this procedure, a lateral extension of the quadriceps incision is made that may then be reflected inferiorly somewhat if needed to allow the quadriceps mechanism to evert laterally in an open-book fashion. This will also improve visualization of the lateral gutter and improve access to tight soft tissues in this area.

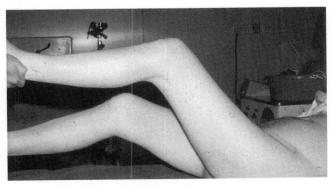

FIG. 4. Ankylosed knee in flexed position.

Once the knee can be flexed to 90 degrees, appropriate bone cuts may be made on the tibia, femur, and patella to allow insertion of trial components. The knee must then be evaluated for stability and motion. Often, if radical releases are necessary, there is persistent instability in a medial-lateral plane or the flexion gap is greater than the extension gap, leading to instability in flexion. Attempts should be made to achieve medial-lateral symmetry of soft tissues by additional release on the tighter side of the joint. If asymmetric laxity persists and is greater than 1 cm, a constrained condylar-type implant should be used. In the stiff knee with a significant flexion contracture, the extensive posterior soft tissue release from the tibia and femur may lead to a flexion gap that may be greater than the extension gap. This leads to flexion instability when an anterior force is applied to the tibia in flexion during the trial reduction. This can be addressed by several methods: (a) selecting a constrained condylar implant, which provides increased anteroposterior stability, (b) increasing flexion stability by posteriorly translating the femoral component, and (c) increasing the size of the femoral component. Simply increasing the thickness of the tibial component makes the knee tight in flexion but produces excessive tightness in extension and results in a flexion contracture. The technique of reducing the flexion gap by posterior translation of the femoral component as much as possible may require downsizing the diameter of the femoral stem to move the femoral component more posterior in the femur. To decrease the flexion gap by increasing the size of the femoral component is useful if there is not prosthetic overhang medially and laterally. This may lead to painful soft tissue impingement postoperatively and should be avoided.

In the most extreme circumstances in which there is complete ligamentous insufficiency or marked flexion or extension instability, a rotating hinge–type prosthesis may be necessary. These implants provide absolute knee instability at the expense of increased interface stress at the bone implant junction. Segmental additions may be used on these hinge implants to accommodate severe bone loss.

EXTENSOR MECHANISM MANAGEMENT

Even in the most severely contracted knees, it is possible to expose and mobilize the knee with subperiosteal radical soft tissue releases. The knee can be flexed to 90 degrees and the appro-

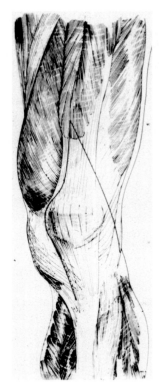

FIG. 6. Quadriceps incision for quadricepsplasty.

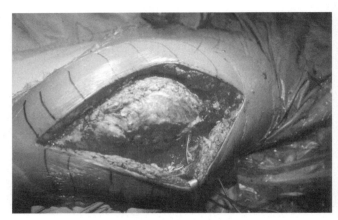

FIG. 7. Quadricepsplasty after closure.

priate bone cuts completed. If the surgeon is careful and thorough with these releases, aside from an occasional "quadriceps snip" there is no need to do anything to the quadriceps tendon or tibial tubercle. After trial reduction, however, the knee may have severe limitation of flexion because of persistent contracture of the extensor mechanism. This tightness can be managed by procedures to lengthen the extensor mechanism proximally or distally. In my experience, the contracture of the extensor mechanism is proximal in the quadriceps muscle and tendon, and therefore lengthening procedures should be used to address the pathology in this proximal area. Procedures that elevate the tibial tubercle and allow it to slide proximally do not address the location of the soft tissue contracture in the quadriceps mechanism and therefore have a more limited role in knees that are stiff in extension.

A number of methods can be used to produce a lengthening of the quadriceps tendon (2,3). Knees that can be flexed to 60 to 70 degrees of flexion passively after trial components have been inserted may be treated by a simple transverse release of the tight bands in the quadriceps tendon. This procedure is performed by palpating the quadriceps tendon and inserting a No. 11 blade transversely into the substance of the tendon in the area of maximum contracture. The blade is rotated 90 degrees, and the tight band is released. This can be performed at multiple levels (usually three or four) of the tendon and at different depths. The knee is flexed, and lengthening and elongation occurs through these tenotomy areas. This procedure is similar to that performed for lengthening of the Achilles tendon. Passive knee flexion of 100 to 110 degrees should be possible at the conclusion of this procedure.

If passive knee flexion is less than 45 degrees after trial component implantation, a more formal quadricepsplasty is necessary. A

modified inverted V-Y–type quadricepsplasty may be performed, basing the V proximally (Fig. 6). The lateral limb of the quadriceps incision is continued distally for 2 to 3 cm. This procedure is a progression of the "lateral snip" described previously and allows distal movement of the tendon with lengthening of the quadriceps mechanism. In the most severe cases of contracture, the lateral quadriceps tendon incision may have to be continued more distally to allow sufficient laxity in the quadriceps tendon. Once final implantation of the components has been performed, the quadriceps tendon is sutured, with the knee flexed between 35 and 45 degrees (Fig. 7). A lengthening of 2 to 3 cm in the tendon is usually adequate for mobilization of the knee. If the tendon is sutured with the knee in greater flexion an extensor lag may persist although knee flexion is achieved more easily. If the tendon is sutured in less flexion, motion is more limited.

Aglietti et al. (4) reported on a series of 22 total knee arthroplasties with preoperative range of motion of less than 50 degrees. Eleven of these patients required V-Y quadricepsplasty. Preoperative range of motion was 32 degrees, and postoperative range of motion increased to 78 degrees. An extensor lag was noted in the majority that resolved significantly with time. In a review of the most severely limited knees, Naranja et al. (5) reviewed 37 knees that were ankylosed or arthrodesed preoperatively. These patients improved their motion to a range of 7 to 62 degrees postoperatively. However, the complication rate was high, with a 14% infection rate and 35% of patients having major complications. Only 29% of this ankylosed group had no pain and unlimited ambulation.

In a review of 82 total knee replacements in 71 patients with less than 50 degrees of motion, Montgomery et al. (6) found that by using radical soft tissue releases range of motion improved from an average of 36 degrees (range of 0 to 50) preoperatively to 93 degrees (range of 35 to 130) postoperatively. There were two patients with peroneal palsies in this group who had severe valgus deformities, and both resolved.

A proximal tibial osteotomy is best reserved for exposure in patients with cemented stemmed prostheses requiring revision knee surgery. Whiteside has advocated its use in the stiff knee and performs it by elevating an osteotomized fragment of proximal tibia 5 to 6 cm in length, leaving soft tissues attached laterally (17). Proximal migration of the fragment is allowed, and then the osteotomy is fixed with cerclage wires. Problems of nonunion, fracture through the proximal tibia, and painful hardware have been described using this technique. More important, proximal tibial osteotomy does not change the contracted nature of the quadriceps tendon proximally where the pathology is present.

POSTOPERATIVE REHABILITATION

In patients in whom a formal quadricepsplasty has not been performed early, mobilization of the knee is key to achieving successful postoperative knee motion. The protocol I have used is to maintain epidural anesthesia and analgesia for 48 to 72 hours postoperatively. This requires coordination with the pain management and anesthesia services. The constant passive motion (CPM) machine is used immediately after surgery, and the knee is flexed maximally from 110 to 120 degrees in the machine. It is important to remember that the degree of knee flexion in these devices is often inaccurate, and in fact only 100 to 105 degrees of flexion may be the actual extent of knee flexion despite the measurement of the machine gauge. Pain management is crucial to the success of postoperative rehabilitation in these patients, and maintenance of adequate levels of epidural analgesia must be continued during the postoperative period. Patients are continued in CPM at these levels, and vigorous twice-daily physical therapy is instituted. Patients are mobilized from bed on day 2 and may require a knee immobilizer for ambulation if elevated levels of epidural analgesia are needed. Hospital stay is longer than that for routine total knee replacement patients, and most patients remain in hospital for 7 to 10 days and are discharged with 90 to 100 degrees of flexion. Most patients are discharged to a rehabilitation unit for continued aggressive management.

In patients in whom a formal inverted V-Y quadricepsplasty has been performed, the CPM machine is still used postoperatively, but motion is restricted to 45 degrees initially. A knee immobilizer is used in these patients for ambulation. Motion beyond 45 degrees is begun gradually and usually not for 7 to 10 days after surgery. Increase in flexion continues slowly to prevent disruption of the repair of the quadricepsplasty. Most patients achieve 70 to 85 degrees of flexion by 6 weeks from surgery. All patients have an extensor lag after quadricepsplasty, but this tends to improve with time. At 6 months after surgery, only a minor lag persists. In a personal series of 13 patients who underwent quadricepsplasty for severe knee stiffness in extension, resultant range of motion was 82 degrees of flexion (45 to 110), with a persistent extensor lag of 15 degrees (0 to 45).

STIFF TOTAL KNEE REPLACEMENT

Limitation of motion after total knee replacement is a major source of dissatisfaction to the patient and may lead to a need for revision surgery. In a review of 102 patients undergoing revision total knee replacement, 17% were reoperated for knee stiffness (7). Therefore, it is important to discuss with the patient preoperatively the expectations in terms of resultant motion. This is particularly true in patients who have severe limitation of knee flexion preoperatively. Despite all of the techniques discussed previously, knees that are invested with severe periarticular fibrosis and at times heterotopic ossification are at risk to have significant limitation of motion postoperatively. Although

motion is generally unchanged or slightly improved after total knee replacement because most current implant designs have average flexion arcs of 115 to 120 degrees, patients are expecting at least these degrees of flexion. If motion is more limited, the patient may be disappointed, and therefore preoperative education of reasonable expectations is important. Aside from preoperative stiffness, there are other causes of limited motion after total knee replacement that should be defined, and the management of the limited motion varies depending on the cause of the stiffness.

CAUSES OF KNEE STIFFNESS AFTER TOTAL KNEE REPLACEMENT

In addition to limited preoperative motion as a cause of knee stiffness after total knee replacement, a number of intraoperative mechanical factors and postoperative complications can produce loss of motion. Implant malposition may lead to knee stiffness and require revision knee replacement. Nicholls and Dorr (8) found implant malposition in 8 of 13 stiff total knee replacements that were revised. In addition, in most of these patients the patella was inferiorly positioned, which further decreased motion. Implant size can influence knee motion, particularly if the implant is oversized for the dimensions of the joint. Although both femoral and tibial components play a role, it is the femoral component that most influences the flexion gap. If a femoral implant is chosen that is greater than the anteroposterior dimension of the native femur, flexion tightness results (Fig. 8). Daluga et al. (9) reviewed 60 osteoarthritic patients undergoing 94 total knee replacements who required manipulation under

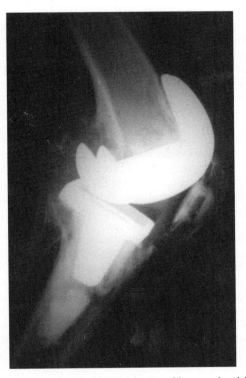

FIG. 8. Radiograph of stiff total knee with oversized femoral component.

anesthesia for stiffness postoperatively. In this study, there was a strong correlation between increased anteroposterior femoral size and need for manipulation when compared with a controlled group of patients. In a similar study, Ellis et al. (10) found the same tendency toward increased femoral anteroposterior dimension in those patients requiring manipulation for stiffness after total knee replacement.

Selection of a tibial polyethylene component that is too thick also limits flexion and increases tension in the flexion gap. Anteriorly, if there is inadequate patellar resection or if a patellar component is used that is thicker than the amount of patellar bone resected, flexion can be limited through a tight patellofemoral articulation. Therefore it is important to assess carefully the sizing of the components and the ease of flexion with trial components in place. If reduction of the implant in flexion is difficult, it may be indicative of oversizing of the components or of failure to release the soft tissues adequately in flexion. This is particularly true when there is a flexion contracture in combination with angular deformity.

If a posterior cruciate ligament (PCL)-retaining prosthesis is used, persistent tightness of the PCL may lead to restriction of knee flexion. The tight PCL acts as a tether and prevents knee flexion. When trial components have been inserted and passive knee flexion performed, if there is a tendency for anterior levering with lifting of the prosthesis from the tibia anteriorly, a tight PCL must be suspected. Williams et al. (11) described ten patients with PCL-retaining total knee replacements with limited flexion. Preoperative motion was 4 to 74 degrees in these patients. All underwent arthroscopic release of the PCL, with a postoperative increase in motion of 1 to 112 degrees.

As a rule, flexion laxity should be present when the knee is tested for anteroposterior stability. However, the tibia should not dislocate anteriorly to the femoral component, but there should be easy anterior translation of the tibia. This will ensure that the flexion gap is not too tight and that implant sizing is correct.

Failure to slope the tibial cut posteriorly also may predispose the knee to tightness in flexion. A 5- to 10-degree posterior inclination of the tibial osteotomy allows easier clearance posteriorly during knee flexion. Additionally, inaccuracy regarding position of the joint line may reduce the degree of knee flexion. Current instrumentation makes joint line position more reproducible, but in the revision knee replacement accurate placement may be more complex. Posterior osteophytes on the femoral and tibial surfaces must be removed during bony preparation, as these can interfere with knee flexion. Laminar spreaders may be used to distract the flexion space, and curved osteotomes can remove these posterior femoral osteophytes. The posterior tibial osteophytes are usually removed when the tibial cut is sloped posteriorly.

Patients who have had prior surgery are also at risk of having increased stiffness after total knee replacement. Radiographs should be evaluated carefully in these patients, and it is important to document the location of the patella. Patients who have patella infera (baja) often have severe fibrosis of the infrapatellar fat pad, and, despite release at surgery, the patella often remains fixed inferiorly. This lower position of the patella and the fibrosis in this area may lead to limitation of knee flexion.

Postoperative complications can also be responsible for periprosthetic fibrosis and stiffness after knee replacement. Development of a hemarthrosis that is tense and not draining may severely interfere with postoperative motion. The mechanical restriction of flexion by the volume of the hemarthrosis, and the severe pain on flexion that often accompanies these severe bleeds, prevents postoperative motion. If motion remains limited for 4 to 6 weeks, fibrosis may ensue with marked difficulty in achieving flexion. Anticoagulation must be monitored carefully to lessen the incidence of this complication.

MANAGEMENT OF STIFF TOTAL KNEE REPLACEMENT

If motion is severely limited by a postoperative intraarticular hematoma, aspiration should be performed. If aspiration proves unsuccessful, surgical evacuation of the hematoma is recommended, with lavage of the joint and cautery of any persistent bleeding sites. Anticoagulation should be resumed slowly and levels maintained at the lower end of acceptable limits.

Manipulation under anesthesia is a useful technique when knee flexion is not progressing postoperatively. The need for manipulation has lessened significantly due to earlier and more aggressive therapy. Despite conflicting literature, the use of a CPM machine appears to speed knee flexion and reduce knee swelling, which may impede motion (12). Manipulation is usually performed in patients with limited motion at 6 to 12 weeks after knee replacement. The indication for manipulation is a patient who has reached a plateau in his or her knee flexion that is unacceptable (less than 70 degrees at 6 weeks postoperatively). If improvement is documented, manipulation may be delayed beyond 3 months. The need to manipulate a knee replacement is less than 5% in total knee replacement patients, and this is markedly reduced from the 30% level 15 years ago.

Manipulation is performed under regional anesthesia and should be performed by exerting only mild to moderate flexion force. It is important in manipulation of a total knee replacement that cephalad force be exerted under the thigh to allow the tibial component to roll beneath the femoral component when the knee is flexed. Repetitive and progressive flexion should be performed until adhesions are disrupted and knee flexion is possible from 110 to 120 degrees. The degree of flexion is influenced by the amount of preoperative knee flexion, and 120 degrees may not be possible when less than 90 degrees of motion was present preoperatively. Once manipulation has been completed CPM is applied at maximum flexion, and this is kept in place for 4 to 6 hours. The patient begins physical therapy the next day to maintain the degree of flexion achieved at the time of the manipulation. The CPM machine may be given to the patient to use at home if there is significant tightness.

Maintenance of flexion achieved after manipulation has been controversial. Esler et al. (13) found that in 467 total knee replacements the need to manipulate was in 47 knees. The preoperative motion averaged 62 degrees in this group of patients, and, at 1 year after manipulation, motion was 95 degrees. In a group of 21 patients with similar motion who refused manipulation, the gain of motion was 3 degrees at 1 year postoperatively.

Manipulation is not without risk and should be performed with care. Fracture of the femur and disruption of the extensor mechanism proximally and distally (Fig. 9) are possible if forcible manipulation is performed in a knee that has established and mature periprosthetic fibrosis (14).

If a mechanical or prosthetic factor is determined that is preventing knee flexion revision, knee surgery should be considered. If prosthetic sizing is inaccurate, revision knee replacement by downsizing the implants often leads to restora-

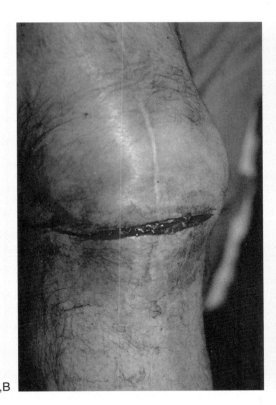
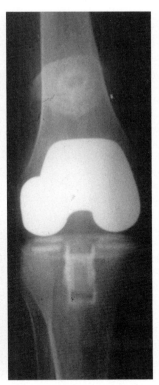

A,B

FIG. 9. A: Disruption of skin and avulsion of patellar tendon after manipulation. **B:** Radiograph of proximally displaced patella after patellar tendon avulsion.

tion of motion. During revision, laxity should be present in the flexion space, and, to prevent risk of subluxation, a constrained condylar implant may be used. Proper alignment, implant position, tibial sloping, and patellofemoral adjustment can also be treated surgically if these are the causes of knee stiffness. If PCL tightness is the cause of limitation of motion, release of this ligament may be performed with or without revision to a posterior-stabilized design. Because periprosthetic fibrosis accompanies these mechanical causes of knee stiffness, it is necessary to perform a wide and aggressive release of this scar, and postoperative rehabilitation should include the maximum flexion technique with the CPM machine and regional anesthesia and analgesia described earlier.

In patients in whom periprosthetic scar has developed with limitation of motion without mechanical cause, a resection of scar technique has been used without implant revision. This has been used in a small group of patients who have developed marked knee stiffness after total knee replacement due to scar formation that has resulted from a poor rehabilitative program, poor patient compliance, or periarticular or intraarticular fibrosis secondary to hemarthrosis or other etiology. In these patients, radical removal of all periarticular and intraarticular scar is performed, with complete mobilization of medial and lateral gutters. Peripatellar scar is excised as well as posterior fibrosis. The infrapatellar fat pad, which is often fibrotic and contracted, is excised. The tourniquet is removed, and hemostasis is obtained meticulously. Intraoperative passive flexion must be accomplished from 110 to 120 degrees before closure. All soft tissue mechanical impediments to knee flexion are removed. It may be necessary to use the multiple transverse tenotomy technique at multiple levels of the quadriceps tendon. In flexing the knee, there is a lengthening effect of the quadriceps tendon, but the tendon remains intact. Care must be taken that these transverse tendon releases do not pass through the entire thickness of the tendon.

The postoperative regimen in these patients is to maintain epidural anesthesia and analgesia and maximum knee flexion in the CPM machine. Postoperative radiation (700 rads) has been used in these patients on the day after the operative procedure. Patients are discharged home when 100 to 110 degrees of flexion can be obtained easily. Physical therapy commences immediately at home three to four times weekly. Patients are given a CPM machine and spend 6 to 8 hours at maximum flexion. Quadriceps exercise programs are stressed also because there is a tendency for an extensor lag to develop as the extensor mechanism has been elongated during and after the operative procedure. Patients are monitored at 3 to 4 weeks after surgery, and, if motion is not being maintained, early manipulation of the knee under anesthesia is performed. Nine patients have undergone this technique since the early 1990s. Preoperative motion averaged 45 to 50 degrees. Average increase in motion in this group of patients was 53 degrees, with a range of 32 to 75.

Techniques for management of the stiff total knee replacement regarding the extensor mechanism when revision knee replacement is necessary are similar to the primary stiff knee described previously. Ries and Badalamente (15) reported on a group of six patients (four with PCL-retaining knee replacements) with a preoperative range of motion of 36 degrees (range of 20 to 70 degrees). At surgery they found no implant malposition or oversizing but, in performing soft tissue release with revision total knee replacement, postoperative motion improved to 86 degrees (range of 70 to 110 degrees). Heterotopic ossification was noted in five of the patients postoperatively.

Quadricepsplasty has provided satisfactory results in a number of series of revision for knee stiffness (4,6,8). Tibial tubercle osteotomy has been a useful adjunct for exposure of the difficult knee during revision and Whiteside has reported encouraging results with this technique (17). Fracture is a complication that has been reported with this procedure, and this procedure should be restricted to only those knees in which exposure is not possible by soft tissue procedures (16,17).

Management of the stiff knee is complex and requires careful preoperative evaluation and surgical management. As important is the postoperative rehabilitation, which must be carefully supervised by the surgeon to prevent suboptimal motion after arthroplasty in these patients. Patients should be carefully counseled that resultant motion will not be as good when preoperative knee stiffness is present. This is a common source of discontent after knee arthroplasty and is best avoided by a frank discussion with the patient preoperatively. Complications are greater in these patients due to the increased need for soft tissue dissection and balancing. If a mechanical problem is the cause of knee stiffness after total knee arthroplasty, it is best addressed surgically and expeditiously to prevent mature periprosthetic fibrosis from developing, which compromises the end result. In most patients, improved motion is possible and increases significantly the function of the patient. However, these are technically demanding procedures and require extensive experience in knee arthroplasty to effect a satisfactory result.

REFERENCES

1. Harvey IA, Barry K, Kirby SP, et al. Factors affecting the range of movement of total knee arthroplasty. *J Bone and Joint Surg Br* 1993;75:950–955.
2. Barrack R. Surgical exposure of the stiff knee. *Acta Orthop Scand* 200;71:85–89.
3. Sculco TP. Complex reconstructions in total knee arthroplasty. *Am J Knee Surg* 1997;10:28–35.
4. Aglietti P, Windsor RE, Buzzi R, et al. Arthroplasty for the stiff or ankylosed knee. *J Arthroplasty* 1989;4:1–5.
5. Naranja RJ, Lotke TA, Pagnano MW, et al. Total knee arthroplasty in a previously ankylosed or arthrodesed knee. *Clin Orthop* 1996;331:234–237.
6. Montgomery WH, Insall JN, Haas SB, et al. Primary total knee arthroplasty in stiff and ankylosed knees. *Am J Knee Surgery* 1998;11:20–23.
7. Lonner JH, Siliski JM, Scott RD. Prodromes of failure of total knee arthroplasty. *J Arthroplasty* 1999;14:488–492.
8. Nicholls DW, Dorr LD. Revision surgery for stiff total knee arthroplasty. *J Arthroplasty* 1990;5(Suppl):73–77.
9. Daluga D, Lombardi AV, Mallory TH, et al. Knee manipulation following total knee arthroplasty. *J Arthroplasty* 1991;6:119–128.
10. Ellis TJ, Beshires E, Brindley GW, et al. Knee manipulation after total knee arthroplasty. *J South Orthop Assoc* 1999;8:73–79.
11. Williams RJ, Westrich GH, Siegel J, et al. Arthroscopic release of the posterior cruciate ligament for stiff total knee arthroplasty. *Clin Orthop* 1996;331:185–191.
12. Lachiewicz PF. The role of continuous passive motion after total knee arthroplasty. *Clin Orthop* 2000;380:144–150.
13. Esler CN, Lock K, Harper WM, et al. Manipulation of total knee replacement: is the flexion gained retained? *J Bone Joint Surg Br* 1999;81:27–29.
14. Rand JA, Morrey BF, Bryan RS. Patellar tendon rupture after total knee arthroplasty. *Clin Orthop* 1989;244:233–238.
15. Ries MD, Badalamente M. Arthrofibrosis after total knee arthroplasty. *Clin Orthop* 2000;380:177–183.
16. Ritter MA, Carr K, Keating EM, et al. Tibial shaft fracture following tibial tubercle osteotomy. *J Arthroplasty* 1996;11:17–19.
17. Whiteside L. Exposure in difficult total knee arthroplasty using tibial tubercle osteotomy. *Clin Orthop* 1995;321:32–35.

CHAPTER 97

Preventing Wound Complications after Total Knee Arthroplasty

Fred D. Cushner

Proper wound healing is essential for a successful total knee arthroplasty (TKA). Should wound failure occur, complications such as prosthetic infection or wound defects requiring a complex plastic surgery reconstruction may occur. This often results in lengthy hospital stays, decreased function, and failed expectations of both the patient and physician. This chapter not only focuses on the prevention of wound failure but also discusses detection and treatment options.

VASCULAR SUPPLY TO THE KNEE

Under normal circumstances, the blood supply to the anterior aspect of the knee consists of a random plexus of perforating blood vessels. These vessels, the extraosseous parapatellar anastomotic ring (1–5), are formed by six main perforating arteries originating from the popliteal artery (Fig. 1). In addition, three extrinsic vessels contribute to the blood supply of the knee. The first extrinsic vessel consists of the branches of the profunda femoris and the vessel supplying the rectus femoris, vastus intermedius, and vastus lateralis, which, via a dermal plexus, supplies the inferior aspect of the knee.

Second, supreme genicular vessels originate from the superficial femoral artery and develop into the musculoarticular branch and the saphenous artery. Whereas the musculoarticular branch supplies the medial aspect of the joint as well as the medial superior skin, it is the saphenous artery that terminates to supply the area of skin just below the medial plateau. The third extrinsic vessel is a recurrent branch of the anterior tibial artery supplying the skin lateral to the patellar tendon.

PREVENTION OF WOUND COMPLICATIONS

From the previous discussion, it can clearly be seen that the skin surrounding the knee has both a medial and lateral distribution. The musculoarticular branches supply the medial skin, whereas the anterior tibial artery has lateral distribution.

As can be seen, a random, plentiful blood supply exists, and, under most circumstances, the skin around the knee can tolerate a single midline incision such as that required for TKA. However, many factors exist that can compromise proper wound healing. These factors, discussed in the next sections, can be divided into patient systemic factors, local factors, surgical technique factors, and postoperative factors.

Systemic Factors

It goes without saying that a thorough history and physical examination are required before performing the indicated TKA. Although often the emphasis is on the patient's cardiac or pulmonary status, equally important is the wound healing potential of the individual patient. Of utmost importance is the vascular status of the involved limb. Because of the ambulatory limitations of an arthritic knee, claudication symptoms may not be present despite significantly impaired blood flow. Therefore, not only should physical examination include evaluation of the skin around the knee, but a thorough vascular examination of the limb should also be performed. Atrophic changes, decreased hair growth, inadequate pulses, and presence of skin discoloration should be noted. The preoperative x-rays may also provide

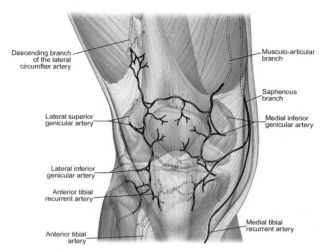

FIG. 1. Blood supply of the knee demonstrating the extraosseous parapatellar anastomotic ring.

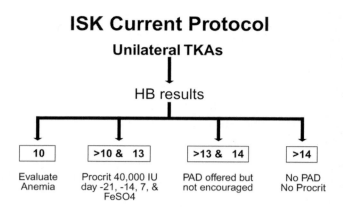

FIG. 2. Preoperative protocol currently recommended at the author's institution. An emphasis is made on maximizing the patient's blood levels before surgery. FeSO4, ferrous sulfate; HB, hemoglobin; ISK, Insall-Scott-Kelly; PAD, preoperative autologous donations; TKA, total knee arthroplasty.

a clue. Although emphasis is often on the degree of deformity or amount of joint space remaining, calcified blood vessels and evidence of arterial sclerosis may also be present.

A vascular surgery consult may be necessary to evaluate for the potential of vascular reconstruction, and, in some instances, changes in the normal TKA protocol may also be required. For example, in some instances, the use of an arterial tourniquet may be contraindicated; in other instances, preoperative intravenous heparin may be required to aid in maintaining the patency of previously reconstructed vessels. In other instances, preoperative arteriograms may be required to document adequate blood flow or normal anatomy. For example, in congenital absence of the patella, a preoperative arteriogram is helpful to document adequate vessel development before surgical intervention to ensure adequate vessel development and skin vascularization.

Another factor to consider before surgery is anemia. Although debatable, anemia has been thought to play a role in wound healing (6,7), with wounds in patients with hematocrits of less than 35% thought to be in jeopardy (9) because of a decrease in oxygen tension at the skin edges of the surgical wound (8,9). This may be multifactorial in that the preoperative anemia may also be related to malnourishment resulting in the apparent anemia. It should be noted that not all researchers agree on the importance of preoperative anemia in wound healing (10). Although Heughan et al. concluded that anemia is well tolerated and that mild to moderate anemia does not adversely impair oxygen delivery in wound healing (10), this does not mean that preoperative anemia should be ignored. In fact, it is now protocol in our institution to evaluate a patient's hemoglobin level before performing the indicated TKA. This is a patient-specific approach, with those with preoperative anemia receiving erythropoietin supplementation before surgery. Patients with hemoglobin levels of more than 10 and less than 13 receive 40,000 units of erythropoietin 3 weeks, 2 weeks, and 1 week before surgery in conjunction with iron supplementation (Fig. 2). This approach is an attempt to maximize preoperative blood levels, thus limiting exposure to potential infections associated with allogeneic transfusions. Research suggests it may play a role in avoiding wound complications. Kendall et al. demonstrated immune suppression after allogeneic transfusion (11), whereas other authors have shown increased joint infections when allogeneic transfusions are received (12).

Preexisting medical conditions should also be of concern to the examining physician. Not only should conditions such as chronic venostasis be noted on physical examination, but also a history of venous ulceration. Human immunodeficiency virus infection should also be noted. Lehman et al. noted increased infection in human immunodeficiency virus patients undergoing total joint arthroplasty (13). Although human immunodeficiency virus should not prevent TKA, discussion should take place before TKA regarding increased evidence of wound failure potential. These authors noted a 14% joint infection rate with intravenous drug–abuser patients, demonstrating an infection in 25% of the cases.

A patient's nutritional status may also play a role in wound healing potential. Albumin levels (less than 3.5 g per dL) as well as total lymphocyte count (less than 1,500) may make a patient more prone to wound failure (14,15). Once a decreased nutritional status is noted, these deficiencies should be corrected, if possible, before surgery.

Another nutritional factor that may place a patient at increased risk for wound failure is obesity (16,17). Certainly, exposure in a morbidly obese patient is technically more difficult because of the abundant adipose tissue as well as physical limitations on knee flexion and joint exposure. Because of these limitations, more vigorous skin retraction may be required. Obese patients have demonstrated increased wound drainage postoperatively (16). Despite these findings, obesity is not a contraindication for TKA. Stern and Insall (18), at our institution, showed no difference in wound complications with TKA and obese patients. This same cohort of patients was examined at 10-year follow-up, and, once again, no increase in wound difficulties was noted (19).

However, little can be done to reduce preoperative obesity; thus, emphasis should be on proper tissue handling in the obese patient. Heavy-tooth forceps and crushing clamps should be avoided, as should excessive skin retraction. Retraction should be intermittent, when applied, to avoid local edema, which may complicate blood flow to the wound edges.

One factor that can be controlled is cigarette smoking. By inhibiting skin microcirculation, cigarette smoking can compromise skin circulation (20–22). Because of the lengthy vasoconstrictor effects, cessation of smoking must occur more than 3 weeks before surgery for a benefit to occur (20–22). Although cessation of smoking is encouraged for all patients, it is a necessity for those who are treated with preoperative tissue expanders.

Of course, certain medical conditions may interfere with wound healing due to several factors. For example, healing of the diabetic patient may be multifactorial, related not only to the diabetes but also to the obesity associated with some diabetic patients. Wong et al. demonstrated delay in wound healing in the diabetic patient, with increased wound separation, erythema, and swelling noted (23). These healing delays may be secondary to delayed collagen synthesis that results in delayed wound tensile strength. Peripheral vasoconstriction in both large and small vessels may also contribute. This does not preclude a TKA procedure. Wilson and associates found no increased risk for infection after TKA in diabetic patients (16). Controversy also exists with regard to wound healing and rheumatoid arthritic patients. Although Wong and associates (23) found a 30% complication rate in rheumatoid arthritis compared with osteoarthritic patients, this conflicts with the data of Garner and associates (24), in which no delay in wound healing was noted. Perhaps the corticosteroids used to treat rheumatoid arthritis interfere with wound healing rather than the disease itself. Wilson et al. demonstrated wound healing difficulty in rheumatoid arthritis patients but only in those treated with corticosteroids (16). No difference in wound healing was noted when corticosteroids were not used. It has been our experience that rheumatoid arthritic skin is fragile and caution should be exercised in tissue handling as well as with the placement and removal of adherent drapes.

As can be seen, many factors can influence wound healing. Recognition of systemic factors before surgery can aid in their correction, thus improving wound healing potential.

Local Factors

Although systemic patient conditions may play a role in wound healing, local factors may also be important. Wound healing potential includes not only the location of previously placed skin incisions but other factors such as the degree of deformity, rotation element of deformity, skin adherence, or history of previous trauma such as burns. Numerous studies have shown increased wound healing problems in knees with numerous incisions (2,25). Problems arise when an avascular bridge exits between the new and previous incision. Not all complications occur in knees with multiple incisions. Any knee with decreased subcutaneous tissue has decreased skin elasticity, which may put a wound at risk. This includes patients with significant long-bone trauma or a history of burns to the anterior aspect of the knee. Large rotary deformities may also place a patient at risk for wound failure, with inadequate skin available for closure after the rotary and varus-valgus deformities are corrected.

Surgical Technique Factors

Although local factors can be identified but not always modified, surgical technique factors can be modified to enhance wound healing potential. To begin, an adequate skin exposure should be chosen. Obviously, even though the patient and physician want to avoid long incisions, the incision should be extensive enough to avoid excessive skin retraction. In addition, the skin should be handled gently to preserve the subcutaneous fascial layer. Large flaps should be avoided, and, really, no lateral flaps should be required. Occasionally, adhesions may result in the subcutaneous layer of valgus deformities, thus requiring release. This should be done only on an as-needed basis. If a flap becomes necessary, it should be minimal and as deep as possible to help preserve the blood flow to this dermal plexus.

The occurrence of lateral release is important, because studies have shown that patients having a lateral release have a decrease in the skin oxygen at the wound healing edges, and this can result in wound healing complications (8). With the use of proper component position, proper patella thickness, and correct component rotation, the lateral release rate can be decreased. Despite this, a lateral release may be required. This results in disruption of the superior genicular vessels, and some skin healing problems cannot be avoided. Johnson and Eastwood (8) noted a decrease in skin oxygen tension when the lateral release was performed. As a result of this lateral release, the rate of superficial drainage and infection rates were also increased in those patients. At the author's institution, if a lateral release is required, a lateral flap is avoided. We prefer an all-inside approach from the middle flap to help seal the postoperative hematoma into the joint. If a large flap is performed in conjunction with a lateral release, the postoperative hematoma is allowed to go through the lateral release site to just below the subcutaneous level. This may present increased pressure on the skin and may lead to prolonged postoperative drainage. In these cases, a subcutaneous drain should be considered.

With no previous incision, the midline approach is preferred. Johnson et al. (26,27) evaluated skin oxygen tension for a variety of incisions and concluded that a medial-side circulation predominance existed in the cutaneous circulation. The more lateral the wound, the lower the skin oxygen tension noted. By postoperative day 8, preoperative levels returned to normal, which is another factor why lateral incisions should be avoided. Previously placed skin incisions make initial incisions more difficult. If avoidance is not possible, we attempt to incorporate the new incision within the old. Transverse incisions can be crossed, in most instances, at 90-degree angles with really no threat to the local skin blood supply (28–30). If a wide scar with minimal subcutaneous tissue is present, the knee may be at risk because it disrupts the underling dermal plexus (28). If this occurs, treatment should include soft tissue expanders as discussed below.

Of importance during surgical technique is the distance between previous incisions. If this skin bridge is less than 2.5 cm, tissue expanders should be considered. Skin bridges of less than 2 cm may result in tissue necrosis between the previous incisions and the new incision (Fig. 3).

Other technical factors include repair of the medial retinaculum. It is commonplace in our institution to perform flexion of the knee after closing the retinaculum to evaluate the suture integrity. Should the sutures break under direct visualization, these can be replaced before closure of the more superficial layers. If this is difficult at the time of surgery, new skin closure systems are available. Sure-Closure (Zimmer, Warsaw, IN) is helpful in increasing elasticity, allowing easier skin closure (Fig. 4).

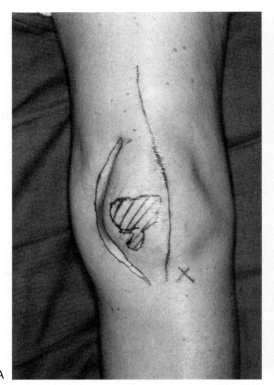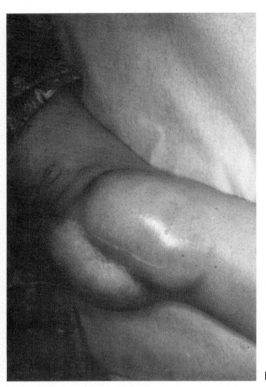

FIG. 3. Fifty-year-old woman with numerous previous incisions as well as a potential avascular skin bridge. **A:** Patient before tissue expander. **B:** Tissue expander in place.

Postoperative Factors

As with surgical factors, postoperative factors can be manipulated to aid in wound healing potential. Avoiding hemarthrosis is of utmost concern to both the surgeon and patient, as a large hematoma can serve as a culture medium for infection and may also lead to local skin compromise because of the tension placed on the subcutaneous tissue. In an attempt to avoid hemarthrosis, some authors deflate the tourniquet before the closure. This has not been a universal technique to decrease blood loss. Other authors have concluded that intraoperative tourniquet deflation actually leads to increased blood loss compared with a tourniquet deflated at the close of the case (28).

Postoperative drains may also play a role in preventing postoperative drainage. Holt and coworkers examined blood loss and wound problems in both drained and undrained TKAs (31). In this study, 40% of the undrained knees and 0% of the drained knees required dressing reinforcement. The undrained knees also had a higher incidence of ecchymosis, and these authors concluded that drains are effective in preventing the accumulation of blood in the surrounding soft tissues. This is not universal. Crevoisier and colleagues (32) concluded, after they examined 32 patients, that there was no advantage of closed-suction drainage. This is a small study of only 32 patients, and it is probably of insufficient size to derive a conclusion on the risk of wound infections that occur in less than 1% of cases. Ovadia and associates evaluated 58 patients after TKA placed into drained and undrained groups (33). Although there was little difference in the rate of infection, there was more serous discharge in the undrained group. At our institution, we use postoperative drainage, which we believe not only avoids hemarthrosis but also provides reinfusion benefits. With the use of reinfusion drains, the allogeneic transfusion rate has been reduced to approximately 2% to 3% for the unicompartmental knee (34). The drain is removed on postoperative day 1, and postoperative antibiotics are used for the 24 hours while the drain is in place. This is important because Drinkwater and Neil have shown an increase in bacterial colonization with drains left in for longer than 24 hours (35).

Concerns have been raised over bleeding complications with postoperative deep venous thrombosis prophylaxis. It should be noted that bleeding complications occurred even before low-molecular-weight heparins were used for deep venous thrombosis prophylaxis. For example, Stulberg and associates (36), looking at 638 TKAs, saw a wound complication rate of 18.1% and a drainage rate of 10.6%. Studies using low-molecular-weight heparin note bleeding complication rates of 2% to 5% in the literature (37–39). It should be noted that bleeding problems are multifactorial. Some wound complications can be avoided with careful hemostasis, proper dosing of anticoagulation agents, and meticulous closure. Review of these papers shows that the bleeding complications are poorly defined and are often not separated out with regard to presence or absence of lateral release, presence or absence of varus release, timing of medications, and the dose. Certainly, the presence of postoperative hematoma is multifactorial and can be related to the type of closure. In our experience with a watertight closure in the subcutaneous layer in conjunction with aggressive stapling of the skin edges, postoperative hematoma and wound complications have not been a problem with the use of low-molecular-weight heparin (enoxaparin).

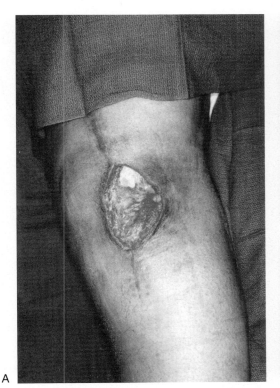

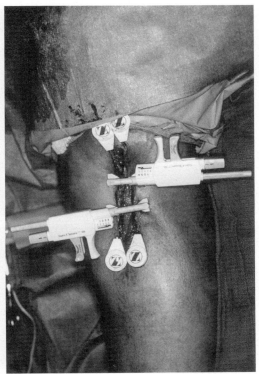

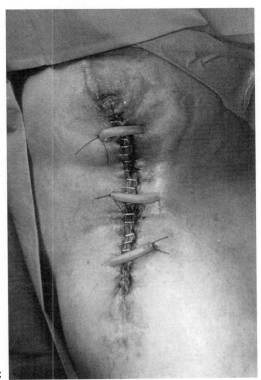

FIG. 4. Use of wound stretching device to aid in closure. **A:** Skin defect with exposed extensor tendons. **B:** Stretching device applying traction to the skin edges. **C:** Closure obtained without excessive tension.

Another postoperative modality that has raised concern for wound healing potential is the continuous passive motion (CPM) machine. Johnson (20) showed a decrease in oxygen tension when the CPM machine was past 40 degrees during the first 3 days (40). Although skin oxygen tension was noted to be decreased, our experience with an aggressive CPM protocol showed no increase in wound complications noted. Yashar (41) also found no increase in problems with an accelerated flexion program. In this case, 70 to 100 degrees was used immediately in the recovery room, with no increase in wound complications noted. Although the average patient can probably tolerate a CPM machine on a high-flexion program, in the patient with a

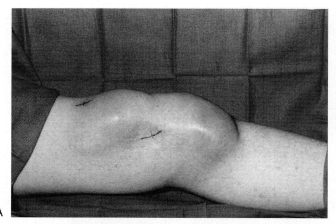

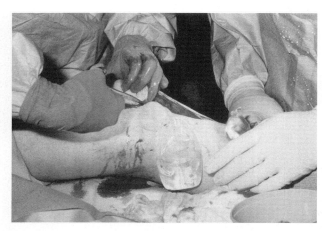

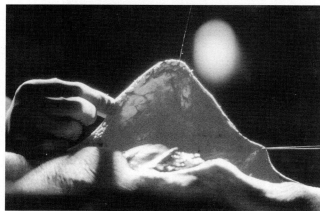

FIG. 5. Sixty-seven-year-old woman after completing the tissue expansion process. **A:** Expander in place. **B:** Expander easily removed at the time of total knee arthroplasty. **C:** Abundant skin with enhanced vasculature noted.

history of potential wound complications, perhaps CPM machine use should be modified. It can be seen that wound complications can be prevented or decreased by understanding the vascular anatomy that exists in this area and by manipulating systemic, local, surgical, and postoperative factors. Maximizing each of these factors may lead to prevention of wound healing problems.

TREATMENT

Treatment of wound healing failures obviously depends on the condition noted. The best form of treatment is the prevention of wound problems before they occur. Despite noting all systemic factors and local factors and initiating postoperative protocols to enhance wound healing, a small number of patients still demonstrate wound healing failure. When this occurs, the surgeon is left with treating the wound complication and at the same time maintaining the prosthesis. This is more complicated in that not only does the prosthesis have to remain in place, but it also needs to function at an acceptable range of motion. Treatment therefore depends on the type of wound complication seen. Wound complications are divided into serous drainage, tense hematoma, superficial tissue necrosis, and full-thickness necrosis. These conditions can occur with or without the presence of infection or with or without prosthesis exposure. Obviously, when dealing with any wound compromise, infection must be ruled out or treated before picking coverage options.

Because not all factors can be corrected before surgery, even the best of surgeons cannot erase the effects of previously placed incisions or local changes from previous trauma. There-

fore, prevention at our institution often involves the use of a soft tissue expander, and we reported our initial results (42). The skin was gradually expanded for an average of 64.5 days before the indicated TKA. All wounds healed without incident. A long-term follow-up of the use of soft tissue expanders around the knee was recently report by Manifold and Cushner (43). In this study, soft tissue expanders were used on 29 knees in 27 patients before TKA and followed up at 34 and 44 months. The average Knee Society score for these patients was 83.7. Although one major wound complication occurred during tissue expansion, necessitating abandonment of the planned arthroplasty, no major wound complications occurred in those patients who underwent knee arthroplasty. Based on this study, we continue to use soft tissue expanders when the potential for wound healing failure exists, such as knees with numerous previous incisions, significant varus rotational angulations, posttraumatic injury, decreased skin elasticity, or decreased subcutaneous tissue. In short, we use this technique in any knee we think has a potential to fail. During this long-term study we have begun using subcutaneous drains at the time of TKA because two knees were taken back for hematoma. The drain evacuation is left in place until the drainage significantly decreases. Since adding this to our protocol, no further evacuation of postoperative hematoma has been needed. The criteria of soft tissue expanders may be subjective, but any patient with adherent immobile skin or anyone with a previous skin incision is considered a candidate for this procedure. Only mild complications have been noted using this technique, and it continues to be our mainstay for those knees with high wound failure potential.

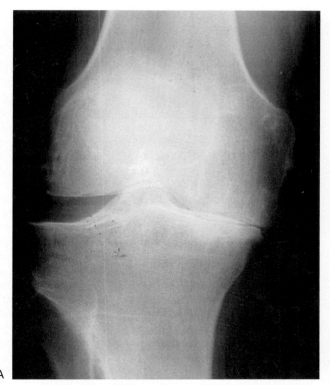

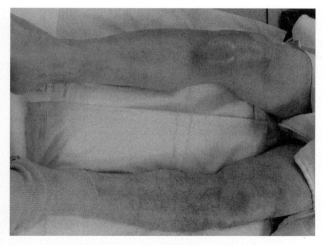

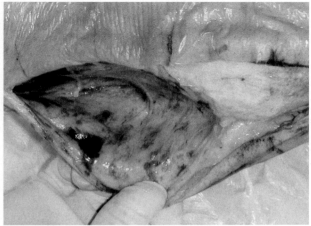

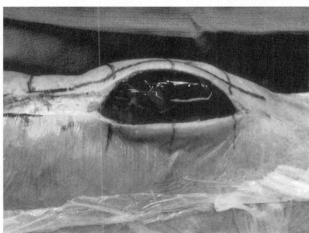

FIG. 6. **A:** Preoperative x-rays demonstrating rotational varus deformity. **B:** Clinical appearance of limb demonstrating a rotary deformity as well as varus alignment. **C:** Preoperative photo after tissue expander placement. **D:** Pseudomembrane that forms secondary to tissue expander use.

Before development of this technique, a sham incision was used. This was reported in the past for those patients thought to have high wound necrosis potential. This incision consists of a midline incision to the depth of the subcutaneous tissue. Skin flaps were elevated and the wound closed in a standard fashion. The wound was then observed to see if skin healed without incident. It was thought that if the wound could heal without incident, a TKA could be performed safely. Obviously, if the wound failed, local measures could be used to obtain healing without the increased pressure of an exposed prosthesis. The sham incision is mentioned for historical reasons and is no longer used at our institution.

TECHNIQUE OF TISSUE EXPANSION

For those patients we believe would benefit from soft tissue expansion, this procedure is performed before performing the TKA in the operating room (Fig. 5). The first step is to inject the subcutaneous space with fluid. In essence, this is a hydrodissection and separates the subcutaneous planes from the skin above. We currently use a mixture of lidocaine (Xylocaine) (0.05%) and 1/1,000,000 epinephrine. Usually, 300 mL is injected into the subcutaneous space. Injection is continued until the subcutaneous tissue is noted to blanch. A small incision is then made in line with the planned TKA. Based on the location of the adherent skin or previous incisions, two tissue expanders are used. If two expanders are used, they can be placed at 90-degree angles to each other, and each expander typically has a 200-mm capacity. The placement of the tissue expanders can be adjusted according to the patient's specific needs. Using blunt dissection, a subcutaneous pocket is created, and the expander balloon is inserted. Currently, we admit the patient for 24 hours and place him or her in a knee immobilizer for 1 week. When this week is completed, gradual expansion is begun, and, on average, 10% of the expanded volume is injected weekly. Injection speed is based on the patient's comfort as well as the presence of capillary refill of 5 seconds or less over the expander surface. As long as the patient tolerates the expansion, expander volume can be increased. Surgery is performed 2 weeks after the last expansion injection. These expanders do not present a problem when removed at the time of surgery (Fig. 6). Based on previous experience, our current recommendations are the placement of drains in the deep, as well as subcutaneous, pouches left by the tissue expander. With regard to skin incision and expansion, the choice exists of using the old incision or creating a new one. When possible, the incision deemed more adequate is used. We have found that tissue expanders enhance the vascularity of the flap in the old incision; therefore, if the prior incision is not adequate, a new longitudinal incision is chosen. If excessive skin is present after tissue expansion, although theoretically the skin bridge between the prior incision and new incision can be excised, the remaining edges are reapproximated. We have often found this is necessary. Certainly, the elastic skin contracts with time and in most cases no skin débridements are required.

This technique has been reported by other authors, mostly in case reports with revision TKA (44,45). While allowing primary closure without tension, standard TKA protocols can be followed with the emphasis on postoperative range of motion and function. More important, invasive procedures, such as free flaps, can be avoided. Although potential complications such as hematoma and infection of prosthesis, as well as prosthesis failure, exist with this technique, they can be limited. Benefits of tissue expansion include primary closure without tension, immediate range of motion, ability to use CPM, and the avoidance of disfiguring and reconstructive procedures such as flap coverage.

One type of wound failure noted after TKA is prolonged serous drainage. The question that remains for all surgeons is when to explore a chronically draining wound if excessive erythema or purulence is not present. When these are not present, the wounds can initially be observed. The etiology of this prolonged drainage may be secondary to a large hematoma, and if drainage is not resolved in 5 to 7 days, evacuation may become necessary. It is thought that hematoma can adversely affect the wound, placing increased tension on the skin edges. Possible breakdown of the hematoma may also play a role in wound healing. When prolonged drainage occurs, physical therapy and CPM may be limited or halted. Suspicion exists for infection because 17% to 50% of chronically draining wounds show later evidence of infection (46–48). It is for this reason that not all authors agree with the observation of prolonged draining of wounds. Weiss and Krackow (46) reported on early intervention with eight draining TKAs. These authors concluded that with early intervention, infection could perhaps be avoided (49).

DEEP TISSUE HEMATOMA

When a deep hematoma that is not draining occurs, the patient can be observed. With any signs of local skin compromise, increased pain, or limited range of motion, surgical exploration may become necessary. In our experience, early intervention for painful, limiting hematomas often allows a patient an early return to normal TKA protocols.

SUPERFICIAL SOFT TISSUE NECROSIS

Superficial necrosis is a vague term encompassing numerous conditions. It can describe a benign stitch abscess that improves with suture débridement and dressing changes and may even be used to describe the superficial soft tissue infection secondary to cellulitis. The term *superficial* is essentially used to describe complications that do not extend to the level of the prosthesis and bone. These superficial infections should be treated aggressively, and cultures should be obtained before initiating any antibiotic treatment. Should a superficial infection or soft tissue necrosis occur, CPM as well as physical therapy should be discontinued until wound appearance improves. It is difficult to differentiate from a deep necrosis and superficial necrosis, so surgical exploration may be needed to appropriately treat the lesion.

With aggressive treatment of superficial infections, skin necrosis can still occur. It is thought that skin necrosis smaller than 3 cm in size can be treated with local débridements and limb immobilization (50). Paramount to successful treatment of these infections is adequate débridement. Necrotic and nonviable tissue must be removed at the time of surgical exploration and débridement. If at the time of surgical exploration the infection is noted to be superficial, local wound débridements may be effective, and prosthesis salvage remains possible. If the prosthesis becomes exposed during the débridement, necrosis is no longer just superficial, and treatment for a major skin necrosis should be initiated.

Treatment of a superficial necrosis begins with local wound care. This includes local débridement as well as appropriate antibiotic coverage (2). Often, eschars are noted to develop on the anterior aspect of the leg, with no evidence of infection. This eschar can be observed until it is separated from the surrounding skin edges. Contracture occurs during this time, and eventual coverage may be less of a burden due to the constricting nature of the wound. Although small wounds may be allowed to heal by secondary intention, this allows the benefit of not undergoing another surgical procedure and continued range of motion once the wound appearance is stabilized. Skin grafting is indicated when the time for the untreated healing is longer than the healing of a routine skin grafting in the postoperative 5 to 7 days that accompany it. Once the skin graft is placed, the knee immobilizer is required to allow penetration of the vascular buds and the underlying wound. Obviously, infection should be controlled for a skin graft to be effective. Skin grafts are effective for treating soft tissue defects. For coverage of prosthesis, tendon, or bone, this is not successful.

A third option in treatment for superficial necrosis is local fasciocutaneous flap. Hallock (50) reported on six patients in whom coverage was successfully performed using this fasciocutaneous technique. Once again, the diagnosis of infection must be ruled out for this technique to be effective.

FULL-THICKNESS SOFT TISSUE NECROSIS

Full-thickness soft tissue necrosis is the most serious of wound complications. By definition, this involves deep penetration of the soft tissue and includes exposure of not only the bone and joint below, but also of the prosthesis that was placed, requiring coverage options and major surgical reconstructions. Although these major reconstructions are successful in maintaining the limb in an established prosthesis, there is a toll with regard to function. Adam et al. (51) reported long-term functional results of an exposed TKA treated by flap coverage. Although the wound was essentially covered, in 76% of the cases functional score was not as good as those with primary wound healing. Other options include advancement of local tissue or the transfer of distant tissue in the form of free flap (46,47). However, because of the complex nature of this problem, the prosthesis is often removed to treat the soft tissue difficulties, and early intervention from plastic surgery consultation cannot be overemphasized (52). The use of the gastrocnemius flap is well described in the orthopedic and plastic surgery literature (53–56). Using this technique, the medial head of the gastrocnemius muscle is used because of its wide arc of motion. It is detached from its insertion on the Achilles and then rotated proximally. The lateral gastrocnemius can also be used for lateral wound difficulties, but it is the medial gastrocnemius that is used for defects around the patella and tibial tubercle. These flaps are effective for covering the two-thirds of the tibia, whereas distal coverage requires free flap, free muscle transfer.

In cases in which gastrocnemius flaps are inadequate, a free muscle transfer, such as one using the latissimus dorsi muscle, the rectus abdominis muscle, or a scapular free flap, may be used. All these methods are well described and are reliable in obtaining coverage (2). Gerwin and coworkers (57) describe 12 patients who had an exposed prosthesis with a medial gastrocnemius flap, and 90% healing was achieved. Markovich et al. noted similar experience with muscle flap coverage (58). These authors described the results of five latissimus dorsi free flaps, six medial gastrocnemius rotational flaps, and two rectus abdominis free flaps, with 100% wound vascularization noted. In this series, prosthesis retention was achieved in 83% of the cases. It should come as no surprise that in evaluating the results, decreased knee function was noted when an infection along with necrosis occurred. Recently, Nahabedian and associates described their 10-year results with 35 complex TKA wounds (59). These patients were treated with aggressive wound management, and a 97% limb salvage rate was achieved. These authors emphasize the success of an aggressive approach to wound failures. We know that these were complex cases, with secondary plastic procedures required in 23% of patients. Secondary orthopedic procedures were required in 15% of the patients. The treatment options are based on the nature, size, location, and depth of the wound.

CONCLUSION

Wound problems are not always avoided with TKA procedures. Despite meticulous surgical technique and appropriate closure, wound failure can occur. The key to prevention of these lesions is twofold. By identifying those patients at risk, many wound failures can be avoided. When wound failure does occur, aggressive treatment is needed. With this approach, the prosthesis can be retained, and acceptable long-term function can be achieved.

REFERENCES

1. Scapinelli R. Studies on the vasculature of the human knee. *Acta Anat* 1968;70:305.
2. Craig SM. Soft tissue considerations in the failed total knee arthroplasty. In: Scott WN, ed. *The knee*, vol. 2. St. Louis: Mosby-Yearbook, 1994:1279.
3. Abbott LC, Carpenter WF. Surgical approaches to the knee joint. *J Bone Joint Surg* 1945;227:277.
4. Bjorkstom S, Goldie IF. A study of the arterial supply of the patella in the normal state, in chondromalacia patellae and in osteonecrosis. *Acta Orthop Scand* 1980;51:63.
5. Waisbrod H, Treiman N. Intra-osseous venography in patellofemoral disorders: a preliminary report. *J Bone Joint Surg Br* 1980;62:454.
6. Arey LB. Wound healing. *Physiol Rev* 1966;16:327.
7. Glenn F, Moore SW. The disruption of abdominal wounds. *Surg Gynecol Obstet* 1941;72:1041.
8. Johnson DD, Eastwood DM. Lateral patellar release in knee arthroplasty: effect on wound healing. *J Arthroplasty* 1992;7(Suppl):407.
9. Archauer BM, Black KS, Litke DK. Transcutaneous PO2 in flaps: a new method of surgical prediction. *Plast Reconstr Surg* 1980;65:738.
10. Heughan C, Chir B, Grislis G, et al. The effect of anemia on wound healing. *Ann Surg* 1974;179:163.
11. Kendall SJL, Weir J, Aspinall R, et al. Erythrocyte transfusion causes immunosuppression after total hip replacement. *Clin Orthop* 2000;381:145.
12. Murphy P, Heal JM, Blumberg N. Infection or suspected infection after total hip replacement surgery with autologous or homologous blood transfusion. *Transfusion* 1991;31:212.
13. Lehman CR, Ries MD, Paiement GD, et al. Infection after total joint arthroplasty in patients with human immunodeficiency virus or intravenous drug use. *J Arthroplasty* 2001;16:330.
14. Ecker ML, Lotke PA. Postoperative care of the total knee patient. *Orthop Clin North Am* 1989;20:55.
15. Dickhaut SC, DeLee JL, Pase CP. Nutritional statistics. Importance in predicting wound healing after amputation. *J Bone Joint Surg Am* 1984;66:71.
16. Wilson MG, Kelley K, Thornhill TS. Infection as a complication of total knee replacement arthroplasty: risk factors and treatment in sixty-seven cases. *J Bone Joint Surg Am* 1990;72:878.
17. Cruse PJ, Foord R. A five-year prospective study of 23,649 surgical wounds. *Arch Surg* 1973;107:206.
18. Stern SH, Insall JN. Total knee arthroplasty in obese patients. *J Bone Joint Surg Am* 1900;72:1400.
19. Griffin FM, Scuderi GR, Insall JN, et al. Total knee arthroplasty in patients who were obese with 10 years follow-up. *Clin Orthop* 1998;356:28.
20. Benowitz NL, Jacob P III. Daily intake of nicotine during cigarette smoking. *Clin Pharmacol Ther* 1984;35:494.
21. Benowitz NL, Kuyt F, Jacob P. Influence of nicotine on cardiovascular and hormonal effects of cigarette smoking. *Clin Pharmacol Ther* 1984;36:74.
22. Benowitz NL. Cotinine disposition and effects. *Clin Pharmacol Ther* 1983;34:664.
23. Wong R, Lotke P, Ecker M. Factors influencing wound healing after total knee arthroplasty. *Orthop Trans* 1986;10:497.
24. Garner RW, Mowot AG, Hazleman BL. Wound healing after operations on patients with rheumatoid arthritis. *J Bone Joint Surg Br* 1973;55:134.
25. Grogan TJ, Dores F, Rolling J, et al. Deep sepsis following total knee arthroplasty. *J Bone Joint Surg Am* 1986;68:226.
26. Johnson DD. Midline or parapatellar incision for knee arthroplasty. A comparative study of wound viability. *J Bone Joint Surg Br* 1988;70:656.
27. Johnson DD, Houshton TA, Redford P. Anterior midline or medial parapatellar incision for arthroplasty of the knee. A comparative study. *J Bone Joint Surg Br* 1986;68:812.
28. Dennis PA. Wound complications in total knee arthroplasty. *Instr Course Lect* 1997;46:165.
29. Ecker ML, Lotke PA. Wound healing complications. In: Rand JA, ed. *Total knee arthroplasty*. New York: Raven Press, 1993:403.
30. Windsor RE, Insall JN, Vince KE. Technical consideration of total

knee arthroplasty after proximal tibial osteotomy. *J Bone Joint Surg Am* 1988;70:547.

31. Holt BT, Parks NL, Ensh GA, et al. Comparison of closed reduction drainage and no drainage after primary total knee arthroplasty. *Orthopedics* 1997;20:1121.

32. Crevoisier XM, Reber P, Noesberger B. Is suction drainage necessary after total knee joint arthroplasty? A prospective study. *Arch Orthop Trauma Surg* 1998;117:121.

33. Ovadia D, Luger E, Bickels J, et al. Efficacy of closed wound drainage after total joint arthroplasty. A prospective randomized study. *J Arthroplasty* 1997;12:317.

34. Cushner FD, Scott WN. Evolution of blood management for a busy knee practice. *Orthopedics* 1999;22:S-145.

35. Drinkwater CJ, Neil MJ. Optimal timing of wound drain removal following total joint arthroplasty. *J Arthroplasty* 1995;10:185.

36. Stulberg RN, Insall JN, Williams GW, et al. Deep-vein thrombosis following total knee replacement. *J Bone Joint Surg Am* 1984;2:194.

37. Levine MN, Gent M, Hirsh J, et al. Ardeparin (low molecular weight heparin) vs. graduated compression stockings for the prevention of venous thromboembolism. A randomized trial in patients undergoing knee surgery. *Arch Intern Med* 1996;156:851.

38. Leclere JR, Geerts WN, DesJardins L, et al. Prevention of venous thromboembolism (WTE) after knee arthroplasty—a randomized double-blind trial comparing a low molecular-weight heparin fragment (enoxaparin) to warfarin. *Blood* 1992;84:246a.

39. Spiro TE, Fitzgerald RH, Trowbridge AA, et al. Enoxaparin—a low molecular weight heparin and warfarin for the prevention of venous thromboembolic disease after elective knee replacement surgery. *Blood* 1994;84:246a.

40. Faralli VJ, Lotke PA, Orenstein E. *Blood loss after total knee replacement: effects of early motion.* Presented at the 55th annual meeting of the American Academy of Orthopaedic Surgeons, New Orleans, February 1998.

41. Yashar AA. Continuous passive motion with accelerated flexion after total knee arthroplasty. *Clin Orthop* 1997;345:38.

42. Gold DA, Scott SC, Scott WN. Soft tissue expansion prior to arthroplasty in the multiply operated knee—a new method of preventing catastrophic skin problems. *J Arthroplasty* 1996;11:512.

43. Manifold SG, Cushner FD, Scott SC, et al. Long-term results of total knee arthroplasty after the use of soft tissue expanders. *Clin Orthop* 2000;380:133.

44. Santore RF, Kaufman D, Robbins AJ, et al. Tissue expansion prior to revision total knee arthroplasty. *J Arthroplasty* 1997;12:475.

45. Namba RS, Diao E. Tissue expansion for staged reimplantation of infected total knee arthroplasty. *J Arthroplasty* 1997;12:471.

46. Weiss AP, Krackow KA. Persistent wound drainage after primary total knee arthroplasty. *J Arthroplasty* 1993;8:285.

47. Bergstrom S, Kruston K, Lidgren I. Treatment of infected knee arthroplasty. *Clin Orthop* 1989;245:173.

48. Insall J, Aglietti P. A five to seven-year follow-up of unicondylar arthroplasty. *J Bone Joint Surg Am* 1980;62:1329.

49. Sculco TP. Local wound complications after total knee arthroplasty. In Ranawat C, ed. *Total condylar knee arthroplasty.* New York: Springer-Verlag, 1985.

50. Hallock GG. Salvage of total knee arthroplasty with local fasciocutaneous flaps. *J Bone Joint Surg Br* 1990;72:1236.

51. Adam RR, Watson SF, Jarratt JW, et al. Outcome after flap coverage for exposed total knee arthroplasties. A report of 25 cases. *J Bone Joint Surg Br* 1994;76:750.

52. Bergstrom S, Carlsson A, Relander M, et al. Treatment of the exposed knee prosthesis. *Acta Orthop Scand* 1987;58:662.

53. Eckhardt JJ, Lesavoy MA, Dubrow TJ, et al. Exposed endo-prosthesis. *Clin Orthop* 1990;251:220.

54. Hemphill CS, Ebert FR, Muench AG. The medial gastrocnemius muscle flap in the treatment of wound complications following total knee arthroplasty. *Orthopedics* 1992;15:477.

55. Peled IJ, Franki U, Wexler MR. Salvage of exposed knee prosthesis by gastrocnemius myocutaneous flap coverage. *Orthopedics* 1983;6:1320.

56. Salibian AH, Sanford HA. Salvage of an infected total knee prosthesis with medial and lateral gastrocnemius muscle flaps. *J Bone Joint Surg Am* 1983;6:681.

57. Gerwin M, Rothaus KU, Windsor RE, et al. Gastrocnemius muscle flap coverage of exposed or infected knee prosthesis. *Clin Orthop* 1993;286:64.

58. Markovich G, Door LD, Klein NE, et al. Muscle flaps in knee arthroplasty. *Clin Orthop* 1995;321:122.

59. Nahabedian ML, Orlando JL, Delanois RE, et al. Salvage procedures for complex soft tissue defects of the knee. *Clin Orthop* 1998;356:119.

CHAPTER 98

Extensor Mechanism Rupture

Raj K. Sinha and Harry E. Rubash

Total knee arthroplasty (TKA) has enjoyed worldwide success in treating the debilitated knee. Despite excellent results for most patients, complications of the patellofemoral joint continue to be a major source of dissatisfaction for both surgeons and patients. Complications may include such undesirable results as painless crepitus with range-of-motion movements, persistent anterior knee pain, patellar subluxation or dislocation, patellar clunk, patellar component loosening, patellar component wear, patellar fracture, and patellar tendon rupture. This chapter addresses the rare but potentially catastrophic complication of extensor mechanism disruption. Rorabeck et al. (1), have reviewed other patellofemoral complications, many of which are discussed elsewhere in this text.

QUADRICEPS TENDON DISRUPTION

Rupture of the quadriceps tendon after TKA is rare. Lynch et al. (2) reported that quadriceps tendon rupture occurred in 3 of 281 patients (1.1%) after TKA. Fernandez-Baillo et al. reported a single case (3) and Grace and Sim reported a single quadriceps tendon rupture postpatellectomy after treatment of a patella fracture after TKA (4).

Because the complication is rare, it is unclear which conditions may predispose a TKA patient to quadriceps rupture. Rheumatoid arthritis was implicated by Fernandez-Baillo (3), whereas Lynch et al. (2) and Grace and Sim (4) suggested that a technical error such as overresection of the patella or violation of the quadriceps tendon was causative. Additional potential causes include poor preoperative range of motion, poor exposure necessitating a rectus snip or V-Y turndown with subsequent incomplete healing, postoperative manipulation, or trauma.

Fernandez-Baillo et al. (3) performed a primary quadriceps tendon repair with proximal turndown over the repair and supplementation with Dacron tape, followed by treatment in a long-leg cast with the knee in extension for 6 weeks. After follow-up of 1 year, the functional result was reported to be good. We have attempted primary repair and an Achilles tendon allograft reinforcement. Both techniques have been less than optimal, although a slightly better functional outcome resulted after the allograft reconstruction.

Treatment of quadriceps rupture after TKA remains difficult and should be prevented with meticulous surgical technique and careful attention to preservation of the blood supply during primary or revision TKA.

PATELLAR FRACTURE

Traumatic and stress fractures of the patella after TKA have been reported in several series (2,4–13). The reported incidence varies from 0.3% to 5.4% (Table 1). Clayton and Thirupathi (7) reported 6 fractures in 111 total condylar TKAs within 18 months of surgery. Five required additional surgery. Of the five patients requiring surgery, only three had a satisfactory result. Similarly, Insall et al. reported four patellar fractures at an average 6.6-year follow-up in a study of 88 total condylar TKAs (9). Despite treatment, the patellar fractures resulted in a poorer outcome after TKA. After duopatellar TKA, Scott et al. (11) noted that the incidence of patellar fractures was 0.5% (6 in 1,213). Three of the six patients were treated nonsurgically with good results. However, two of three surgical patients eventually went on to require a patellectomy. In a series by Grace and Sim (4), 12 of 8,249 TKAs (0.15%) were associated with a patellar fracture. Eight patients had operative treatment, three of whom had

TABLE 1. *Incidence of extensor mechanism rupture*

Quadriceps tendon	
Fernandez-Baillo et al. (3)	1 case report
Lynch et al. (2)	3/281 (1.1%)
Patellar fractures	
Scott et al. (11)	
Resurfaced	5/372 (1.3%)
Unresurfaced	1/841 (0.12%)
Clayton (7)	6/111 (5.4%)
Lynch et al. (2)	5/281 (1.8%)
Webster (31)	1/366 (0.27%)
Insall (9)	4/88 (5.4%)
Ritter (16)	
Lateral release	1/84 (1.2%)
No lateral release	17/471 (3.6%)
Brick et al. (6)	15/2,887 (0.52%)
Grace and Sim (4)	
Resurfaced	9/2,719 (0.33%)
Unresurfaced	3/5,530 (0.05%)
Boyd et al. (5)	
Resurfaced	3/396 (0.76%)
Unresurfaced	0/495
Tria et al. (13)	18/504 (3.6%)
Healy et al. (8)	5/211 (2.4%)
Patellar tendon	
Wilson and Venteers (24)	3/54 (5.6%)
Deburge (26)	5/292 (1.7%)
Lettin et al. (22)	2/100 (2.0%)
Yamamoto (28)	1/170 (0.59%)
Wilson et al. (25)	1/62 (1.6%)
Hui and Fitzgerald (27)	2/77 (2.6%)
Kaufer and Matthews (44)	1/82 (1.2%)
Lettin et al. (23)	1/20 (5.0%)
Oglesby and Wilson (18)	4/160 (2.5%)
Townley (12)	2/532 (0.38%)
Webster and Murray (31)	1/366 (0.27%)
Lynch et al. (2)	4/281 (1.4%)
Grace and Rand (35)	2/25 (8.0%)
Rand et al. (30)	17/8,288 (0.21%)
Boyd et al. (5)	
Resurfaced	3/396 (0.76%)
Unresurfaced	2/495 (0.40%)
Healy et al. (8)	1/211 (0.47%)

TABLE 2. *Etiology of extensor mechanism ruptures*

Technical issues
Lateral release
Component malalignment
Patellar subluxation
Overresection of patellar bone
Overstuffing of anterior compartment
Total fat pad excision
Thermal necrosis from cement
Excessive pressure from use of patellar clamps
Inset patellar components
Revision surgery
Devascularization
Mechanical impingement
Patellar instability
Implant choices
Resurfacing
Cementless fixation
Hinged total knee prosthesis
Posterior stabilized components
Patient factors
Revision total knee arthroplasty
Previous patellar fracture
Manipulation
Excessive early range of motion
Male gender
Osteoporosis
Subchondral cysts
Rheumatoid arthritis
Chronic steroid use
Collagen vascular diseases
Diabetes mellitus
Trauma
Infection

---

significant complications, including quadriceps rupture, sepsis, and refracture. Brick and Scott (6) reported 15 fractures in 2,887 cases (0.52%), nine of which were treated with repeat surgery. Seven of these patients had significant complications that resulted in a poorer outcome. Thus, despite its low incidence, patellar fracture adversely affects the results of TKA.

Factors that may increase the chance of patellar fracture (Table 2) include patellar resurfacing (1,4,5), lateral release (1,8,14), use of press-fit patellar components (8,14), revision surgery (4), malalignment of the arthroplasty components (12,15), aggressive excision of the fat pad (7), overresection leading to a thin patellar remnant (1,4,7,14), the use of patellar clamps (14), improper size and orientation of the fixation pegs (1,14), thermal necrosis induced by cement (4,7), osteoporosis (6), osteoarthritic cysts (6), patellar subluxation (4), incorrect patellar component size (4), postoperative manipulation (1), previous patellar fracture (1), hinged TKA (16), male gender (14), excessive early flexion (17), use of posterior stabilized femoral components (14), use of inset patellar components (14),

increased thickness of the patella, and excessive anterior displacement of the femoral component (18). Of the many possible causes of patellar fracture, a few have been shown to have statistical significance. For example, Grace and Sim (4) reported that fractures occurred in 9 of 2,719 resurfaced patellae (0.33%), but in only 3 of 5,530 unresurfaced patellae (0.05%) (p <.05). Similarly, Scott et al. (11) showed that 5 of 372 resurfaced patellae (1.3%) went on to fracture, whereas only 1 of 841 unresurfaced patellae (0.12%) did. In addition, the series of Boyd et al. (5) reported that 3 of 396 resurfaced patellae (0.76%) fractured, and 0 of 495 unresurfaced patella fractured. Thus, fractures appear to occur more commonly after patella resurfacing performed as part of the TKA.

Another commonly implicated cause of fracture is lateral retinacular release with subsequent devascularization of the patella (19). Healy et al. (8) reported that four of five fractures occurred after lateral release (p <.04). Scott et al. found a similar incidence (11). In addition, Tria et al. (13) determined that 18 of 18 patellar fractures followed a lateral release, although 82% of all cases required lateral release. Ritter and Campbell (16), however, specifically addressed the question of lateral release and patellar fracture in a prospective study. These authors found a higher incidence of patellar fracture in TKAs not requiring lateral release (3.6%) than in those requiring lateral release (1.4%), even though no attempt was made to preserve the superior lateral geniculate artery. Regardless of these conflicting studies, most authors agree that the benefits of lateral release to balance the patella and improve patellofemoral mechanics outweigh the risk of avascularity, although preservation of the superior lateral geniculate artery is preferred.

Another predisposing factor for patellar fracture is revision TKA. Patella fracture occurred in 3 of 495 revision TKAs (0.61%), compared with 9 of 7,754 primary TKAs (0.12%) (p <.05) (4). Similarly, four of five fractures occurred after the use of cementless patellar components versus one of five fractures after placement of cemented components (20). Tria et al. (13) showed that minor malalignment of the TKA (15) may have contributed to 17 of 18 patellar fractures. In addition, minor malalignment may cause more severe patellar fractures compared with neutral alignment (15). The other suggested predisposing factors listed in Table 2 are based on individual authors' experience but have not been shown statistically to increase the incidence of patellar fracture.

The poorer quality of bone in patients with rheumatoid arthritis than in those with osteoarthritis suggests that patellar fracture should occur more often in TKA patients with rheumatoid arthritis. Scott et al. (11), however, noted fractures in 2 of 286 rheumatoid arthritis patients (0.7%) and in 3 of 86 of osteoarthritis patients (3.5%). In addition, Ritter and Campbell (16), Grace and Sim (4), and Brick and Scott (6) found no increased incidence of patellar fracture in patients with rheumatoid arthritis. This may be the result of lower demand on the TKA and the decreased flexion seen in rheumatoid arthritis patients.

Classification and Treatment

Goldberg et al. (20) attempted to classify and describe the natural history of various types of patellar fractures that were treated in 36 patients. They identified five categories: type I—no involvement of the implant/cement composite or quadriceps mechanism; type II—involvement of the implant/cement composite or quadriceps mechanism; type IIIA—inferior pole fractures with patellar tendon rupture; type IIIB—inferior pole fractures without patellar tendon rupture; and type IV—fractures-dislocations.

The authors treated 14 type I fractures nonoperatively with resulting good or excellent functional scores and no pain, locking, or mechanical symptoms. All six patients with type II midbody fractures had surgery to revise loose components and to repair the quadriceps tendon. Four knees had unsatisfactory results. Two of two type IIIB fractures treated nonoperatively had no superior migration with acceptable results. Eight type IIIA fractures were identified, and surgery was recommended for all patients to repair the ruptured patellar tendon. Five of seven operated knees had poor outcomes, and the one patient who refused surgery had a poor outcome also. Nine patients had type IV fractures, and all had surgical treatment. Four patients had unsatisfactory results. Overall, 13 of 22 surgically treated knees had unsatisfactory results.

Hozack et al. (21) treated 21 periprosthetic patellar fractures and reviewed the outcomes. A wide variety of treatments were rendered to their heterogeneous group of patients. Seven patients had a nondisplaced fracture, five of which were comminuted. Four of these patients were treated with a patellectomy and had eventual good range of motion, no extensor lag, and good functional knee scores. Three of four patients, however, had decreased quadriceps strength. Three patients with nondisplaced fractures

were treated in a cylinder cast. One patient had a poor result due to limited flexion after treatment. Fourteen patients had displaced fractures. Six were treated with a patellectomy, with only two having a satisfactory outcome. The remaining patients had decreased quadriceps strength and residual extensor lags. Open reduction and internal fixation of two displaced inferior pole fractures failed. Two patients treated nonoperatively had satisfactory results in terms of extensor lag, quadriceps strength, and range of motion. Of the four patients treated by fragment excision, two had favorable results and two had poor results. Based on these findings, Hozack et al. recommended treatment of nondisplaced fractures and displaced fractures with no extensor lag nonoperatively with casting or bracing in extension. Results are poor for displaced fractures with extensor lag, and distal fragment excision should be considered. Patellectomy should be reserved for all failed interventions.

Authors' Preferred Treatment

We have identified several criteria that determine treatment and reflect outcome after a periprosthetic patellar fracture. These criteria include extensor mechanism integrity, fracture displacement, loosening of the patellar component, and vascularity of the patella. We have established a useful treatment algorithm based on these criteria (Fig. 1).

When a patient presents with a patellar fracture, the integrity of the extensor mechanism is assessed first. If the patient is able to fully extend the limb against gravity or perform a straight leg raise, then the extensor mechanism is considered to be intact. These patients usually have a nondisplaced fracture that does not involve the quadriceps or patellar tendon and can be treated reliably with a long-leg cast or brace in extension for 6 weeks or until the fracture shows radiographic signs of healing. Once the fracture heals, patellar component stability is assessed. If the fracture did not disrupt the component-bone interface, physical therapy to work on range of motion can be instituted. If the fracture heals but the component has become loose (typically seen with comminuted fractures), the quality of remaining bone and the extent of its vascularity determine whether revision or resection would be appropriate. If the fracture does not heal, then component fixation determines the next step. Displaced fractures not involving the component-bone interface (typically vertical and marginal fractures) may progress to nonunion, which leads to later fragment excision. If the nonunited fracture results in component loosening, the quality and vascularity of the remaining patellar bone determine the next step. The presence of good-quality bone allows open reduction and internal fixation of the fracture with component revision. The presence of poor-quality bone should lead the surgeon to resect the remnants, perform a primary repair, and possibly supplement the extensor mechanism with an Achilles tendon or extensor mechanism allograft.

Displaced transverse fractures often lead to component loosening and disrupt the extensor mechanism, and thus require operative intervention. If the component is stable (an unusual circumstance) and the patellar bone is vascular and sufficiently thick, then open reduction and internal fixation is appropriate. If the component is loose and the patella has sufficient bone stock and vascularity, then open reduction and internal fixation with component revision is performed. If the patella is avascular, too thin, or too ectatic for

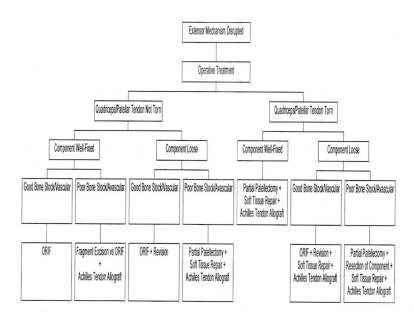

FIG. 1. Algorithm for treatment of patellar fractures after total knee arthroplasty. ORIF, open reduction, internal fixation.

resurfacing, or if the patellar or quadriceps tendon is ruptured, we prefer partial or total patellectomy, coupled with primary repair and Achilles tendon allograft augmentation. In addition, the same algorithmic approach is used for displaced chronic fractures with loss of extensor mechanism function.

An important caveat when treating patellar fractures associated with ruptured extensor mechanisms is that the patient may not be a suitable candidate for operative treatment. Elderly patients with minimal ambulatory potential, patients with poor skin that would compromise wound healing, and patients with debilitating medical comorbidities, among others, may be better treated with a brace despite the residual extensor lag.

Another important surgical issue to address is component alignment and rotational position. When operative treatment is required, the femoral and tibial component orientation must be addressed, with revision of one or more components as indicated. Failure to address component orientation may result in recurrent patellar fracture, maltracking, or subluxation.

PATELLAR TENDON RUPTURE

Incidence

Like patellar fracture, patellar tendon rupture after TKA is a potentially devastating complication (Fig. 2). Despite the low incidence of patellar tendon rupture, most large series that discuss the results of TKA using a variety of prosthesis types report some such ruptures (summarized in Table 1).

For example, a review of the Stanmore hinged prosthesis by Lettin et al. (22) noted two patellar tendon avulsions at the time of surgery and two subsequent ruptures (4% incidence). Both of the latter patients required ambulatory aids after the complication. The same authors reported one additional rupture (5% incidence) in the 20 patients followed longer than 10 years (23). With the Walldius hinged prosthesis, 3 of 54 patients (5.6%) had a patellar tendon rupture (24). Similarly, in a study comparing the Walldius hinged and the Geometric knee prostheses (25), 1 of 62 TKAs (1.6%) using hinged devices was complicated by a

patellar ligament rupture 4 months after surgery. After primary repair, the patient developed deep sepsis and an eventual 35-degree extensor lag. Another comparative study between the Walldius, Geometric, and total condylar knees (18) revealed 5 of 160 ruptures (3.1%), 4 of which occurred in the Walldius group. All four patellar tendon ruptures were treated with a primary repair, but patients had residual extensor lags of 10 to 35 degrees. Using the Guepar hinged prosthesis, Deburge (26) reported an incidence of 5 in 292 (1.7%) tendon ruptures. Furthermore, a Mayo Clinic series using hinged Walldius and Guepar prostheses showed a 2.6% incidence (2 of 77 TKAs) of patellar tendon rupture (27).

Patellar tendon rupture has also been reported with other knee designs. Yamamoto (28) found patellar tendon avulsion from the tibial tubercle during surgery in 1 of 170 TKAs (0.59%). The tendon was successfully reattached with a staple. Two of 532 TKAs using Townley prostheses (0.38%) were complicated by patellar tendon rupture or avulsion (12). Lynch et al. (2) reported a 1.4% incidence (4 of 281), whereas Boyd et al. (5) reported a 0.56% incidence (5 of 891). Similarly, Cadambi and Engh (29) found a 0.55% incidence in their series, Healy et al. (8) reported 1 of 211 (0.5% incidence), and Rand et al. (30) reported a 0.17% incidence of patellar tendon rupture in 8,288 TKAs. Thus, the reported incidence of patellar tendon rupture varies from 0.17% to 5.6% after primary TKA.

As with quadriceps tendon ruptures, the low incidence of patellar tendon ruptures after TKA makes it difficult to delineate specific predisposing factors. Several authors have outlined possible causes, however (summarized in Table 2). For example, Rand et al. (30) suggested that attempts to gain exposure during revision TKA were the most common cause. In addition, chronic steroid use (24,29,31), trauma (32), multiple surgeries (2), devascularization of the tendon (33,34), and mechanical impingement by the tibial or patellar components (33,34) have been implicated. Infection may result in patellar tendon rupture (24,25). In the study of Cadambi and Engh (29), five of seven patients had systemic conditions such as diabetes mellitus and rheumatoid arthritis. These authors also suggested that collagen vascular diseases may be a predisposing factor. In addition,

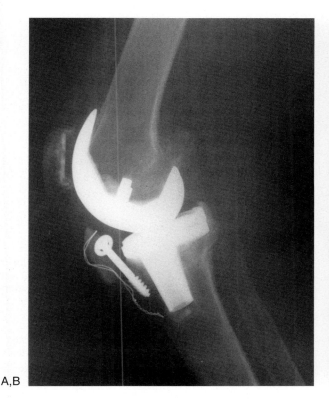
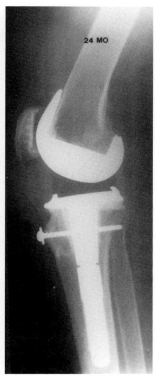

A,B

FIG. 2. A: Radiograph of patellar tendon rupture after total knee arthroplasty (TKA) and tibial tubercle osteotomy. **B:** Radiograph of revision TKA and extensor mechanism reconstruction using an Achilles tendon allograft.

Grace and Rand noted that two tendon ruptures occurred after 25 realignment procedures for patellar instability (35). Also, hinged TKAs appear to be more likely to cause a patellar tendon rupture because of the increased constraint (25). A slightly increased predisposition to rupture after patellar resurfacing (0.76% versus 0.40% with no resurfacing) (5) may be present. Finally, dislocation of a knee prosthesis may be the result of a ruptured patellar tendon (36).

Treatment and Results

As discussed earlier, initial attempts at primary repair of the ruptured patellar tendon were fraught with unpredictable results. One exception may be when the tendon peels off at the tibial tubercle at the time of surgery. In our experience, if the periosteal sleeve is intact, the tendon may be reattached with a suture anchor or through drill holes. The TKA is usually unaffected, even with standard rehabilitation protocols. Repair of late ruptures or avulsions, however, presents a different treatment quandary.

Wilson and Venteers (24) used the plantaris tendon to repair midsubstance patellar tendon ruptures. Both patients achieved full active extension, although no details of the repair technique or of the postoperative regimen were provided. More recently, Rand et al. (30) reviewed their results after treating 18 tendon ruptures. All nine patients who were treated with primary suture repair failed to gain full active extension. Four patients had staple fixation of tendon avulsions, which was successful in two patients. One patient had a primary suture repair with semitendinosus tendon augmentation, which also failed. Two other patients had xenograft reconstructions, both of which were successful. The final two patients were treated with a cast, and nei-

ther was able to achieve full extension. Thus, of 18 treated patellar tendon ruptures, a successful outcome occurred in only four cases, and the mean flexion was only 81 degrees. This study underscores the difficulty in treating patellar tendon ruptures with primary repair.

Emerson and associates first reported an allograft technique in 1990 (33) and later reported intermediate-term follow-up results in 1994 (34). In their technique, the graft included the quadriceps tendon, patella with cemented prosthesis, patellar tendon, and tibial tubercle. The tubercle was keyed into the host tibia at an anatomic location and secured with a screw or cerclage wire. The patella was placed on the anterior flange of the femoral prosthesis and tensioned, whereas the quadriceps tendon was attached to the host tendon with nonabsorbable sutures to allow 60 degrees of flexion with minimal tension. Postoperatively, the patient was allowed limited flexion for several weeks, followed by a gradual increase in range of motion. At an average follow-up of 23 months in ten patients, two graft ruptures and one patellar fracture were noted, all of which led to failure of the reconstruction. In the remaining seven patients, all the tubercles and quadriceps tendon repairs healed. Nine patients were further followed for a mean of 4.1 years (34). Six patients gained full active extension, and three had extensor lags ranging from 20 to 40 degrees. The average flexion was 106 degrees. There were no additional graft ruptures, but two patellar prostheses became loose and required reoperation. Thus, the authors saw no need to resurface the patella. Overall, this technique was thought to be a reasonable option for extensor-mechanism-deficient TKAs, particularly in patients with low-demand activities, although longevity was a concern.

Two other groups of authors have reported their results with the technique of Emerson et al. Leopold et al. (37) reported on seven patients who underwent extensor mechanism reconstruc-

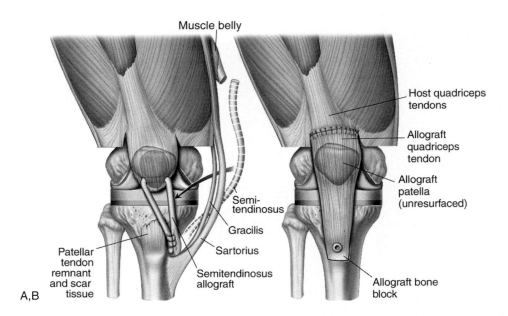

FIG. 3. Schematic representation of the Cadambi and Engh **(A)** and Emerson **(B)** techniques for extensor mechanism reconstruction.

tion with strict adherence to the technique described by Emerson et al. At a mean follow-up of 39 months, all patients had an extensor lag of more than 30 degrees, with a mean of 59 degrees. Knee scores improved only from 50 to 52. There was no apparent improvement in function in any patient. Meanwhile, Nazarian and Booth (38) reported their results with the Emerson technique. In 36 patients, 15 had resultant extensor lags, with a mean of 13 degrees. Twenty-three patients had no extensor lag, and the average range of motion for the entire group was 1.4 degrees of extension to 98 degrees of flexion. Knee scores improved from 37 to 68, and at mean of 3.6 years of follow-up, 34 of 36 patients were satisfied with the procedure. Importantly, although Leopold et al. followed the technique of Emerson et al. strictly, Nazarian and Booth performed the repair of the allograft with the knee in full extension and immobilized the knee in a brace postoperatively. Thus, slight modifications in the technique and rehabilitation protocols may account for the differences in reported results.

Cadambi and Engh (29) used a semitendinosus tendon to reconstruct seven ruptured patellar tendons. The tendon was divided at its proximal muscle junction, routed along the medial edge of the ruptured patellar tendon, through a drill hole in the distal pole of the patella, and then sutured to itself at the distal insertion. The knee was flexed to 90 degrees to ensure that the graft was free of excessive tension. Immediate full weightbearing in a knee immobilizer was allowed. After 6 weeks, limited flexion to 60 degrees was allowed for an additional 6 weeks. A knee immobilizer was required for ambulation. Among these seven patients, the average extension lag was 10 degrees, with an average flexion of only 79 degrees. Four patients required a cane to walk. The authors concluded that the autogenous graft technique was superior to primary repair or allograft reconstruction, and that sufficient quadriceps strength and motion of the knee were restored.

Jaureguito and associates (39) used a medial gastrocnemius muscle flap to reconstruct six patellar tendon ruptures after TKA. The flap was mobilized and sutured transversely to the anterior muscle compartment at the level of the tubercle. The patellar tendon was then sutured to the gastrocnemius flap. Post-operatively, patients were placed in a long-leg cast in full extension for 6 weeks, followed by a hinged knee brace for 8 weeks, with progressive flexion allowed by the brace. At an average 26-month follow-up, the average extensor lag was 24 degrees, and the average range of motion was 100 degrees. The ambulatory ability of all patients improved, with two each requiring no aids, a cane, or a walker. There were two complications. One postoperative manipulation led to a 30-degree extensor lag, and one patient required a skin graft for a small area of skin. The authors concluded that a medial gastrocnemius flap was a reliable option for reconstructing ruptured patellar tendons and simultaneously improved soft tissue coverage.

Several case reports describe other methods to treat ruptured patellar tendons after TKA. For example, Abril et al. (40) used Bunnell repairs with nonabsorbable suture placed through two drill holes in the tubercle to treat two patellar tendon avulsions. A figure-of-eight wire placed through the quadriceps tendon and around a screw in the tubercle protected the repair. Both patients gained full active extension, 85 and 95 degrees of flexion, and could ambulate with no walking aids. Similarly, Zanotti et al. (32) used a bone–patellar tendon–bone allograft, such as are used for anterior cruciate ligament reconstructions. The allograft was secured to the patella proximally by interference fit and distally by an interference screw. The leg was held in an extension cast for 12 weeks, and flexion was gradually increased. At 2 years, the patient had full active extension but required a knee-foot-ankle orthosis to control 5 to 10 degrees of chronic hyperextension. Flexion was not mentioned. Alternatively, Chiou et al. (41) reported satisfactory results after using an autogenous lateral gastrocnemius–Achilles tendon graft to reconstruct a patellar tendon rupture with an accompanying skin defect. Finally, Kempenaar and Cameron (42) described a patellotibial fusion for a chronic patellar tendon rupture. The patient's active range of motion was −20 to 90 degrees. Although each of these techniques may be a potential option, additional experience with longer follow-up is necessary.

Figure 3 is a schematic representation of the common methods to reconstruct a ruptured patellar tendon after TKA.

Authors' Method for Achilles Tendon Allograft Reconstruction

Drawing from the experience of various authors, we chose to use a fresh frozen Achilles tendon allograft with os calcis bone block to reconstruct patellar and quadriceps tendon ruptures and to supplement fixation of patellar fractures, as outlined in Figure 1. This is based on several observations:

1. Simple primary repairs often result in an extensor lag with the need for ambulatory aids.
2. Freeze-dried allografts are mechanically inferior to fresh frozen allografts (33,34).
3. Securely fixed bony allografts appear to heal to the tibia without difficulty (33,34).
4. Allograft tendon heals reliably to the quadriceps myofascia and tendon when nonabsorbable suture is used (33,34).
5. Autograft tendons are unreliable in length, thickness, strength, and integrity (29).
6. Use of autogenous muscle-tendon autografts is technically very challenging and carries the chance of avoidable donor-site morbidity (39,41).

There are several important points to remember when using this technique:

1. Fresh-frozen allograft is used rather than freeze-dried allograft.
2. Minimal autogenous tissue is removed, and primary repairs are performed if possible.
3. The tendinous portion of the allograft is handled with no crushing instruments.
4. The bony portion of the allograft is maintained thick enough so as not to predispose to its fracture.
5. Atraumatic tapered needles should be used.
6. Thick skin and subcutaneous flaps must be created and closed with minimal tension.
7. Strict adherence to postoperative rehabilitation protocols is required.

Postoperatively, the patient is maintained in a hinged knee brace locked at full extension with touch-down weightbearing and isometric exercises. After 1 month, the patient can progress to 50% weightbearing, with the brace set to allow 0 to 40 degrees total range of motion. Active and passive range-of-motion and quadriceps-strengthening exercises are instituted within the limitations of the brace parameters. After the second month, the brace is reset to allow 90 degrees of flexion. Weightbearing may be advanced to full weightbearing. At the end of the third month, the brace is discontinued. Physical therapy continues for an additional 6 to 12 weeks.

Our preliminary results with this technique were reported (43). Results were described for ten patients at an average follow-up of 30 months. The average preoperative extensor lag was 40 degrees. Postoperatively, two patients had 5-degree extensor lags and, significantly, eight patients had no extensor lag. The average flexion was 101 degrees, which was improved from 89 degrees preoperatively. All patients improved their ambulation status, with seven requiring a cane and three requiring a walker. Three complications occurred. The first patient fell, acutely hyperflexed his knee, and dislodged the bony block. The block was surgically resecured, and the patient achieved full active extension and 110 degrees of flexion. The second patient sustained a tibial shaft fracture at the allograft fixation site 14 months after the index operation. After revision of the tibial tray with a long stem that bypassed the nonunion site, the fracture healed and the patient had no extensor lag with 110 degrees of flexion.

CONCLUSION

Ruptures of extensor mechanisms after TKA can be devastating injuries. In the absence of TKA, these injuries are much easier to diagnose and treat. After TKA, however, extreme disability can result. Thus, a systematic approach for treatment is necessary. Two decades of experience suggest that surgery is not always indicated. When surgery is required, however, primary repair is usually insufficient and should not be attempted. A grafting procedure is usually required to supplement the repair and to restore functional outcomes. TKA patients represent a difficult population with multiple comorbidities. Thus, minor complications are fairly frequent, and treatment must be tailored to the patient. With the appropriate approach, however, good outcomes can be achieved consistently.

REFERENCES

1. Rorabeck CH, Angliss RD, Lewis L. Fractures of the femur, tibia, and patella after total knee arthroplasty: decision making and principles of management. *Instr Course Lect* 1998;47:449.
2. Lynch AF, Rorabeck CH, Bourne RB. Extensor mechanism complications following total knee arthroplasty. *J Arthroplasty* 1987;2:135.
3. Fernandez-Baillo N, Garay EG, Ordonez JM. Rupture of the quadriceps tendon after total knee arthroplasty. *J Arthroplasty* 1993;8:331.
4. Grace JN, Sim FH. Fracture of the patella after total knee arthroplasty. *Clin Orthop* 1988;230:168.
5. Boyd AD, Ewald FC, Thomas WH, et al. Long-term complications after total knee arthroplasty with or without resurfacing of the patella. *J Bone Joint Surg Am* 1993;75:674.
6. Brick GW, Scott RD. The patellofemoral component of total knee arthroplasty. *Clin Orthop* 1988;231:163.
7. Clayton ML, Thirupathi R. Patellar complications after total condylar arthroplasty. *Clin Orthop* 1982;170:152.
8. Healy WL, Wasilewski SA, Takei R, et al. Patellofemoral complications following total knee arthroplasty. *J Arthroplasty* 1995;10:197.
9. Insall JN, Hood RW, Flawn LB, et al. The total condylar knee prosthesis in gonarthrosis. *J Bone Joint Surg Am* 1983;65:619.
10. Reuben JD, McDonald L, Woodard PL, et al. The effect of patella thickness on patella strain following total knee arthroplasty. *J Arthroplasty* 1991;6:251.
11. Scott RD, Turoff N, Ewald FC. Stress fracture of the patella following duopatellar knee arthroplasty with patellar resurfacing. *Clin Orthop* 1982;170:147.
12. Townley CO. The anatomic total knee resurfacing arthroplasty. *Clin Orthop* 1985;192:82.
13. Tria AJ, Harwood DA, Alicea JA, et al. Patellar fractures in posterior stabilized knee arthroplasties. *Clin Orthop* 1994;299:131.
14. Roffman M, Hirsh DM, Mended DG. Fracture of the resurfaced patella in total knee replacement. *Clin Orthop* 1980;148:112.
15. Figgie HE, Goldberg VM, Figgie MP, et al. The effect of alignment of the implant on fractures of the patella after condylar knee arthroplasty. *J Bone Joint Surg Am* 1989;71:1031.
16. Ritter MA, Campbell ED. Postoperative patellar complications with or without lateral release during total knee arthroplasty. *Clin Orthop* 1987;219:163.
17. Insall JN, Haas SB. Complications of total knee arthroplasty. In: Insall JN, Windsor RE, Scott WN, eds. *Surgery of the knee.* New York: Churchill Livingstone, 1993:891.
18. Oglesby JW, Wilson FC. The evolution of knee arthroplasty. *Clin Orthop* 1984;186:96.

19. Scuderi G, Scharf SC, Meltzer LP. The relationship of lateral releases to patella viability in total knee arthroplasty. *J Arthroplasty* 1987;2:209.

20. Goldberg VM, Figgie HE, Inglis AE, et al. Patellar fracture type and prognosis in condylar total knee arthroplasty. *Clin Orthop* 1988;236:115.

21. Hozack WJ, Goll SR, Lotke PA, et al. The treatment of patella fractures after total knee arthroplasty. *Clin Orthop* 1988;236:123.

22. Lettin AWF, DeLiss LJ, Blackburne JS, et al. The Stanmore hinged knee arthroplasty. *J Bone Joint Surg Br* 1978;60:327.

23. Lettin AWF, Kavanagh TG, Scales JT. The long-term results of Stanmore total knee replacement. *J Bone Joint Surg Br* 1984;66:349.

24. Wilson FC, Venteers GC. Results of knee replacement with the Walldius prosthesis. *Clin Orthop* 1976;120:39.

25. Wilson FC, Fajgenbaum DM, Venteers GC. Results of knee replacement with Walldius and Geometric prostheses. *J Bone Joint Surg Am* 1980;62:497.

26. Deburge A, Guepar. Guepar hinge prosthesis: complications and results with two years' follow-up. *Clin Orthop* 1976;120:47.

27. Hui FC, Fitzgerald RH. Hinged total knee arthroplasty. *J Bone Joint Surg Am* 1980;62:513.

28. Yamamoto S. Total knee replacement with the Kodama-Yamamoto prosthesis. *Clin Orthop* 1979;145:60.

29. Cadambi A, Engh GA. Use of a semitendinosus tendon autogenous graft for rupture of the patellar ligament after total knee arthroplasty. *J Bone Joint Surg Am* 1992;74:974.

30. Rand JA, Morrey BF, Bryan RS. Patellar tendon rupture after total knee arthroplasty. *Clin Orthop* 1989;244:233.

31. Webster DA, Murray DG. Complications of variable axis total knee arthroplasty. *Clin Orthop* 1985;193:162.

32. Zanotti RM, Freiberg AA, Matthews LS. Use of patellar allograft to reconstruct a patellar tendon-deficient knee after total joint arthroplasty. *J Arthroplasty* 1995;10:271.

33. Emerson RH, Head WC, Malinin TI. Reconstruction of patellar tendon rupture after total knee arthroplasty with an extensor mechanism allograft. *Clin Orthop* 1990;260:154.

34. Emerson RH, Head WC, Malinin TI. Extensor mechanism reconstruction with an allograft after total knee arthroplasty. *Clin Orthop* 1994;303:79.

35. Grace JN, Rand JA. Patellar instability after total knee arthroplasty. *Clin Orthop* 1988;237:184.

36. Sharkey PF, Hozack WJ, Booth RE, et al. Posterior dislocation of total knee arthroplasty. *Clin Orthop* 1992;278:128.

37. Leopold SS, Greidanus N, Paprosky WG, et al. High rate of failure of allograft reconstruction of the extensor mechanism after total knee arthroplasty. *J Bone Joint Surg Am* 1999;81:1574.

38. Nazarian DG, Booth RE. Extensor mechanism allografts in total knee arthroplasty. *Clin Orthop* 1999;367:123.

39. Jaureguito JW, Dubois CM, Smith SR, et al. Medial gastrocnemius transposition flap for the treatment of disruption of the extensor mechanism after total knee arthroplasty. *J Bone Joint Surg Am* 1997;79:866.

40. Abril JC, Alvarez L, Vallejo JC. Patellar tendon avulsion after total knee arthroplasty. *J Arthroplasty* 1995;10:275.

41. Chiou HM, Chang MC, Lo WH. One-stage reconstruction of skin defect and patellar tendon rupture after total knee arthroplasty. *J Arthroplasty* 1997;12:575.

42. Kempenaar JW, Cameron JC. Patellotibial fusion for patellar tendon rupture after total knee arthroplasty. *J Arthroplasty* 1999;14:115.

43. Crossett LC, Zimmerman GW, Fada R, et al. Patellar tendon reconstruction using tendon allograft following total knee arthroplasty. *Final program of the 65th annual meeting of the American Academy of Orthopaedic Surgeons.* Rosemont, IL: American Academy of Orthopaedic Surgeons, 1998:168.

44. Kaufer H, Matthews LS. Spherocentric arthroplasty of the knee. *J Bone Joint Surg Am* 1981;63:545.

CHAPTER 99

Periprosthetic Fractures after Total Knee Arthroplasty

M. Gavan McAlinden, Bassam A. Masri, Donald S. Garbuz, Nelson V. Greidanus, and Clive P. Duncan

Fractures around a total knee replacement prosthesis, like those in association with hip prostheses, have become an increasing problem in recent years. This is because of the increased numbers and older age of the at-risk population and the increase in the number of patients with multiply revised joints (1). Fractures during or after total knee arthroplasty are less common than those associated with hip replacement. Data from the Mayo Clinic Joint Registry suggest that approximately 2% of knees undergoing total knee arthroplasties, primary and revision, experience a femoral or tibial fracture (1). This patient population included those in whom early implant designs, which have been reported to have a higher overall fracture rate, were used (2,3). It is expected that the prevalence of these fractures will be lower when modern implants are used.

Fractures occur intraoperatively or, more commonly, postoperatively. Femoral, tibial, and patellar fractures have all been described. Patellar fractures are discussed in a separate chapter (Chapter 98). The occurrence and treatment of both intraoperative and postoperative fractures of the femur and tibia are discussed in turn.

PATIENT FACTORS

The management of periprosthetic fractures depends not just on the time of occurrence, location, and type of fracture sustained, but also on the status of the implant before fracture and on the general health status of the individual who has sustained the fracture. A more conservative approach may be adopted in the elderly, frail patient, particularly if the patient is nonambulatory. For example, Figure 1 illustrates a supracondylar fracture sustained in an elderly, nonambulatory woman with dementia. We elected to treat this fracture conservatively, avoiding an extensive revision procedure.

INTRAOPERATIVE FEMORAL FRACTURES AND MANAGEMENT

Intraoperative fractures of the femur can be divided into two subtypes: femoral shaft (diaphyseal) fractures and metaphyseal fractures. These are uncommon injuries in the primary total knee

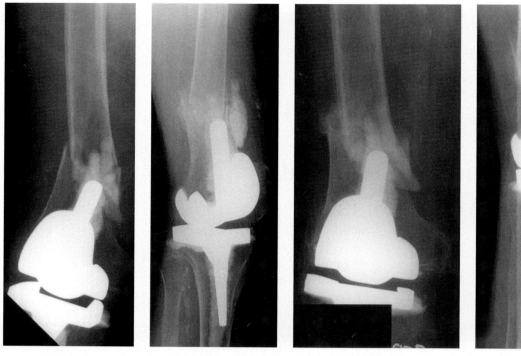

A,B   C,D

FIG. 1. Anteroposterior **(A)** and lateral **(B)** radiographs of the knee of a frail, demented 85-year-old wheel-chair-bound woman who sustained a type II supracondylar fracture of her femur above a short-stemmed total knee arthroplasty. Three months after stabilization in a soft splint, callus can be seen around both cortices on both the anteroposterior **(C)** and lateral **(D)** views. Although there is an obvious malunion, satisfactory pain relief had been attained. Had she had better premorbid function, the result would have been clearly suboptimal.

arthroplasty, occurring in as few as 0.1% of patients (1) but increasing to a frequency as high as 0.9% in the revision setting (1).

Femoral Diaphyseal Fractures

Femoral diaphyseal fractures are usually due either to perforation of the femoral shaft at the time of introduction of the intramedullary femoral guide or to anterior impingement of a femoral press-fit stem (Fig. 2). Perforation of the femoral shaft is technique dependent and should be preventable.

In most knee replacement systems, a sharp-tipped drill bit is used to enter the medullary canal of the femur, in preparation for the introduction of the intramedullary femoral guide. The correct entry point is medial to the midline, just anterior to the femoral origin of the posterior cruciate ligament. This is the point through which the anatomic axis of the femur runs and is therefore the point that should correlate with the line of an intramedullary referencing rod. Eccentric placement of the entry hole can lead not only to malalignment of the femoral component but also to perforation of the femoral cortex.

To prevent a cortical perforation, the authors recommend that the guide drill be introduced gently by hand, without power and without drilling, once a slightly oversized entry point into the distal femur has been made. If the drill cannot be introduced by hand without drilling, then the site of the entry hole should be reevaluated. To this end, a long, standing film of the knee from the hip to the ankle is invaluable, in that it can show the surgeon the correct entry point, determined by lining up the center of the

medullary canal of the femur with the knee joint. In cases of a previous osteotomy, fracture, or deformity secondary to congenital problems, such as multiple hereditary exostoses or epiphyseal and metaphyseal dysplasias, the guide rod may not pass easily up the medullary canal. If it is impossible to introduce the guide rod into the distal femur without drilling farther than the entry point, it should be introduced slowly and preferably under image-intensifier guidance to avoid a cortical perforation. If a cortical perforation is recognized, and it is distal enough that it may be bypassed with a stem, use of a stemmed femoral component will suffice to prevent a fracture. The stem should bypass the perforation by at least two to three cortical diameters. If the perforation is not recognized until after the operation, then the patient should have restricted weightbearing for 6 weeks to prevent a fracture.

Femoral Metaphyseal Fractures

Metaphyseal fractures may occur intraoperatively, particularly with posterior stabilized designs (4). These fractures may present during insertion or extraction of either trial or definitive components. If the notch cut is asymmetric, with the femoral component displaced excessively in a lateral or, particularly, a medial direction, one condyle will be significantly smaller, with a tenuous bony connection to the metaphysis. In implant designs with a deep box cut, the smaller condyle may fracture due to transmission of stresses during impaction. Angular insertion of components may cause a fracture by a similar mechanism.

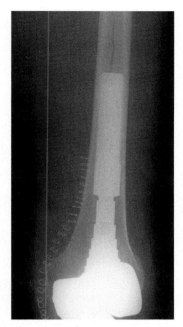

FIG. 2. Postoperative anteroposterior radiograph of the knee of a 45-year-old man after insertion of an S-ROM rotating-hinge revision total knee arthroplasty. A longitudinal linear split is evident. The fracture was managed with 6 weeks of protected weightbearing. The patient experienced no further consequences from the fracture. In retrospect, overreaming of the canal by 0.5 to 1.0 mm might have prevented the fracture.

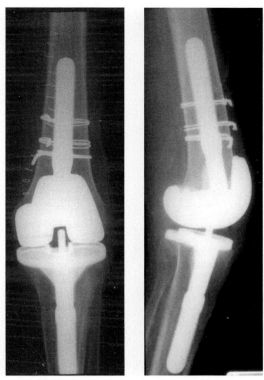

FIG. 3. Anteroposterior **(A)** and lateral **(B)** radiographs of the knee of a 74-year-old man after reimplantation of a knee replacement for infection in a two-stage manner. The cuts were made for a PFC posterior stabilized femoral component; however, a TC-3 femoral component was opened and handed to the surgeon. The TC-3 implant was inserted, and, after complete seating, an undisplaced fracture of the metaphysis was noted. This was treated with cerclage wiring, because a stem was already used. Great care must be taken in passing circumferential cerclage wires in this area to avoid neurovascular injury.

Angular extraction of a component may lever the susceptible condyle from the metaphysis. The authors recommend the use of a trial component extractor and a slap hammer to ensure that only forces in line with the axis of the component are applied. Another rare or unusual cause of an intraoperative metaphyseal femoral fracture is the insertion of a component with a deeper box after the initial box cut has been made for a component with a shallower box. In some implant systems, a more constrained femoral component, such as the constrained condylar knee (Zimmer, Warsaw, IN) or TC-3 (Johnson & Johnson, Warsaw, IN), is available in addition to the standard posterior stabilized femoral component (Insall-Burstein II or PFC Sigma). If the box cut is made for the standard component and the more constrained component with a larger box is inserted forcibly, a longitudinal fracture from the superior aspect of the box cut to either the medial or lateral cortex will occur (Fig. 3).

In a report of 898 arthroplasties using Insall-Burstein posterior stabilized condylar II knees, 40 distal femoral intercondylar fractures were noted (4). Of these, 35 were undisplaced and five were displaced. Undisplaced fractures were noted only on the immediately postoperative radiograph, whereas displaced fractures were noted and treated intraoperatively. The occurrence of these fractures not only may be dependent on use of posterior stabilized components, but also may be implant dependent. The same authors reported on the insertion of 532 Maxim posterior stabilized knees, with the occurrence of only one displaced intercondylar fracture. The difference between the two groups was significant ($p < .0001$). It is worth noting that the surgical technique used with the Maxim knee included use of an intercondylar sizing guide to check resection size and that the

Maxim series followed the Insall-Burstein-II series, with an increased awareness of the complication.

An unrecognized, undisplaced intercondylar fracture can be safely treated expectantly. All 34 patients (35 knees) in the series of Lombardi et al. (4) were managed with no change in postoperative physiotherapy or rehabilitation regimens. Displaced fractures should be managed by internal fixation with two screws and use of a stemmed component or with screws only. The screws can be inserted anterior and posterior to a stem, when used. Routine physiotherapy and rehabilitation can also be used in this group.

Fractures occurring after insertion of a large-box component can also be treated with a cerclage wire and use of a stemmed component. In this area, the passage of a cerclage wire is risky, and careful subperiosteal dissection is recommended to make sure that the site of passage of the cerclage wire is distal to the vastoadductor interval and therefore away from the popliteal artery. Furthermore, the wire passer should be in contact with the posterior aspect of the femur at all times, to avoid neurovascular injury (Fig. 3).

The long-term prognosis for these fractures, when treated with internal fixation, is excellent. These patients have been

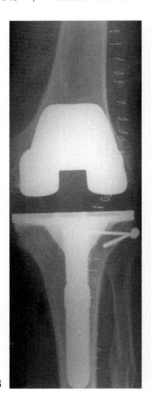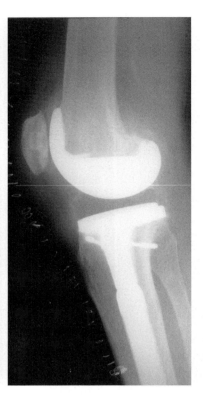

A,B

FIG. 4. Anteroposterior **(A)** and lateral **(B)** radiographs of the knee of an 87-year-old man. At the time of primary knee replacement, an undisplaced fracture of the lateral tibial plateau was caused by the keel punch. This was fixed with two 3.5-mm screws, and the fixation of the tibial component was augmented with a press-fit stem. There was no further displacement despite immediate weightbearing.

reported to have no significant differences in postoperative Hospital for Special Surgery knee scores or pain scores when compared to a similar group of patients who did not sustain an intraoperative fracture (4).

In cases in which there is very poor bone stock, allograft replacement of the fractured metaphysis may have to be considered. This is explored later in the chapter.

INTRAOPERATIVE TIBIAL FRACTURES AND MANAGEMENT

A displaced fracture may occur at the time of removal of a solidly fixed tibial component, when the cement-prosthesis interface is debonded anteriorly but not posteriorly and the stem or keel remains solidly fixed. As the component is being extracted from below and remains attached posteriorly, a coronal fracture may occur, particularly if bone stock is deficient.

Fractures of the tibial plateau can occur at the time of insertion of a keeled tibial component. Although such fractures may occur in the primary setting, they represent a greater problem in a revision situation, particularly if the component has to be placed eccentrically. If the center of the medullary canal of the tibia does not line up with the center of the tibial plateau and offset stems are not available, the keel may transmit stress to the tibial cortex during impaction and cause a fracture. These fractures are often undisplaced and occur in a vertical direction. If they are undisplaced, they frequently require no specific treatment, except for a 6-week period of protected weightbearing. If a displaced fracture occurs, it can be reduced and fixed with one or two screws directed away from the keel and stem. Fracture fixation should be augmented with a stemmed component, so that the fracture is bypassed (Fig. 4).

POSTOPERATIVE STRESS FRACTURES

Stress fractures of both the pubic rami and femoral neck have been reported after total knee arthroplasty. Common to both types of fracture is delay in presentation and delay and difficulty in diagnosis. These fractures usually present within 1 year in patients who had severe restriction in mobility preoperatively.

Pubic Ramus Fractures

Four cases (in three patients) of pubic ramus stress fractures have been reported after total knee arthroplasty (5–7). All patients were female and had severe rheumatoid arthritis. They presented with severe groin and hip pain between 6 months and 8 years after surgery. In all patients, initial radiographic findings were interpreted as negative and tomography or radioisotope scans were required to aid diagnosis. All of the cases were managed conservatively, with one pubic ramus nonunion occurring (7).

Femoral Neck Fractures

At least 16 stress fractures of the femoral neck have been reported after a knee replacement (8–13). Although the incidence is thought to be low, there is no clear evidence of the actual prevalence. In the largest series, the reported prevalence was 1.4% of the authors' entire experience with total knee arthroplasty, although this may reflect the authors' use of a hinged prosthesis (12).

These fractures occur more often in female patients (12 out of 14 cases in which gender was specified). In the series of McElwaine and Sheehan (72), six out of seven fractures occurred in patients with rheumatoid arthritis who had received long-term steroid therapy. The majority of the other reported cases, however, were patients who had osteoarthritis before operation. The fractures usually present in the first year after surgery (at an average of 7 months) with complaints of groin pain. Delay in presentation and diagnosis is common and may result in displacement of an initially undisplaced fracture. A common theme in these patients is severe restriction of activity preoperatively, and it has been suggested that the fractures may result from postoperative relief of pain and increased activity in patients who have developed disuse osteoporosis due to their knee arthritis.

Although the total reported number of cases is low, the diagnosis is an important one to bear in mind in a previously immobile patient who presents with sudden onset of hip or groin pain in the year after total knee arthroplasty. Indeed, the actual incidence of this complication may be much higher as these fractures may be considered insufficiency fractures, unrelated to the arthroplasty surgery. Successful conservative management of such fractures has been reported, although this was because of delay in diagnosis with clinical improvement (10). Failed conservative management has also been seen (12). Treatment should therefore be operative, as dictated by the fracture pattern, with the aims of preventing fracture displacement and preserving the patient's own hip.

POSTOPERATIVE INTERPROSTHETIC FRACTURES OF THE FEMUR

Fractures of the femoral shaft between a total hip prosthesis and a total knee prosthesis are rare. Delport et al. (14) reported successful conservative management of a displaced interprosthetic fracture with initial traction followed by cast bracing. Kenny et al. (15) described their experience in surgically treating three fractures above a stemmed total knee prosthesis and one above a resurfacing total knee prosthesis. Only the fracture between a total hip prosthesis and a resurfacing knee implant was successfully treated. In the remaining two cases, single or double femoral plates failed within months of surgery. As a salvage procedure, revision total hip and knee arthroplasties have been performed on an implanted total femoral allograft (16). No reports have been published on the use of cable plates and allograft struts in these complex cases, but they may have a role to play.

POSTOPERATIVE SUPRACONDYLAR FRACTURES OF THE FEMUR

Definition, Incidence, and Classification of Supracondylar Fractures

The brief initial report of four cases of supracondylar fracture after total knee arthroplasty contained much of what is still held to be true about this injury (17). All four patients were osteopenic and sustained the injury in a minor fall. The place of surgical management of the unstable fracture was highlighted. The possible relationship between anterior femoral notching and supracondylar fractures was also emphasized.

There is little consensus as to what defines a supracondylar fracture above a total knee implant. Supracondylar femoral fractures have variously been defined as fractures occurring within

TABLE 1. *Neer et al. classification of supracondylar fractures*

Type	Definition
I	Undisplaced
II	Displaced
a	Medial displacement of femoral condyles
b	Lateral displacement of femoral condyles
III	Conjoined supracondylar and shaft fractures

From Neer CS II, Grantham SA, Shelton ML. Supracondylar fracture of the adult femur: a study of one hundred and ten cases. *J Bone Joint Surg Am* 1967;49:591–613, with permission.

15 cm or 5 cm proximal to a stemmed component of a total knee prosthesis (18,19), within 9 cm of the joint line (20), or within 2 cm of the component (21).

Supracondylar fractures have been reported to occur in 0.6% (26 of 4,596) of primary total knee arthroplasties and 1.6% (10 of 637) of revision procedures (22). Other authors have reported a fracture rate as high as 38% after revision (23) and as low as 0.3% (2 of 670) after primary surgery (24). The true prevalence is probably difficult to determine, as few centers treat all fracture complications of their own patients. These prevalence rates must, therefore, be considered minimal figures.

Many of the published works on supracondylar femoral fractures after total knee arthroplasty base their categorization on the Neer classification of supracondylar fractures (25). This was developed for fractures occurring in the absence of a total knee arthroplasty and is based on the fracture displacement or association with a diaphyseal fracture (Table 1). Neer et al. did not define displacement, but it has subsequently been defined as less than 5 mm displacement or 5-degree angulation or both (26).

Chen et al. (27) rationalized Neer's classification (Table 1) for application to periprosthetic fractures: Type I fractures are undisplaced (Figs. 5 and 6), and type II fractures are displaced or comminuted (Figs. 1, 7, and 8). This classification does not take account of fixation of the femoral component, a factor that has important implications for management. Therefore, the authors' recommended classification system is that described by Rorabeck, Angliss, and Lewis (28) and summarized in Table 2. There are three types: Types I and II fractures are the same as those of Chen et al. (27), provided the component is solidly fixed. Displacement is defined as more than 5 mm or displacement or 5 degrees of angulation or both. Type III fractures are those in which a component is loose, regardless of fracture displacement. The majority of femoral fractures occur with well-fixed components.

Risk Factors

Both systemic and local factors influence the risk of developing a supracondylar periprosthetic fracture. Virtually every series reporting this injury has noted a high incidence of patients with osteoporosis or osteopenia among the fracture population. In particular, patients with rheumatoid arthritis, especially more severe disease with osteopenia and steroid use, have consistently been demonstrated to be at a higher risk of fracture.

Patients with neurologic disorders are also at risk. Patients with illnesses such as seizure disorders, cerebellar ataxias, Parkinson's disease, myasthenia gravis, cerebral palsy, polio, Char-

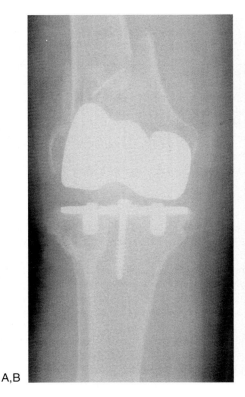
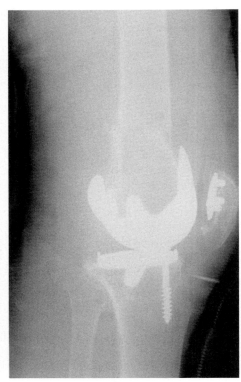

A,B

FIG. 5. Anteroposterior **(A)** and lateral **(B)** radiographs of the knee of a 73-year-old woman showing a type I supracondylar fracture above a resurfacing total knee implant. As the radiographs show, this fracture is being treated in a cylinder (stovepipe) cast. Considering the lack of displacement and the osteopenic bone stock, this is appropriate management, but displacement should be detected by frequent follow-up.

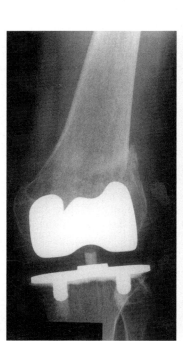
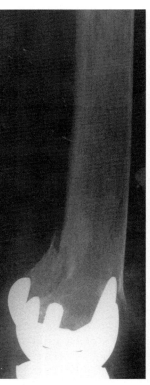
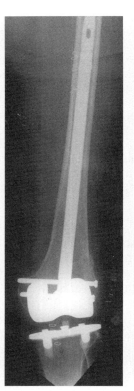
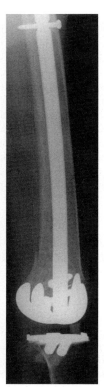

A,B

C,D

FIG. 6. Radiographs of the knee of a 53-year-old woman with severe rheumatoid arthritis who sustained a type I supracondylar fracture above a cruciate-retaining total knee implant. **A, B:** Anteroposterior and lateral radiographs of the initial fracture position. **C, D:** Anteroposterior and lateral radiographs after closed reduction and fixation with a rigid intramedullary nail. A long nail has been used with interlocking screws proximally and distally, which gives a long isthmic working distance. Early range-of-motion exercises can begin.

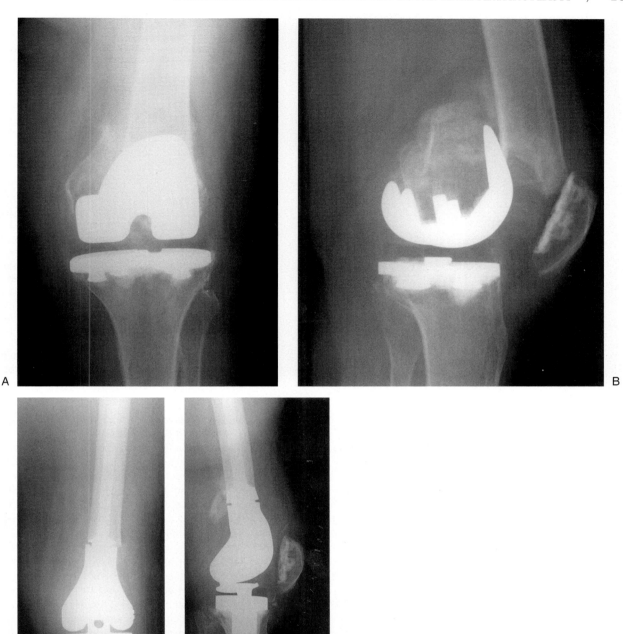

FIG. 7. Anteroposterior **(A)** and lateral **(B)** radiographs of the knee of a 69-year-old man who sustained a type II supracondylar fracture above a cruciate-retaining total knee implant. Bone quality, particularly as noted in the lateral view **(B)**, was thought to preclude internal fixation due to osteolysis, which was confirmed at the time of operation. **C, D:** This fracture was treated with a revision total knee arthroplasty to an oncologic rotating-hinge prosthesis.

cot joints (undefined neuropathic arthropathy), or cervical spondylosis with myelopathy made up 28% (17 of 61 cases) of patients who sustained supracondylar fractures in one series. In these patients, falls secondary to gait disturbance or seizures combined with osteopenia due to relative immobility are the probable mechanisms for an increased risk of fracture (20).

Local factors that compromise the biomechanical integrity of the femur can also predispose to fracture. Fractures have been described in relation to old screw holes (29) and to anterior femoral notching (30,31). Local osteolysis, by weakening bone, can also put the supracondylar region at risk. There is no clear association between component malalignment and subsequent fracture.

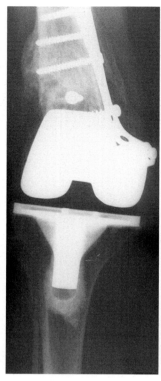 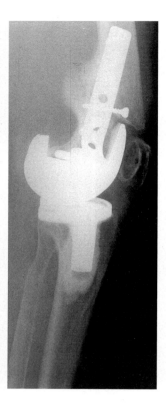

A,B

FIG. 8. Anteroposterior **(A)** and lateral **(B)** radiographs of the knee of a 65-year-old obese woman with severe rheumatoid arthritis who experienced a type II periprosthetic fracture of the distal femur secondary to notching of the distal femur at the time of a total knee arthroplasty. Despite an anatomic reduction at the time of open reduction, internal fixation with a condylar buttress plate, and bone grafting with allograft bone, the fracture displaced within 2 weeks from the time of surgery. It was elected to treat her fracture with further immobilization in a brace because of her poor bone stock and limited activity demands. The fracture healed with marked displacement, as can be seen on the anteroposterior **(A)** and lateral **(B)** radiographs.

Anterior Femoral Notching

Anterior femoral notching has proven to be controversial as an etiologic factor. For example, it has been suggested that a notch of smaller than 3 mm should be considered as a "blend" rather than a notch (32). It seems that the value of 3 mm has been selected on the basis that this is the smallest notch that can be reliably measured on a lateral radiograph (20). There is biomechanical evidence supporting the view that notching predisposes to a fracture (33). In some series, however, notching has not been seen to be associated with any supracondylar fractures (29), nor has a significant association been found between notching and fractures (34).

In an elegant laboratory study, Lesh and coworkers (33) examined the biomechanical effect of creating a 3-mm anterior notch in femora while inserting a femoral component. Twelve pairs of femora were tested for bending and torsional strength after application of the femoral component of a total knee arthroplasty. One of each pair had a notch created while inserting the component. Bending strength was reduced by 18% ($p = .0034$) and torsional strength by 39.2% ($p = .01$). In the notched femora, the fracture was seen to originate from the notch. This reduction in torsional strength is close to the 29.2% predicted by Culp et al. (20) in a mathematical model. The cadaver study may explain early supracondylar fractures, but it does not take into account the cortical remodeling that is observed to occur clinically after anterior notching.

Healy et al. (35) reported a series of 20 distal femoral fractures proximal to total knee arthroplasties. In only 2 of the 20 cases was anterior cortical notching noted. They surmised that notching was not a major factor in supracondylar fractures and focused instead on the preponderance of osteoporotic female patients with concomitant disease in their series. No reference was made to the incidence of notching in the overall arthroplasty population. Aaron and Scott (30) reported on a series of 250 duopatellar total knee arthroplasties in which five patients experienced postoperative supracondylar fractures. Only 12 of the 250 knees had an "excessively deep resection"; however, all five knees with a supracondylar fracture had anterior notching. The authors concluded that anterior notching predisposed to fracture. It should be noted that all of the fracture patients had moderate to severe rheumatoid arthritis and osteoporosis.

Ritter et al. (34) studied 670 posterior cruciate–retaining condylar total knee arthroplasties. One hundred eighty knees had a notched femur, and in 138 the notch was deeper than 3 mm. At a follow-up of between 2 and 10 years, only two fractures had occurred, one in a notched femur and one in a normal femur. In both, the fracture originated at the junction between the anterior femoral component flange and the femur, which led the authors to conjecture that stress shielding from the flange, rather than notching, may explain the anatomic pattern of many

TABLE 2. *Rorabeck, Angliss, and Lewis classification of supracondylar periprosthetic fractures proximal to knee arthroplasty*

Type	Definition
I	Undisplaced fracture: prosthesis intact
II	Displaced fracture: prosthesis intact
III	Displaced or undisplaced fracture: prosthesis loose or failing (polyethylene wear or instability)

From Rorabeck CH, Angliss RD, Lewis PL. Fractures of the femur, tibia, and patella after total knee arthroplasty: decision making and principles of management. *Instr Course Lect* 1998;47:449–458, with permission.

supracondylar fractures. In subsequent correspondence with Scott (36), the authors conceded that notching might predispose to a fracture in an osteopenic individual.

The incidence of anterior femoral notching should be reduced in more recent arthroplasty surgery with the availability of more sophisticated instrumentation systems and larger femoral components with an increased anteroposterior dimension. Despite this, a surgeon's attention to this detail remains important in preventing notching. At present, with careful attention to technical detail, notching should be preventable, and regardless of whether it is an independent factor in postoperative fracture or whether it acts in combination with osteopenia as a risk factor, it is best prevented. If a notch is recognized intraoperatively, it may be prudent to bypass it with a canal-filling stem.

Malalignment

Merkel and Johnson (22) in their series of 36 supracondylar fractures found that pre-injury component alignment was similar to that in previous series of total knee arthroplasties. This suggests that postoperative component alignment may not be a major factor in the risk of developing a fracture.

Osteolysis

It would seem obvious that the process of osteolysis secondary to polyethylene wear with resultant cortical thinning could result in periprosthetic fractures. Perhaps surprisingly, only two reports focus on this as a causal agent (37,38). Rand (38) reported that 12 of a series of 267 porous-coated anatomic total knee arthroplasties were revised due to polyethylene wear. Only 25% of knees (3 of 12) showed significant periarticular osteolysis and, of these, just one had undergone a fracture. In contrast, in total hip arthroplasty, polyethylene wear–induced osteolysis is now the principal cause of periprosthetic fractures.

Treatment of Supracondylar Fractures of the Femur

The goals of treating supracondylar fractures are obtaining fracture union, maintaining alignment of the extremity, preserving range of motion, and restoring the patient to the premorbid level of function, without compromising outcome with treatment complications. Nonoperative and surgical management of these difficult fractures have been used with variable success. The frequency with which these fractures occur in patients with marked osteoporosis, often accompanying rheumatoid arthritis or neurologic disease, limits the surgeon's ability to achieve rigid fixation of the fracture. Alternatively, conservative management may also entail restricted patient mobility, prolonged bed rest with its medical and economic implications, and the possibility of local skin problems.

Nonoperative versus Operative Treatment

Healy at al. (35) reviewed the literature on closed and open management of supracondylar fractures of the femur and found 173 such fractures. They reported that results were excellent or good in 68% of the 95 patients who had been treated nonopera-

TABLE 3. *Results of treatment of supracondylar periprosthetic fractures*

Treatment method	No. treated	No. of good or successful outcomes	Percentage of good or successful outcomes
Closed treatment, including traction, cast bracing, and casting	132	79	59.8
Open reduction and internal fixation with plate and screws	96	69	71.9
External fixation	12	10	83.3
Flexible intramedullary nail	28	23	82.1
Rigid intramedullary nail	78	70	89.7
Revision prosthesis	21	18	85.7
Structural allograft with prosthesis	26	23	88.5

Data from refs. 14, 15, 17, 20, 22, 29, 31, 35, 39–58, 60, 61, and 63–66.

tively and in 68% of the 78 patients who had been treated surgically. Chen et al. (27) reviewed many of the same papers, along with some additional series, and identified 195 cases. They concluded that conservative management of closed fractures resulted in a satisfactory outcome in 83% of patients with type I fractures (25 out of 30 cases), but this fell to 67% (28 out of 41 cases) for those with type II fractures. Surgical management of type II fractures resulted in a satisfactory outcome in 61% of patients (20 out of 33 cases). These investigators did note, however, that a more successful outcome was seen in 10 of 11 cases treated with revision arthroplasty (93%) and in both patients treated with intramedullary nailing. McLaren et al. (21) reviewed information on 223 cases reported between 1980 and 1991 and found that satisfactory results were achieved in 57% of cases treated with closed methods and 67% of those treated with open reduction.

When the results of conservative and surgical management in 393 patients reported in the English language are examined, the superiority of surgical management becomes apparent (Table 3). Conservative management is associated with a successful outcome in fewer than 60% of cases, although the results are better for type I fractures. Intramedullary nailing, both flexible and rigid, and revision arthroplasty with or without structural allograft all achieve a successful outcome in more than 80% of cases. Although some reports of open reduction and internal fixation, using plates and screws, approach these figures, this technique appears less consistent in its ability to provide a good outcome, and fracture nonunions and deep infection are not uncommon complications.

Results of Nonoperative Management

At least 132 cases of supracondylar fracture that have been conservatively managed have been reported (14,17,20,22,31,39–46). In only 79 instances was treatment deemed to be successful.

Merkel and Johnson (22) found that 65% (9 out of 26 cases) initially treated by a variety of conservative measures, including traction, cast bracing, or casting, had a successful outcome. The remaining nine cases required surgical management for failure of conservative treatment: four for nonunion, two each for malunion and loose prosthesis, and one for limited motion. The authors thought that this success rate justified their assertion that conservative management should be attempted in most patients.

Moran et al. (43) reported the experience at the Brigham and Women's Hospital. Fourteen of a series of 29 supracondylar fractures (five undisplaced, nine displaced) were treated conservatively. All of the undisplaced fractures healed satisfactorily, whereas all of the nine displaced fractures thus treated healed with a malunion and two required revision surgery. None of the displaced fractures had a satisfactory outcome. Garnavos et al. (42) reported a similar experience with five undisplaced fractures, which had a good outcome, and seven displaced fractures, all of which resulted in malunion or nonunion.

Conservative management is not without significant local complications. Bogoch et al. (39) noted skin breakdown or ulceration in four out of eight patients treated conservatively. Although traditionally this was the treatment of choice, the morbidity of prolonged traction and bed rest is no longer justified given the availability of safe and effective surgical techniques. Perhaps the only indication at present for nonoperative treatment would be the presence of a type I fracture in an elderly patient who is a poor surgical candidate (Figs. 1, 5), either for functional reasons or because of marked osteopenia and minimal displacement. In the authors' experience, these cases are few.

Results of Operative Management

Open Reduction and Internal Fixation

Open reduction and internal fixation of supracondylar fractures has been reported using a variety of devices, including fixed-angle blade plates, condylar screw plates, condylar buttress plates, clamp-on plates (15,47,48), and fork plates (49) designed to fit around the lugs of femoral components. Out of 96 cases reviewed, 69 had a good or satisfactory result (17,20, 22,31,35,39–45,49,50). Rigid internal fixation allows early return of motion and mobilization with protected weightbearing. Complications commonly reported include malunion, despite the theoretical advantage of anatomic reduction, delayed union or nonunions, and deep infections (Fig. 8).

Culp et al. (20) included 20 supracondylar fractures treated with open reduction and plating in their series of 60 fractures treated by a variety of open and closed methods. In two patients fractures healed with a malunion and one fracture failed to unite. One additional patient treated with multiple percutaneous pinnings ultimately underwent amputation for sepsis. Figgie et al. (41) noted that fractures in five out of ten patients treated by open reduction and internal fixation with plates and screws healed with a malunion. Moran et al. (43) described the outcome of open reduction and plating in 15 patients with displaced fractures. Five patients had an adverse outcome from surgery; in three cases this was attributed to an error in surgical technique. Two patients healed with a malunion; three had a nonunion, which required repeat internal fixation in one and salvage with a long-stemmed femoral component in two.

The findings of Healy et al. (35), who reported a 90% success rate in the treatment of 20 fractures by a number of surgeons,

illustrate that it is possible to obtain results superior to those with conservative treatment using open reduction and plating. In their series, two nonunions were treated by an additional procedure with ultimate healing of the fractures. At an average follow-up of 27 months (range, 12 to 96 months), the average Knee Society scores and Knee Society function scores had returned to pre-injury levels. The success of these authors may be a result of their use of bone graft in 15 of the 20 cases.

The Mennen plate (CH Medical, Exeter, UK) is a paraskeletal clamp-on plate that holds the reduced fracture, with the aim of allowing fracture healing. It does not require screw insertion and therefore has a theoretical advantage in the presence of a total hip prosthesis above a stemmed total knee prosthesis. Use of this device has been described in a handful of cases of periprosthetic supracondylar fractures related to total knee arthroplasties (15,47,48). In only one of these cases, however, was treatment successful (47). Failure in one of the other two cases ultimately resulted in use of an above-knee replacement for that patient (15). This device should probably not be used for fixation of periprosthetic fractures adjacent to total knee prostheses.

Intramedullary Fixation: Rush Pins and Retrograde Nailing

Intramedullary fixation of fractures carries with it biomechanical load-sharing advantages compared to extramedullary side plate fixation (51). Attempts have been made to stabilize supracondylar, periprosthetic fractures with both flexible (31,39,44,52) and rigid intramedullary devices (21,29,51,53–58,73). Flexible intramedullary rods (Rush rods) have met with varying degrees of success, whereas rigid supracondylar nails appear to produce a more consistent outcome.

Cain et al. (31) reported on three cases treated with Rush rods. In only one was treatment a success, with nonunion or malunion occurring in the others. Rush rods have also been reported to lose fixation and back out of osteoporotic bone (39). In contrast, Ritter et al. (52) reported on the long-term follow-up of 22 patients with displaced fractures, which had been treated with Rush rods. Two patients developed a malunion due to intraoperative technical errors. No other significant complications were noted. Nielsen et al. (44) have also reported two cases in which Rush rods were used without complication.

In perhaps the first reported case of the use of a rigid intramedullary nail to treat a supracondylar fracture, a segment cut from an intramedullary nail was used. This was inserted in an antegrade fashion and was engaged on the stem of a Guepar prosthesis. Supplementary fixation was provided with a plate, screws, and cerclage wires (57). Sekel and Newman (58), who engaged an antegrade Huckstepp intramedullary nail (Down Surgical, Mitcham, Surrey, England) on the stem of the femoral component, also described a similar technique. Hanks et al. (53) also used an antegrade technique: In their three cases, a Brooker-Wills nail was inserted to stabilize fractures above resurfacing components. One of three fracture patients lost 5 degrees of movement compared to the pre-injury range, whereas the others had no loss of movement. Despite their success, the authors noted that this technique was limited to fractures more than 8 cm from the joint. A novel approach to fracture fixation in the modular constrained condylar knee was described by Peyton and Booth (3). By inserting a custom tool through the intercondylar box of the femoral component to "capture" an intramedullary stem inserted into the proximal femur, they reduced and stabilized the fracture by cables. This technique, although of interest, is not applicable in the majority of supracondylar fractures.

The development of the supracondylar nail allowed retrograde nailing with a rigid implant. The nail is a closed-section stainless steel implant with an outer diameter of 11, 12, or 13 mm. The device has an 8-degree bend 38 mm from the driving end. Holes for screw interlocking are 20 mm apart, except for the two most distal screws, which are 15 and 30 mm from the driving end. Interlocking is performed with the aid of an alignment guide and uses 5-mm cortical screws (51).

Supracondylar, retrograde nailing has been used successfully, even in patients with marked osteopenia and those with distal fractures within 2 cm of the prosthesis (21). McLaren et al. (21) used this device, exposing the fracture to allow direct reduction. Of seven fractures, six had bridging callus at 6 weeks and the seventh at 12 weeks. These authors stressed avoidance of early strengthening exercises and weightbearing until fracture union is achieved. Closed reduction of the fracture, with intramedullary stabilization, has not been associated with any reported increase in fracture malunion (29,55,56). Jabczenski and Crawford (29) recommended closed rather than open reduction to preserve fracture hematoma and reduce operative blood loss. Evidence in support of this practice came from Henry (51). In a large multicenter series, 29 patients were treated with open reduction and intramedullary nailing, and 19 were treated with closed reduction and percutaneous intramedullary nailing. The percutaneous group had a shorter mean operative time than the open reduction group (74 minutes vs. 110 minutes), less operative blood loss (126 mL vs. 250 mL), and a greater postoperative range of motion (106 degrees of flexion vs. 91 degrees of flexion).

As with any fracture implant, use of the supracondylar nail may be complicated by infection or by loss of fracture fixation. Migration of a supracondylar nail back through the intercondylar region has been reported (59), with a recommendation to use bone graft or bone cement in cases with poor bone quality. Fracture malalignment has not been rigorously assessed in studies of supracondylar nailing, but use of the longest nail possible has been recommended to reduce this likelihood (51).

External Fixation

Few authors have reported on the use of external fixation for treating supracondylar fractures. External fixation carries the disadvantages of tethering the quadriceps and inhibiting early mobilization, and percutaneous pin fixation adjacent to the knee prosthesis carries the risk that pin site infection will generate a prosthetic infection. Some initial reports were discouraging. Culp et al. (20) reported that the only patient in their series thus treated lost 50 degrees of movement and healed with a 20-degree malunion. Figgie et al. (41) treated one of their series of 22 patients with external fixation. The patient developed a deep infection and required removal of the prosthesis with revision to an arthrodesis.

On the other hand, Merkel and Johnson (22) reported on three fractures treated by external fixation and reviewed at an average of 45 months. Function, motion, and alignment were assessed. Results for two of the patients were rated as excellent and results for one as good. Biswas et al. (60) reported on five cases of supracondylar fractures above Stanmore total knee arthroplasties treated with external fixation. All five healed within 16 weeks, with recovery of a prefracture range of motion. No comment was made regarding malunion, but no major complications were encountered. The indications for external fixation were extended by a report of the use of an Ilizarov-type ring external fixator in a patient whose bone quality was felt to preclude internal fixation (61). At a 19-month follow-up, the patient had maintained her range of motion and had experienced no complications as a result of surgery.

Allograft and Stemmed Components

Use of an allograft-prosthesis composite has been considered a salvage procedure in patients whose bone loss is considered a contraindication to fracture fixation or in those for whom fracture fixation had already failed. Despite the recipient patient population, a successful outcome has been obtained in 88% of reported cases. Figgie et al. (41) described two cases, Harris et al. (62) described six cases, and Engh et al. (63) described a further two cases thus treated. All of these ten cases had a successful outcome. Kraay et al. (64) noted no mechanical failures in five of seven cases treated with a composite of allograft and semiconstrained components. Two of these patients had died of unrelated causes within 2 years of surgery. Although care was taken to preserve the soft tissue envelope, a further two patients had ongoing knee instability requiring use of a knee brace. Only one allograft showed full union to host bone and one was partially united. Ghazavi et al. (65) reported on nine additional cases. A delayed union at the graft-host junction occurred in one; the remaining eight cases had a successful outcome at 24 to 60 months.

Stemmed Revision Components

Like the use of allograft-prosthesis composites, the use of stemmed revision components and tumor prostheses can be considered a salvage procedure. The technique has not been the subject of any large studies, although a small number of cases have been reported in isolation or as part of a larger series. Kress et al. (66) reported three cases of supracondylar fracture nonunions above total knee replacements. Two cases had been managed with traction and casting, and one had had internal fixation with subsequent infection. They were revised to custom total knee replacements with press-fit intramedullary stems. At a follow-up ranging from 1.2 to 11.6 years, all three patients had recovered function to a level approaching their pre-injury status.

Culp et al. (20) included five cases of a supracondylar fracture above a total knee prosthesis managed with a revision arthroplasty. They reported that there were no nonunions or malunions in this group but that one patient subsequently underwent an above-knee amputation. Cordeiro et al. (40) reported on four patients who had revision from standard to stemmed components for supracondylar fractures. With range of motion used as an indication of outcome, three attained at least 0 to 90 degrees of flexion and the fourth, who had rheumatoid arthritis with multiple joint involvement, attained a range of 0 to 70 degrees. The authors considered all four to have had a good outcome.

Merkel and Johnson (22) reported on nine patients who had initially undergone conservative treatment of a supracondylar fracture but who required a revision arthroplasty procedure for persistent nonunion, malunion, loose prosthesis, or limited range of motion. One required an above-knee amputation for fulminant infection. Of the remaining eight patients, seven had a range of motion greater then 0 to 85 degrees of flexion and the eighth had a range of 0 to 65 degrees of flexion. In only one case did postoperative Knee Society scores drop more than 10 points compared to the preoperative score, where this was known.

Authors' Preferred Management of Supracondylar Fractures

Types I and II

In frail elderly patients who are not candidates for surgical treatment, particularly those with a type I fracture, conservative treatment is our preferred approach. In all other patients with type I and II fractures, these may be treated with internal fixation. With the introduction of supracondylar and retrograde femoral intramedullary nails, the treatment of these fractures has been greatly simplified (Fig. 6). A closed reduction can be achieved on a radiolucent table, with a wedge-shaped post, bolster, or a rolled-up pillow placed behind the knee. The knee should rest at 45 to 55 degrees of flexion. An arthrotomy is performed and the patellar tendon is split. Medial or lateral retraction of the patellar tendon compromises the approach to the intercondylar notch and puts the tibial tubercle at risk of a partial or complete avulsion (55). The entry point for the awl is in the femoral notch area or through the box of a posterior cruciate–sacrificing design of prosthesis. Any cement within the notch is removed. After an entry point is made, the femoral canal can be enlarged with sequential reaming to accept a nail. In this patient population, however, reaming rarely is necessary due to osteopenia. The nail is introduced into the femur in a retrograde fashion. The most distal portion of the nail should not protrude into the joint, to avoid impingement. Reduction of the fracture can now be checked again. The nail should be locked distally first, using the outrigger guide, to allow final adjustment of the fracture position. The nail is then locked proximally, again using the guide. All interlocking screws should be checked for position with fluoroscopy after insertion, as it is possible to miss the screw holes, even with the help of the guide. One caveat is that the width of the notch must match the diameter of the femoral nail. Therefore, the surgeon should compare the specifications of the femoral component with the diameter of the femoral nail before proceeding. The intercondylar gap of some commonly used components is shown in Table 4.

In some posterior stabilized designs, the femoral box obscures the notch area. This may be removed with a metal-cutting burr before proceeding (54). It is important to remove the tibial insert for exposure, and therefore the surgeon should ensure that a new tibial insert is available. The authors who describe this technique also recommend applying an adhesive barrier drape to the femoral component and covering the tibial component with a moist laparotomy sponge. Furthermore, the joint should be copiously irrigated to remove all metal fragments and avoid third-body wear.

For very distal fractures, it may be difficult to achieve distal fixation while leaving the distal end of the nail flush with the

TABLE 4. *Intercondylar distance of commonly used femoral components*

Manufacturer	Component	Intercondylar distance of smallest femoral component (mm)
Johnson & Johnson/ DePuy (Warsaw, IN)	AMK	20
	PFC Sigma	20
Zimmer (Warsaw, IN)	Insall-Burstein I	16
	Insall-Burstein II (posterior stabilized or constrained condylar)	15
	Miller-Galante I	
	Small/small +	11
	Regular/regular +	12.5
	Large/large +	15
	Large ++	18
	Miller-Galante II	13
Biomet (Warsaw, IN)	AGC	18
	Universal	18
Dow Corning Wright (Arlington, IN)	Whitesides modular	20
Stryker-Howmedica-Osteonics (Rutherford, NJ)	Porous-coated anatomic	18.5
Intermedics (Austin, TX)	Natural	14
Kirschner (Timonium, MD)	Performance	14

From Rolston LR, Christ DJ, Halpern A, et al. Treatment of supracondylar fractures of the femur proximal to a total knee arthroplasty. A report of four cases. *J Bone Joint Surg Am* 1995;77:924–931, with permission.

component. In these cases, the nail may be left proud, interlocked, and the protruding metal removed with a metal-cutting burr (21). Again, it is important to remove all metal fragments.

If a femoral nail cannot be used, the fracture can be fixed with a condylar buttress plate, condylar screw plate, blade plate, or the newly released Synthes less invasive stabilization system. In patients with osteopenic bone, this can be complicated by hardware failure. Consideration should be given to using polymethylmethacrylate bone cement to augment screw fixation. Cement should be kept away from the fracture site, to avoid delayed union or nonunion. If the fracture is opened, it should be bone-grafted.

Type III

If the implant is loose, it should be revised, regardless of the degree of displacement of the fracture. The fracture may be reduced and fixed with an intramedullary stem extension. With these fractures, it is important to bone-graft and to avoid cement

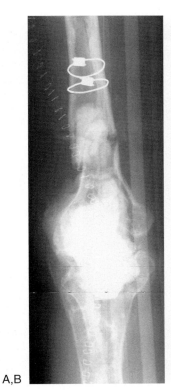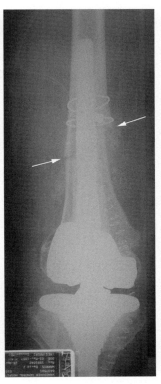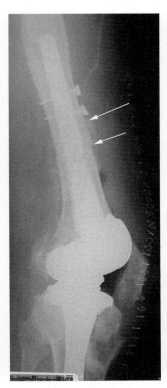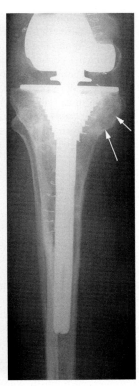

A,B   C,D

FIG. 9. A 45-year-old man presented for a revision of a hinged cemented knee replacement for aseptic loosening of the tibial component. At the time of cement removal on the femoral side, a comminuted fracture of the distal femur was noted. An attempt at fixation with cerclage cables failed, and, therefore, the surgeon inserted an antibiotic-loaded cement spacer and referred the patient for further managements. **A:** Anteroposterior radiograph. Due to the severe comminution of the distal femur, a reconstruction with an allograft-prosthesis composite on the femoral side was performed, and a hinged S-ROM knee prosthesis was used. **B, C:** Postoperative anteroposterior and lateral radiographs, respectively. The white arrows point to the step-cut junction, which was used to stabilize the allograft-host junction. **D:** Due to marked bone loss on the tibia, tibial bone stock was augmented with a structural femoral head allograft (*white arrows*).

intrusion into the fracture. Occasionally, comminution is worse than predicted by the radiographs, or bone loss due to osteoporosis or osteolysis is considerable. In these cases, revision with an allograft-prosthesis composite may be performed in younger patients (Fig. 9). Alternatively, in older patients or those with low-demand activities, an oncology prosthesis can be used to replace the distal femur (Fig. 7). It is therefore important to have access to structural allograft or oncology prostheses before embarking on a revision in such a complex fracture case.

The technique for use of an allograft-prosthesis composite has been well described (12,67). A standard revision approach should be used. Preservation of the soft tissue envelope is of paramount importance. The medial and lateral collateral ligaments may be preserved either by osteotomizing the epicondyles with a substantial fragment of bone (larger than 2 cm) or by splitting the femur distal to the fracture in an anteroposterior plane. A step cut is made in the host femur at the level of the fracture, if this bone can provide a healthy, strong site for allograft incorporation. The donor femur is prepared on the back table. The allograft can be held in a holder. The distal allograft is fashioned with cutting jigs for the intended revision component. A trial stemmed component should be inserted into the graft to allow an approximation of the level of proximal resection of the allograft. Proximally, a step cut is made to correspond to host

femur. It is better to be conservative with this cut initially, which allows later fine-tuning. Care must be taken when making the step cut to ensure that the distal femur and component are positioned in the correct orientation. The definitive component should be cemented into the allograft, but no cement should be allowed to come into contact with the host-graft junction. The step cut should be secured with circumferential wires or cables. If the femur was bivalved, the two halves, with attached ligaments, can be secured around the allograft, also with wires. If the epicondyles have been osteotomized, they can be reattached to the allograft with heavy sutures, after the epicondylar areas are removed with a saw.

It is possible to reconstruct the knee joint with an allograft and posterior stabilized components, but constrained and hinged components should be available should instability dictate otherwise.

POSTOPERATIVE FRACTURES OF THE TIBIA

Incidence and Classification of Tibial Fractures

Individual series of tibial periprosthetic fractures have reported a tibial fracture rate as high as 6.6% (5 of 76 patients)

(2). However, the largest report of tibial periprosthetic fractures gives some indication of the true incidence of this relatively rare complication of total knee arthroplasty (68). Out of 17,727 total knee arthroplasties performed at the Mayo Clinic between 1970 and 1995, 19 intraoperative fractures (0.1%) and 71 postoperative fractures (0.4%) occurred. Intraoperative fractures were more common in revision cases (occurring in 0.36% of cases) than in primary cases (0.07%). Similarly, postoperative fractures were slightly more common after revision surgery (0.48%) than after primary surgery (0.39%).

Risk Factors

Preoperative deformity, postoperative component malposition, and use of components inserted without cement have been described as important risk factors for tibial periprosthetic fractures. Fractures in association with loose components appear to be more common than is the case for supracondylar fractures. In a series of 76 Geometric total knee arthroplasties followed at 3 years, five patients had experienced fractures of the medial tibial plateau (2). Four of the five patients had the tibial component positioned in varus. In a separate series, 15 patients of a total of 705 who had received a Geometric prosthesis (1.7%) experienced a tibial fracture (69). Risk factors for these patients were thought to be postoperative malalignment, particularly in marked varus, and malpositioning of the component in a flexed position.

Thompson et al. (70) reported seven cases of early proximal tibial plateau fractures out of a population of 971 patients who had had insertion of a Low Contact Stress total knee prosthesis (DePuy, Leeds, UK) without cement. All patients had postoperative radiographs taken between 6 days and 1 year after surgery and before their fracture, which showed no component malalignment. By comparison, none of 1,105 patients who had Low Contact Stress total knee prostheses inserted with cement sustained a similar fracture. In addition to a change to components inserted without cement, these authors felt that the main risk factors for this fracture pattern were female gender, osteopenia, and preoperative valgus alignment. Four of these seven patients required revision to a stemmed total knee prosthesis.

Fractures can occur at any stage of arthroplasty and may be technique dependent. Intraoperative fractures have been reported while removing cement or a prosthesis during a revision operation, while retracting or preparing bone, during trial reductions, or while seating the tibial component (68). A tibial tubercle osteotomy, used for exposure in difficult revision cases, may be associated with an increased risk of tibial shaft fracture. Ritter et al. (24)

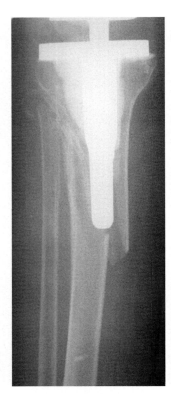

FIG. 10. This fracture at the tip of a revision hinged tibial component occurred after a minor fall in this 88-year-old woman. At the time of revision arthroplasty, a cortical defect was noted as the cause of the fracture.

reported two cases of tibial shaft fracture occurring in patients within 2 months of tibial tubercle osteotomies. A total of nine tibial tubercle osteotomies had been performed at their institution over the same time period. Both cases healed without surgical intervention, but one healed with malunion for which a tibial osteotomy was being considered. Arredondo et al. (71) reported on the case of a 67-year-old man who sustained a tibial shaft fracture after a tibial tubercle osteotomy with a subsequent nonunion, which required surgical treatment.

Rand and Coventry (69) noted that patient body weight, the presence of contralateral joint disease, and steroid use were not significantly related to the occurrence of tibial stress fractures.

Classification

Felix et al. (68) reviewed the Mayo Clinic experience over 25 years (102 fractures) in an attempt to classify fracture patterns and assess the outcome of various treatment methods. This Mayo Clinic classification system (Table 5) takes into consideration the anatomic location (types I through IV) as well as the status of fixation of the components and the time of injury (subcategories A, B, and C).

Type I or condylar fractures were most common fracture type (61 out of 102 fractures). In this series, these fractures occurred either intraoperatively (type IC, 11 patients) (Fig. 4) or in patients with loose components (type IB, 50 patients). They tended to be associated with minimal trauma and more often occurred with early component designs (predominantly Geo-

TABLE 5. *Felix, Stuart, and Hanssen classification of periprosthetic tibial fractures*

Major anatomic pattern	Subcategory
I. Tibial plateau	A. Prosthesis well fixed
II. Adjacent to stem	B. Loose prosthesis
III. Distal to prosthesis	C. Intraoperative
IV. Tibial tubercle	

From Felix NA, Stuart MJ, Hanssen AD. Periprosthetic fractures of the tibia associated with total knee arthroplasty. *Clin Orthop* 1997;345:113–124, with permission.

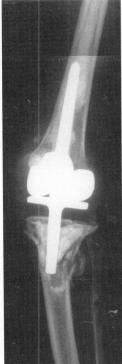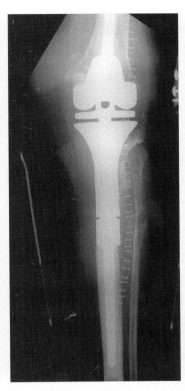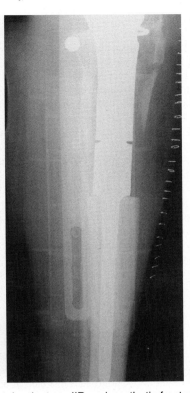

A,B   C

FIG. 11. Radiographs of the knee of an 87-year-old woman who sustained a type IIB periprosthetic fracture of the tibia. **A:** Anteroposterior radiograph of the initial fracture. Marked osteolysis and loosening of the total knee implant can be appreciated. As the patient already had a rotating-hinge implant in place, it was possible to revise the tibial component without revising the femoral component by converting the tibia to a segmental replacement tibial component. **B:** Postoperative anteroposterior radiograph. **C:** Postoperative lateral radiograph. It can be seen that the extensor mechanism has been preserved and reattached to the prosthesis.

metric and polycentric knees) (69). Collapse of the medial plateau (55 cases) occurred more often in tibial components that were positioned in varus.

Type II fractures, located in the metaphysis or proximal diaphysis, adjacent to the prosthesis stem, were the next most common fracture type, occurring in 22 out of 102 cases. As with type I fractures, most were the result of relatively minor trauma. Fractures with well-fixed prostheses (type IIA) (Fig. 10) were associated with modern component designs, whereas fractures with loose components (type IIB) occurred adjacent to long-stemmed components (Fig. 11). The presence of extensive osteolysis seemed to be an important factor in development of the fracture. Intraoperative (type IIC) fractures occurred during component removal (one out of seven cases), cement removal (two out of seven cases), or insertion of a long-stemmed component (four out of seven cases).

Type III fractures distal to the component were almost as common as type II fractures (17 cases). Most occurred in association with a well-fixed component (15 out of 17 cases). Type IV fractures occurred in only two patients, both in association with well-fixed components (type IVA).

Treatment of Postoperative Tibial Fractures

Unlike postoperative supracondylar periprosthetic fractures, there is no large pool of evidence to guide the clinician in man-

agement of postoperative tibial fractures. The authors' preferred methods of treatment are therefore presented.

Type I

Type I fractures almost never occur without loosening of the tibial component, and therefore it may be assumed that type IA fractures do not occur. The treatment of type IB fractures is therefore revision total knee arthroplasty. The region of the fracture generally has sufficient bone loss that internal fixation is rarely, if ever, adequate. In most cases, revision with modular augments or bone graft for larger defects is required. As in most revision operations with poor bone stock, use of a stem is necessary.

Type IC fractures may be treated conservatively, with bracing and protected weightbearing, if they appear stable intraoperatively. If unstable, they should be treated using a stemmed component that bypasses the fracture, with or without screw fixation of the fracture fragment.

Type II

Management of type IIA fractures depends on the nature of the fracture. If the fracture is undisplaced and stable, conservative management with early casting followed by bracing and protective weightbearing produces a satisfactory outcome with no effect on knee function. If the fracture is displaced, closed reduction and casting may be used if an acceptable reduction can be attained. Failing this, open reduction and internal fixation of the fracture should be used.

Associated osteolysis and bone loss dictates the treatment of type IIB fractures. They require revision arthroplasty with a long-stemmed component. Often, there is insufficient bone stock for a revision arthroplasty, and reconstruction with a structural allograft is often necessary. Ghazavi et al. (65) reported success in treatment of three such fractures with proximal tibial allografts. In older patients, a tumor prosthesis may be used to allow expedient rehabilitation.

Intraoperative type II fractures must be assessed for stability. If the fracture is stable, a successful outcome can be expected by treating conservatively, in the same manner as type IIA fractures. If the fracture is unstable, revision to a long-stemmed component bypassing the fracture should be performed. Any cortical defects should be bone-grafted.

Type III

Type IIIA and rare type IIIC fractures can be treated in a similar fashion. If the fracture is undisplaced and stable, immobilization in a cast, followed by bracing with protected weightbearing can be expected to be successful. Displaced fractures may also be reduced and treated in a cast, if an acceptable reduction can be achieved and maintained. If not, these fractures need to be treated independently of the knee replacement with open reduction and internal fixation, as the presence of a knee replacement precludes intramedullary nailing.

Type IIIB fractures are challenging fractures whose treatment needs to be individualized depending on the patient and the fracture. Occasionally, osteosynthesis to reestablish an intact tibia should be done initially, followed by revision total knee arthroplasty after fracture healing, if the fracture is very distal to the knee. If the fracture is proximal enough to be bypassed with a stem, revision arthroplasty with a long stemmed component is the treatment of choice.

Type IV

There is little guidance on how to treat type IV fractures. Even in the series of Felix et al. (68), only two such fractures were identified. One patient was treated with extension immobilization and had a good functional result and range of motion 11 years after the injury. The other patient was treated with screw fixation of the fracture. This patient also had an excellent outcome at 18 months. If there is any doubt about the ability to hold the tubercle in place, the fracture should probably be treated with secure internal fixation.

REFERENCES

1. Berry DJ. Periprosthetic fractures after major joint replacement. Epidemiology: hip and knee. *Orthop Clin North Am* 1999;30:183–190.
2. Lotke PA, Ecker ML. Influence of positioning of prosthesis in total knee replacement. *J Bone Joint Surg Am* 1977;59:77–79.
3. Peyton RS, Booth RE Jr. Supracondylar femur fractures above an Insall-Burstein CCK total knee: a new method of intramedullary stem fixation. *J Arthroplasty* 1998;13:473–478.
4. Lombardi AV, Mallory TH, Waterman RA, et al. Intercondylar distal femoral fracture. An unreported complication of posterior-stabilized total knee arthroplasty. *J Arthroplasty* 1995;10:643–650.
5. Cracchiolo A. Stress fractures of the pelvis as a cause of hip pain following total hip and knee arthroplasty. *Arthritis Rheum* 1981;24:740–742.
6. Smith MD, Henke JA. Pubic ramus fractures after total knee arthroplasty. *Orthopaedics* 1988;11:315–317.
7. Torisu T. Fatigue fracture of the pelvis after total knee replacements. *Clin Orthop* 1980;149:216–219.
8. Cameron HU, Hu C, Vyamont D. Hinge total knee replacement revisited. *Can J Surg* 1997;41:278–283.
9. Fipp G. Stress fracture of the femoral neck following total knee arthroplasty. *J Arthroplasty* 1988;3:347–350.
10. Hardy DCR, Delince PE, Yasik E, et al. Stress fractures of the hip: an unusual complication of total knee arthroplasty. *Clin Orthop* 1992;281:140–144.
11. Lesniewski PJ, Testa NN. Stress fracture of the hip as a complication of total knee arthroplasty. *J Bone Joint Surg Am* 1982;64:304–306.
12. McAuley JP, Sanchez FL. Knee: role and results of allografts. *Orthop Clin North Am* 1999;30:293–303.
13. Rawes ML, Patsalis T, Gregg PJ. Sub-capital stress fractures of the hip complicating total knee replacement. *Injury* 1995;26:421–423.
14. Delport PH, Van Audekercke R, Martens M, et al. Conservative treatment of ipsilateral supracondylar femoral fracture after total knee arthroplasty. *J Trauma* 1984;24:846–849.
15. Kenny P, Rice J, Quinlan W. Interprosthetic fracture of the femoral shaft. *J Arthroplasty* 1998;13:361–364.
16. Urch SE, Moskal JT. Simultaneous ipsilateral revision total hip arthroplasty and revision total knee arthroplasty with entire femoral allograft. *J Arthroplasty* 1998;13:833–836.
17. Hirsh DM, Bhalla S, Roffman M. Supracondylar fracture of the femur following total knee replacement. Report of four cases. *J Bone Joint Surg Am* 1981;63:162–163.
18. DiGioia AM 3rd, Rubash HE. Periprosthetic fractures of the femur after total knee arthroplasty. A literature review and treatment algorithm. *Clin Orthop* 1991;271:135–142.
19. Booth RE Jr. Supracondylar fractures: all or nothing. *Orthopedics* 1995;18:921–922.
20. Culp RW, Schmidt RG, Hanks G, et al. Supracondylar fracture of the femur following prosthetic knee arthroplasty. *Clin Orthop* 1987;222:212–222.
21. McLaren AC, Dupont JA, Schroeber DC. Open reduction internal fixation of supracondylar fractures above total knee arthroplasties using the intramedullary supracondylar rod. *Clin Orthop* 1994;302:194–198.
22. Merkel KD, Johnson EW Jr. Supracondylar fracture of the femur after total knee arthroplasty. *J Bone Joint Surg Am* 1986;68:29–43.
23. Inglis AE, Walker PS. Revision of failed knee replacements using fixed-axis hinges. *J Bone Joint Surg Br* 1991;73:757–761.
24. Ritter MA, Carr K, Keating EM, et al. Tibial shaft fracture following tibial tubercle osteotomy. *J Arthroplasty* 1996;11:117–119.
25. Neer CS II, Grantham SA, Shelton ML. Supracondylar fracture of the adult femur: a study of one hundred and ten cases. *J Bone Joint Surg Am* 1967;49:591–613.
26. Rorabeck CH, Taylor JW. Periprosthetic fractures of the femur complicating total knee arthroplasty. *Orthop Clin North Am* 1999;30:265–277.
27. Chen F, Mont MA, Bachner RS. Management of ipsilateral supracondylar femur fractures following total knee arthroplasty. *J Arthroplasty* 1994;9:521–526.
28. Rorabeck CH, Angliss RD, Lewis PL. Fractures of the femur, tibia, and patella after total knee arthroplasty: decision making and principles of management. *Instr Course Lect* 1998;47:449–458.
29. Jabczenski FF, Crawford M. Retrograde intramedullary nailing of supracondylar femur fractures above total knee arthroplasty. A preliminary report of four cases. *J Arthroplasty* 1995;10:95–101.
30. Aaron RK, Scott R. Supracondylar fracture of the femur after total knee arthroplasty. *Clin Orthop* 1987;219:136–139.
31. Cain PR, Rubash HE, Wissinger HA, et al. Periprosthetic femoral fractures following total knee arthroplasty. *Clin Orthop* 1986;208:205–214.

32. Dorr LD. Fractures following total knee arthroplasty. *Orthopedics* 1997;20:848–850.

33. Lesh ML, Schneider DJ, Deol G, et al. The consequences of anterior femoral notching in total knee arthroplasty. A biomechanical study. *J Bone Joint Surg Am* 2000;82:1096–1101.

34. Ritter MA, Faris PM, Keating EM. Anterior femoral notching and ipsilateral supracondylar femur fracture in total knee arthroplasty. *J Arthroplasty* 1988;3:185–187.

35. Healy WL, Siliski JM, Incavo SJ. Operative treatment of distal femoral fractures proximal to total knee replacements. *J Bone Joint Surg Am* 1993;75:27–34.

36. Scott RD. Anterior femoral notching and ipsilateral supracondylar femur fracture in total knee arthroplasty [letter]. *J Arthroplasty* 1988;3:381.

37. Benevenia J, Lee FY, Buechel F, et al. Pathologic supracondylar fracture due to osteolytic pseudotumor of knee following cementless total knee replacement. *J Biomed Mater Res* 1998;43:473–477.

38. Rand JA. Supracondylar fracture of the femur associated with polyethylene wear after total knee arthroplasty. A case report. *J Bone Joint Surg Am* 1994;76:1389–1393.

39. Bogoch E, Hastings D, Gross A, et al. Supracondylar fractures of the femur adjacent to resurfacing and MacIntosh arthroplasties of the knee in patients with rheumatoid arthritis. *Clin Orthop* 1988;229:213–220.

40. Cordeiro EN, Costa RC, Carazzato JG, et al. Periprosthetic fractures in patients with total knee arthroplasties. *Clin Orthop* 1990;252:182–189.

41. Figgie MP, Goldberg VM, Figgie HE 3rd, et al. The results of treatment of supracondylar fracture above total knee arthroplasty. *J Arthroplasty* 1990;5:267–276.

42. Garnavos C, Rafiq M, Henry AP. Treatment of femoral fracture above a knee prosthesis. 18 cases followed 0.5–14 years. *Acta Orthop Scand* 1994;65:610–614.

43. Moran MC, Brick GW, Sledge CB, et al. Supracondylar femoral fracture following total knee arthroplasty. *Clin Orthop* 1996;324:196–209.

44. Nielsen BF, Petersen VS, Varmarken JE. Fracture of the femur after knee arthroplasty. *Acta Orthop Scand* 1988;59:155–157.

45. Short WH, Hootnick DR, Murray DG. Ipsilateral supracondylar femur fractures following knee arthroplasty. *Clin Orthop* 1981;158:111–116.

46. Sochart DH, Hardinge K. Nonsurgical management of supracondylar fracture above total knee arthroplasty. Still the nineties option. *J Arthroplasty* 1997;12:830–834.

47. Dave DJ, Koka SR, James SE. Mennen plate fixation for fracture of the femoral shaft with ipsilateral total hip and knee arthroplasties. *J Arthroplasty* 1995;10:113–115.

48. Hagroo GA, Qurashi V, Butt MS. Breakage of Mennen femur device. *Injury* 1996;27:593–595.

49. Ochsner PE, Pfister A. Use of the fork plate for internal fixation of periprosthetic fractures and osteotomies in connection with total knee replacement. *Orthopedics* 1999;22:517–521.

50. Zehntner MK, Ganz R. Internal fixation of supracondylar fractures after condylar total knee arthroplasty. *Clin Orthop* 1993;293:219–224.

51. Henry SL. Supracondylar femur fractures treated percutaneously. *Clin Orthop* 2000;375:51–59.

52. Ritter MA, Keating EM, Faris PM, et al. Rush rod fixation of supracondylar fractures above total knee arthroplasties. *J Arthroplasty* 1995;10:213–216.

53. Hanks GA, Mathews HH, Routson GW, et al. Supracondylar fracture of the femur following total knee arthroplasty. *J Arthroplasty* 1989;4:289–292.

54. Maniar RN, Umlas ME, Rodriguez JA, et al. Supracondylar femoral fracture above a PFC posterior cruciate–substituting total knee arthroplasty treated with supracondylar nailing. A unique technical problem. *J Arthroplasty* 1996;11:637–639.

55. Murrell GA, Nunley JA. Interlocked supracondylar intramedullary nails for supracondylar fractures after total knee arthroplasty. A new treatment method. *J Arthroplasty* 1995;10:37–42.

56. Rolston LR, Christ DJ, Halpern A, et al. Treatment of supracondylar fractures of the femur proximal to a total knee arthroplasty. A report of four cases. *J Bone Joint Surg Am* 1995;77:924–931.

57. Roscoe MW, Goodman SB, Schatzker J. Supracondylar fracture of the femur after GUEPAR total knee arthroplasty. A new treatment method. *Clin Orthop* 1989;241:221–223.

58. Sekel R, Newman AS. Supracondylar fractures above a total knee arthroplasty. A novel use of the Huckstepp nail. *J Arthroplasty* 1994;9:445–447.

59. Engh GA, Ammeen DJ. Periprosthetic fractures adjacent to total knee implants: treatment and clinical results. *J Bone Joint Surg Am* 1997;79:1100–1113.

60. Biswas SP, Kurer MH, Mackenney RP. External fixation for femoral shaft fracture after Stanmore total knee replacement. *J Bone Joint Surg Br* 1992;74:313–314.

61. Simon RG, Brinker MR. Use of Ilizarov external fixation for a periprosthetic supracondylar femur fracture. *J Arthroplasty* 1999;14:118–121.

62. Harris AI, Poddar S, Gitelis S, et al. Arthroplasty with a composite of an allograft and a prosthesis for knees with severe deficiency of bone. *J Bone Joint Surg Am* 1995;77:373–386.

63. Engh GA, Herzwurm PJ, Parks NL. Treatment of major defects of bone with bulk allografts and stemmed components during total knee arthroplasty. *J Bone Joint Surg Am* 1997;79:1030–1039.

64. Kraay MJ, Goldberg VM, Figgie MP, et al. Distal femoral replacement with allograft/prosthetic reconstruction for treatment of supracondylar fractures in patients with total knee arthroplasty. *J Arthroplasty* 1992;7:7–16.

65. Ghazavi MT, Stockley I, Yee G, et al. Reconstruction of massive bone defects with allograft in revision total knee arthroplasty. *J Bone Joint Surg Am* 1997;79:17–25.

66. Kress KJ, Scuderi GR, Windsor RE, et al. Treatment of non-unions about the knee utilizing custom total knee arthroplasty with press-fit intramedullary stems. *J Arthroplasty* 1993;8:49–55.

67. Wong P, Gross AE. The use of structural allografts for treating periprosthetic fractures about the hip and knee. *Orthop Clin North Am* 1999;30:259–264.

68. Felix NA, Stuart MJ, Hanssen AD. Periprosthetic fractures of the tibia associated with total knee arthroplasty. *Clin Orthop* 1997;345:113–124.

69. Rand JA, Coventry MB. Stress fractures after total knee arthroplasty. *J Bone Joint Surg Am* 1980;62:226–233.

70. Thompson NW, McAlinden MG, Breslin E, et al. Periprosthetic tibial fractures following cementless Low Contact Stress total knee arthroplasty. *J Arthroplasty* 2001;16(8):984–990.

71. Arredondo J, Worland RL, Jessup DE. Nonunion after a tibial shaft fracture complicating tibial tubercle osteotomy. *J Arthroplasty* 1998;13:958–960.

72. McElwaine JP, Sheehan JM. Spontaneous fractures of the femoral neck after total replacement of the knee. *J Bone Joint Surg Br* 1983;64:323–325.

73. Smith WJ, Martin SL, Mabrey JD. Use of a supracondylar nail for treatment of a supracondylar fracture of the femur following total knee arthroplasty. *J Arthroplasty* 1996;11:210–213.

CHAPTER 100

Instability after Total Knee Arthroplasty

M. Shannon Moore and James P. McAuley

Symptomatic knee instability after total knee arthroplasty (TKA) is a source of chronic pain and disability for the patient and a source of frustration and remorse for the surgeon. Most revision knee series report instability as the second or third most common reason for revision of the primary implant (1–4). It is with some trepidation that most surgeons undertake the revision of a radiographically well-aligned and well-fixed implant. It is, therefore, imperative to approach such a revision with a clear understanding of the pattern of instability present in the individual patient. The plan for intervention should specifically address the particular pattern of instability without resorting to excessive constraint. The surgeon must ensure the availability of a full range of implants that provide various levels of inherent stability before embarking on the revision of an unstable primary knee.

A primary cause of knee instability after TKA is malalignment (5). Almost no degree of bony resection plane malalignment is tolerated in the weightbearing knee after TKA. Minor degrees of instability tolerated in the well-aligned knee may become grossly symptomatic in the malaligned knee. The sequence of off-center loading, loosening, and late instability has been described well, as has the logical remedial measure of correcting the angle of the resection plane (5). Addressing this challenge in the setting of bone defects is the subject of other portions of this book. There is a greater diagnostic challenge in dealing with the knee that exhibits symptomatic instability despite adequate alignment, and this is the focus of this chapter. For ease of discussion, we first address instability occurring between the patella and femur and then instability between the femur and tibia.

PATELLOFEMORAL INSTABILITY

Etiology

Patellar stability is a function of numerous interrelated variables, including axial alignment, quadriceps muscle group vectors and relative strength, retinacular tension, component position and rotation, design of the patellofemoral sulcus and patellar implant, patellar thickness, femoral component size, and dynamic stability at the tibiofemoral articulation. In general terms, patellar instability results from one of two mechanisms of failure: (a) lateralization of the extensor mechanism in relation to the prosthetic femoral sulcus and (b) problems with retinacular balancing.

Lateralization of the extensor mechanism relative to the femoral sulcus alters patellar tracking. This occurs in the excessively valgus knee and with internal rotation or medialization of the femoral or tibial components. Each of these factors shifts the quadriceps summation vector (acting in a line through the quadriceps tendon, patella, patellar tendon, and tibial tubercle) laterally relative to the femoral sulcus. The imbalance becomes more obvious when the patient applies quadriceps force. It is important to note that, although this mechanism is referred to as *quadriceps imbalance* or *lateralization of the extensor mechanism*, the problem is described more accurately as *medial displacement of the femoral sulcus*, resulting from limb malalignment or component malposition. Only in rare cases of tibial tubercle malunion or iatrogenic alteration of quadriceps alignment does the problem lie in the quadriceps itself.

To illustrate rotational issues that must be assessed in an unstable TKA, it is worthwhile to review the landmarks commonly used in component positioning.

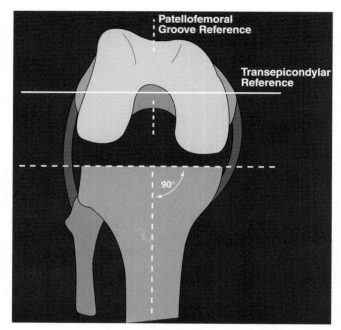

FIG. 1. Landmarks used in rotational orientation of the femoral component: the transepicondylar axis, the patellofemoral groove reference, and the proximal tibial resection (flexion gap).

Looking first at femoral component orientation, three axes are used with the knee flexed 90 degrees. All three—the transepicondylar axis, the plane of proximal tibial resection (flexion space), and the patellofemoral groove reference (Fig. 1)—have inherent limitations and should be used in combination to double- and triple-check appropriate femoral component rotation. Ideally, the resections should result in the transverse axis of the component being parallel to the transepicondylar axis and perpendicular to the patellofemoral reference, and producing a rectangular flexion gap (symmetric soft tissue balance). Appropriate position of a femoral cutting block is illustrated in Figure 2A. External rotation of the component (Fig. 2B) results in a looser medial flexion gap and a tighter lateral flexion gap and, most important, laterally displaces the patellofemoral groove of the implant, which is favorable for patellar tracking. More posterior medial bone is often resected in the optimally positioned knee, because the posterior medial femoral condyle usually extends farther posterior to the transepicondylar axis than does the posterior lateral condyle. In addition, external rotation compensates for the normal asymmetric tibial resection that occurs when the tibia is resected at 90 degrees to its long axis. Conversely, internal rotation has the opposite effect on the flexion space and results in medialization if the patellar groove (Fig. 2C), which adversely affects patellar tracking. This can occur in the valgus knee when resections are based on posterior bone referencing of the hypoplastic lateral condyle. It also can occur in a varus knee after an excessive medial release has been performed and resections are based only on the creation of a rectangular flexion space.

On the tibial side, three landmarks are frequently used for rotational orientation: the transmalleolar axis (which varies greatly in the normal population), the transverse axis of the proximal tibia, and the tibial tubercle (Fig. 3A). Internal rotation of the tibial

component (Fig. 3B) results in lateral displacement of the tibial tubercle, which effectively increases the quadriceps angle of the knee and is detrimental to optimum patellar tracking.

With retinacular imbalance, tension in the lateral retinaculum exceeds the static and dynamic forces acting to medialize the patella. The problem may be an inherently tight or contracted lateral retinaculum. Soft tissue contracture and muscle atrophy in the arthritic knee may give rise to a tight lateral retinaculum, weak vastus medialis, and patellar maltracking before TKA. In the series reported by Brick and Scott (6), 40% of patients with symptomatic patellar instability after TKA had preoperative patellar dislocation or abnormal tracking. If the tight retinaculum remains unaddressed at the time of the initial procedure, maltracking is likely to persist.

In some cases, insufficiency of the medial retinacular tissues results in imbalance. Conlan et al. found the medial patellofemoral ligament to be the major stabilizer of medial soft tissue in the native joint, providing 53% of the total medial restraining force (7). Postoperative trauma or hematoma can disrupt the medial parapatellar repair, which leaves an uncompensated lateral tether.

The morphology of the patella itself or of the resurfaced patella and femoral construct may create imbalance. Any change in the articulation that increases the lateral retinacular tension also increases the likelihood of instability. This occurs with large peripheral patellar osteophytes, patellar underresection, overstuffing of the patellofemoral joint with a thick patellar button, oblique resection of the patella (particularly lateral underresection) (8), lateral placement of the patellar resurfacing component, oversizing or anteriorization of the femoral component, or use of a design with a shallow femoral sulcus. A strong vastus medialis obliquus may act to dynamically offset the imbalance; therefore, retinacular imbalance is best assessed with the quadriceps relaxed.

Clinical Presentation

Symptomatic instability of the patella after TKA occurs with a reported incidence ranging from 1% to 20% (9) and can occur with or without resurfacing of the patella (10). Subluxation is more common than dislocation (6). The reoperation rate for patellofemoral instability remains less than 1% in most large series. Patellofemoral instability usually results from errors in surgical technique, although trauma and problems with prosthetic design may contribute.

The patient with patellar maltracking after TKA may present with recurrent or fixed dislocation but more commonly describes episodic subluxation with complaints of "giving way" or buckling of the knee, anterior or poorly localized knee pain, and crepitus (6,11). Over time, recurrent episodes may lead to component wear or failure (11), loosening, or patellar fracture.

It is imperative that the surgeon understand the mechanism of failure before intervention. Alignment and patellar tilt are evaluated with careful clinical examination and plain films, including patellar axial or "sunrise" views (Fig. 4). The subluxed patella may exhibit 20% to 90% displacement of the patella over the lateral femoral condyle (patellar overhang) (11). In some cases, axial computed tomography (CT) may be useful. CT has been demonstrated to be more sensitive than plain radiography in evaluating patellofemoral congruence in the native joint (12).

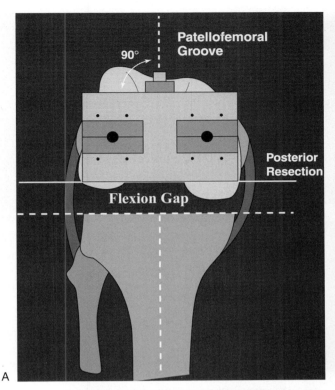

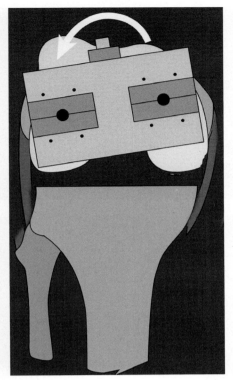

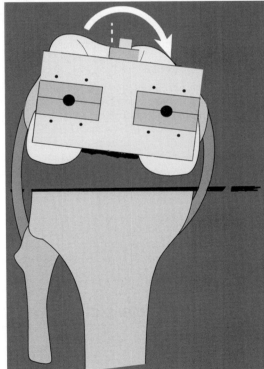

FIG. 2. A: An appropriately positioned femoral resection block. **B:** External rotation results in an increased medial flexion gap, decreased lateral gap, and lateralization of the patellar groove of the implant. **C:** Internal rotation produces the opposite effect on the flexion space and has the undesirable effect of medialization of the patellar groove.

CT also has advantages in the setting of TKA. CT allows axial imaging in initial knee flexion (less than 20 degrees). It also provides a means to assess the rotational alignment of the femoral component with respect to the transepicondylar axis and of the tibial component with respect to the tibial tubercle, posterior tibial axis, or transtibial axis (13–15). Cadaver studies have con-

firmed the accuracy of CT for assessing rotational alignment (15). Other investigators have confirmed the usefulness of CT in the planning of TKA revision for patellofemoral problems. In particular, CT not only confirms the presence of rotational malalignment but also localizes the rotational problem to the femoral component, the tibial component, or both (13).

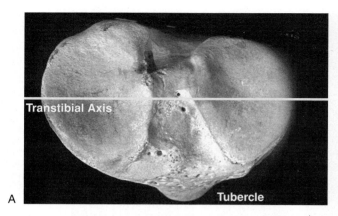

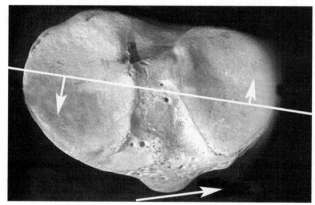

FIG. 3. A: Landmarks for rotational orientation of the tibial component. **B:** Internal rotation of the tibial component results in lateral rotational displacement of the insertion of the patellar tendon, which effectively increases the quadriceps angle of the knee.

Treatment

Intervention for patellar maltracking depends on symptom severity and mechanism of failure (Table 1). Patients who are mildly symptomatic may benefit from a course of physical therapy directed toward vastus medialis obliquus strengthening. This may slightly medialize the quadriceps force vector and provide a dynamic counterbalance to lateral retinacular tightness. In cases of dislocation or severe subluxation, nonsurgical means rarely are sufficient.

Ideally, surgical intervention should address the specific cause of patellar maltracking. At times, success can be attained when the mechanism of failure is addressed adequately without correcting the primary cause. For example, a proximal or distal realignment procedure may compensate for a malrotated tibial component that produces patellofemoral instability but otherwise retains satisfactory tibiofemoral kinematics. On the other hand, an intervention that does not address the primary mechanism may not work. For example, an isolated lateral release for instability secondary to lateralization of the quadriceps vector is doomed to failure.

Patellofemoral instability due to retinacular imbalance may be treated with lateral release alone or in combination with patellar or femoral component revision. Asymmetric patellar

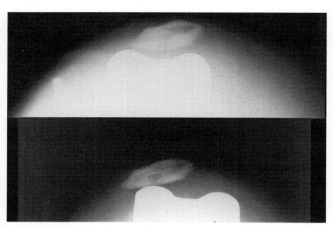

FIG. 4. "Sunrise view" radiographs reveal lateral patellar subluxation with increasing flexion.

cuts or underresection of the patella should be corrected by patellar revision.

Success in addressing quadriceps malalignment has been reported with proximal, distal, and combined realignment procedures (6,8,9,16). Proximal realignment is accomplished through vastus medialis obliquus advancement or imbrication or by V-Y quadricepsplasty, usually in combination with a lateral release. Distal realignment can be performed at the level of the patellar ligament (Roux-Goldthwait procedure) or via medial transposition of the tibial tubercle. Advocates of tibial tubercle transposition cite the advantages of precise realignment and the ability to address patella baja or alta without compromising the power of the quadriceps (18). Nevertheless, tibial tubercle transposition, particularly in the setting of revision surgery, has a high complication rate (16). Wolff et al. reported a 23% major complication rate in 26 tibial tubercle osteotomies performed during TKA (18). Of their 11 patients who had a tibial tubercle osteotomy during revision surgery, four had major complications, including a ruptured patellar tendon and wound problems at the region of the osteotomy requiring muscle flap coverage. Distal and combined procedures should be undertaken with great caution.

In some patients, there are elements of both retinacular imbalance and quadriceps instability, and both must be addressed. Instability secondary to axial malalignment should be treated with component revision and restoration of proper alignment.

TABLE 1. *Management options for patellofemoral instability*

Retinacular imbalance	Physical therapy to strengthen the vastus medialis obliquus
	Lateral release
	Medial imbrication/vastus medialis obliquus advancement
Patellar asymmetry	Patellar revision
Quadriceps malalignment	Proximal realignment
	Distal realignment
	Combined procedures
	Femoral/tibial revision

TIBIOFEMORAL INSTABILITY

The patterns of instability after TKA are best divided into three groups: (a) flexion space or anteroposterior instability, (b) varus or valgus instability, and (c) global instability.

Flexion Space (Anteroposterior) Instability

Anteroposterior instability in the post-TKA knee is most commonly manifest in flexion. Most modern designs sacrifice the anterior cruciate ligament and display some degree of anterior laxity, which is usually limited by the conformity of the implant in the sagittal plane. Indeed, a biomechanical study of several TKA designs concluded that at least 5 mm of anteroposterior laxity is necessary to avoid impairment of the range of motion regardless of the design (19). Various approaches have been taken to address the posterior cruciate ligament (PCL). Some cruciate-sacrificing implants substitute for the function of the PCL via curved or dished tibial polyethylene, which increases conformity and anteroposterior constraint. Posterior stabilized implants substitute for the PCL with a central tibial post and femoral cam mechanism. Although there can be gross flexion space instability or design problems (an overly anterior or short keel), which allow dramatic tibiofemoral dislocation in flexion, these problems are rare with modern posterior stabilized designs. In contrast, posterior instability in a knee with a cruciate retaining design may present in a subtle fashion. Although the problem of posterior instability after TKA has long been recognized, details of the clinical picture were not fully elucidated until recently.

Clinical Presentation

The patient with flexion space instability may present with a spectrum of symptoms, ranging from obvious dislocation to vague, nonspecific complaints. Symptoms may begin during the initial postoperative rehabilitation, if the instability was created intraoperatively, or they may begin late, particularly with late attritional rupture of the PCL. Regardless of when the symptoms begin, the pattern remains consistent. Waslewski et al. have characterized the constellation of subjective complaints from patients with posteriorly unstable knee arthroplasties as a triad: anterior knee pain, swelling, and giving way (20). Some patients describe diffuse pain whereas others describe localized pain in the anterior knee, particularly in the pes anserinus tendons and retinacular tissues (21). There is a subjective sense of dissatisfaction sometimes described as giving way or as the need to "get the knee in gear" before walking (20). Patients often have particular difficulty climbing or descending stairs. They describe knee swelling that fluctuates with activity but never completely resolves.

On examination, the knee may demonstrate an effusion. Fehring and Valadie found a predominance of red blood cells in the aspirates from unstable TKAs with an average of 64,000 red cells per mm^3 (22). Palpation reveals anterior soft tissue tenderness. On passive examination a posterior sag or drawer is present. The flexed knee demonstrates reduction of the tibia from a posteriorly subluxed resting position to a neutral or slightly anterior position beneath the femur as the patient contracts his or her quadriceps. A quadriceps-active test is the manifestation of this reduction during static contraction of the quadriceps. An active anterior drawer sign is the dynamic manifestation during which the tibia sometimes reduces dramatically when the patient actively extends the knee from 90 degrees of flexion (20). The overall anteroposterior laxity on examination is greater in cases of a large flexion gap, because laxity of the collateral and capsular structures in flexion precludes the sagittal constraint normally provided by tibiofemoral conformity. This is particularly evident when the patient sits on the examination table with the foot off the floor. The knee also may exhibit posterolateral rotatory instability if the arcuate complex is absent or compromised. The presence of this sign is highly dependent on component conformity and design. Lateral radiographs taken in flexion may demonstrate posterior subluxation or dislocation of the tibia and at a minimum show decreased femoral rollback (Fig. 5A).

Etiology

Posterior instability after TKA is almost always the result of one of three errors in surgical technique: (a) the creation of an excessively large flexion space, (b) the loss of PCL/popliteal function, or (c) the creation of an excessively tight flexion space that results in late PCL rupture during attempts to regain flexion. Insall et al. emphasize the importance of balancing the flexion and extension gaps (23), and this concept is particularly critical to the success of a cruciate-retaining implant. To some extent, a posterior stabilized implant can compensate for an excessive flexion gap; most patients tolerate some varus or valgus instability in flexion if the components are well aligned and the stability in extension is good. Insufficiency or iatrogenic injury of the PCL that goes unrecognized and, therefore, unaddressed at the time of the index arthroplasty may result in symptomatic instability. An intact popliteus and arcuate complex can provide femoral rollback, particularly in the lateral portion of the joint. The action of the popliteus combined with a somewhat conforming tibial polyethylene may provide a functional, asymptomatic knee, even if the PCL is incompetent. When both the PCL and the popliteus have failed, however, there is no effective check rein to posterior translation of the tibia in flexion, and this function must be substituted by the prosthetic design.

Treatment

Conservative treatment for posterior instability is appropriate only in the setting of acute tibiofemoral dislocation of a posterior stabilized implant. In one of two patients with this complication, Gebhard et al. reported success with brace treatment after closed reduction (24). Lombardi et al. (25) successfully treated 11 of 15 dislocations with reduction, cast immobilization, and intensive quadriceps rehabilitation, and a gradual flexion program. Sharkey et al. treated three of seven cases with closed reduction and immobilization; of these, two were successful (26). All other symptomatic forms of posterior instability require surgical intervention for resolution (Table 2).

If instability is the result of a mismatch of the flexion-extension gap, surgical options include an exchange of the tibial insert to a thicker polyethylene or a revision to a posterior stabi-

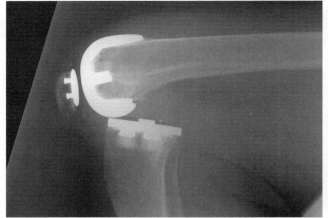

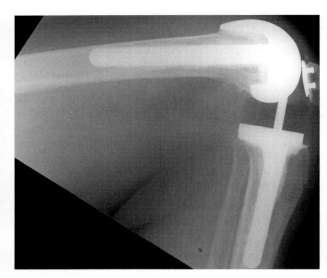

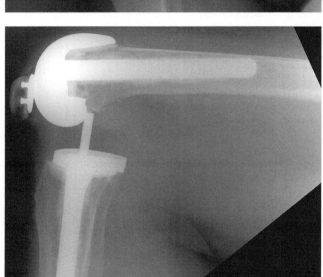

FIG. 5. A: Lateral radiograph of a cruciate-retaining implant demonstrating posterior instability. **B:** Revision to a posterior stabilized implant initially provides good mechanical femoral rollback. **C:** Six years after revision, the same patient demonstrates dislocation of the cam over the femoral post. The clinical examination showed global instability that resulted from polyethylene wear and attrition of the collateral ligaments.

lized or varus-valgus constrained (VVC) implant. Although polyethylene exchange has the appeal of simplicity, it does not address the problem of mismatched flexion and extension. Usually, revision to a posterior stabilized system entails revising the femoral component to one with a cam mechanism, as well as exchanging the tibial insert to one with a keel (Fig. 5B). Atten-

TABLE 2. Management options for tibiofemoral instability

Flexion space insta- bility	Use of thicker tibial insert
	Revision to a PS implant
	Revision to a VVC implant
Varus-valgus instability	Correction of malalignment
	Revision to a VVC implant
	Ligament reconstruction or advancement
	Revision to a linked hinged implant
Global instability	Revision to a PS implant with a thicker tibial insert
	Revision to a VVC implant
	Revision to a linked hinged implant
	Fusion

PS, posterior stabilized; VVC, varus-valgus constrained.

tion to the proper size and position of the revised femoral component can restore the flexion-extension balance at the same time. If the PCL and popliteus are insufficient but the flexion-extension gaps are in balance, then revision to a posterior stabilized implant will provide stability.

To address anteroposterior instability, we have found that insert exchange is unpredictable, whereas revision to a posterior stabilized or VVC insert is more successful. At our institution, we revised 20 cases for isolated flexion instability. We managed eight with exchanges to thicker tibial inserts; of these, four achieved stability after revision. Twelve were revised to a posterior stabilized or VVC implant, nine of which achieved stability (Fig. 5).

Varus or Valgus Instability

Clinical Presentation

Patients with varus or valgus instability also present with chronic pain, effusion, and lateral or medial giving way of the knee. They may return to the clinic wearing a brace. In general, the patient can tolerate collateral deficiency on the lateral side

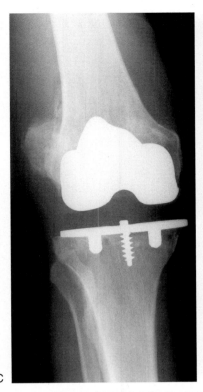
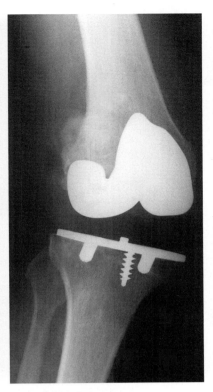

A,C

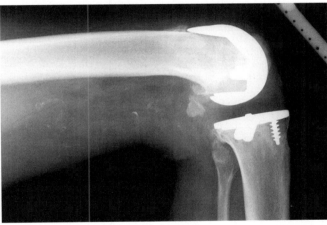

B

FIG. 6. Anteroposterior **(A)** and lateral **(B)** radiographs of a primary cruciate–retaining implant with lateral patellar dislocation. The patient had sustained a gunshot wound to the left distal thigh during World War II but had no symptoms of patellar instability before surgery. Shortly after the primary total knee arthroplasty, he developed patellar dislocation with extensor mechanism weakness. Neurologic evaluation revealed a femoral neuropathy with medial quadriceps weakness that was believed to be present, but subclinical, before the arthroplasty procedure. Revision surgery revealed a failed medial parapatellar repair. **C:** Anteroposterior valgus stress radiograph of the same patient demonstrates incompetence of the medial collateral structures.

better than on the medial side, in part because of the normal valgus alignment of the knee. This is not the case in a knee with varus malalignment. Radiographs may demonstrate coronal subluxation or gaping on the side of the knee with collateral failure. In a knee with both good alignment and a failed collateral ligament, stress radiographs can be more helpful than weight-bearing films (Fig. 6). When the knee is examined in full extension, tension in the structures of the posterior capsule causes the prosthetic joint surfaces to abut. This diminishes the sense of varus-valgus instability and provides a false sense of collateral competence. Therefore, it is best to examine the knee in slight flexion. When the knee is slightly flexed, the posterior capsule becomes lax, insufficiency of one or both of the collateral ligaments is unmasked, and midflexion instability is demonstrated. Varus or valgus instability is evident in 90 degrees of flexion, although hip rotation makes clinical assessment more difficult in this position (5).

Treatment

The causes of varus or valgus instability include iatrogenic ones, such as bony resection error and inappropriate ligament release, as well as problems of a more insidious onset, such as component subsidence and wear. All of these problems necessitate revision to restore alignment and stability (Table 2). Ligament disruption can occur intraoperatively or postoperatively. When recognized, intraoperative disruption of the medial collateral ligament can be treated successfully with primary repair or ligament reattachment to bone with protective postoperative bracing (27). On occasion, a medial epicondylar osteotomy is performed for exposure or ligament balancing. If the bony fragment migrates or fails to achieve osseous or fibrous union, medial instability can result.

Varus or valgus instability that is secondary to polyethylene wear may be treated with polyethylene exchange if it adequately

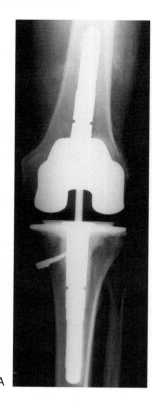

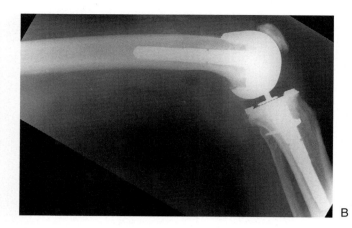

FIG. 7. Anteroposterior (A) and lateral (B) radiographs after revision to a varus-valgus constrained implant with medial collateral ligament (MCL) advancement, lateral parapatellar release, and imbrication of the insertion of the vastus medialis. Normal patellar tracking and valgus stability was restored. The MCL advancement was protected by a brace for 2 months postoperatively. The knee remained stable until the patient's death 5 years after revision.

restores ligament tension and balance. If the polyethylene wear was premature, however, then it is essential to correct the underlying cause of the premature wear at the same time. Malalignment, oxidized polyethylene, or a poor locking mechanism allowing backside wear dooms isolated polyethylene exchange to a postrevision survival time even shorter than the life of the original failed implant.

Surgical options to address collateral insufficiency include attempts at ligament advancement, which have been reported with primary arthroplasty but not for revisions (28,29). Other options are

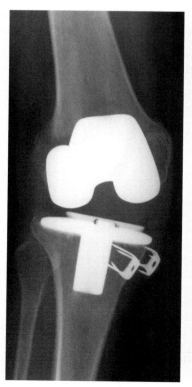
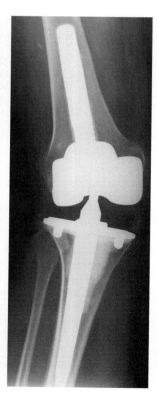

FIG. 8. A: Knee with primary cruciate-retaining implant demonstrates valgus instability. The staples were placed as part of a failed secondary medial collateral ligament reconstruction. B: Valgus instability remains despite revision to a varus-valgus constrained implant.

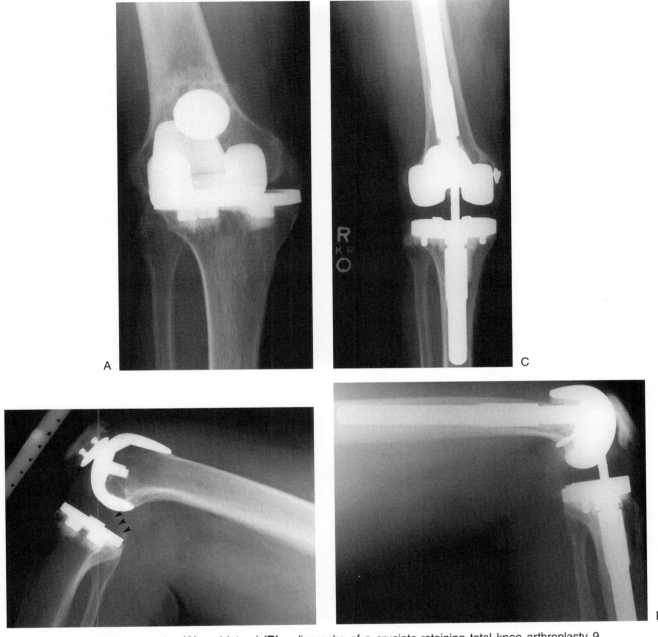

FIG. 9. Anteroposterior **(A)** and lateral **(B)** radiographs of a cruciate-retaining total knee arthroplasty 9 years after primary surgery. Note the posterior polyethylene wear. Physical examination demonstrated both anteroposterior and varus-valgus instability. The global instability resulted from a combination of posterior cruciate ligament attritional failure and polyethylene wear that led to laxity rather than failure of the collateral ligaments. **C, D:** Revision arthroplasty to a posterior stabilized implant with restoration of the joint line and of ligamentous tension with a relatively thick tibial base plate and polyethylene insert. Integrity of the collateral ligaments obviated the need for further constraint.

allograft ligament reconstruction or revision to a VVC or linked hinged implant (Fig. 7). In knees with varus or valgus instability, revision to a posterior stabilized component alone is inadequate. Peters et al. reported on 57 knee revisions, of which 16 were done for instability; four revisions failed—three partly because of residual instability from the retention of a posterior stabilized design (4).

Reports on revisions using VVC implants are limited in number and duration of follow-up. In most series, only a sub-

set of revisions was performed for symptomatic instability, and few authors comment on the resolution of instability within this population. The reported results of revision to a VVC implant for varus-valgus instability have been mixed. Friedman et al. reported on 137 patients undergoing revision, of whom 45% had mediolateral instability preoperatively, which was subsequently addressed with increased constraint (1). Postoperatively, the incidence of symptomatic instability

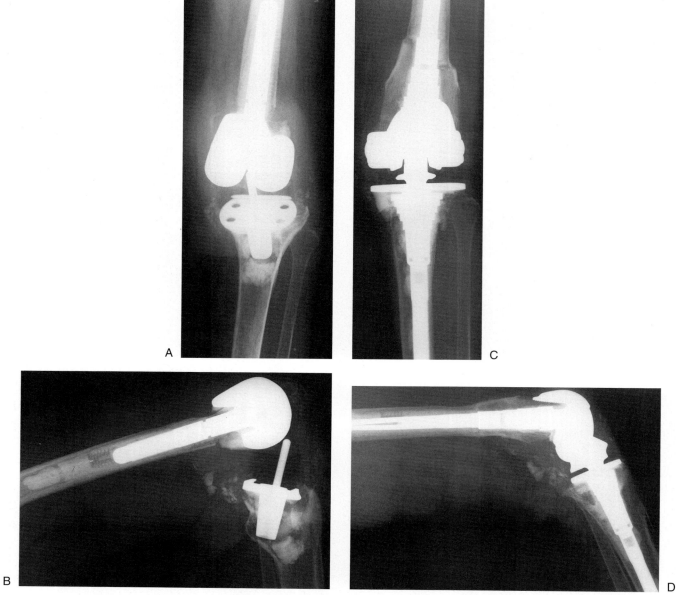

FIG. 10. Anteroposterior **(A)** and lateral **(B)** radiographs demonstrate catastrophic failure of a posterior cruciate ligament–substituting implant due to subsidence. Hardware displacement resulted in global instability. **C, D:** Revision to a rotating hinged implant restored clinical stability. A distal femoral allograft and a femoral head allograft to the central tibia were used to restore bone stock and reestablish the joint line.

was reduced to 20%. Rosenberg et al. reported on 36 revisions using the Total Condylar III (Johnson & Johnson, Raynham, MA) VVC implant. They achieved stability in two knees that were revised for symptomatic instability (30). Rand reported 4-year results for 21 knees, nine of which underwent revision, at least in part, for instability (31). Of the knees revised for instability, none achieved an excellent postoperative Hospital for Special Surgery knee score and only one achieved a good score. Hartford et al. (32) reported 5-year results for 16 Zimmer constrained condylar knee–type VVC revision implants; eight revisions were done for reasons other than infection. The stated success rate for his overall series was 80%, but the pre-

operative incidence of instability and postoperative success in resolving instability were not reported.

In our experience, VVC implants cannot fully substitute for absent collateral ligaments in active patients. We revised five knees with medial instability and three knees with lateral instability to a VVC component; only one in each group achieved long-term stability (Fig. 8). A linked hinged implant may be an acceptable option, but a high complication rate and poor long-term survival limit its applicability. Whether by advancement or allograft reconstruction, every attempt to restore ligamentous stability should be undertaken when using a VVC implant (Fig. 7).

Global Instability

Global instability occurs in both flexion and extension and is a combination of anteroposterior and varus or valgus laxity. A deficiency in quadriceps function, such as motor dysfunction or extensor mechanism disruption, often contributes to this mode of instability. Marked polyethylene wear (Figs. 9A and B) or implant migration can produce gross ligamentous and capsular laxity (Figs. 10A and B). Clinical conditions that involve dysfunction or disruption of multiple ligaments, such as rheumatoid arthritis or collagen vascular disorders, can result in global laxity. The use of implant designs with minimal congruity (i.e., components with relatively flat polyethylene bearing surfaces) compound global instability.

Clinical Presentation

As in flexion space and varus or valgus instability, the patient may present with an effusion, along with symptoms of instability and pain. In global instability, the observed laxity is more pronounced, and frequently the knee demonstrates recurvatum. A quadriceps lag may occur primarily, as a result of extensor mechanism dysfunction, or secondarily, as a result of component migration with a decrease in resting muscle tension.

Treatment

Management options include insertion of a thicker insert in an attempt to restore ligamentous and capsular tension, revision to a more constrained component (posterior stabilized, VVC, or linked implant), or knee fusion (Table 2). We reviewed the records of the 12 patients treated at our institution for global instability. Stability was achieved in neither of two patients managed with insertion of a thicker tibial insert, in two of three undergoing revision to a posterior stabilized implant (Figs. 9C and D), in three of three undergoing revision to a VVC implant, and in one of one undergoing revision to a linked implant (Figs. 10C and D). In the two remaining patients, one knee was fused successfully, and one knee that was managed with a brace experienced treatment failure. Overall, revision surgery using constrained or linked implants was successful in the short term for management of global instability. In the revision procedure, it is essential to reconstruct the extensor mechanism and to eliminate recurvatum by reestablishing the joint line and re-creating posterior soft tissue tension. If these elements cannot be restored, fusion is the most predictable and functional procedure.

CONCLUSION

The evaluation and treatment of knee instability after TKA is challenging. To have any hope of long-term success, the surgical intervention must address the cause of the instability. Increasing component constraint with revision surgery also increases stress transmission to the prosthesis-host interface. Therefore, the surgeon should select the least constrained implant that adequately addresses the pattern of instability. Intervention must be individualized; stability considerations must be integrated into an overall knee construct that optimizes alignment, restores bone stock, and provides secure attachment of the prosthesis to bone.

REFERENCES

1. Friedman RJ, Hirst P, Poss R, et al. Results of revision total knee arthroplasty performed for aseptic loosening, *Clin Orthop* 1990;255:235–241.
2. Goldberg VM, Figgie MP, Figgie HE, et al. The results of revision total knee arthroplasty. *Clin Orthop* 1988;226:86–92.
3. Knutson K, Lindstrand A, Lidgren L. Survival of knee arthroplasties: a nation-wide multicentre investigation of 8000 cases. *J Bone Joint Surg Br* 1986;68:795–803.
4. Peters CL, Hennessey R, Barden RM, et al. Revision total knee arthroplasty with a cemented posterior-stabilized or constrained condylar prosthesis: a minimum three-year and average five-year follow-up study. *J Arthroplasty* 1997;8:896–903.
5. Moreland JR. Mechanisms of failure in total knee arthroplasty. *Clin Orthop* 1988;226:49–64.
6. Brick GW, Scott RD. The patellofemoral component of total knee arthroplasty. *Clin Orthop* 1988;231:163–178.
7. Conlan T, Garth WP, Lemons JE. Evaluation of the medial soft-tissue restraints of the extensor mechanism of the knee. *J Bone Joint Surg Am* 1993;75:682–693.
8. Briard J-L, Hungerford DS. Patellofemoral instability in total knee arthroplasty. *J Arthroplasty* 1989;4(Suppl):S87–S97.
9. Merkow RL, Soudry M, Insall JN. Patellar dislocation following total knee replacement. *J Bone Joint Surg Am* 1985;67:1321–1327.
10. Rand JA. The patellofemoral joint in total knee arthroplasty. *J Bone Joint Surg Am* 1994;76:612–620.
11. Mochizuki RM, Schurman DJ. Patellar complications following total knee arthroplasty. *J Bone Joint Surg Am* 1979;61:879–883.
12. Inoue M, Shino K, Hirose H, et al. Subluxation of the patella: computed tomography analysis of patello-femoral congruence. *J Bone Joint Surg Am* 1988;70:1331–1337.
13. Berger RA, Crossett LS, Jacobs JJ, et al. Malrotation causing patellofemoral complication after total knee arthroplasty. *Clin Orthop* 1998;356:155–163.
14. Akagi M, Matsusue Y, Mata T, et al. Effect of rotational alignment on patellar tracking in total knee arthroplasty. *Clin Orthop* 1999;366:155–163.
15. Jazrawi LM, Birdzell L, Kummer FJ, et al. The accuracy of computed tomography for determining femoral and tibial total knee arthroplasty component rotation. *J Arthroplasty* 2000;15:761–766.
16. Grace JN, Rand JA. Patellar instability after total knee arthroplasty. *Clin Orthop* 1988;237:184–189.
17. Reference deleted in text.
18. Wolff AM, Hungerford DS, Krackow KA, et al. Osteotomy of the tibial tubercle during total knee replacement: a report of twenty-six cases. *J Bone Joint Surg Am* 1989;71:848–852.
19. Warren PJ, Olanlokun TK, Cobb AG, et al. Laxity and function in knee replacements: a comparative study of three prosthetic designs. *Clin Orthop* 1994;305:200–208.
20. Waslewski GL, Marson BM, Benjamin JB. Early, incapacitating instability of posterior cruciate ligament–retaining total knee arthroplasty. *J Arthroplasty* 1998;13:763–767.
21. Pagnano MW, Hanssen AD, Lewallen DG. Flexion instability after primary posterior cruciate retaining total knee arthroplasty. *Clin Orthop* 1998;356:38–46.
22. Fehring TK, Valadie AL. Knee instability after total knee arthroplasty. *Clin Orthop* 1994;299:157–162.
23. Insall JN, Easley ME. Surgical techniques and instrumentation in total knee arthroplasty. In: Insall JN, Scott WN, eds. *Surgery of the knee.* New York: Churchill Livingstone, 2001:1553–1620.
24. Gebhard JS, Kilgus DJ. Dislocation of a posterior stabilized total knee prosthesis: a report of two cases. *Clin Orthop* 1990;254:225–229.
25. Lombardi AV, Mallory TH, Vaughn BK, et al. Dislocation following primary posterior-stabilized total knee arthroplasty. *J Arthroplasty* 1993;8:633–639.
26. Sharkey PF, Hozack WJ, Booth RE, et al. Posterior dislocation of total knee arthroplasty. *Clin Orthop* 1992;278:128–133.

27. Leopold SS, McStay C, Klafeta K, et al. Primary repair of intraoperative disruption of the medial collateral ligament during total knee arthroplasty. *J Bone Joint Surg Am* 2001;83:86–91.

28. Krackow KA, Jones MM, Teeny SM, et al. Primary total knee arthroplasty in patients with fixed valgus deformity. *Clin Orthop* 1991;273:9–18.

29. Healy WL, Iorio R, Lemos DW. Medial reconstruction during total knee arthroplasty for severe valgus deformity. *Clin Orthop* 1998;356:161–169.

30. Rosenberg AG, Verner JJ, Galante JO. Clinical results of total knee revision using the Total Condylar III prosthesis. *Clin Orthop* 1991;273:83–90.

31. Rand JA. Revision total knee arthroplasty using the Total Condylar III prosthesis. *J Arthroplasty* 1991;6:279–284.

32. Hartford JM, Goodman SB, Schurman DJ. Complex primary and revision total knee arthroplasty using the condylar constrained prosthesis: an average five-year follow-up. *J Arthroplasty* 1991;6:341–350.

CHAPTER 101

Miscellaneous Complications

William W. Colman and Michael D. Ries

Complications that may occur during the early postoperative period after total knee arthroplasty include deep venous thrombosis (DVT), pulmonary embolism, fat embolism, nerve palsy, vascular injury, skin necrosis, infection, stiffness, and reflex sympathetic dystrophy (RSD). Some patients may be at increased risk for developing these complications and should be counseled about the potential risks before surgery if possible. Early recognition and treatment of the complications can improve the outcome of the joint replacement.

THROMBOEMBOLIC DISEASE

Thromboembolic disease (TED) is common after total knee arthroplasty. The prevalence of venographically proven DVT is as high as 45% in patients receiving prophylaxis and as high as 80% in untreated patients (1). DVT itself can cause significant morbidity by producing calf pain, swelling, or the postphlebitic syndrome, and can lead to pulmonary embolism. Intraoperative factors contributing to the formation of clot include vascular trauma, systemic initiation of the coagulation cascade, and local vascular stasis changes. Other factors that put the patient at increased risk for TED include both primary and secondary hypercoagulable states. Primary states include antithrombin III deficiency, protein C deficiency, protein S deficiency, and activated protein C resistance. Secondary states include nursing home confinement, major surgery, trauma, malignant neoplasm,

chemotherapy, neurologic disease with paresis, the presence of a central venous catheter or pacemaker, varicose veins, prolonged immobility, obesity, congestive heart failure, prior TED, nephrotic syndrome, inflammatory bowel disease, and estrogen use (2–5). To allow better determination of a patient's risk of developing DVT and appropriate prophylaxis, the American College of Chest Physicians (ACCP) in its most recent consensus statement on antithrombotic therapy agreed on a DVT rating system. A number and a letter are provided that signify the risk-benefit assessment of the regimen and the quality of the studies supporting the regimen, respectively. A grade of "1A" indicates the highest recommendation (6).

Tourniquet Use

The use of a tourniquet has been suggested as a possible means for the promotion of clot formation because of increased venous stasis and venous hypoxia (7,8). Other studies have challenged this concept by demonstrating that total knee replacement (TKR) surgery results in activation of coagulation reflected by increased thrombin production (9). Tourniquet use is associated with increased fibrinolysis, a finding that has been corroborated by several studies (10–13). Randomized prospective studies, however, have not identified a difference between groups undergoing surgery with and without tourniquet use (14,15). In one prospective study, higher rates of DVT were

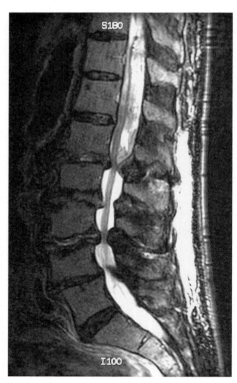

FIG. 1. Epidural hematoma. Sagittal magnetic resonance image of a patient who received low-molecular-weight heparin within 12 hours after epidural anesthesia for a joint replacement procedure.

observed with the use of a tourniquet (16). For patients who are at high risk for DVT, it may be beneficial to limit the use of a tourniquet when possible and inflate it only during cementing of the components.

Prevention

Chemical Prophylaxis

Warfarin Sodium

Warfarin sodium is a commonly used form of anticoagulation therapy after knee replacement. It is an oral anticoagulant that affects the production of vitamin K–dependent coagulation factors and therefore inhibits the initiation of the coagulation cascade. Warfarin impedes the propagation of an existing clot but does not decrease the rate of DVT (17). It is dosed to prolong the international normalized ratio to up to twice normal, but the exact figure varies with different investigators. This method of prophylaxis requires more frequent international normalized ratio monitoring than other methods. Bleeding complications may result if drug effects are not closely monitored.

Low-Molecular-Weight Heparins

Low-molecular-weight heparins (LMWHs) are fractionated forms of heparin with consequently lower molecular weights

than heparin, in the range of 4,000 to 6,000 d. Currently, four LMWHs (dalteparin sodium, enoxaparin sodium, nadropin calcium, and tinzaparin sodium) are available in the United States, and there are no data supporting the use of one particular drug over the others (18). Enoxaparin is the only LMWH that is approved by the U.S. Food and Drug Administration for DVT prophylaxis after TKR surgery. LMWH has been studied extensively and is an effective prophylaxis after TKR surgery (19–27). Enoxaparin prophylaxis does not require laboratory monitoring, and the drug is administered as a subcutaneous injection. The initial postoperative prophylactic dose should be delayed until hemostasis is assured. Current recommended dosing is 30 mg twice daily starting 12 to 24 hours postoperatively (18). Bleeding complications associated with enoxaparin have been a concern and can occur at any site during therapy with enoxaparin (28,29). An unexplained fall in the hematocrit or blood pressure should lead to a search for a bleeding site. Neuraxial hematomas have been reported when LMWH is used in combination with spinal or epidural anesthesia. Symptoms of hematoma include lower extremity neurologic deficit and low back pain, with surgical intervention being the mainstay of treatment. Negative sequelae have included permanent paralysis. LMWH should be used with caution in combination with an indwelling epidural catheter or after multiple epidural punctures (30,31) (Fig. 1). The ACCP 2001 consensus conference gave LMWH a designation of 1A (18).

Mechanical Prophylaxis

Intermittent pneumatic compression devices function by decreasing stasis by periodically raising venous pressure in the lower extremity. They have been found to be an effective means of DVT prophylaxis either in the form of continuous passive motion (CPM) (32,33), sequential compression boots, or intermittent compression stockings (34–37). These devices include compression leggings, boots, and stockings with inflatable bladders. Ideally, they should be worn preoperatively and until the patient is fully ambulatory. They have been shown to reduce the rate of DVT after TKR, but their effectiveness may be limited by nonuse during physical therapy, patient intolerance, and the inability to continue prophylaxis after hospital discharge (34,35,38–40). Intermittent pneumatic compression devices may provide additional benefit as an adjunct to chemical prophylaxis regimens (41).

Choice of Anticoagulant

Low-dose heparin sodium (24) or aspirin prophylaxis (25) is relatively ineffective compared with other prophylactic regimens. Several studies comparing warfarin with LMWH (20–23,26) using discharge venography to diagnose DVT suggest that warfarin is less effective than LMWH after total knee arthroplasty. However, postoperative DVT rates in these studies range from 38% to 55% and almost all were asymptomatic. Because studies examining the role of warfarin therapy in symptomatic DVT (42) have identified very low rates of symptomatic DVT (0.8%), it is safe to conclude that the vast majority of asymptomatic DVT detected by venography does not become symptomatic and that adjusted-dose warfarin therapy is safe and effective as DVT prophylaxis after TKR surgery (21,41). However, the venographically determined prevalence of DVT among TKR patients receiving LMWH prophylaxis remains substantial at 25% to 45%. In a recent cohort study of TKR patients (n = 842) receiving LMWH prophylaxis for a mean duration of 9 days, the overall 84-day incidence of symptomatic TED and fatal pulmonary embolism was only 3.9% and 0.4%, respectively (43). Bleeding complications (20) and a significant increase in blood loss and transfusion requirements (21,23,27) among patients receiving LMWH prophylaxis as compared with adjusted-dose warfarin are a drawback to the use of LMWHs. Prospective randomized studies comparing LMWH with warfarin for DVT prophylaxis after TKR taking symptomatic, objectively documented TED as the primary end point still need to be performed. The 2001 ACCP consensus conference recommends warfarin or LMWH for TED prophylaxis after total knee arthroplasty. Mechanical prophylaxis remains an alternate choice (18). For patients with additional risk factors, a combined regimen of intermittent pneumatic compression and either warfarin or LMWH should be considered. The ACCP conference gave adjusted-dose warfarin and LMWH a 1A rating. It rated intermittent pneumatic compression prophylaxis as an alternative option and gave it a 1B rating because of the comparatively few trials and small sample sizes (18).

Duration of Treatment

As inpatient length of stay decreases the necessity for postdischarge DVT prophylaxis has increased. Studies examining the rates of DVT in total hip arthroplasty patients have found high rates of DVT for up to 2 months after discharge (44–47). Recent studies have found that the incidence of asymptomatic DVT after hospital discharge was substantial and was significantly reduced by LMWH prophylaxis (48–50). The current recommended duration of DVT prophylaxis is controversial, and the recommendation of the current ACCP consensus conference is 7 to 10 days (18).

Diagnosis

Deep Venous Thrombosis

The diagnosis of DVT by physical examination is in general unreliable. The gold standard for the detection of DVT in the thigh or calf is the contrast venogram. It loses accuracy above the inguinal ligament where significant thrombi may originate (51). However, the test is invasive, expensive, and painful, and can precipitate an anaphylactoid reaction. Ultrasonography is safe, carries low morbidity, and is fairly accurate for diagnosing proximal DVT. Like venography it does not detect clots proximal to the inguinal ligament and also is poor at detecting partial clots and fresh clots. The incompressibility by ultrasonography of the vein in question is the best criteria for diagnosing DVT, and in low-risk patients a negative compression ultrasonographic finding can reliably rule out a thrombus in the thigh (51). This method is technician dependent, however, and has a steep learning curve. The addition of Doppler studies to ultrasonography may increase the diagnostic accuracy compared with ultrasonography alone. Ultrasonographic screening after

total joint arthroplasty remains controversial. A recent randomized study found no benefit to ultrasonographic screening in patients treated with warfarin prophylaxis after total knee or total hip arthroplasty (42). As many as 50% of thrombi originate in the pelvic region where contrast venography and ultrasonography are less accurate. Magnetic resonance venography may be the best choice for diagnosing thrombus in this region, but cost and experience have limited its use thus far (52).

Pulmonary Embolism

The diagnosis of pulmonary embolism by physical examination alone is also unreliable, but most patients with pulmonary embolism have at least one of the following symptoms: sudden dyspnea, tachypnea, and chest pain (53). Measurement of arterial blood gases often shows a reduced PaO_2 and $PaCO_2$ due to hyperventilation, but these changes are nonspecific. Chest radiograph and electrocardiogram changes may occur but are also nonspecific. Ventilation-perfusion ($\dot{V}/\dot{Q}$) scanning is a noninvasive test that has a relatively high sensitivity but low specificity, so that a normal $\dot{V}/\dot{Q}$ scan essentially excludes the diagnosis of a clinically relevant pulmonary embolism. $\dot{V}/\dot{Q}$ scan results can be categorized as either high-probability, intermediate-probability, low-probability, or normal. If the results of the scan are in the high-probability category, the positive predictive value is higher than 85%. Most patients with clinically suspected pulmonary embolism, however, have either low- or intermediate-probability scan results. In this subset of patients the prevalence of pulmonary embolism is approximately 25%, and thus the positive predictive value is lower (53). Computed tomography is increasingly being used in the clinical setting because it is faster, less complex, and less operator-dependent than other evaluation methods. There is better interobserver agreement in the interpretation of computed tomographic scans than in the interpretation of scintigraphic scans, and in addition alternative diagnoses, for example, pulmonary masses, pneumonia, or pleural effusion, can be considered. Additional research is required before computed tomography is used routinely in clinical practice. Pulmonary angiography is still considered the gold standard, with both high sensitivity and specificity. It has limited availability, however, and a small (less than 0.3%) but definite risk of mortality. It should be considered when results of other tests are inconclusive and cardiovascular collapse or hypotension is present (53).

Treatment

The treatment of proximal DVT and pulmonary embolism must be weighed against the possible drawbacks of the treatment being considered. Morbidity resulting from untreated DVT includes postphlebitic syndrome, pulmonary hypertension, proximal propagation of the clot, and possible pulmonary embolus (17,54). Treatment options include pharmacologic anticoagulation and vena caval filters. The pharmacologic options include unfractionated heparin, LMWHs, and warfarin. Until recently, administration of unfractionated heparin followed by long-term warfarin therapy was the mainstay of treatment. LMWHs have been found to be as safe and efficacious as unfractionated heparin and warfarin with a more predictable dose-response relationship and fixed administration dosage (55–59). These properties make treatment of patients in an outpatient setting feasible (60,61). The decision to treat must be weighed against the possible deleterious consequences in the setting of increased bleeding or risk of bleeding. In addition to the aforementioned pharmacologic treatment, supportive medical therapy may be required. The treatment of DVT of the calf after TKR is controversial. Evidence exists that calf thrombi do propagate proximally, so that some investigators recommend treatment with low-dose warfarin (17,54). If no anticoagulation therapy is instituted, then follow-up ultrasonography is highly recommended.

Pulmonary Embolism

Although all the aforementioned methods for detecting thrombus in the deep veins do not establish the diagnosis of pulmonary embolism, the confirmation of DVT is of major importance in management decisions. The logic of leg vein imaging is that many patients with pulmonary embolism have residual proximal clot even in the absence of clinical evidence of DVT, itself an indication for treatment even if there is no direct proof of pulmonary embolism. If there is no thrombosis in the proximal leg or pelvic veins, the chance of a further significant pulmonary embolism is low; therefore, even if a small pulmonary embolism has occurred already, anticoagulation therapy can be omitted. This approach requires caution if the patient has inadequate cardiorespiratory reserve or is likely to remain immobile, or if there could be an embolic source elsewhere (e.g., the right atrium or vena cava) (53).

Future Directions

With respect to DVT prophylaxis, several new treatments have promise both in increasing efficacy and in reducing bleeding complications. Antithrombotics pose a risk of bleeding and other side effects, including heparin-induced thrombocytopenia. Indirect and direct thrombin inhibitors both promise decreased side effects. New indirect thrombin inhibitors include pentasaccharides and the heparinoid danaparoid sodium. These agents may offer reduced risk of bleeding while maintaining efficacy compared with current regimens and may prove valuable in the management of heparin-induced thrombocytopenia. Direct thrombin inhibitors may offer even greater antithrombotic effects because direct thrombin inhibitors inhibit both free and clot-bound thrombin (62).

FAT EMBOLISM

Embolization of marrow elements and thrombus during total knee arthroplasty can cause hypotension, hypoxia, cardiac arrest, and, occasionally, sudden death (63–74). Clinical manifestations of these acute embolic events have been reported in association with the use of intramedullary alignment rods during resurfacing total knee arthroplasty and when long-stemmed components are cemented (75–84).

Although embolization of marrow elements, including fat, appears to occur commonly during total knee arthroplasty, fat embolism syndrome is rarely observed. Fat embolism syndrome develops more often after long bone fracture, 24 to 72 hours

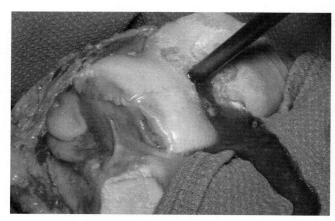

FIG. 2. Overdrilling of the intramedullary rod entry hole decompresses the distal femur when the rod is inserted and allows marrow elements to exit into the knee wound.

after embolization of marrow elements. Patients with fat embolism syndrome usually present with respiratory distress, tachycardia, petechiae, and mental status changes (85,86).

Fahmy et al. (87) observed a decrease in oxygen saturation, arterial oxygen tension, and end-tidal carbon dioxide tension after an 8-mm-diameter intramedullary alignment rod was inserted into the femur. The cardiopulmonary changes were completely eliminated after the entry hole for rod insertion was overdrilled to 12.7-mm diameter. Marrow element embolization is associated with an increase in intramedullary pressure when the rod is inserted. Overdrilling the entry hole for the rod helps decompress the intramedullary canal and permits marrow elements to exit into the knee wound (Fig. 2) (87–90). Although overdrilling the rod entry hole decreases pressures in the distal femur, however, pressures at the tip of the rod when it is inserted past the femoral isthmus may still be high (Fig. 3). Proximal intramedullary pressures with use of a 10-mm-diameter round rod can exceed 1,000 torr even when the entry hole is overdrilled to a 12.7-mm diameter (91). The intramedullary pressure is significantly reduced with the use of a fluted rather than a round rod (91). Flutes may allow marrow elements to travel along the rod and exit into the knee wound. Techniques to evacuate marrow elements from the intramedullary canal before rod insertion, including suction and irrigation as well as slow rod insertion, may further decrease the amount of embolic material.

The embolic load and risk of fat embolism would be expected to be increased when intramedullary alignment is used for both the femur and tibia and with bilateral compared to unilateral total knee arthroplasty. Dorr et al. (92) reported clinical fat embolism syndrome, including one death, in 8 of 65 patients who underwent bilateral simultaneous TKR when both femoral and tibial intramedullary alignment were used. Ritter et al. (93) observed a significantly higher 30-day mortality rate for a large population of Medicare patients who underwent simultaneous bilateral TKR than for those undergoing sequential staged replacements. Lane et al. (94) reported a three times greater incidence of cardiopulmonary complications and four times greater incidence of postoperative confusion in patients with simultaneous bilateral procedures than in those with unilateral TKR. Other authors, however, have reported no higher morbidity or mortality for patients having

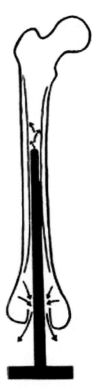

FIG. 3. Overdrilling of the intramedullary rod entry hole may decompress the distal femur, but when the rod is inserted past the isthmus, proximal pressures may still be high.

simultaneous bilateral total knee arthroplasty than for those having unilateral procedures provided that a fluted femoral alignment rod is used, the femoral rod entry hole is overdrilled, and extramedullary tibial alignment is used (95,96). Even with these techniques to reduce embolism of marrow contents, there is still a trend toward greater pulmonary shunting in simultaneous bilateral than in unilateral TKR (91). Embolization of some marrow elements may be well tolerated by most patients who do not have significant underlying medical disorders. Lynch et al. (97) found a higher incidence of postoperative cardiovascular and neurologic complications in patients older than age 80 years who underwent simultaneous bilateral knee replacement than in those undergoing unilateral replacement. Simultaneous bilateral TKR is also associated with a longer operative time and greater blood loss than unilateral TKR (95–97). For elderly patients or those with significant cardiopulmonary disease, staged unilateral TKRs may be more appropriate than simultaneous bilateral TKR.

The specific composition of the embolized material is also not clear. It may represent marrow fat, air, blood, bone, or polymethylmethacrylate (98–105). Several studies using transesophageal echocardiography during total knee arthroplasty have demonstrated showers of echogenic emboli in the central venous circulation, particularly after tourniquet deflation (99,106,107). Berman et al. (99) identified fresh venous thrombus in blood aspirated from pulmonary artery catheters in five of ten patients who underwent total knee arthroplasty with transesophageal echocardiac monitoring. Markel et al. (108) performed histologic analyses of the lungs of dogs after total knee arthroplasty. Sustained transesophageal echogenic showers were also observed. The

authors found emboli consisting of fat cells and hematopoietic marrow elements interspersed with free fat globules, which obstructed the pulmonary vasculature. Morawa et al. (107) observed transesophageal echocardiac showers in patients who underwent total knee arthroplasty with use of a fluted femoral intramedullary alignment rod, overdrilling of the rod entry hole, and extramedullary tibial alignment. The authors found a dramatic decrease in transesophageal echocardiac showers when extramedullary femoral alignment was used; this suggests that the echogenic material originated from the intramedullary canal, which is consistent with marrow element embolization.

Use of extramedullary rather than intramedullary femoral alignment would be expected to further minimize the risk of acute embolic events during total knee arthroplasty. Conventional methods to identify the femoral head and properly orient the femoral bone cuts in extramedullary femoral alignment are relatively imprecise, however, and better alignment is achieved with intramedullary alignment (109). Recent developments in computer-assisted techniques and image-guided surgery may permit accurate alignment without use of intramedullary alignment rods (78). However, outcome studies that include examination of the effects on length of surgery and complications, and cost-benefit analyses will be required to fully assess the safety and efficacy of this technology.

Acute cardiopulmonary collapse can also occur when cemented long-stemmed components are used during total knee arthroplasty (79,81). In total hip arthroplasty, intraoperative and postoperative pulmonary shunt is greater when a cemented femoral stem is inserted than when an uncemented stem is used (110). Sudden death has occurred after cementing of the components in place (111,112). Circulating methacrylate monomer has been implicated as a possible cause because the monomer has a direct myocardial depressant effect (113–115). The measured serum levels of methacrylate monomer are not high enough to cause the physiologic changes, however (116). A more likely mechanism is increased intramedullary pressure during cementing of the stem, which causes embolization of marrow contents. The cardiopulmonary changes can be minimized by thorough irrigation of the intramedullary canal to remove blood and marrow elements before the stem is cemented (117).

INFECTION

Infection after TKR can be classified by chronology into early and late, and by anatomic location into superficial and deep. This section covers early infections, including both superficial and deep infections. Early infections generally occur less than 4 weeks after the index procedure and are thought to result from contamination during the procedure. Superficial infections usually involve only the skin and subcutaneous tissues, whereas deep infections invade the joint space and involve the total knee components. Superficial infection poses a theoretical risk to the implants through inward tracking to cause a deep infection, but this is difficult to predict in practice.

One study of primary hip and knee arthroplasty found a superficial infection rate of 10.5% for knees and 14.3% for hips. No correlation with late infection or ultimate outcome was found in these patients (118). Of 4,171 total knee arthroplasties that were performed, Wilson (119) found 67 that were followed by deep infection. Of these, eight (0.2%) occurred within 3 months. Acute infection may be more common in patients with diabetes. Papagelopoulos found 2.5% early infections (120), and others have found rates of 12% with either limited wound drainage or mild skin necrosis during the perioperative period in diabetic patients (121,122).

Perioperative antibiotic prophylaxis has been found to reduce the incidence of acute infection in total joint surgery (123–131). Although there are no absolute recommendations for the choice and duration of antibiotics, the most common prophylactic regimen consists of a first-generation cephalosporin given for 24 to 48 hours after surgery. The first dose is administered before tourniquet inflation. The unfavorable effects of antibiotic prophylaxis, such as the expense, drug-related side effects, and possible emergence of drug-resistant bacteria can be limited by restricting the duration of antibiotic use (132).

Postoperative urinary tract infection has been shown to correlate with deep sepsis after total joint replacement (133–135). Postoperative lower urinary tract infections and urinary retention can be prevented by the use of a Foley catheter inserted preoperatively under sterile conditions and removed at 24 to 48 hours (136,137). This protocol is better in preventing distention than are intermittent catheterization protocols (138).

Preoperative urine analysis can potentially alert the surgeon to the possibility of lower urinary tract infection. In cases of asymptomatic bacteriuria, the literature supports proceeding with total joint replacement (139). Routine perioperative antibiotics should be used in this setting. If the urine culture results are subsequently positive, treatment should commence with administration of organism-specific antibiotics for 10 days. The literature neither supports nor proscribes proceeding with total joint replacement in the setting of symptomatic bacteruria (139).

Emergence of Resistant Strains

The use of vancomycin hydrochloride to treat infections of methicillin-resistant *Staphylococcus aureus* has contributed to the increase in the number of vancomycin-resistant *Enterococcus* species. One study documented two cases of early postoperative infection with vancomycin-resistant *Enterococcus* that ultimately required fusion in one patient and resection arthroplasty in the other (140). Judicious use of perioperative antibiotics may help to decrease but not prevent emergence of resistant strains.

Clinical Presentation

The patient with an acute infection usually presents with at least one of the following symptoms: pain, swelling, stiffness, persistent drainage, and wound breakdown. Range of motion may be painful above and beyond the level expected in the normal postoperative course.

Laboratory Evaluation

Radiography, determination of erythrocyte sedimentation rate, and measurement of C-reactive protein levels are usually not helpful in the early postoperative period. Aspiration for Gram staining and culture may be helpful, but the cell count is unreliable in the early postoperative period.

Diagnosis

Diagnosis is usually made clinically, and a high index of suspicion is important in these patients. Persistent worsening wound drainage may indicate early postoperative infection. It may not be apparent if the infection is superficial or deep until the decision is made to explore the knee for an irrigation and débridement procedure.

Treatment

Surgical Débridement

If the diagnosis of superficial infection can be made with a high degree of certainty, then a course of intravenous antibiotics followed by oral antibiotics may be warranted. Because the agents of these infections are usually intraoperative contaminants, anti-*Staphylococcus* antibiotics are appropriate. If a deep infection is suspected and the prosthesis is well fixed, provided it is within 2 to 4 weeks of the index procedure, then débridement with polyethylene insert exchange is appropriate (119,141–145). Key elements of a successful procedure include complete synovectomy, polyethylene insert exchange, and adequate irrigation with copious amounts of sterile saline. Arthroscopic management precludes polyethylene exchange and has been found to be less effective than open débridement; it is not recommended unless the patient has an abnormal coagulation profile or is medically unfit for an open procedure (146). Postoperative drains should be used, and organism-specific antibiotics should be administered for a minimum of 6 weeks.

The results of débridement are difficult to assess because of the variability in time to treatment, the number of débridements performed, antibiotic management, species of bacteria, implant choice and fixation, and criteria for success in reported studies. Success rate reported in the literature has ranged from 25% to 100% for débridement carried out before 4 weeks (147).

Other Procedures

If surgical débridement fails, then other procedures for treating late infection such as one- or two-stage revision, fusion, resection arthroplasty, or, in rare circumstances, amputation may be indicated. These procedures are covered elsewhere in the text.

SKIN AND WOUND COMPLICATIONS

Skin necrosis after total knee arthroplasty can rapidly lead to infection of the prosthetic components. Risk factors for the development of skin necrosis include rheumatoid arthritis, steroid use, immunosuppression, malnutrition, peripheral vascular disease, and the presence of multiple prior scars. Lengthy tourniquet times, particularly in patients with other risk factors for developing wound complications, may also be a contributing factor (16).

The preoperative nutritional status can influence the risk of wound complications. Greene et al. found that total joint arthroplasty patients with a preoperative lymphocyte count of less than 1,500 cells per mm^3 had a five times greater frequency of

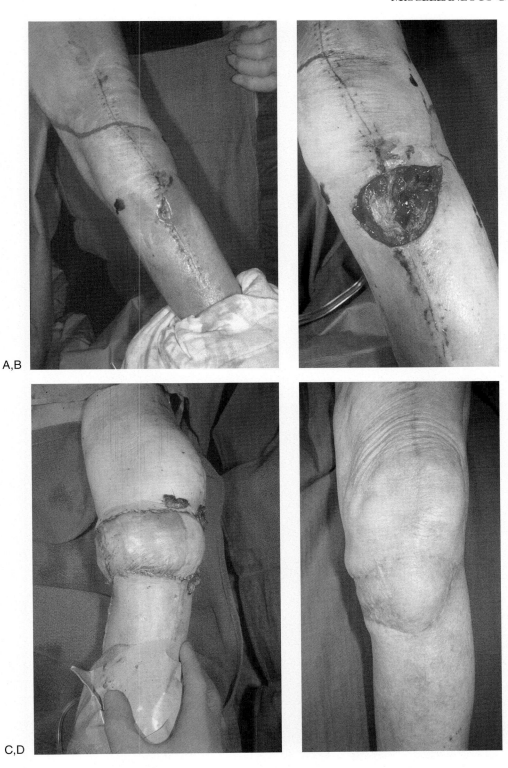

FIG. 4. A: Skin necrosis directly over tibial tubercle in a 72-year-old woman after revision total knee replacement. **B:** Nonviable skin over tibial tubercle débrided. **C:** Medial gastrocnemius flap coverage and skin grafting. **D:** One year after surgery, knee range of motion is 0 to 90 degrees, and the wound is well healed.

developing major wound complications and patients with an albumin level of less than 3.5 g per dL had a seven times greater frequency (148).

Vascularity of the skin over the knee affects the rate of healing postoperatively and the risk of necrosis. Johnson measured transcutaneous skin oxygen tension and found that the oxygen tension decreases for the first 2 to 3 days after surgery and then increases (149). In addition, the lateral skin edge is more hypoxic than the medial edge (149). This suggests that, when multiple prior scars are present, the most vertical lateral incision should be used to minimize skin hypoxia.

Skin tension can also affect the vascularity. The medial parapatellar incision is relatively parallel to the skin cleavage lines compared to the vertical midline incision and is associated with

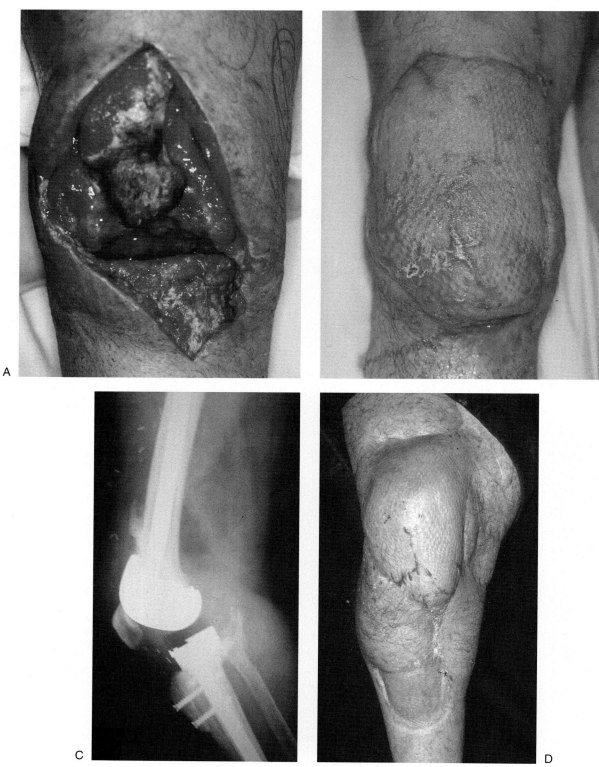

FIG. 5. A: Extensive necrosis of the skin and extensor mechanism developed after primary total knee replacement in a 63-year-old man with diabetes and previous surgical scars. The prosthetic components have been removed, and the patellar tendon is not present. The patella was necrotic and was later débrided. **B:** The patient refused amputation, and after placement of an antibiotic-impregnated cement spacer, the knee wound was covered with a free latissimus muscle flap. Serous drainage developed from the inferior edge of the wound, requiring further débridement and medial gastrocnemius muscle flap coverage. **C:** The extensor mechanism was reconstructed with a patellar tendon allograft. **D:** One year after revision total knee arthroplasty, the wound is well healed.

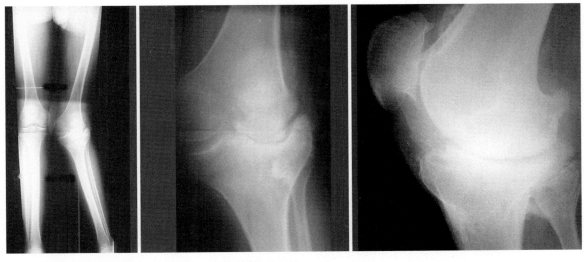

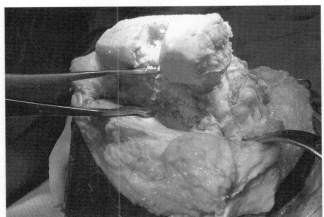

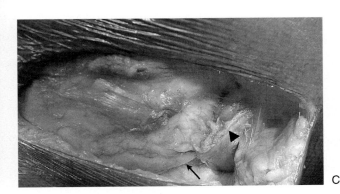

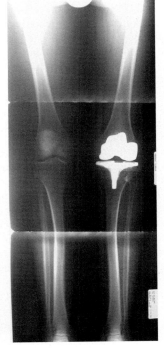

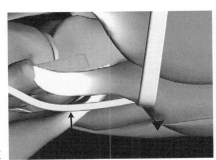

FIG. 6. A: Radiograph of a 45-year-old man with posttraumatic arthritis, 40 degrees of fixed varus, and 35 degrees of fixed flexion contracture. **B:** Release of the fibular collateral ligament, posterolateral capsule, popliteus tendon, posterior cruciate ligament, and lateral gastrocnemius tendon was required to correct soft tissue contracture. **C:** The peroneal nerve (*arrow*) was exposed through a second posterolateral incision with an adequate skin bridge maintained between it and the anterior midline incision. The biceps tendon (*arrowhead*) was released and peroneal nerve tension monitored during correction of valgus and flexion deformity. **D:** Schematic of the peroneal nerve (*arrow*) shown in the same orientation as in the intraoperative photograph in **C**. Note that it appears from underneath the muscle belly of the biceps femoris muscle and then courses around the head of the fibula distally. **E:** One year after total knee arthroplasty, the patient is pain free and ambulates without support. Knee motion is 0 to 120 degrees. Peroneal nerve function is normal. The knee is stable in extension with moderate laxity to varus stress in flexion.

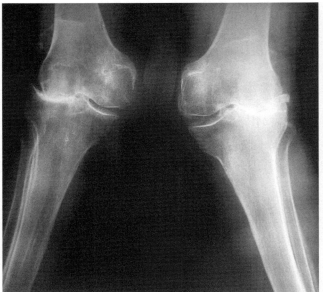
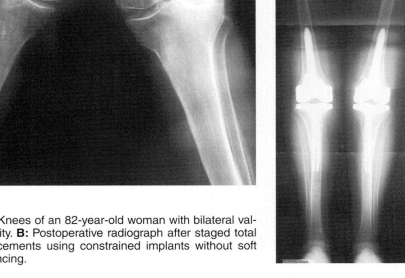

FIG. 7. A: Knees of an 82-year-old woman with bilateral valgus deformity. **B:** Postoperative radiograph after staged total knee replacements using constrained implants without soft tissue balancing.

less tension during flexion (150). However, the midline approach requires a smaller soft tissue flap to expose the lateral side of the knee. Constant passive motion further decreases skin oxygen tension (149). Yashar et al. reported that high-flexion constant passive motion of 70 to 100 degrees of flexion started in the recovery room was associated with increased knee motion during the hospitalization, but wound necrosis requiring medial gastrocnemius coverage occurred in 1 of 104 patients (151). Kim et al. observed skin necrosis in 13 of 27 patients who underwent total knee arthroplasty for bony ankylosis (152). Particularly for patients with multiple risk factors for developing wound complications, avoidance or delayed use of constant passive motion and early range-of-motion exercises may be beneficial in reducing the development of skin necrosis.

If skin necrosis does occur after total knee arthroplasty, early recognition of the problem and treatment minimizes the risk of deep infection of the prosthetic components. Necrosis of the proximal wound, including the area over the patella, may be treated by local wound care and skin grafting. Necrosis over the tibial tubercle or patellar tendon, however, requires muscle flap coverage to prevent infection involving the patellar tendon (Fig. 4). If the patellar tendon is not viable and the extensor mechanism is disrupted, the medial gastrocnemius flap can also be used to augment the extensor mechanism (153). The tendon of the gastrocnemius is repaired to the quadriceps tendon, with continuity maintained between the tibia and extensor mechanism.

If necrosis of both the proximal skin and extensor mechanism occurs, the gastrocnemius flap is usually not sufficient to achieve adequate coverage, and a free flap is necessary (Fig. 5). Both flaps may be needed, as well as reconstruction of the extensor mechanism, to restore some knee function. The limitations of such a salvage procedure may outweigh the potential benefits, however, and amputation should be considered as an appropriate option.

NERVE INJURY

Nerve injury after total knee arthroplasty is an uncommon complication. Asp and Rand reported 26 peroneal nerve palsies in 8,998 total knee arthroplasties (0.3%) (154). Nerve injury typically occurs from direct compression during retraction but may also result from limb lengthening (155). The peroneal nerve is peripheral to the operative field during TKR and would not be expected to be injured from retraction or direct trauma. However, the peroneal nerve is tethered at the fibular head, and particularly during correction of fixed valgus and flexion deformities, it may be lengthened. Peroneal nerve palsy rates of 3% to 4% have been reported for correction of valgus deformity (156–158) and rates of up to 8% after a correction of severe flexion contracture of more than 60 degrees (159).

Severe valgus and flexion deformities may be treated with extensive lateral and posterior soft tissue release using an unconstrained posterior stabilized implant (Fig. 6). The convex posterolateral size of the deformity is lengthened to balance medial soft tissue tension in both flexion and extension. The peroneal nerve can be visualized through a posterolateral skin incision to assess nerve tension during correction of the deformity. However, routine exposure of the peroneal nerve during correction of valgus deformity is unnecessary.

After correction of valgus deformity, the neurovascular status of the extremity should be carefully assessed. Nerve tension may be decreased during knee flexion. After routine splinting of the knee in flexion following valgus deformity correction, Miyasaka et al. reported transient nerve palsy in only 1 of 160 cases (0.6%) (160).

Valgus deformities may also be corrected by medial collateral ligament advancement. The ligament is advanced either distally (156) or proximally (161). This avoids lengthening the lateral

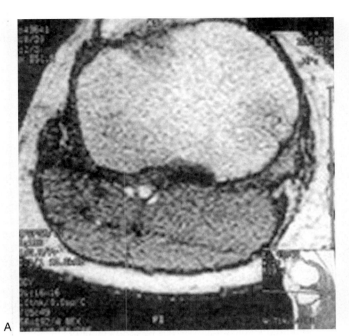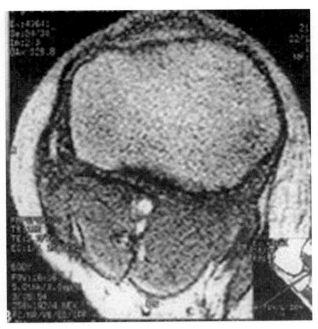

A   B

FIG. 8. Sections at the total knee replacement cross-sectional level. **A:** Magnetic resonance image obtained with the knee in full extension showing the proximity of the artery and accompanying veins to the joint in the extended position. **B:** Magnetic resonance image obtained with the knee at 90 degrees of flexion showing posterior movement of the artery and especially of the veins.

side of the knee but requires stable fixation of the ligament repair. Alternatively, severe valgus deformities can be treated with use of a fully constrained implant without soft tissue balancing. This may be most appropriate for elderly patients with limited activity demands (Fig. 7).

Idusuyi and Morrey reviewed 32 cases of peroneal nerve palsy after total knee arthroplasty and identified risk factors other than preoperative valgus deformity, including previous laminectomy, prior high tibial osteotomy, and use of epidural anesthesia (162). The authors suggested that use of epidural anesthesia for postoperative pain control can lead to decreased sensation postoperatively, and positioning the limb in an unprotected state may be a factor in the development of late nerve palsy. Horlocker et al. reviewed eight cases of peroneal nerve palsy and observed that the use of epidural anesthesia may cause a delay in diagnosis (163). In addition to valgus deformity of more than 10 degrees, preoperative neuropathy, tourniquet time longer than 120 minutes, and postoperative bleeding complications were associated with an increased risk of developing peroneal nerve palsy. Unwin and Thomas used a magnetic stimulator to monitor peroneal nerve function during total knee arthroplasty (164). Loss of signal from the nerve was observed 25 minutes after tourniquet inflation. Lengthy tourniquet times, particularly in patients with other risk factors for nerve palsy, may contribute to the development of this complication.

If peroneal palsy does develop and nerve recovery does not occur, surgical treatment may be beneficial. Mont et al. reported favorable results of nerve decompression in 31 patients with peroneal nerve palsy who had been managed nonoperatively for at least 2 months (165). Epineural fibrosis and bands of fibrous tissue constricting the nerve at the fibular head and proximal origin of the peroneus longus muscle were found intraoperatively.

VASCULAR COMPLICATIONS

Vascular injury at the time of surgery—in particular, popliteal vessel injury—is a serious complication that can result in acute ischemia, compartment syndrome, and amputation. The incidence of popliteal injury is likely underreported and has been shown to be as high as 5% in one study (166). Because the popliteal vessels are not tethered at the level of the joint line, knee flexion moves the vessels in a posterior direction and thus imparts some safety when total knee arthroplasty is performed with the knee in flexion (167,168). Despite this posterior movement, however, the popliteal artery is an average of 9 mm (range, 6 to 15 mm) posterior to the posterior aspect of the tibial plateau at 90 degrees of flexion (Fig. 8) (168). With knee flexion, the popliteal artery lies anterior to the popliteal vein and is therefore more likely to be injured by a saw blade or scalpel penetrating from the anterior direction (168).

An abnormally high origin of the anterior tibial artery leading to the anterior passage of the same vessel to the popliteus muscle has been reported in approximately 2% of the population (169). Although uncommon, this anomaly could theoretically present a problem during TKR.

Magnetic resonance imaging and duplex sonography studies have challenged the concept that flexion offers protection to popliteal vessel injury and have shown that knee flexion variably affects the position of the popliteal artery (168,170). Ninomiya and coworkers (171) identified the location of the popliteal artery in knees using both magnetic resonance imaging and arteriography, and found the popliteal artery to be consistently located lateral to the midline of the tibial plateau. They found that hyperflexion produced kinking and hyperextension produced predictable tenting of the popliteal artery against the posterior tibial plateau. They advocate placing posterior retractors medial to the midline to avoid injury to the popliteal artery.

Based on these imaging studies, it appears that knee flexion does not always guarantee posterior displacement of the vascular structures away from potential harm during total knee arthroplasty.

When necessary, débridement of the posterior compartment should be performed under direct vision to minimize the risk of vascular injury.

STIFFNESS

The patient with a knee that is excessively stiff or painful or both in the early postoperative period can be a diagnostic challenge. The problem is often multifactorial, and its causes include inadequate physical therapy, insufficient pain control, RSD, inadequate releases, oversized femoral component, infection, referred pain, an increased tendency for arthrofibrosis, and muscle spasm (172,173). Heterotopic ossification after primary TKR also correlates with a limitation in postoperative knee flexion (174). The reported incidence of heterotopic ossification after TKR has ranged from 3.8% (175) to 26% (174).

Manipulation

Manipulation in the acute setting after TKR is best suited for the patient who has been unwilling or unable to perform physical therapy. The decision to manipulate is not absolute and no strict guidelines can be stated, but manipulation probably should be performed before 3 months when the scar has begun to consolidate (173). It is unrealistic to expect better motion after manipulation than was achieved at the time of surgery. The likelihood of heterotopic bone is increased if quadriceps adhesions are present and are ruptured at the time of manipulation (176).

Reflex Sympathetic Dystrophy

RSD is uncommon after total knee arthroplasty. It is poorly understood, difficult to diagnose, and problematic to treat. There have been many proposed mechanisms explaining the pathophysiology of RSD, but it is generally agreed that the pathologic mechanism involves an abnormal sympathetic discharge that occurs in response to injury or trauma, and the abnormal prolongation of sympathetic outflow escalates the underlying symptoms. If left untreated, this process leads to RSD, which may continue until there is permanent dysfunction of the extremity (177).

The incidence of RSD after total knee arthroplasty is relatively low and was reported to be 0.8% in one series (178). The classic presentation of RSD includes disproportionate pain, atrophic skin changes with decreased skin temperature, swelling, and stiffness. The diagnosis is rarely straightforward but should be considered in any postoperative TKR patient with unexplained pain or stiffness (179). The most consistent sign is pain out of proportion to the symptoms.

A treatment algorithm for RSD of the knee was presented by Cooper and DeLee (177) and has a reasonable application to the post-TKR patient. This includes a trial of nonsteroidal antiinflammatory drugs, contrast soaks, muscle stimulation, gentle physical therapy, and weightbearing. If this regimen is not suc-

cessful, then a diagnostic sympathetic block is performed. If results are positive, then an in-hospital epidural blockade is instituted combined with CPM and manipulation for 5 to 7 days. Psychological evaluations should also be considered.

Role of Continuous Passive Motion

CPM after total knee arthroplasty has been extensively examined (33,149,151,180–201). Most investigations, both retrospective and prospective randomized studies, fail to show any long-term benefits in terms of range of motion, Knee Society scores, or rates of serious complications. Reported disadvantages of CPM include quadriceps weakness, increased bleeding, greater frequency of wound complications, and increased hospital costs (185,201,202). Opponents of the use of CPM argue that it leads to no improvements in range of motion, no change in the rate of DVT, and no change in the length of hospital stay (185,195). The reported benefits of CPM after total knee arthroplasty include increased range of motion, a decreased rate of knee manipulation, less postoperative pain, less DVT, shorter hospital stay, and decreased costs (33,180,183,189,192,196).

A definite indication to use CPM would be in the presence of inadequate physical therapy, either because of patient noncompliance or inadequate resources.

Pain Management

In the immediately postoperative period, limited recovery of motion is most commonly related to postsurgical pain. The use of either patient-controlled analgesia, postoperative epidural analgesia, or both is extremely helpful to ensure adequate pain relief and allow immediate motion. Overaggressive physical therapy or activity may actually be detrimental and cause stiffness due to pain or inflammation. Femoral blocks are becoming more widely used for postoperative pain management. In addition, preemptive anesthesia instituted before surgery has been demonstrated to decrease pain medication requirements (203,204).

Revision Total Knee Replacement for the Stiff Knee

A revision procedure to treat a stiff and painful knee after TKR usually results in improved range of motion, reduced pain, and higher Knee Society scores (205,206). Results improve if the cause of the stiffness is malpositioned components or a primary diagnosis of osteoarthritis (207). If stiffness is secondary to an overly tight posterior cruciate ligament, then arthroscopic release has been shown to be beneficial (208). Notably, revision for unexplained pain in the setting of a normal range of motion is usually unsuccessful (209).

REFERENCES

1. Clagett GP, Anderson FA Jr, Heit J, et al. Prevention of venous thromboembolism [see comments]. *Chest* 1995;108(4[Suppl]): 312S–334S.
2. Heit JA, Silverstein MD, Mohr DN, et al. Risk factors for deep vein thrombosis and pulmonary embolism: a population-based case-control study. *Arch Intern Med* 2000;160(6):809–815.

3. Coon WW. Venous thromboembolism. Prevalence, risk factors, and prevention. *Clin Chest Med* 1984;5(3):391–401.

4. Coon WW. Epidemiology of venous thromboembolism. *Ann Surg* 1977;186(2):149–164.

5. Lowe GDO, Greer IA, Cooke TG. Risk of and prophylaxis for venous thromboembolism in hospital patients. *BMJ* 1992;305:567–574.

6. Guyatt G, Schunemann H, Cook D, et al. Grades of recommendation for antithrombotic agents. *Chest* 2001;119(1):3S–7S.

7. Parmet JL, Berman AT, Horrow JC, et al. Thromboembolism coincident with tourniquet deflation during total knee arthroplasty [see comments]. *Lancet* 1993;341(8852):1057–1058.

8. Ogawa S, Gerlach H, Esposito C, et al. Hypoxia modulates the barrier and coagulant function of cultured bovine endothelium. Increased monolayer permeability and induction of procoagulant properties. *J Clin Invest* 1990;85(4):1090–1098.

9. Aglietti P, Baldini A, Vena LM, et al. Effect of tourniquet use on activation of coagulation in total knee replacement. *Clin Orthop* 2000;371:169–177.

10. Holemans HR. Increase in fibrinolytic activity by venous occlusion. *J Appl Phys* 1963;18:1123–1128.

11. Fahmy NR, Patel DG. Hemostatic changes and postoperative deep-vein thrombosis associated with use of a pneumatic tourniquet. *J Bone Joint Surg Am* 1981;63(3):461–465.

12. Klenerman L, Chakrabarti R, Mackie I, et al. Changes in haemostatic system after application of a tourniquet. *Lancet* 1977;1(8019):970–972.

13. Petaja J, Myllynen P, Myllyla G, et al. Fibrinolysis after application of a pneumatic tourniquet. *Acta Chir Scand* 1987;153(11–12):647–651.

14. Wakankar HM, Nicholl JE, Koka R, et al. The tourniquet in total knee arthroplasty. A prospective, randomised study. *J Bone Joint Surg Br* 1999;81(1):30–33.

15. Harvey EJ, Leclerc J, Brooks CE, et al. Effect of tourniquet use on blood loss and incidence of deep vein thrombosis in total knee arthroplasty. *J Arthroplasty* 1997;12(3):291–296.

16. Abdel-Salam A, Eyres KS. Effects of tourniquet during total knee arthroplasty. A prospective randomised study. *J Bone Joint Surg Br* 1995;77(2):250–253.

17. Mosca PJ, Haas SB. Thromboembolic disease. In: Fu FH, Harner CD, Vince KG, eds. *Knee surgery*, 1st ed, vol 2. Baltimore: Williams and Wilkins, 1994:1493–1506.

18. Geerts W, Heit J, Clagett GP, et al. Prevention of venous thromboembolism. *Chest* 2001;119(1):132S–175S.

19. Blanchard J, Meuwly JY, Leyvraz PF, et al. Prevention of deep-vein thrombosis after total knee replacement. Randomised comparison between a low-molecular-weight heparin (nadroparin) and mechanical prophylaxis with a foot-pump system. *J Bone Joint Surg Br* 1999;81(4):654–659.

20. Group RHA. RD heparin compared with warfarin for prevention of venous thromboembolic disease following total hip or knee arthroplasty. *J Bone Joint Surg Am* 1994;76:1174–1185.

21. Heit JA, Berkowitz SD, Bona R, et al. Efficacy and safety of low molecular weight heparin (ardeparin sodium) compared to warfarin for the prevention of venous thromboembolism after total knee replacement surgery: a double-blind, dose-ranging study. Ardeparin Arthroplasty Study Group. *Thromb Haemost* 1997;77(1):32–38.

22. Hull R, Raskob G, Pineo G, et al. A comparison of subcutaneous low-molecular-weight heparin with warfarin sodium for prophylaxis against deep-vein thrombosis after hip or knee implantation [see comments]. *N Engl J Med* 1993;329(19):1370–1376.

23. Spiro TE, Fitzgerald RH Jr, Trowbridge AA, et al. Enoxaparin, a low molecular weight heparin, and warfarin for the prevention of venous thromboembolic disease after elective knee replacement surgery. *Blood* 1994;84[Suppl 1]:246A.

24. Colwell CW Jr, Spiro TE, Trowbridge AA, et al. Efficacy and safety of enoxaparin versus unfractionated heparin for prevention of deep venous thrombosis after elective knee arthroplasty. Enoxaparin Clinical Trial Group. *Clin Orthop* 1995;321:19–27.

25. Lotke PA, Palevsky H, Keenan AM, et al. Aspirin and warfarin for thromboembolic disease after total joint arthroplasty [see comments]. *Clin Orthop* 1996;324:251–258.

26. Leclerc JR, Geerts WH, Desjardins L, et al. Prevention of venous thromboembolism after knee arthroplasty. A randomized, double-blind trial comparing enoxaparin with warfarin [see comments]. *Ann Intern Med* 1996;124(7):619–626.

27. Leclerc JR, Geerts WH, Desjardins L, et al. Prevention of deep vein thrombosis after major knee surgery—a randomized, double-blind trial comparing a low molecular weight heparin fragment (enoxaparin) to placebo. *Thromb Haemost* 1992;67(4):417–423.

28. Antonelli D, Fares L, Anene C. Enoxaparin associated with huge abdominal wall hematomas: a report of two cases. *Am Surg* 2000;66(8):797–800.

29. Montoya JP, Pokala N, Melde SL. Retroperitoneal hematoma and enoxaparin. *Ann Intern Med* 1999;131(10):796–797.

30. Lumpkin MM. FDA public health advisory. *Anesthesiology* 1998;88(2):27A–28A.

31. Wysowski DK, Talarico L, Bacsanyi J, et al. Spinal and epidural hematoma and low-molecular-weight heparin [letter]. *N Engl J Med* 1998;338(24):1774–1775.

32. Lynch AF, Bourne RB, Rorabeck CH, et al. Deep-vein thrombosis and continuous passive motion after total knee arthroplasty. *J Bone Joint Surg Am* 1988;70(1):11–14.

33. Vince KG, Kelly MA, Beck J, et al. Continuous passive motion after total knee arthroplasty. *J Arthroplasty* 1987;2(4):281–284.

34. Hull R, Delmore TJ, Hirsh J, et al. Effectiveness of intermittent pulsatile elastic stockings for the prevention of calf and thigh vein thrombosis in patients undergoing elective knee surgery. *Thromb Res* 1979;16(1–2):37–45.

35. McKenna R, Galante J, Bachmann F, et al. Prevention of venous thromboembolism after total knee replacement by high-dose aspirin or intermittent calf and thigh compression. *BMJ* 1980;280(6213):514–517.

36. Haas S, Haas P, Creutzig A. Therapy of venous thromboembolism with low-molecular-weight heparins [in German]. *Vasa* 2000;29(1):5–10.

37. Lynch JA, Baker PL, Polly RE, et al. Mechanical measures in the prophylaxis of postoperative thromboembolism in total knee arthroplasty. *Clin Orthop* 1990;260:24–29.

38. Hui AC, Heras-Palou C, Dunn I, et al. Graded compression stockings for prevention of deep-vein thrombosis after hip and knee replacement. *J Bone Joint Surg Br* 1996;78(4):550–554.

39. Levine MN, Gent M, Hirsh J, et al. Ardeparin (low-molecular-weight heparin) vs graduated compression stockings for the prevention of venous thromboembolism. A randomized trial in patients undergoing knee surgery [see comments]. *Arch Intern Med* 1996;156(8):851–856.

40. Haas SB, Insall JN, Scuderi GR, et al. Pneumatic sequential-compression boots compared with aspirin prophylaxis of deep-vein thrombosis after total knee arthroplasty. *J Bone Joint Surg Am* 1990;72(1):27–31.

41. Clagett GP, Anderson FA Jr, Geerts W, et al. Prevention of venous thromboembolism [see comments]. *Chest* 1998;114(5[Suppl]):531S–560S.

42. Robinson KS, Anderson DR, Gross M, et al. Ultrasonographic screening before hospital discharge for deep venous thrombosis after arthroplasty: the post-arthroplasty screening study. A randomized, controlled trial [see comments]. *Ann Intern Med* 1997;127(6):439–445.

43. Leclerc JR, Gent M, Hirsh J, et al. The incidence of symptomatic venous thromboembolism during and after prophylaxis with enoxaparin: a multi-institutional cohort study of patients who underwent hip or knee arthroplasty. Canadian Collaborative Group. *Arch Intern Med* 1998;158(8):873–878.

44. Sikorski JM, Hampson WG, Staddon GE. The natural history and aetiology of deep vein thrombosis after total hip replacement. *J Bone Joint Surg Br* 1981;63(2):171–177.

45. Lotke PA, Steinberg ME, Ecker ML. Significance of deep venous thrombosis in the lower extremity after total joint arthroplasty. *Clin Orthop* 1994;299:25–30.

46. Pellegrini VD, Clement D, Lush-Ehmann C, et al. The John Charnley Award. Natural history of thromboembolic disease after total hip arthroplasty. *Clin Orthop* 1996;333:27–40.

47. Trowbridge A, Boese CK, Woodruff B, et al. Incidence of posthospitalization proximal deep venous thrombosis after total hip arthroplasty. A pilot study. *Clin Orthop* 1994;299:203–208.

48. Planes A, Vochelle N, Darmon JY, et al. Risk of deep-venous thrombosis after hospital discharge in patients having undergone total hip

replacement: double-blind randomised comparison of enoxaparin versus placebo. *Lancet* 1996;348(9022):224–228.

49. Bergqvist D, Benoni G, Bjorgell O, et al. Low-molecular-weight heparin (enoxaparin) as prophylaxis against venous thromboembolism after total hip replacement. *N Engl J Med* 1996;335(10):696–700.

50. Dahl OE, Andreassen G, Aspelin T, et al. Prolonged thromboprophylaxis following hip replacement surgery—results of a double-blind, prospective, randomised, placebo-controlled study with dalteparin (Fragmin). *Thromb Haemost* 1997;77(1):26–31.

51. Fraser JD, Anderson DR. Deep venous thrombosis: recent advances and optimal investigation with US. *Radiology* 1999;211(1):9–24.

52. Lonner JH, Lieberman JR. Coagulation and thromboembolism in orthopaedic surgery. In: Koval KJ, ed. *Orthopaedic knowledge update*, vol 7. Rosemont, IL: American Academy of Orthopaedic Surgeons, 2001.

53. Riedel M. Acute pulmonary embolism 1: pathophysiology, clinical presentation, and diagnosis. *Heart* 2001;85(2):229–240.

54. Haas SB, Tribus CB, Insall JN, et al. The significance of calf thrombi after total knee arthroplasty [see comments]. *J Bone Joint Surg Br* 1992;74(6):799–802.

55. Hull RD, Raskob GE, Pineo GF, et al. Subcutaneous low-molecular-weight heparin compared with continuous intravenous heparin in the treatment of proximal-vein thrombosis. *N Engl J Med* 1992;326(15):975–982.

56. Low-molecular-weight heparin in the treatment of patients with venous thromboembolism. The Columbus Investigators. *N Engl J Med* 1997;337(10):657–662.

57. Prandoni P. Unfractionated heparin and low-molecular-weight heparin for the initial treatment of acute venous thromboembolism. *Haemostasis* 1998;28[Suppl S3]:85–90.

58. Hull RD, Pineo GF. Treatment of venous thromboembolism with low-molecular-weight heparin. *J Thromb Thrombolysis* 1995;1(3):279–284.

59. Hettiarachchi RJ, Prins MH, Lensing AW, et al. Low molecular weight heparin versus unfractionated heparin in the initial treatment of venous thromboembolism. *Curr Opin Pulm Med* 1998;4(4):220–225.

60. Levine M, Gent M, Hirsh J, et al. A comparison of low-molecular-weight heparin administered primarily at home with unfractionated heparin administered in the hospital for proximal deep-vein thrombosis. *N Engl J Med* 1996;334(11):677–681.

61. Koopman MM, Prandoni P, Piovella F, et al. Treatment of venous thrombosis with intravenous unfractionated heparin administered in the hospital as compared with subcutaneous low-molecular-weight heparin administered at home. The Tasman Study Group. *N Engl J Med* 1996;334(11):682–687.

62. Pini M. Future prospects of prophylaxis for deep vein thrombosis. *Blood Coagul Fibrinolysis* 1999;10[Suppl 2]:S19–S27.

63. Cohen CA, Smith TC. The intraoperative hazard of acrylic bone cement: report of a case. *Anesthesiology* 1971;35(5):547–549.

64. Dandy DJ. Fat embolism following prosthetic replacement of the femoral head. *Injury* 1971;3(2):85–88.

65. du Toit HJ, Erasmus FR, Taljaard JJ, et al. Early recognition of pulmonary dysfunction during intramedullary orthopaedic surgery. *S Afr Med J* 1982;62(27):1027–1029.

66. Esemenli BT, Toker K, Lawrence R. Hypotension associated with methylmethacrylate in partial hip arthroplasties. The role of femoral canal size. *Orthop Rev* 1991;20(7):619–623.

67. Hagley SR, Lee FC, Blumbergs PC. Fat embolism syndrome with total hip replacement. *Med J Aust* 1986;145(10):541–543.

68. Kim KC, Ritter MA. Hypotension associated with methyl methacrylate in total hip arthroplasties. *Clin Orthop* 1972;88:154–160.

69. Lachiewicz PF, Ranawat CS. Fat embolism syndrome following bilateral total knee replacement with total condylar prosthesis: report of two cases. *Clin Orthop* 1981;160:106–108.

70. Modig J, Busch C, Olerud S, et al. Arterial hypotension and hypoxaemia during total hip replacement: the importance of thromboplastic products, fat embolism and acrylic monomers. *Acta Anaesthesiol Scand* 1975;19(1):28–43.

71. Newens AF, Volz RG. Severe hypotension during prosthetic hip surgery with acrylic bone cement. *Anesthesiology* 1972;36(3):298–300.

72. Phillips H, Cole PV, Lettin AW. Cardiovascular effects of implanted acrylic bone cement. *BMJ* 1971;3(772):460–461.

73. Powell JN, McGrath PJ, Lahiri SK, et al. Cardiac arrest associated with bone cement. *BMJ* 1970;3(718):326.

74. Watson JT, Stulberg BN. Fat embolism associated with cementing of femoral stems designed for press-fit application. *J Arthroplasty* 1989;4(2):133–137.

75. Bisla RS, Inglis AE, Lewis RJ. Fat embolism following bilateral total knee replacement with the Guepar prosthesis. A case report. *Clin Orthop* 1976;115:195–198.

76. Caillouette JT, Anzel SH. Fat embolism syndrome following the intramedullary alignment guide in total knee arthroplasty. *Clin Orthop* 1990;251:198–199.

77. Deburge A, Guepar. Guepar hinge prosthesis: complications and results with two years' follow-up. *Clin Orthop* 1976;120:47–53.

78. Delp SL, Stulberg SD, Davies B, et al. Computer assisted knee replacement. *Clin Orthop* 1998;354:49–56.

79. Enneking FK. Cardiac arrest during total knee replacement using a long-stem prosthesis [clinical conference]. *J Clin Anesth* 1995;7(3):253–263.

80. Monto RR, Garcia J, Callaghan JJ. Fatal fat embolism following total condylar knee arthroplasty. *J Arthroplasty* 1990;5(4):291–299.

81. Orsini EC, Richards RR, Mullen JM. Fatal fat embolism during cemented total knee arthroplasty: a case report. *Can J Surg* 1986;29(5):385–386.

82. Samii K, Elmelik E, Goutalier D, et al. Hemodynamic effects of prosthesis insertion during knee replacement without tourniquet. *Anesthesiology* 1980;52(3):271–273.

83. Samii K, Elmelik E, Mourtada MB, et al. Intraoperative hemodynamic changes during total knee replacement. *Anesthesiology* 1979;50(3):239–242.

84. Zimmerman RL, Kroner LF, Blomberg DJ, et al. Fatal fat embolism following total knee arthroplasty. *Minn Med* 1983;66(4):213–216.

85. Levy D. The fat embolism syndrome. A review. *Clin Orthop* 1990;261:281–286.

86. Lindeque BG, Schoeman HS, Dommisse GF, et al. Fat embolism and the fat embolism syndrome. A double-blind therapeutic study. *J Bone Joint Surg Br* 1987;69(1):128–131.

87. Fahmy NR, Chandler HP, Danylchuk K, et al. Blood-gas and circulatory changes during total knee replacement. Role of the intramedullary alignment rod. *J Bone Joint Surg Am* 1990;72(1):19–26.

88. Hofmann S, Hopf R, Huemer G, et al. Modified surgical technique for the reduction of bone marrow spilling in knee endoprosthesis [in German]. *Orthopade* 1995;24(2):144–150.

89. Ries MD. Fat embolism associated with intramedullary alignment during total knee arthroplasty. *Contemp Orthop* 1994;28:211.

90. Ries MD, Lynch F, Raucher LA, et al. Pulmonary function during and after total knee arthroplasty: the effect of overdrilling the femoral intramedullary alignment rod hole. *Am J Knee Surg* 1994;7:57.

91. Ries MD, Rauscher LA, Hoskins S, et al. Intramedullary pressure and pulmonary function during total knee arthroplasty. *Clin Orthop* 1998;356:154–160.

92. Dorr LD, Merkel C, Mellman MF, et al. Fat emboli in bilateral total knee arthroplasty. Predictive factors for neurologic manifestations. *Clin Orthop* 1989;248:112–118; discussion 118–119.

93. Ritter MD, Mamlin LA, Melfi CA, et al. Outcome implications for the timing of bilateral total knee arthroplasties. *Clin Orthop* 1997;345:99–105.

94. Lane GJ, Hozack WJ, Shah S, et al. Simultaneous bilateral versus unilateral total knee arthroplasty. Outcomes analysis. *Clin Orthop* 1997;345:106–112.

95. Jankiewicz JJ, Sculco TP, Ranawat CS, et al. One-stage versus 2-stage bilateral total knee arthroplasty. *Clin Orthop* 1994;309:94–101.

96. Kolettis GT, Wixson RL, Peruzzi WT, et al. Safety of 1-stage bilateral total knee arthroplasty. *Clin Orthop* 1994;309:102–109.

97. Lynch NM, Trousdale RT, Ilstrup DM. Complications after concomitant bilateral total knee arthroplasty in elderly patients [see comments]. *Mayo Clin Proc* 1997;72(9):799–805.

98. Adolph MD, Fabian HF, el-Khairi SM, et al. The pulmonary artery catheter: a diagnostic adjunct for fat embolism syndrome. *J Orthop Trauma* 1994;8(2):173–176.

99. Berman AT, Parmet JL, Harding SP, et al. Emboli observed with use of transesophageal echocardiography immediately after tourniquet release during total knee arthroplasty with cement. *J Bone Joint Surg Am* 1998;80(3):389–396.

100. Fong J, Gadalla F, Pierri MK, et al. Are Doppler-detected venous emboli during cesarean section air emboli? [published erratum appears in *Anesth Analg* 1990;71(5):574]. *Anesth Analg* 1990;71(3):254–257.

101. Heinrich H, Kremer P, Winter H, et al. Embolic events during total hip replacement. An echocardiographic study. *Acta Orthop Belg* 1988;54(1):12–17.

102. Marshall PD DD, Henry L. Transesophageal echocardiographic visualization of pulmonary embolism from pneumatic tourniquet use during orthopaedic surgery. *Anaesthesia* 1992;77[Suppl]: A1080(abst).

103. Sikorski JM, Bradfield JW. Fat and thromboembolism after total hip replacement. *Acta Orthop Scand* 1983;54(3):403–407.

104. Spiess BD, Sloan MS, McCarthy RJ, et al. The incidence of venous air embolism during total hip arthroplasty. *J Clin Anesth* 1988;1(1):25–30.

105. Svartling N. Detection of embolized material in the right atrium during cementation in hip arthroplasty. *Acta Anaesthesiol Scand* 1988;32(3):203–208.

106. McGrath BJ, Hsia J, Boyd A, et al. Venous embolization after deflation of lower extremity tourniquets. *Anesth Analg* 1994;78(2):349–353.

107. Morawa LG, Manley MT, Edidin AA, et al. Transesophageal echocardiographic monitored events during total knee arthroplasty. *Clin Orthop* 1996;331:192–198.

108. Markel DC, Femino JE, Farkas P, et al. Analysis of lower extremity embolic material after total knee arthroplasty in a canine model. *J Arthroplasty* 1999;14(2):227–232.

109. Cates HE, Ritter MA, Keating EM, et al. Intramedullary versus extramedullary femoral alignment systems in total knee replacement. *Clin Orthop* 1993;286:32–39.

110. Ries MD, Lynch F, Rauscher LA, et al. Pulmonary function during and after total hip replacement. Findings in patients who have insertion of a femoral component with and without cement. *J Bone Joint Surg Am* 1993;75(4):581–587.

111. Duncan JA. Intra-operative collapse or death related to the use of acrylic cement in hip surgery [see comments]. *Anaesthesia* 1989;44(2):149–153.

112. Kepes ER, Undersood PS, Becsey L. Intraoperative death associated with acrylic bone cement. Report of two cases. *JAMA* 1972;222(5):576–577.

113. Pahuja K, Lowe H, Chand K. Blood methyl methacrylate levels in patients having prosthetic joint replacement. *Acta Orthop Scand* 1974;45(5):737–741.

114. Park WY, Balingit P, Kenmore PI, et al. Changes in arterial oxygen tension during total hip replacement. *Anesthesiology* 1973;39(6): 642–644.

115. Schuh FT, Schuh SM, Viguera MG, et al. Circulatory changes following implantation of methylmethacrylate bone cement. *Anesthesiology* 1973;39(4):455–457.

116. Homsy CA, Tullos HS, Anderson MS, et al. Some physiological aspects of prosthesis stabilization with acrylic polymer. *Clin Orthop* 1972;83:317–328.

117. Byrick RJ, Bell RS, Kay JC, et al. High-volume, high-pressure pulsatile lavage during cemented arthroplasty. *J Bone Joint Surg Am* 1989;71(9):1331–1336.

118. Gaine WJ, Ramamohan NA, Hussein NA, et al. Wound infection in hip and knee arthroplasty. *J Bone Joint Surg Br* 2000;82(4):561–565.

119. Wilson MG, Kelley K, Thornhill TS. Infection as a complication of total knee-replacement arthroplasty. Risk factors and treatment in sixty-seven cases. *J Bone Joint Surg Am* 1990;72(6):878–883.

120. Papagelopoulos PJ, Idusuyi OB, Wallrichs SL, et al. Long term outcome and survivorship analysis of primary total knee arthroplasty in patients with diabetes mellitus. *Clin Orthop* 1996;330:124–132.

121. England SP, Stern SH, Insall JN, et al. Total knee arthroplasty in diabetes mellitus. *Clin Orthop* 1990;260:130–134.

122. Serna F, Mont MA, Krackow KA, et al. Total knee arthroplasty in diabetic patients. Comparison to a matched control group. *J Arthroplasty* 1994;9(4):375–379.

123. Pollard JP, Hughes SP, Scott JE, et al. Antibiotic prophylaxis in total hip replacement. *BMJ* 1979;1(6165):707–709.

124. Hill C, Flamant R, Mazas F, et al. Prophylactic cefazolin versus placebo in total hip replacement. Report of a multicentre double-blind randomised trial. *Lancet* 1981;1(8224):795–796.

125. Ericson C, Lidgren L, Lindberg L. Cloxacillin in the prophylaxis of postoperative infections of the hip. *J Bone Joint Surg Am* 1973;55(4):808–813, 843.

126. Carlsson AK, Lidgren L, Lindberg L. Prophylactic antibiotics against early and late deep infections after total hip replacements. *Acta Orthop Scand* 1977;48(4):405–410.

127. Nelson CL, Green TG, Porter RA, et al. One day versus seven days of preventive antibiotic therapy in orthopedic surgery. *Clin Orthop* 1983;176:258–263.

128. Pavel A, Smith RL, Ballard A, et al. Prophylactic antibiotics in clean orthopaedic surgery. *J Bone Joint Surg Am* 1974;56(4):777–782.

129. Pavel A, Smith RL, Ballard A, et al. Prophylactic antibiotics in elective orthopedic surgery: a prospective study of 1,591 cases. *South Med J* 1977;70[Suppl 1]:50–55.

130. Norden CW. Antibiotic prophylaxis in orthopedic surgery. *Rev Infect Dis* 1991;13[Suppl 10]:S842–S846.

131. Periti P, Mazzei T, Periti E. Prophylaxis in gynaecological and obstetric surgery: a comparative randomised multicentre study of single-dose cefotetan versus two doses of cefazolin. *Chemioterapia* 1988;7(4):245–252.

132. Williams DN, Gustilo RB. The use of preventive antibiotics in orthopaedic surgery. *Clin Orthop* 1984;190:83–88.

133. D'Ambrosia RD, Shoji H, Heater R. Secondarily infected total joint replacements by hematogenous spread. *J Bone Joint Surg Am* 1976;58(4):450–453.

134. Cruess RL, Bickel WS, von Kessler KL. Infections in total hips secondary to a primary source elsewhere. *Clin Orthop* 1975;106:99–101.

135. Hall AJ. Late infection about a total knee prosthesis. Report of a case secondary to urinary tract infection. *J Bone Joint Surg Br* 1974;56(1):144–147.

136. Michelson JD, Lotke PA, Steinberg ME. Urinary-bladder management after total joint-replacement surgery. *N Engl J Med* 1988;319(6):321–326.

137. Oishi CS, Williams VJ, Hanson PB, et al. Perioperative bladder management after primary total hip arthroplasty. *J Arthroplasty* 1995;10(6):732–736.

138. Carpiniello VL, Cendron M, Altman HG, et al. Treatment of urinary complications after total joint replacement in elderly females. *Urology* 1988;32(3):186–188.

139. David TS, Vrahas MS. Perioperative lower urinary tract infections and deep sepsis in patients undergoing total joint arthroplasty. *J Am Acad Orthop Surg* 2000;8(1):66–74.

140. Ries MD. Vancomycin resistant *Enterococcus* infected total knee arthroplasty. A report of two cases. *J Arthroplasty* 2001;16(6):802–805.

141. Hartman MB, Fehring TK, Jordan L, et al. Periprosthetic knee sepsis. The role of irrigation and debridement. *Clin Orthop* 1991;273:113–118.

142. Wasielewski RC, Barden RM, Rosenberg AG. Results of different surgical procedures on total knee arthroplasty infections. *J Arthroplasty* 1996;11(8):931–938.

143. Rand JA, Bryan RS, Morrey BF, et al. Management of infected total knee arthroplasty. *Clin Orthop* 1986;205:75–85.

144. Rand JA. Alternatives to reimplantation for salvage of the total knee arthroplasty complicated by infection. *Instr Course Lect* 1993;41:341–347.

145. Bengston S, Knutson K, Lidgren L. Treatment of infected knee arthroplasty. *Clin Orthop* 1989;245:173–178.

146. Waldman BJ, Hostin E, Mont MA, et al. Infected total knee arthroplasty treated by arthroscopic irrigation and debridement. *J Arthroplasty* 2000;15(4):430–436.

147. Mont MA, Waldman B, Banerjee C, et al. Multiple irrigation, debridement, and retention of components in infected total knee arthroplasty. *J Arthroplasty* 1997;12(4):426–433.

148. Greene KA, Wilde AH, Stulberg BN. Preoperative nutritional status of total joint patients. Relationship to postoperative wound complications. *J Arthroplasty* 1991;6(4):321–325.

149. Johnson DP. The effect of continuous passive motion on wound-healing and joint mobility after knee arthroplasty. *J Bone Joint Surg Am* 1990;72(3):421–426.

150. Johnson DP. Midline or parapatellar incision for knee arthroplasty. A comparative study of wound viability. *J Bone Joint Surg Br* 1988;70(4):656–658.

151. Yashar AA, Venn-Watson E, Welsh T, et al. Continuous passive motion with accelerated flexion after total knee arthroplasty. *Clin Orthop* 1997;345:38–43.

152. Kim YH, Cho SM, Kim JS. Total knee arthroplasty in bony ankylosis in gross flexion. *J Bone Joint Surg Br* 1999;81(2):296–300.

153. Rhomberg M, Schwabegger AH, Ninkovic M, et al. Gastrocnemius myotendinous flap for patellar or quadriceps tendon repair, or both. *Clin Orthop* 2000;377:152–160.

154. Asp JP, Rand JA. Peroneal nerve palsy after total knee arthroplasty. *Clin Orthop* 1990;261:233–237.

155. Schmalzried TP, Noordin S, Amstutz HC. Update on nerve palsy associated with total hip replacement. *Clin Orthop* 1997;344:188–206.

156. Krackow KA, Jones MM, Teeny SM, et al. Primary total knee arthroplasty in patients with fixed valgus deformity. *Clin Orthop* 1991;273:9–18.

157. Laurencin CT, Volatile TB, Gebhardt EM, et al. Total knee replacement in severe valgus deformity. *Am J Knee Surg* 1992;5:135.

158. Ranawat CS, Rich DS. Total condylar knee arthroplasty for valgus and combined valgus flexion deformity of the knee. *Instr Course Lect* 1984;33:414–417.

159. Lu S, Lin J, Kou B. Total knee replacement of severe flexion contracture deformities greater than 60 degree [in Chinese]. *Chung Hua Wai Ko Tsa Chih* 1997;35(7):414–417.

160. Miyasaka KC, Ranawat CS, Mullaji A. 10- to 20-year followup of total knee arthroplasty for valgus deformities. *Clin Orthop* 1997;345:29–37.

161. Healy WL, Iorio R, Lemos DW. Medial reconstruction during total knee arthroplasty for severe valgus deformity. *Clin Orthop* 1998;356:161–169.

162. Idusuyi OB, Morrey BF. Peroneal nerve palsy after total knee arthroplasty. Assessment of predisposing and prognostic factors. *J Bone Joint Surg Am* 1996;78(2):177–184.

163. Horlocker TT, Cabanela ME, Wedel DJ. Does postoperative epidural analgesia increase the risk of peroneal nerve palsy after total knee arthroplasty? *Anesth Analg* 1994;79(3):495–500.

164. Unwin AJ, Thomas M. Intra-operative monitoring of the common peroneal nerve during total knee replacement. *J R Soc Med* 1994;87(11):701–703.

165. Mont MA, Dellon AL, Chen F, et al. The operative treatment of peroneal nerve palsy. *J Bone Joint Surg Am* 1996;78(6):863–869.

166. Rush JH, Vidovich JD, Johnson MA. Arterial complications of total knee replacement. The Australian experience. *J Bone Joint Surg Br* 1987;69(3):400–402.

167. Farrington WJ, Charnley GJ, Harries SR, et al. The position of the popliteal artery in the arthritic knee. *J Arthroplasty* 1999;14(7):800–802.

168. Smith PN, Gelinas J, Kennedy K, et al. Popliteal vessels in knee surgery. A magnetic resonance imaging study. *Clin Orthop* 1999;367:158–164.

169. Trotter M. The level of termination of the popliteal artery in the white and the negro. *Am J Phys Anthropol* 1940;27:109–118.

170. Zaidi SH, Cobb AG, Bentley G. Danger to the popliteal artery in high tibial osteotomy. *J Bone Joint Surg Br* 1995;77(3):384–386.

171. Ninomiya JT, Dean JC, Goldberg VM. Injury to the popliteal artery and its anatomic location in total knee arthroplasty. *J Arthroplasty* 1999;14(7):803–809.

172. Ellis TJ, Beshires E, Brindley GW, et al. Knee manipulation after total knee arthroplasty. *J South Orthop Assoc* 1999;8(2):73–79.

173. Lonner JH, Lotke PA. Aseptic complications after total knee arthroplasty. *J Am Acad Orthop Surg* 1999;7(5):311–324.

174. Furia JP, Pellegrini VD Jr. Heterotopic ossification following primary total knee arthroplasty. *J Arthroplasty* 1995;10(4):413–419.

175. Harwin SF, Stein AJ, Stern RE, et al. Heterotopic ossification following primary total knee arthroplasty. *J Arthroplasty* 1993;8(2):113–116.

176. Daluga D, Lombardi AV Jr, Mallory TH, et al. Knee manipulation following total knee arthroplasty. Analysis of prognostic variables. *J Arthroplasty* 1991;6(2):119–128.

177. Cooper DE, DeLee JC. Reflex sympathetic dystrophy of the knee. *J Am Acad Orthop Surg* 1994;2(2):79–86.

178. Katz MM, Hungerford DS. Reflex sympathetic dystrophy affecting the knee. *J Bone Joint Surg Br* 1987;69(5):797–803.

179. Tietjen R. Reflex sympathetic dystrophy of the knee. *Clin Orthop* 1986;209:234–243.

180. Lachiewicz PF. The role of continuous passive motion after total knee arthroplasty. *Clin Orthop* 2000;380:144–150.

181. MacDonald SJ, Bourne RB, Rorabeck CH, et al. Prospective randomized clinical trial of continuous passive motion after total knee arthroplasty. *Clin Orthop* 2000;380:30–35.

182. Wasilewski SA, Woods LC, Torgerson WR Jr, et al. Value of continuous passive motion in total knee arthroplasty. *Orthopedics* 1990;13(3):291–295.

183. Verevereli PA, Sutton DC, Hearn SL, et al. Continuous passive motion after total knee arthroplasty. Analysis of cost and benefits. *Clin Orthop* 1995;321:208–215.

184. Nielsen PT, Rechnagel K, Nielsen SE. No effect of continuous passive motion after arthroplasty of the knee. *Acta Orthop Scand* 1988;59(5):580–581.

185. Ritter MA, Gandolf VS, Holston KS. Continuous passive motion versus physical therapy in total knee arthroplasty. *Clin Orthop* 1989;244:239–243.

186. Kusswetter W, Sell S. Continuous passive motion in the after care of knee joint prostheses [in German]. *Orthopade* 1991;20(3):216–220.

187. Goletz TH, Henry JH. Continuous passive motion after total knee arthroplasty. *South Med J* 1986;79(9):1116–1120.

188. Shih KZ, Liu TK. The role of continuous passive motion following total knee arthroplasty. *J Formos Med Assoc* 1990;89(12):1077–1080.

189. McInnes J, Larson MG, Daltroy LH, et al. A controlled evaluation of continuous passive motion in patients undergoing total knee arthroplasty. *JAMA* 1992;268(11):1423–1428.

190. Kumar PJ, McPherson EJ, Dorr LD, et al. Rehabilitation after total knee arthroplasty: a comparison of 2 rehabilitation techniques. *Clin Orthop* 1996;331:93–101.

191. Nadler SF, Malanga GA, Zimmerman JR. Continuous passive motion in the rehabilitation setting. A retrospective study. *Am J Phys Med Rehabil* 1993;72(3):162–165.

192. Colwell CW Jr, Morris BA. The influence of continuous passive motion on the results of total knee arthroplasty. *Clin Orthop* 1992;276:225–228.

193. Chiarello CM, Gundersen L, O'Halloran T. The effect of continuous passive motion duration and increment on range of motion in total knee arthroplasty patients. *J Orthop Sports Phys Ther* 1997;25(2):119–127.

194. Gose JC. Continuous passive motion in the postoperative treatment of patients with total knee replacement. A retrospective study. *Phys Ther* 1987;67(1):39–42.

195. Montgomery F, Eliasson M. Continuous passive motion compared to active physical therapy after knee arthroplasty: similar hospitalization times in a randomized study of 68 patients. *Acta Orthop Scand* 1996;67(1):7–9.

196. Romness DW, Rand JA. The role of continuous passive motion following total knee arthroplasty. *Clin Orthop* 1988;226:34–37.

197. Chen B, Zimmerman JR, Soulen L, et al. Continuous passive motion after total knee arthroplasty: a prospective study. *Am J Phys Med Rehabil* 2000;79(5):421–426.

198. Jordan LR, Siegel JL, Olivo JL. Early flexion routine. An alternative method of continuous passive motion. *Clin Orthop* 1995;315:231–233.

199. Basso DM, Knapp L. Comparison of two continuous passive motion protocols for patients with total knee implants [published erratum appears in *Phys Ther* 1987;67(6):979]. *Phys Ther* 1987;67(3):360–363.

200. Maloney WJ, Schurman DJ, Hangen D, et al. The influence of continuous passive motion on outcome in total knee arthroplasty. *Clin Orthop* 1990;256:162–168.

201. Pope RO, Corcoran S, McCaul K, et al. Continuous passive motion after primary total knee arthroplasty. Does it offer any benefits? *J Bone Joint Surg Br* 1997;79(6):914–917.

202. Lotke PA, Faralli VJ, Orenstein EM, et al. Blood loss after total knee replacement. Effects of tourniquet release and continuous passive motion. *J Bone Joint Surg Am* 1991;73(7):1037–1040.

203. Allen HW, Liu SS, Ware PD, et al. Peripheral nerve blocks improve analgesia after total knee replacement surgery. *Anesth Analg* 1998;87(1):93–97.

204. Mulroy MF, Larkin KL, Batra MS, et al. Femoral nerve block with 0.25% or 0.5% bupivacaine improves postoperative analgesia following outpatient arthroscopic anterior cruciate ligament repair. *Reg Anesth Pain Med* 2001;26(1):24–29.

205. Ries MD, Badalamente M. Arthrofibrosis after total knee arthroplasty. *Clin Orthop* 2000;380:177–183.

206. Aglietti P, Windsor RE, Buzzi R, et al. Arthroplasty for the stiff or ankylosed knee. *J Arthroplasty* 1989;4(1):1–5.

207. Nicholls DW, Dorr LD. Revision surgery for stiff total knee arthroplasty. *J Arthroplasty* 1990;5[Suppl]:S73–S77.

208. Williams RJ 3rd, Westrich GH, Siegel J, et al. Arthroscopic release of the posterior cruciate ligament for stiff total knee arthroplasty. *Clin Orthop* 1996;331:185–191.

209. Mont MA, Serna FK, Krackow KA, et al. Exploration of radiographically normal total knee replacements for unexplained pain. *Clin Orthop* 1996;331:216–220.

CHAPTER 102

Evaluation of the Symptomatic Total Knee Replacement

David C. Ayers

Total knee replacement (TKR) is a reliable surgical procedure that provides predictable pain relief and restoration of knee function for the vast majority of patients. A minority of patients have persistent symptoms after surgery or develop new postoperative symptoms. A comprehensive history and thorough physical examination are crucial to accurately diagnose the cause of a patient's symptoms (1). Often, it is helpful to examine the patient on more than one occasion to ensure consistency in the history and physical findings. Some patients have symptoms severe enough to define the knee replacement as a failure. Radiographs are a routine part of the evaluation of a failed TKR (2). Selective use of diagnostic tests supplement the information gathered from the history, physical examination, and routine radiographs and typically allow for an accurate diagnosis in patients with a symptomatic TKR (1). A specific diagnosis and treatment plan are mandatory before undertaking any additional surgical procedure (1,3).

HISTORY

A comprehensive history is crucial when evaluating patients with complaints after TKR. All problems that preceded the knee replacement should be documented, including antecedent operations, date of the index TKR, and any perioperative problems or delays in recovery or rehabilitation. Persistent swelling or drainage after the knee replacement raises the index of suspicion for infection (4). It is important to determine whether primary wound healing occurred and whether the patient had an initial period of pain relief after the TKR surgery. It is helpful to determine whether the patient's presenting symptoms are the same as the symptoms before the TKR. If the patient's current symptoms are identical to the preoperative symptoms, the original diagno-

sis of the knee being the cause of the patient's pain must be carefully reevaluated. Medical comorbidities should be determined, including the presence of diabetes mellitus, a neurologic or vascular disease, a septic focus, and an immunocompromised state.

One must initially establish the exact nature of the patient's complaint. Although pain is typically given as the chief complaint, specific questioning may reveal that the problem is actually weakness, giving way, or swelling. Giving way may be a sign of ligamentous instability, patellofemoral instability, component malalignment, or muscle weakness or inhibition. Weakness may be a result of spinal stenosis or muscle atrophy. After pain has been established as the principal problem, the exact location of the pain should be sought and localized as precisely as possible. Radicular pain may arise from lumbar spine disease. Medial knee pain may result from hip disease. Pain in the thigh or calf can be of vascular or neurologic origin. Pain that is well localized to the anterior portion of the knee is often of patellofemoral origin. Posterior knee pain may be related to a popliteal cyst, deep venous thrombosis, or pseudoaneurysm. Pain that is consistently localized to a small area may result from a neuroma (5) or chronic bursitis. Typically the pain is described as related to the knee joint in the region of the medial and lateral joint lines.

Factors that aggravate or alleviate the pain should be sought. Pain associated with weightbearing activities may indicate mechanical loosening. Pain that is constant, that is unrelated to activity, and that occurs at night may be related to infection. Start-up pain that worsens with the first few steps is typical of loosening and may represent inadequate ingrowth of a cementless prosthesis or early loosening of a cemented prosthesis. Pain associated with inadequate ingrowth of a cementless prosthesis is often present within the first year, whereas pain associated with loosening of a well-aligned noninfected cemented prosthesis occurs much later (6).

The patient should be questioned regarding functional activities. The distance or time a patient reports being able to walk should be recorded, along with the use of ambulatory devices. It is helpful to ask about the patient's ability to ascend and descend stairs and to know which leg is used to go up or down first. The ability of the patient to arise from a chair and symptoms typical of instability during walking are important to question the patient about.

The patient should be queried regarding his or her expectations after knee replacement. The patient's problems preoperatively should be compared with his or her anticipated results and current symptoms and function. The patient's employment history should be recorded and taken into consideration. Patients receiving workers' compensation benefits have been reported to have less predictable results after TKR. Any ongoing or pending legal action regarding the patient's knee condition should be questioned and recorded. Underlying depression or psychiatric disease should be evaluated. Current or previous treatment with antidepressants or other neuropsychiatric medications should be recorded. Patients with a preoperative mental composite score of less than 50 on the Short Form-36 Questionnaire are at increased risk for less improvement in their physical function score after TKR.

PHYSICAL EXAMINATION

A thorough physical examination of the patient with pain after TKR should not be limited to the knee, as knee pain can be associated with lumbar spine, hip, or retroperitoneal pathology. Therefore, examination of the spine, hip, and abdomen is necessary in addition to the knee. It is useful to begin the examination with examination of the extrinsic causes of knee pain. Careful examination of the lumbar spine is particularly important if there is any radicular component to the patient's pain. Examination of the hip is mandatory and should include range of motion and whether motion of the hip reproduces pain in the knee. Gait abnormalities, limb length inequality, hip girdle weakness, or fixed deformity of the hip should be sought. If range of motion of the hip is limited or other aspects of the hip examination are abnormal, radiographic examination of the hip is required. In some instances, injection of local anesthetic into the hip and determining whether this alleviates the patient's knee pain can be helpful. Examination of the patient's feet should include evaluation for evidence of peripheral neuropathy. Hypersensitivity of the limb associated with cool, shiny skin may indicate reflex sympathetic dystrophy. Absence of ankle deep tendon reflexes may indicate lumbar spine disease. Absent pulses may indicate peripheral vascular disease and often warrant noninvasive arterial duplex scanning. Finally, be sure to examine the foot and ankle alignment, as hindfoot or forefoot deformities can place increased stresses on the knee.

Examination of the knee joint often begins while observing the patient's walk with and without supportive aids. Varus or valgus alignment of the knee may indicate ligamentous instability, component loosening or subsidence, or component malpositioning. Patients with hyperextension when weightbearing may have posterior cruciate insufficiency or excessive wear of the posterior aspect of the polyethylene insert. The knee should be evaluated for erythema, edema, or an intraarticular effusion. Point tenderness to palpation at the joint line may be indicative of impingement of an underlying prominence such as an unresected osteophyte, a cementophyte, or an overhanging implant. Point tenderness and inflammation about the medial aspect of the tibia are often indicative of pes anserine bursitis. Point tenderness away from the joint line, with a positive Tinel's sign, and elimination of the point tenderness by a local injection indicate a neuroma (5).

Active and passive range of motion of the knee replacement should be recorded. The maximum flexion and extension should be compared with preoperative values measured before the index knee replacement. The presence of crepitus with motion should be noted. The knee should be examined for a fixed flexion contracture or an extensor lag. An audible pop that occurs as the knee moves from flexion into extension is termed *patellar clunk syndrome* and results from a soft tissue nodule at the superior pole of the patella (7). The audible pop results from the soft tissue nodule popping into the trochlear groove (7).

Knee stability is determined by static ligament testing. A TKR typically approximates the stability of a normal knee with mild anterior cruciate instability (8). Ligament competence in full extension and at 30 degrees and 90 degrees of flexion should be evaluated. Laxity to stress testing is typically recorded as 1+, 2+, and 3+, with notation of whether there is a firm end point. Sagittal plane laxity (anterior and posterior translation of the tibia on the femur to stress) should also be evaluated. Pseudolaxity is created by component collapse and should not be confused with ligament insufficiency.

In patients with symptoms after TKR, a detailed examination of the patellofemoral joint is important because patellofemoral pathology is the most common cause of additional surgery after TKR (9). Determine the competence of the extensor mechanism by evaluating the strength of knee extension and the presence of an extensor lag. Patellar tracking should be observed during passive motion and active motion. The presence of patellar tilting, crepitus, or clunking should be sought. Patellar mobility should be assessed in full extension and slight flexion. A positive apprehension sign is indicative of patellar instability, whereas decreased patellar mobility may be associated with patella baja or fibrosis and scar formation. The medial and lateral aspects of the patella should be palpated for patellar tenderness. Rotational abnormal alignment of the femoral or tibial components may be difficult to observe during examination of the knee (10). If present, malrotation of the components may be manifested by patellofemoral instability.

RADIOGRAPHIC EXAMINATION

A complete radiographic evaluation is necessary to assess a painful TKR. Initial postoperative radiographs should be reviewed for radiolucent lines at the bone–cement interface or the implant–bone interface. A careful review of sequential radiographs is an important part of evaluating a symptomatic TKR. Radiolucent lines are a common finding after cemented TKR (11). Radiolucent lines that are noncircumferential and observed over only a minority of the interface are not diagnostic of loosening (11). Radiographic evidence of loosening is defined as a radiolucency that is progressive in serial x-rays or circumferential and larger than 2 mm at either the cement-prosthesis or bone-cement interface. Component subsidence or change in position is diagnostic of implant loosening. A radiolu-

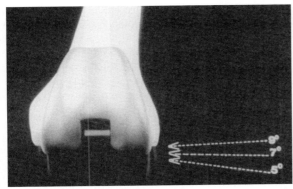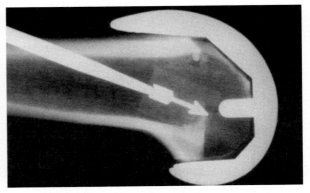

FIG. 1. A: Distal fluoroscopic examination must consider the angle of the distal femoral cut. The x-ray beam must be angled accordingly to evaluate the distal femoral interface. **B:** A lateral fluoroscopic view of the distal femoral interface. The arrow indicates the radiolucency between the distal femur and the implant. (From Fehring TK, McAvoy GM. Fluoroscopic evaluation of the painful total knee arthroplasty. *Clin Orthop* 1996;331:226–233, with permission.)

cent line that is present at only a portion of the interface (especially in zones I and IV of the tibial component), is less than 1 mm in width, and is not progressive on serial radiographs does not indicate loosening of the prosthesis and is most likely not the etiology of the patient's pain. A radiolucency that has developed and progressed over a short period has an entirely different meaning than one that was present on the immediate postoperative x-ray and has not progressed.

Routine radiographic examination should include a minimum of three views: a coronal anteroposterior (AP) view obtained with the patient bearing weight on the limb, a lateral view taken with the knee flexed approximately 30 degrees, and a patellar axial view with the knee flexed between 30 and 45 degrees. The femoral interface is examined best in the lateral view, whereas both the AP and lateral views can be helpful when examining the tibial interface. Many believe that the bone-cement interface is more difficult to assess in cementless TKRs. Fluoroscopic examinations can be quite helpful to ensure optimal visualiza-

tion of the interface by placing the x-ray beam tangential to the interface being examined (Fig. 1) (12). The location of the x-ray beam differs in the lateral plane when examining the femoral interface and the tibial interface (13). Some authors have advocated using fluoroscopy to realign the x-ray beam when examining the interface at the anterior femoral flange and the posterior condyles interface (Fig. 2) (12). Fluoroscopic examination is also helpful to examine the tibial bone interface in the AP plane.

Alignment of the limb and each individual component should be radiographically determined. The femoral component should ideally be aligned 90 degrees to the mechanical axis of the limb. The tibial component should be oriented at 90 degrees to the anatomic axis of the tibia. The anterior flange of the femoral component on the lateral radiograph should be parallel to the anterior cortex of the femur. The orientation of the tibial component on the lateral view differs based on the type of component used. In a posterior cruciate–retaining component, the tibial component typi-

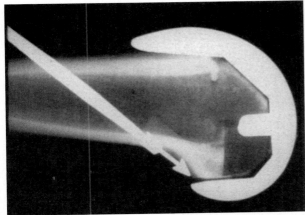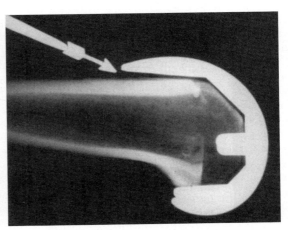

FIG. 2. A: Lateral fluoroscopic view of the posterior condylar interface. The arrow indicates the radiolucency between the posterior runner and the posterior condyle. **B:** A lateral fluoroscopic view of the anterior femoral interface. The arrow indicates the radiolucency between the implant and the anterior femur. (From Fehring TK, McAvoy GM. Fluoroscopic evaluation of the painful total knee arthroplasty. *Clin Orthop* 1996;331:226–233, with permission.)

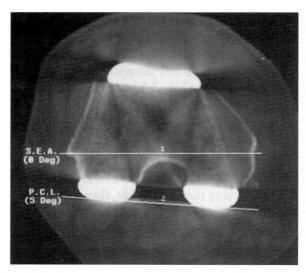

FIG. 3. Axial computed tomographic image of the right femur through the epicondylar axis. The surgical epicondylar axis (S.E.A.) connects the lateral epicondylar prominence and the medial sulcus of the medial epicondyle. The posterior condylar line (P.C.L.) connects the medial and lateral prosthetic posterior condylar surfaces. Deg, degrees. (From Berger RA, Crossett LS, Jacobs JJ, et al. Malrotation causing patellofemoral complications after total knee arthroplasty. *Clin Orthop* 1998;356:144–153, with permission.)

cally has approximately 7 degrees of posterior slope. In a cruciate-substituting component, the tibial component is implanted between 0 degrees and 3 degrees of posterior slope. The rotational alignment of the prosthetic components are difficult to determine with plain radiographic examinations. If malrotation of the femoral or tibial component is suspected, obtaining a computed tomographic scan of the knee can be quite helpful (10). The rotational alignment of the femoral component in relation to the transepicondylar axis (Fig. 3) and the tibial component in relation to the tibial tubercle can be determined (10). This technique provides a noninvasive method for quantitatively determining the rotational alignment of the tibial and femoral components on a standard computed tomographic scanner and can be useful for patients with patellofemoral instability (10).

The lateral radiograph yields much information pertinent to the evaluation of a painful TKR. The size (AP diameter) of the femoral component can be measured and compared with the AP diameter of the contralateral femur. An increase in the AP diameter of the femur may be associated with poor range of motion and stiffness. A decrease in the AP diameter of the femur may be associated with flexion instability. Elevation of the joint line resulting in an acquired patella baja can be detected on the lateral view. An acquired patella baja may result in restriction of flexion of the TKR. The point of contact between the femur and tibial insert is visualized on the lateral radiograph. Excessive rollback of the femoral component may be related to tightness of the posterior cruciate ligament and resultant pain and poor flexion of the TKR. The thickness of the patellar remnant can be assessed on the lateral radiograph. A thick patellar remnant that results in an increased lateral diameter of the patellar can result in decreased knee flexion.

The patellar axial view is particularly useful for evaluating tracking of the patellofemoral joint (9). Patellar tilt or instability is visualized in this view (Fig. 4). Occasionally, radiographs in varying degrees of flexion are useful. In addition, problems related to the polyethylene of the patellar component can often be visualized such as wear-through of metal-backed components or polyethylene dissociation (9). Stress fractures of the patella can also be seen in the skyline view.

The AP radiograph with the patient bearing weight gives information regarding the polyethylene thickness of the tibial insert and ligament balance. Varus and valgus stress views are useful if the patient is unable to bear weight on the limb and for documenting ligamentous instability (8).

NUCLEAR MEDICINE EXAMINATION

After a thorough history, physical examination, and study of serial x-rays, occasionally there still may be uncertainty regarding the fixation of the prosthetic components in a patient with a painful TKR. Radionucleotide studies may be used to aid in the diagnosis of loosening and infection (14–16). One must bear in mind that in asymptomatic knees, increased activity on diphosphonate scanning can be expected for at least 1 year after surgery. Increased activity of the diphosphonate scan after 1 year is present in 89% of tibial and 63% of femoral components in asymptomatic knee replacements (2,15,17). Bone scans must therefore be carefully interpreted as an additional data point in conjunction with the data obtained from the history, the physical examination, and the radiographs (Fig. 5) (18). A negative bone scan is in many respects more helpful than a positive scan. If a diphosphonate scan has normal uptake in a patient with a painful TKR, the pain is unlikely to originate from loosening or infection. Conversely, if there is increased uptake about the TKR, the patient does not necessarily have infection or loosening. Other causes of accelerated bone turnover in addition to infection and loosening include trauma and tumor. Technetium diphosphonate scan has a sensitivity of 95% in detecting infection; its specificity is only 20% (14,19).

Gallium citrate is a radioisotope that accumulates in areas of inflammation. On intravenous injection, gallium binds to serum transferrin and is carried to the extracellular space, including sites of infection. Gallium scan sensitivity is high, and a negative scan can reliably rule out infection. However, because gallium may show increased uptake at uninfected sites of bone remodeling, the positive predictive value is 70% to 75% (20–22).

Scans using indium (indium-111) may improve the diagnostic accuracy of radionucleotide scans for infection (17). A sample of the patient's blood is drawn, and the white cells in it are labeled with indium-111. These labeled cells are reinfused. Local areas of increased white cell accumulation in bone as seen on a subsequent scan are suggestive of infection. Using indium-111 to diagnose infection has a reported accuracy of 84%, sensitivity of 83%, and specificity of 85% (Fig. 6) (23). False-positives have been seen in patients with rheumatoid arthritis or osteolysis. An accuracy of 95% has been reported for diagnosing infection in TKR when using indium-111 in combination with technetium diphosphonate scans (21). If both of these nuclear studies are normal, further diagnostic studies, continued observation, and referral for a second opinion are all appropriate treatment options (19,22).

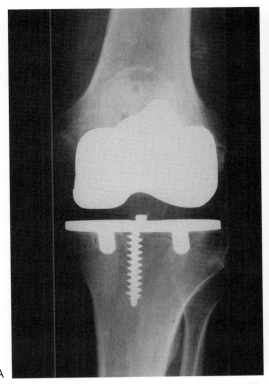

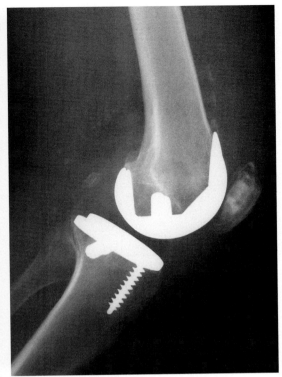

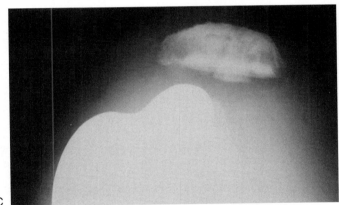

FIG. 4. Anteroposterior **(A)** and lateral **(B)** radiographs of a 76-year-old man 8 years after cementless total knee replacement returned for knee instability after exchange of tibial insert and revision of patellar component. The patellar component was lateralized, resulting in patellar instability seen on the patellar axial view **(C)**.

LABORATORY EVALUATION

Blood studies commonly used to evaluate patients with a painful TKR include a blood cell count and differential, erythrocyte sedimentation rate (ESR), and C-reactive protein. These studies are intended to serve as screening tests for infection (18,24). The white blood cell count is the least useful and is elevated in a minority of patients with an infected TKR (18,24). The sedimentation rate has a sensitivity of 60% to 80% when 30 mm per hour is used as the cutoff level for diagnosing infection (18,24,25). An elevated sedimentation rate is an extremely nonspecific finding and the ESR may remain elevated for several months after surgery in asymptomatic, noninfected TKRs. The C-reactive protein returns to a normal level sooner than the ESR and is therefore more helpful in evaluating a patient with a painful TKR within 3 months of the index surgical procedure (18,25).

Analysis of fluid aspirated from the painful TKR is the standard of care to determine if a prosthetic infection is present. A synovial fluid white blood cell count of greater than 25,000 per µL or a differential with more than 75% polymorphonuclear leukocytes is highly suggestive of infection (19,26–28). Laboratory culture of the joint aspirate can also identify the bacterial species causing the infection and its antibiotic sensitivities (29). A finding of elevated protein and low glucose levels in the aspirated fluid are consistent with deep prosthetic infection (18,29,30). It is important to determine whether the patient had been on antibiotics at the time of the aspirate or in the immediate past, as antibiotic use is a major factor in obtaining false-negative cultures from fluid aspirated from infected TKRs. In patients who have not been on antibiotics, aspiration has been found to be 75% sensitive in detecting infection (26). If a high index of suspicion for infection exists, a second knee aspirate can

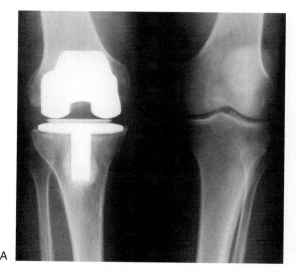

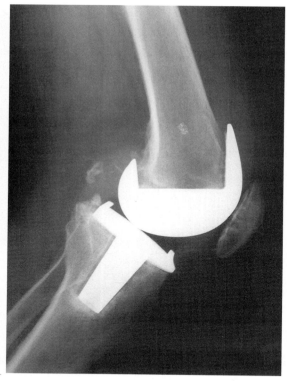

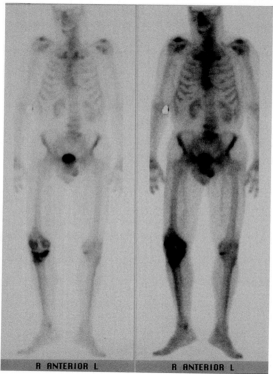

FIG. 5. Seventy-three-year-old man referred for evaluation of a painful total knee replacement 2 years after surgery. X-rays **(A, B)** illustrate loosening of the femoral and tibial components. Bone scans **(C, D)** illustrate increased uptake at both the distal femur and proximal tibia. Aspiration was negative for infection. Cultures obtained at revision surgery were positive for coagulase-negative *Staphylococcus aureus*.

increase the sensitivity to 85% (26). False-negative aspirates are not uncommon and a single negative aspiration does not rule out infection. Aspiration of a TKR must be performed under sterile conditions and without the use of local anesthetics. The preservative added to lidocaine is bactericidal to many bacteria and may lead to false-negative cultures of the aspirated fluid.

Molecular biologic techniques may aid greatly in our ability to diagnose infection in TKRs. Polymerase chain reaction testing of fluid aspirated from a painful TKR is the most sensitive test to detect bacteria in the specimen (31). This test is based on the fact that nearly all bacteria that cause infections after TKR have a gene that encodes the 16S RNA of a small ribosomal subunit of the bacteria. A set of primers is used to target this gene and amplify the production of DNA from these bacteria. The type of bacterial DNA can then be identified. This study is extremely sensitive and may have a high false-positive rate in laboratories not expert in this technique (31). This laboratory investigation is not currently in routine clinical use and is not quantitative but qualitative. Nonetheless this test may be an invaluable aid in diagnosing periprosthetic infections in the future and it has the added benefit that it is not affected by the presence of antibiotics in the synovial fluid.

TOTAL KNEE REPLACEMENT FAILURES

TKR provides the arthritic patient with predictable pain relief and restoration of function of the arthritic joint. There are

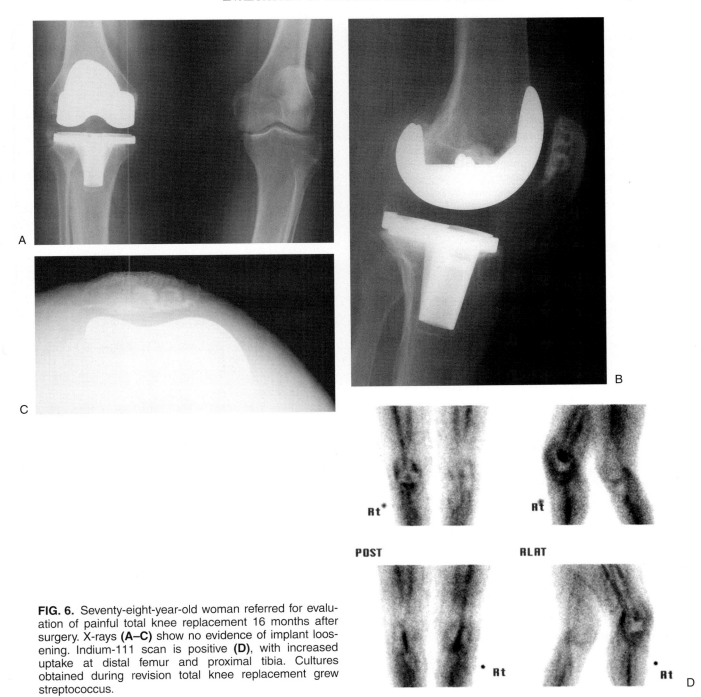

FIG. 6. Seventy-eight-year-old woman referred for evaluation of painful total knee replacement 16 months after surgery. X-rays **(A–C)** show no evidence of implant loosening. Indium-111 scan is positive **(D)**, with increased uptake at distal femur and proximal tibia. Cultures obtained during revision total knee replacement grew streptococcus.

patients who do not obtain this predictable result, and this group can be divided into two categories. The first group contains failures that occur early in the postoperative period, within the first 5 years. The second group, or late failures, includes patients in whom failure occurs after 10 years.

Early failures after TKR are of great concern, as both patients and surgeons have come to expect results far superior to this, with 10 to 15 years of prosthetic function before revision is necessary. A group of 440 patients in whom the index replacement failed and revision was necessary were studied (6). Of the 440 patients evaluated, 279 (63%) had revision surgery within 5 years of their index replacement. In this cohort, 105 of the 279 patients (38%) had revision surgery because of infection; 74 (27%) had revision surgery because of instability; 37 (13%) had revision surgery because of patellofemoral problems; and 21 (7%) had revision surgery because of wear or osteolysis (6). In only eight (3%) patients there was an early revision due to aseptic loosening of the prosthesis. Two major causes of early failure of TKR ultimately requiring revision surgery seen in this series were the failure of cementless fixation and prosthetic instability (6). If all the knee replacements had been cemented routinely and the ligaments balanced carefully, the number of early revisions would have decreased by approximately 40%, and the overall failures would have been reduced by 25% (6). Special care must be given to the soft tissue aspects of the knee replacement procedure to avoid early revision for instability by ensuring careful equalization of the flexion and extension gaps.

No patient with a painful TKR should be offered revision surgery without a diagnosis as to the cause of the patient's pain (1). There is little place for surgical exploration of the painful total knee, either arthroscopically or through an open incision (3). One can determine the etiology of the pain in the vast majority of patients with pain after TKR by carrying out a complete history and a thorough physical examination, reviewing serial and current radiographs, ordering appropriate laboratory examinations, and obtaining occasional radionucleotide scans when appropriate (1,3).

REFERENCES

1. Ayers DC, Dennis DA, Johanson, NA, et al. Common complications of total knee arthroplasty. *J Bone Joint Surg Am* 1997;79:278–311.
2. Schneider R, Soudry M. Radiographic and scintigraphic evaluation of total knee arthroplasty. *Clin Orthop* 1986;205:108–112.
3. Mont MA, Serna FK, Krackow KA. Exploration of radiographically normal total knee replacements for unexplained pain. *Clin Orthop* 1996;331:216–219.
4. Rand JA. Sepsis following total knee arthroplasty. In: Rand JA, ed. *Total knee arthroplasty*. New York: Raven Press, 1993:349–375.
5. Dellon AL, Mont MA, Krackow KA, et al. Partial denervation for persistent neuroma pain after total knee arthroplasty. *Clin Orthop* 1995;316:145–150.
6. Fehring TK, Odum S, Griffin WL. Early failures in total knee arthroplasty. *Clin Orthop* 2001;392:315–318.
7. Beight JL, Yao B, Hozack WJ, et al. The patellar "clunk" syndrome after posterior stabilized total knee arthroplasty. *Clin Orthop* 1994;299:139–142.
8. Fehring TK, Valadie AL. Knee instability after total knee arthroplasty. *Clin Orthop* 1994;299:157–162.
9. Rand JA. The patellofemoral joint in total knee arthroplasty. *J Bone Joint Surg Am* 1994;76:612–620.
10. Berger RA, Crossett LS, Jacobs JJ, et al. Malrotation causing patellofemoral complications after total knee arthroplasty. *Clin Orthop* 1998;356:144–153.
11. Hunter JC, Jattner RS, Murray WR. Loosening of the total knee replacement: correlation with pain and radiolucent lines. A prospective study. *Invest Radiol* 1987;22:891–894.
12. Fehring TK, McAvoy G. Fluoroscopic evaluation of the painful total knee arthroplasty. *Clin Orthop* 1996;331:226–233.
13. Mintz AD, Pilkington DA, Howie DW. A comparison of plain and fluoroscopically guided radiographs in the assessment of arthroplasty of the knee. *J Bone Joint Surg Am* 1989;71:1343–1347.
14. Davis LP. Nuclear imaging in the diagnosis of the infected total joint arthroplasty. *Semin Arthroplasty* 1994;5:147–152.
15. Kantor SG, Schneider R, Insall JN. Radionuclide imaging of asymptomatic versus symptomatic total knee arthroplasties. *Clin Orthop* 1990;260:118–123.
16. Morrey BF, Westholm F, Schoifet S. Long-term results of various treatment options for infected total knee arthroplasty. *Clin Orthop* 1989;248:120–128.
17. Rosenthall L, Lepanto L, Raymone F. Radiophosphate uptake on asymptomatic knee arthroplasty. *J Nucl Med* 1987;28:1546–1549.
18. Levitsky KA, Hozack WJ, Balderston RA. Evaluation of the painful prosthetic joint: relative value of bone scan, sedimentation rate and joint aspiration. *J Arthroplasty* 1991;6:237–244.
19. Hansen AD, Rand JA. Evaluation and treatment of infection at the site of a total hip or knee arthroplasty. *J Bone Joint Surg Am* 1998;80:910–922.
20. Magnuson JE, Brown ML, Hausen JF. In-111 labeled leukocyte scintigraphy in suspected orthopedic prosthesis infection: comparison with other imaging modalities. *Radiology* 1988;168: 235–239.
21. Merkel KD, Brown ML, Dewangee MK. Comparison of indium-labeled-leukocyte imaging with sequential technetium-gallium scanning in the diagnosis of low-grade musculoskeletal sepsis: a prospective study. *J Bone Joint Surg Am* 1985;67:465–476.
22. Windsor RE, Insall JN. Management of the infected total knee arthroplasty. In: Insall JN, ed. *Surgery of the knee*, vol. 2. New York: Churchill Livingstone, 1993:47–71.
23. Rand JA, Brown ML. The value of indium 111 leukocyte scanning in the evaluation of painful or infected total knee arthroplasties. *Clin Orthop* 1990;259:179–182.
24. Aslto K, Osterman K, Peltola H. Changes in erythrocyte sedimentation rate and C-reactive protein after total hip arthroplasty. *Clin Orthop* 1984;184:118–120.
25. Carlsson AS. Erythrocyte sedimentation rate in infected and noninfected total hip arthroplasties. *Acta Orthop Scand* 1978;49:287–291.
26. Barrack RL, Jennings RW, Wolfe MW, et al. The value of preoperative aspiration before total knee revision. *Clin Orthop* 1997;345:8–16.
27. Duff GP, Lachiewicz PL, Kelly SS. Aspiration of the knee joint before revision arthroplasty. *Clin Orthop* 1996;331:132–139.
28. O'Neill DA, Harris WH. Failed total hip replacement: assessment by plain radiographs, arthrograms, and aspiration of the hip joint. *J Bone Joint Surg Am* 1984;66:540–546.
29. Chimento GF, Finger S, Barrack RL. Gram stain detection of infection during revision arthroplasty. *J Bone Joint Surg Br* 1996;78:828–839.
30. Windsor RE, Insall JN, Urs WK. Two-stage reimplantation for the salvage of total knee arthroplasty complicated by infection: further follow-up and refinement of indications. *J Bone Joint Surg Am* 1990;72:272–278.
31. Mariani BD, Martin DS, Levine MJ. Polymerase chain reaction detection of bacterial infection in total knee arthroplasty. *Clin Orthop* 1996;331:11–22.

CHAPTER 103

Preoperative Planning for Revision Total Knee Arthroplasty

Daniel J. Berry

Careful preoperative planning for a complex operation like revision knee replacement provides tremendous benefits to the patient and surgeon by improving the quality and efficiency of the surgery, and by reducing the potential for operative complications. At its best, preoperative planning involves more than just advance consideration of the tools required to remove failed implants and consideration of the design and size of implants that will be implanted: Preoperative planning involves consideration of all the resources that will be needed during surgery and in the postoperative period; preoperative planning involves a mental rehearsal of the planned operation from start to finish, which allows the surgeon to consider the order of steps in which the operation will be performed, and the techniques that he or she must be familiar with to complete each step; and preoperative planning involves considering contingencies for problems that might arise during surgery. Thorough and thoughtful preoperative planning helps the surgeon to have on hand all of the materials necessary for an optimal reconstruction and allows the surgeon to become familiar with and have access to techniques, implants, and tools that could be needed to overcome potential problems. The chance of needing to compromise because a specific implant or tool was not available or because the surgeon was not familiar with a specific useful technique is reduced. Finally, detailed preoperative planning helps the surgeon predict problems that are important to discuss with the patient in advance. The patient, then, is better informed about the risks of surgery and potential problems that may compromise the surgical outcome; such an understanding leads to more realistic patient expectations and ultimately to greater patient satisfaction with the entire process of surgery, regardless of the outcome.

PREOPERATIVE EVALUATION

Patient History and Physical Examination

Identify problems by history and physical examination that will influence what procedure is done and how it is done. Determine if the patient has a history or physical findings of hip problems such as pain or stiffness, known arthritis, or previous fracture or osteotomy of the hip or femur. Determine if the patient has an ipsilateral tibial deformity, or ankle or foot problems. These pieces of information are important to optimize the mechanical axis of the limb at operation. Learn as much as possible about the patient's failed knee replacement. Identify the implant manufacturer, implant design, and implant sizes. If part of the knee implant will be retained intact at operation, all this information is essential to ensure that matching parts are available. Learn whether special design-specific instruments are available for implant extraction or disassembly. Review whether

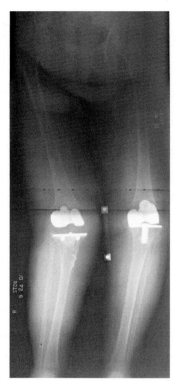

FIG. 1. Long, standing hip-to-ankle radiograph of both lower extremities.

there is anything in the history or examination to suggest infection of the failed total knee arthroplasty (TKA). If so, consider preoperative evaluation with measurement of C-reactive protein level, erythrocyte sedimentation rate, knee aspiration (1,2), and radionuclide scans.

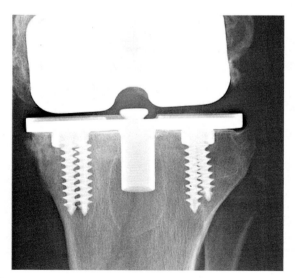

FIG. 2. Fluoroscopically positioned radiograph of an uncemented tibial component demonstrates a complete radiolucent line at the implant-bone interface and osteolysis around the stem of the implant. The implant was not bone ingrown at revision.

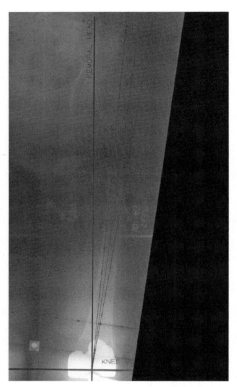

FIG. 3. Template over a long hip-to-ankle radiograph demonstrates that a 7-degree valgus cut on the femur (in combination with a 0-degree cut on the tibia) will restore the mechanical axis of the limb to neutral.

Evaluate the skin and previous skin incisions and find out if the patient has ever had problems with wound healing. Measure the knee range of motion and consider whether stiffness may make an extensile exposure necessary. Determine if there is evidence of ligamentous deficiency or knee instability. Test extensor mechanism power. Evaluate the patient's vascular status. If significant peripheral vascular disease is a concern by history or examination, consider a preoperative vascular medicine or vascular surgery consult, or preoperative noninvasive arterial studies, or both. Ask if the patient has a history of venous thromboembolic problems; if so, plan accordingly for venous thromboembolism prophylaxis and consider whether preoperative evaluation by an internist, vascular medicine specialist, or thrombosis expert would be helpful. Consider the patient's overall medical situation. Make arrangements for an appropriate preoperative medical evaluation and for postoperative support by specialists in internal medicine, cardiology, pulmonology, nephrology, or other medical disciplines if needed. If a large procedure is planned, and if the patient has numerous medical problems, make preoperative arrangements for a postoperative intensive care unit bed. Determine if the patient has experienced unusual bleeding or blood loss problems that may require preoperative hematologic evaluation and special arrangements with the blood bank. By having the patient evaluated in advance by specialists in other disciplines, such as plastic surgery, vascular surgery, or internal medicine, some problems may be avoided. Equally important, if problems do occur intra- or postoperatively, the consultants can deal with them more effectively because they already know the patient.

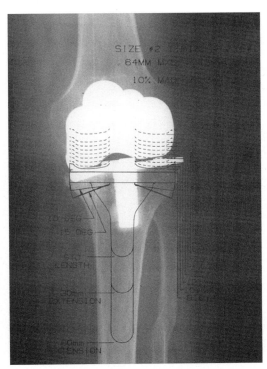

FIG. 4. Template over anteroposterior radiograph of the tibia demonstrating the axis of a 0-degree tibial cut needed to restore the mechanical axis of the limb to neutral. Note that the real tibial resection line would be more superior and would remove less bone (see Fig. 6).

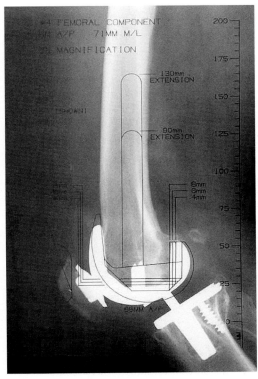

FIG. 6. Osteolysis of the posterior femoral condyles. The femoral template also demonstrates that an offset femoral stem will be needed to avoid impingement of the stem against the posterior femoral cortex.

Likewise, the patient is more likely to take the problem in stride because the potential for such problems was anticipated.

Radiographs

Knee radiographs should include anteroposterior standing films, lateral films, and patellar skyline views. In most cases also obtain a long, standing film from hips to ankles (Fig. 1) (3,4). Stress films occasionally may be helpful to determine the degree of ligament competence. Fluoroscopically positioned radiographs provide views that are perfectly tangential to the implant interface, and most provide detailed information of implant fixation status (Fig. 2). Combine the radiographic information with the rest of the preoperative evaluation to determine the mechanism of previous implant failure. Understanding the failure mechanism helps determine what needs to be done to correct the problem. Determine if the previous implants appear to be well fixed or loose. Determine if the implants are well positioned or malpositioned on an anteroposterior radiograph. Use the radiographs to determine the proper angle of femoral and tibial resection needed to restore the mechanical axis of the limb (Fig. 3). Use the templates to estimate the bone resections needed to place the tibial and femoral components in optimal orientation (Fig. 4). Use templates over the anteroposterior and lateral radiographs to determine the approximate tibial or femoral implant sizes that will be needed. Evaluate the location and severity of tibial and femoral bone loss. Use templates to determine whether metal prosthetic augmentation or bone grafts will be needed (Fig. 5). Examine the

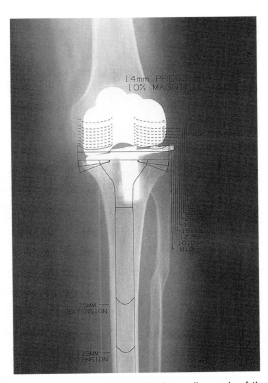

FIG. 5. Template over anteroposterior radiograph of the tibia. The template demonstrates that a medial tibial metal augmentation wedge will be needed to compensate for medial tibial bone defect.

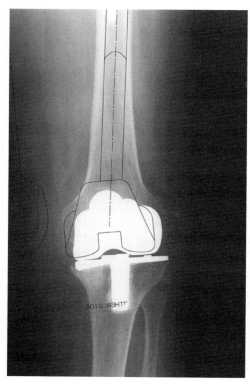

FIG. 7. Template over anteroposterior radiograph of the femur to estimate planned diameter of a press-fit femoral stem.

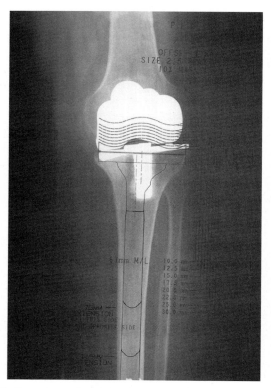

FIG. 8. Template of a tibial component with an offset stem over anteroposterior radiograph of the tibia. Use of an offset stem eliminates the medial overhang of the tibial component seen in Figure 6 (the same case without an offset stem).

distal femur carefully for subtle signs of osteolysis of the condyles, especially posteriorly (Fig. 6). Use templates to determine the length and diameter of planned tibial and femoral implant stems (Fig. 7). Determine whether offset stems are likely to be needed to compensate for unusual bone shape or bone deformity (Fig. 8).

Evaluate the patella. Is the implant metal backed or all polyethylene? Is it loose or well fixed? If the patella needs to be removed, consider whether adequate bone stock remains to allow another implant to be placed. Consider whether there is evidence of tibial or femoral implant malrotation or of patellar maltracking. If the major problem is patellofemoral maltracking, consider evaluating rotation of the implants with a computerized tomographic scan (5).

After obtaining a careful history and physical examination and good radiographs, it is helpful to consider each issue that will affect the operation in a methodical and organized manner. Systematic review of each subject is useful for three reasons: First, it forces the surgeon to consider every aspect of the planned operation—this makes it less likely that a tool or implant will be needed that was not anticipated and therefore is not available. Second, it forces the surgeon to review the planned steps of the operation—in doing so, the surgeon can move through the actual procedure more efficiently. Having conceived the plan in advance, the surgeon will have less need to pause to think about options during surgery. A careful plan forces the surgeon to think through how a decision at one point in the operation will affect the requirements for the rest of the procedure. Finally, by considering each step of the procedure, the surgeon should have in mind a plan A, a plan B, and a plan

C for each contingency: Anticipating challenges and problems blunts their negative impact should they occur at operation.

STEP-BY-STEP PREOPERATIVE CONSIDERATIONS

Skin

Consider the scars already present. If a single midline vertical incision is present, plan to use it. If there are multiple scars, plan which will be best to use. Because much of the cutaneous blood supply comes medially, in general, the most lateral usable previous incision is best. If the risk of skin slough seems high even if precautions are taken, consider having the patient evaluated by a plastic surgeon preoperatively. The plastic surgeon may have useful ideas about how to prevent problems and, if a problem does occur, the patient will have been seen and evaluated in advance. If muscle flaps from previous surgery will be elevated, get information about the location of the vascular pedicle to the flap and consider plastic surgery consultation.

Peripheral Vascular Supply

If the patient has evidence by history or physical examination of significant peripheral vascular disease, consider consultation with a vascular surgeon or vascular medicine expert. Consider noninvasive vascular studies and transcutaneous oximetry to determine if wound healing at the knee level is likely to be a problem. If the patient has marked peripheral vascular disease or previous vascular reconstruction, consider doing most of the procedure, with the exception of exposure and implant cementation, without a tourniquet inflated (6). When the knee is flexed, bleeding often is minimal.

Neurologic Status

Make sure the preoperative neurologic status is evaluated and carefully documented. For patients at high risk for nerve palsy after surgery, set in place a preoperative plan to reduce that risk. Patients with large flexion contractures, valgus knee deformities, and particularly a combination of the two are at risk when the deformity is corrected and the peroneal nerve is placed under tension (7). Avoid the use of long-lasting regional anesthesia or nerve blocks that will make postoperative evaluation of nerve function difficult. A preoperative plan to keep the knee flexed postoperatively until neurologic status is verified is reasonable, and a plan can be set in place to gradually extend the knee while the clinical status of the nerve is evaluated postoperatively.

Exposure

Even though the need for an extensile knee exposure can never be determined with certainty until the operation itself is under way, frequently it can be predicted in advance. The most common situation that requires an extensile exposure is the very stiff knee. The main extensile exposures to the knee are proximal quadriceps snip, V-Y quadricepsplasty, and tibial tubercle osteotomy. Extensile knee exposures are discussed in detail in Chapter 75.

Implant Removal

One of the most important issues to address by preoperative planning is removal of previous implants. Identify the manufacturer, implant design, and size of the failed knee implants. Keep in mind that some implant designs have several design iterations, some of which look remarkably similar radiographically.

It is important to know the type of implant for several reasons. First, if some of the previous components will be retained, compatible components (tibia, femur, patella, tibial insert, tibial insert locking pins, etc.) need to be available. Second, knowing the type of implants in place allows the surgeon to have implant-specific extractors available. Finally, the surgeon can learn in advance about implant-specific methods of disassembly or reassembly.

Consider what tools may be needed to remove the implants from the bone. For cemented implants, have osteotomes, saws, or ultrasonic instruments (8–10) available to cut the prosthesis-cement interface. Have extractors available to remove implants. If the implants have stems, have special instruments available to remove the stem from the canal. If there are large cement columns in the femur or tibia, have special instruments available to remove cement. The instruments designed for cement removal

in revision hip arthroplasty are particularly useful. These include hand instruments, cannulated cement-removal systems, and ultrasonic cement-removal systems.

If the implants are uncemented, have oscillating and Gigli saws available to cut the bone-implant interfaces. Metal-cutting instruments may be needed when there are well-fixed implant stems or pegs that need to be cut free of the implant before extraction (11).

Bone Defects and Templating

Consider the location, severity, and geometry of bone loss. Use templates to determine the planned implant position and implant size. Also use templates to plan for bone defect management. Have metal augmentation for femoral and tibial components available. Have appropriate bone grafts available if they may be needed. Most cavitary and moderate-sized segmental defects can be managed with particulate bone grafts or bulk femoral head grafts. For large defects of the femur or tibia, structural distal femoral grafts or proximal tibial grafts may be needed. Have available internal fixation materials to fix grafts in place.

Consider the implant stems needed to provide added fixation, to off-load stress, and to bypass bone defects. In general, larger defects require longer stems to off-load stress. When possible, bone defects that could lead to fracture, including old screw holes, should be bypassed.

Finally, with templates, determine if any bone deformities will make difficult or compromise ideal implant placement. Determine if offset implant stems or special custom stems may be needed to optimize positioning and sizing of the implants and stems.

Flexion-Extension Gap Balancing and Joint Line Restoration

Consider what will be necessary to balance flexion and extension gaps. When possible, the simultaneous goals of the operation are to balance the flexion and extension gaps and to restore the joint line to a normal level. There is growing understanding, however, that in practice sometimes these two goals are mutually exclusive. Not rarely in revision TKA the flexion gap is considerably larger than the extension gap, and some elevation of the joint line is necessary to balance the knee in flexion and extension.

Study the preoperative radiographs to determine the relative amounts of posterior femoral bone loss and distal femoral bone loss that are present. More posterior femoral bone loss means more posterior femoral build-up will be needed to fill the flexion gap. If there is a great deal of distal femoral bone loss, as measured from the epicondyles, more distal femoral augmentation probably will be required. Physical examination can provide information on the likely relative sizes of the flexion and extension gaps. If the knee is loose in flexion but tight in extension (as evidenced by a flexion contracture), the flexion gap probably will be larger than the extension gap. Likewise, if the knee hyperextends, is lax in extension, or has an extension contracture, then the extension gap may be larger than the flexion gap. Understanding the probable relative sizes of flexion and extension gaps in advance allows the surgeon to consider the measures that will be required to equalize the gaps.

Stability and Ligament Defects

Information obtained by history and the physical examination is important to solve ligament problems. Successful management of ligament problems falls into several categories.

1. Optimization of the limb and implant alignment: This requires viewing long, standing hip-to-ankle films to determine the optimal tibial femoral angle (and thus the angle of the distal femur cut). If the knee has medial ligament insufficiency, make sure not to leave the mechanical axis of the knee lateral to the center of the knee; if the knee has lateral ligament insufficiency, make sure not to leave the mechanical axis medial to the center of the knee.

2. Implant constraint level: For revision TKA, different levels of constraint are needed for different problems. The general tenet is to use the least constraint necessary to solve the problem effectively. Although excessively constrained implants are not desirable, providing a marginally adequate level of constraint often is not in the patient's best interest, particularly if the patient is elderly and cannot tolerate repetitive procedures. Most situations of moderate ligament laxity can be treated with release of tight ligaments coupled with tensioning of loose ligaments. When these measures are not sufficient, use of constrained condylar implants generally can solve the problem. Infrequently, profound ligament deficiency or failure of previous procedures to stabilize an unstable knee requires the use of rotating hinge implants.

Extensor Mechanism

Good function of the extensor mechanism is important for the overall function of the knee.

Determine from physical examination if the extensor mechanism is intact. If it is grossly deficient, consider whether revision TKA is appropriate. Alternatives include external bracing or knee arthrodesis. If revision TKA is deemed appropriate, extensor mechanism reconstruction will be necessary, either with autogenous tissue augmentation (such as with semitendinosus and gracilis tendon) or with an extensor mechanism allograft (12) (either an Achilles tendon allograft with a bone block or a bone–patellar tendon–patella quadriceps tendon allograft). Due to their specialized nature, such allograft materials usually need to be ordered in advance, even in hospitals with a standard bone bank.

Consider how the patella will be managed. Well-functioning patellar implants usually should be preserved. Most dome-shaped patellar components do not need to be removed—even if the new tibial and femoral implants being placed are from a different manufacturer—because the small incongruences that arise from intermanufacturer implant geometry differences usually do not justify the risks of patellar revision. If the patellar implant is loose, determine if sufficient bone remains for patellar reimplantation. When the bone appears too deficient to consider reimplantation, consider other options for patellar management: resection arthroplasty with patelloplasty or impaction grafting of the patella.

Review the patellar skyline radiographs and consider whether efforts to improve patellar or extensor mechanism tracking will be needed.

Closure

Anticipate whether closure is likely to be problematic. Most commonly, wound closure is problematic when patients have extremely woody tissue, a foreshortened limb that will be lengthened (such as one with a long-standing resection arthroplasty), or a limb with a great deal of deformity. Preoperative evaluation by a plastic surgeon can be helpful in these circumstances.

POSTOPERATIVE ISSUES

Venous Thromboembolic Disease

Preoperatively, consider whether the patient is at high risk for postoperative venous thromboembolism. For patients at especially high risk consider a preoperative vascular medicine consultation. Determine in advance the plan for postoperative venous thromboembolism prophylaxis.

Medical Issues

Determine whether special medical problems require special medical management after surgery. Patients with major medical problems and patients anticipated to have extremely large operations may require a postoperative intensive care unit bed, which may be arranged in advance. Make preoperative arrangements to have specific postoperative consultations and support from cardiology, pulmonary, or other groups if the patient has major medical problems in these areas.

Pain Management

Consider whether special pain management measures will be needed postoperatively. Discussion with the anesthesia team before the operation can be helpful, and sometimes epidural blocks, lumbar psoas blocks, or femoral nerve blocks can be used.

Dismissal Plan

Before surgery, discuss the plan for care after the hospitalization with the patient and patient's family. Determine the level of support available in the patient's own home. If the patient will require help beyond that available at home, arrange for a bed in a rehabilitation facility. Securing a bed in advance can optimize the postoperative recovery environment.

REFERENCES

1. Duff G, Lachiewicz P, Kelley S. Aspiration of the knee joint before revision arthroplasty. *Clin Orthop* 1996;331:132.
2. Windsor R, Bono J. Infected total knee replacements. *J Am Acad Orthop Surg* 1994;2:44.
3. Patel DV, Ferrus BD, Aichroth PM. Radiological study of alignment after total knee replacement: short radiographs or long radiographs? *Int Orthop* 1991;15:209.
4. Petersen TL, Engh GA. Radiographic assessment of knee alignment after total knee arthroplasty. *J Arthroplasty* 1988;3:67–72.

5. Berger RA, Crossett LS, Jacobs JJ, et al. Malrotation causing patellofemoral complications after total knee arthroplasty. *Clin Orthop* 1998;356:144–153.

6. Rush JH, Vidovich JD, Johnson MA. Arterial complications of total knee replacement: the Australian experience. *J Bone Joint Surg Br* 1987;69:400.

7. Asp JPL, Rand JA. Peroneal nerve palsy after total knee arthroplasty. *Clin Orthop* 1990;261:233.

8. Caillouette JT, Gorab RS, Klapper RC, et al. Revision arthroplasty facilitated by ultrasonic tool cement removal. *Orthop Rev* 1991;20:353–440.

9. Klapper RC, Caillouette JT. The use of ultrasonic tools in revision arthroplasty procedures. *Contemp Orthop* 1990;20:273–279.

10. Klapper RC, Caillouette JT, Callaghan JJ, et al. Ultrasonic technology in revision joint arthroplasty. *Clin Orthop* 1992;285:147–154.

11. Berry DJ. Component removal during revision total knee arthroplasty. In: Lotke PA, Garino JP, eds. *Revision total knee arthroplasty*. Philadelphia: Lippincott–Raven Publishers, 1998.

12. Emerson RH Jr, Head WC, Malinin TI. Reconstruction patellar tendon rupture after total knee arthroplasty with an extensor mechanism allograft. *Clin Orthop* 1990;260:154.

Hinged Knee Replacement*

Mary I. O'Connor

Hinged knee arthroplasty was first introduced in the 1950s (1,2). The hinged type of implant permitted management of more significant deformity than was possible with other designs of the time such as femoral condyle implants, tibial plates, and unicondylar plates. Failure rates, however, were high with the initial hinge designs. More successful condylar resurfacing implants were developed, and the use of hinged implants dramatically declined. Currently, hinged implants are used most frequently in reconstruction of a skeletal defect after bone sarcoma resection and in a few selected patients without tumors. Contemporary designs and surgical technique have improved results associated with the use of hinged implants. This chapter reviews the evolution and clinical results of the various types of hinged prostheses, as well as indications and surgical considerations for hinged knee arthroplasty.

EVOLUTION AND CLINICAL RESULTS OF HINGED KNEE PROSTHESES

Clinical data regarding hinged prostheses should be interpreted with caution. Because of improvements in implant design, surgical technique, and patient selection, results with early fixed-hinge designs do not reflect current outcomes. Furthermore, many reports of hinged implant arthroplasties included results of combined analyses of both primary and revision procedures, with large variation among patients in bone loss, soft tissue compromise, and number of previous operations.

Fixed-Hinge Designs

Initial hinged knee implants were metal-on-metal articulations with a fixed hinge that permitted motion only in flexion and extension. Significant bone resection was required for implantation (3). Such implants included the Walldius (1) and the Shiers (2) prostheses. In the 1970s, the Stanmore (4) and the Guepar (4) all-metal fixed-hinge implants were also introduced.

Results with early metal-on-metal fixed-hinge implants were poor (5–7). In 1986, data from the Swedish arthroplasty registry showed that the 5- to 6-year survival rate of fixed-hinge knee implants for primary knee arthroplasty in osteoarthritic knees was only 65% compared to 87% for the two- or three-compartment designs used at that time (8). Results for patients with rheumatoid arthritis were more favorable, however; in such patients, the 5- to 6-year survival rate of the hinge implant was 83% compared to 90% for two- or three-compartment prostheses. Failures were due to loosening, infection, fracture, or patellar pain.

Many of the failures were a result of poor implant design. The single nonanatomic fixed axis was load bearing and transmitted stress to the bone-cement interface, which facilitated loosening. The intramedullary stems filled large canals poorly, which resulted in subsidence. Stem fracture also occurred (9), a problem rarely seen with current implants. Patellar resurfacing was not performed, and the trochlear groove of the femoral component was flat. Postoperative effusions occurred in as many as 48% of knees (10). Analysis of synovial fluid in patients with hinged metal-on-metal implants showed high concentrations of metal debris (11), which may cause synovitis and osteolysis.

Even with modification of the metal-on-metal fixed Guepar hinge to include longer stem lengths, results were disappointing. At follow-up of 2 to 13 years in 45 patients with the Guepar II implant, Cameron et al. (12) reported an aseptic loosening rate of only 7%, which they attributed to longer stem lengths and

*Portions of this chapter are from O'Connor M. Linked or hinged total knee arthroplasty. In: Rosenberg AA, ed. *The arthritic knee.* Rosemont, IL: American Academy of Orthopaedic Surgeons, 2000.

improved cementing technique. The percentage of good to excellent results, however, had declined to 38% from an earlier report of 67% at 1 to 7 years of follow-up (13), and extensor mechanism problems and infection continued to be troublesome.

Poor results with metal-on-metal fixed hinges led to redesign of the Stanmore implant to include metal-polyethylene bushings to articulate with the metal implant. In a series of 103 cases in which Stanmore implants were used for both primary and revision procedures, Grimer et al. (14) reported 80% prosthetic retention at an average follow-up of 68 months; only 64% of patients were enthusiastic about their knee implants, and 70% were free of pain. Since then, the Stanmore implant has been further modified to a rotating hinge with metal-on-plastic bearing surfaces.

In Germany, Blauth and Hassenpflug (3) introduced a fixed-hinge implant with interposed polyethylene components that conform to the larger condylar surfaces of the femoral implant. The purpose of this design is to transfer the constrained forces through these large surfaces to adjacent bone and away from the hinge. Some gliding motion is possible, and the patella can be resurfaced. For 422 primary knee arthroplasties in 330 patients with a mean follow-up of 6 years (range, 0 to 20 years), the cumulative rate of implant survival at 20 years was 87% for a worst-case definition of failure, including removal, infection, and patients lost to follow-up (15). The incidence of deep infection was 3.8%; three patients developed aseptic loosening, and four sustained patellar fractures. The Blauth implant remains in use today in Europe.

Rotating-Hinge Designs

Development

Because of concerns about the contribution of a fixed axis of rotation to poor results, implants with rotation about axes other than flexion and extension were developed. Early designs included the spherocentric (16), Sheehan (17), and Herbert (18) knee implants.

The first Noiles rotary-hinge arthroplasty was performed in 1976 (19). Unlike a fixed-hinge implant, this design incorporated a tibia-bearing component that fit into a cemented polyethylene tibial component. The tibia-bearing component was then fixed between the flanges of the femoral component by the axle. The tibia-bearing component could rotate within the cemented polyethylene tibial component up to 20 degrees from neutral without significant prosthetic resistance. Some axial distraction of the tibia-bearing component within the cemented polyethylene component was also possible (19). In theory, permitting rotation and axial distraction would reduce stress at the bone-cement interface (19). Subsequently, several modifications were made, including redesign of the femoral component to a condylar-type implant to prevent subsidence of the femoral component (20,21).

The Noiles rotating-hinge articulation was incorporated by Walker et al. (22) in the Kinematic rotating-hinge implant introduced for clinical use in 1978. Implant modifications have occurred over the years, and the Kinematic rotating-hinge knee system is currently in use in the United States. Other rotating-hinge knee implant systems currently available include the S-ROM Noiles rotating knee system, the Link Endo-Model rotating-hinge knee implant, the Segmental Oncology System (Wright Medical Technology, Arlington, TN), and the Finn Knee.

Clinical Results

In the late 1980s, clinical results with rotating-hinge implants for nonneoplastic indications were variable. Two studies of the use of the Kinematic rotating-hinge implant for treatment of significant ligamentous instability, loss of bone, or both reported satisfactory results in 80% of patients with a primary procedure (23,24) and in 61% (24) to 74% (23) of patients with revision surgery at a mean follow-up of approximately 50 months. Probable loosening observed on radiography was a concern in 10% of knees in one study (23). Progression of radiolucent lines occurred in 26% of knees in that study (23) and in 7% after primary and 20% after revision procedures in the other study (24). The most common complication was instability of the nonresurfaced patella, which occurred in approximately 22% of primary arthroplasties (23,24) and 36% of revision procedures (24). With subsequent improved implant design, resurfacing of the patella, and improved attention to component positioning, patellar complications significantly diminished.

As nonhinged implant systems evolved to include more constrained designs applicable to most cases of ligamentous instability and nonmassive bone loss, use of rotating-hinge implants became much more selective. At Mayo Clinic in Rochester, Minnesota, only 188 (0.01%) of the 15,798 primary and 2,673 revision knee arthroplasty procedures performed between 1980 and 1998 used Kinematic rotating-hinge knee replacements (25). Of these 188 replacements, 111 were for reconstruction after bone tumor resection, and only 69 were for nonneoplastic conditions (severe bone loss, ligamentous instability, acute or nonunited periprosthetic fractures, or combinations thereof). Of the 69 patients with nonneoplastic conditions, 43 received a standard Kinematic rotating-hinge implant, and 26 patients with more extensive bone loss received a modular segmental implant. At mean follow-up of 75 months (range, 24 to 199 months), Knee Society scores improved from a preoperative score of 40.3 to a postoperative value of 77. Complications in these complex cases were numerous (32% of patients) and included deep infection (14.5%), patellar complications (13%), and prosthetic component breakage (10%). At final follow-up, nine patients (13%) had definite loosening of the tibial or femoral component, or both. The authors concluded that this procedure should be reserved as a final salvage option in these difficult cases.

Use of Rotating-Hinge Implants in Revision

Contemporary use of rotating-hinge implants has been predominantly in revision cases. Lombardi et al. (26) reported on a large series in which the Link Endo-Model rotating-hinge implant was used for revision knee arthroplasty; 113 implants were performed for aseptic loosening, periprosthetic supracondylar femur fracture, septic failure, or instability. Allografts were also used, but the type and numbers were not detailed. At early follow-up of 25 months, results were excellent in 16% of cases, good in 51%, fair in 23%, and poor in 10%. Postoperative flexion averaged 95 degrees, and nonprogressive radiolucent lines were noted in 12% of cases. Complications included allograft failure with femoral component loosening (5%), superficial infection (3%), deep infection (2%; these patients had prior infection), femoral-tibial dislocation (2%), patellar fracture (2%), and patellar subluxation (1%). The authors attribute the relatively high rate of complications to the significant deformity and ligamentous instability present in these patients.

The S-ROM Noiles rotating-hinge knee system has also been used in complex revision cases. In 2000, Barrack et al. (27) reported on 14 revisions with 2- to 6-year follow-up in patients considered to be salvage candidates because of multiple previous operations and the need for associated procedures such as structural allografts, creation of muscle flaps, and extensor mechanism reconstructions. The S-ROM implant was selected because the system's modular metaphyseal sleeves were able to fill large intramedullary defects, which were frequent in this series because of failure of previous hinged implants. Results showed improvement in the Knee Society clinical score from a preoperative mean of 41 to a postoperative mean of 131. Knee range of motion improved from a preoperative mean of 78 degrees to a postoperative mean of 93 degrees. No patient had progressive radiolucency, and all patients but one were satisfied with the outcome of the procedure. Complications included one intraoperative femur fracture treated with cable fixation, one patellar instability requiring further surgery, one peroneal nerve palsy, and one incident of slight backing-out of the axle component, which required no intervention. The authors noted that, although further follow-up is needed, clinical and radiographic results were encouraging in these difficult salvage cases.

Jones et al. (28) also noted significant improvement in function after knee arthroplasty using the S-ROM rotating hinge for severe bone loss and instability (15 revisions and one primary procedure, with a minimum of 2 years of follow-up). Knee Society scores for pain, motion, and stability improved from 33.6 preoperatively to 76.5 postoperatively, with no evidence of loosening. Mean knee range of motion was 2 to 84 degrees preoperatively and 2 to 105 degrees postoperatively. Complications included two intraoperative fractures, one recurrent infection, and one postoperative traumatic quadriceps tendon rupture. In this system, the modular metaphyseal sleeves transfer stress from deficient to intact bone. In addition, the authors noted that benefits of this implant system included a more anatomic femoral groove, fluted stems to enhance rotational stability, improved contact area between the femoral and tibial components, and load bearing across both the rotating hinge and the polyethylene tibia-bearing surface.

Megaprostheses

Rotating-hinge articulations are commonly used in implants designed for reconstruction after resection of bone tumors about the knee when marked loss of ligamentous structures has occurred. Such implants are designed to replace the resected large bone segment (e.g., distal femur) and are referred to as *megaprostheses*. Megaprostheses have evolved from nonmodular implants to segmental modular systems with a porous coating at the shoulder of the implant to encourage extracortical bone bridging between the remaining host metadiaphyseal bone and the adjacent portion of the implant. Ward et al. (29) postulated that firm attachment of bone or soft tissue to such a porous coating may retard osteolysis by preventing implant-debris-containing synovial fluid from contacting the bone-prosthesis or bone-cement interface. Modularity of current systems allows for intraoperative determination of appropriate length of the replacement implant.

In 1991, Finn et al. (30) reported on a modification of the rotating-hinge megaprosthesis, which sought to improve patellofemoral kinematics and distribution of weightbearing forces. The femoral component was anatomically designed and reduced in size (to assist with soft tissue closure). The patellar groove was deepened, the center of rotation was anatomically located, and congruent polyethylene was placed between the femoral and tibial components to distribute weight throughout the entire femoral component and not just the axle. A report of preliminary results described aseptic loosening in 3 and patellar complications in 2 of 44 patients at a median of 35 months of follow-up (31). Since the introduction of the Finn knee prosthesis, the femoral components of the Kinematic rotating-hinge implant and other designs have been modified or made smaller, and patellar tracking has been improved.

Several authors have reported results at intermediate follow-up for implantation of megaprostheses after distal femoral resection, and outcomes are influenced by implant design. Early Stanmore fixed-hinge prostheses had a 10-year probability of implant survival of 68% (168 patients) (32). Studies of cemented Kinematic rotating-hinge megaprostheses reported better results. Choong et al. (33) reported 90% implant survival for megaprostheses at 5 years (30 patients), with two-thirds of patients having good or excellent function and flexion of more than 120 degrees. Ward et al. (34) showed 83% implant survival at 6 years (48 patients; 44 with Kinematic and four with Noiles S-ROM rotating-hinge implants).

Problems with rotating-hinge megaprostheses were primarily related to aseptic loosening or extensor mechanism dysfunction. Ward et al. (34) identified greater body weight and lesser knee range of motion as predictors of failure in their series, in which revision was performed in seven of the eight patients with definite radiolucent lines (more than 1 mm). Choong et al. (33) reported nine complications occurring in seven patients, including patellar problems in four, periprosthetic femur fracture in two, aseptic femoral loosening after trauma in one, wound infection in one, and temporary peroneal nerve palsy in one. Four femoral revisions, one patellar revision, and one débridement were required for management of these complications. Because of the patellar complications encountered and the lack of functional difference between patients who had resurfacing of the patella and those who did not, Choong et al. (33) recommended only selective patellar resurfacing.

Megaprostheses have also been used in a press-fit application. Kawai et al. (35) reported 2- to 7-year results with the Finn rotating-hinge knee replacement modified to accept a press-fit application used after resection of the distal femur in 25 patients and of the proximal tibia in seven patients. Unlike in the series reported by Choong et al. (33) and Ward et al. (34), the majority of stems were press-fit. Prosthetic survival at 5 years was 88% for distal femoral replacements but only 58% for proximal tibial replacements. The Hospital for Special Surgery knee score ranged from 64 to 98 (median, 80). Further surgical treatment was required for wound problems or infection (four patients), aseptic femoral loosening (one patient), and articulating component failures (four patients, including two with broken tibial yokes). The tibial yoke component was subsequently thickened, and no further component failures were reported.

The degree of development of extracortical bone bridging at the host bone-megaprosthesis junction has been variable. Choong et al. (33) reported extracortical bone bridging of greater than 25% in 18 of 27 patients with use of a porous-coated implant and bone graft applied at the junction. Kawai et al. (35) also reported variable bone formation in 30 patients but found that, when extracortical bone bridging did occur, function was better. Further studies of extracortical bone bridging are needed, particularly with regard to implant longevity and risk of aseptic loosening. The author of the present paper routinely places allograft and bone substitute materials at the junction of the porous coating and host bone to encourage the formation of extracortical bone bridging.

The extent of bone loss appears to influence implant survival in megaprostheses. In a 1994 study in which 493 distal femoral and 245 proximal tibial Stanmore hinged megaprostheses were implanted, Cobb et al. (36) reported 94% survival of the implant at 10 years with distal resection of less than 40% of the femur, compared to 49% survival with resection of more than 40%. Five-year implant survival for proximal tibial replacements was 100% if less than 40% of the tibia was resected, compared to 83% survival if more than 40% was removed. The authors concluded that "less is more" and that the least amount of bone that provides an adequate tumor margin should be resected. Ward et al. (34) reported on the addition of a cemented interlocking pin through the femoral stem and into the femoral head and neck in patients with extensive resection of the distal and mid femur. This addition augmented fixation in patients who had less than 4 in. of retained diaphysis below the lesser trochanter.

In Vivo *Kinematic Studies*

In vivo investigations of rotating-hinge implants have studied gait, stair stepping, torsional stiffness, and rotational laxity. Draganich et al. (37) investigated the effect of the use of a Finn rotating-hinge knee implant on gait and stair stepping. At a minimum of 1 year of follow-up after surgery, all patients had excellent clinical results. Older patients with a rotating-hinge prosthesis showed significantly different results compared to older controls without arthroplasty and to patients undergoing semiconstrained posterior cruciate–retaining knee arthroplasties. Nevertheless, these older patients were able to complete the evaluated tasks nearly as well as the patients given semiconstrained prostheses. Older patients walked with a stiff-legged gait, apparently locking their knees in full extension at heel strike through midstance. This action would decrease demand on the extensor mechanism. The authors suggested that patients might be compensating for a compromised extensor mechanism. When stepping on a step, older patients placed their feet in an externally rotated position, and this was attributed to the loss of collateral ligaments. The patients tended to externally rotate their bodies as well, which may have reduced torque on the knee and decreased stress at the implant-cement or implant-bone interface. In contrast, younger patients demonstrated gait and stair stepping similar to that of normal controls. External rotation during stair stepping was much less likely than in older patients. The authors suggested that this might have been related to overall better muscle control in young adults.

Kabo et al. (38) reported on *in vivo* rotational stability of the Kinematic rotating-hinge tumor prosthesis after resection of the distal femur. Patients underwent follow-up examinations at a minimum of 1 year after surgery, and their contralateral knee served as the control. Twenty patients were studied, with nine tested at year 1, ten at year 2, and ten at year 3. The authors concluded that, despite the small number of patients, the preliminary results demonstrated the natural course of torsional stiffness and rotatory laxity of the knee with the rotating-hinge implant. The total laxity of the knee was greater than that of the control knee at years 2 and 3, with the peak at year 2. At year 1, the operated knee had 30% less torsional stiffness in external

rotation than the control knee but recovered to normal at year 3. The authors noted that residual soft tissue plays an important role in preventing excessive *in vivo* axial rotation and that strength maturation of the periprosthetic scar may take 2 years. Rotatory laxity and torsional stiffness during the first 3 years did not correlate with subsequent aseptic loosening.

Infections in Hinged Knee Implants

As noted in these clinical series, complications may be significant. Historically, hinged knee implants have been associated with a high rate of infection. In 1980, Hui and Fitzgerald (6) noted an 11.7% rate of infection in 77 patients with fixed Guepar or Walldius implants. Of the nine patients with deep infection, seven had had previous surgery and three had distal wound breakdown. The authors believed that the resultant scarring and poorly vascularized tissue had predisposed these patients to infection. In 1987, Karpinski and Grimer (39) reported a lower infection rate of only 3.8% at an average follow-up of 44.7 months for 52 Stanmore implants used in revision arthroplasty. Reviewing 15 series, with implantation of 3,245 hinged prostheses, Böhm and Holy (15) noted an overall infection rate of 5.7% (range, 2.9% to 23.0%) compared with an overall infection rate of 1.6% (range, 0% to 6.3%) in 20 series, with implantation of 7,944 bicompartmental and tricompartmental prostheses. These authors suggested that the real risk factor associated with the higher incidence of infection might be the amount of implanted foreign material and not the degree of constraint.

For procedures involving megaprostheses currently used for limb salvage reconstruction after tumor resection about the knee, infections were reported in 1 of 32 patients (3%) in one study (33), in 2 of 32 (6%) patients in a second study (35), and in 4 of 48 patients (8%) in a third study (34). Bell (40) suggested that the decreasing infection rates may reflect a learning curve for arthroplasty surgeons. Current surgical technique is now more refined, and management of soft tissues has improved with the use of muscle flaps and, in particularly challenging cases, preoperative tissue expanders (41).

Revision of Hinged Knee Arthroplasty

Revision of failed hinged knee arthroplasties is challenging because of loss of bone and functional soft tissues. As a result of the generous bone resection required for placement of the original hinge, significant structural bone compromise is common in the revision setting. A segmental implant may be required for revision of a failed resurfacing hinged prosthesis (42). Furthermore, revision of a failed fixed-hinge implant to another fixed-hinge implant is not likely to be successful (32,42,43), and a rotating-hinge device should be considered.

Revision of a failed hinged prosthesis with a rotating-hinge implant has been reported in patients treated for neoplasms. In 1999, reviewing only patients who received implants after tumor resection and were followed for an average of 48 months (minimum of 2 years or until death), Wirganowicz et al. (44) reported on 42 failures in 136 distal femoral megaprostheses and 7 failures in 27 proximal tibial implants. Failure was most frequently due to aseptic loosening and was more likely in men and in patients younger than 26 years of age at either initial surgery or revision. Revision of the 42 distal femoral failures resulted in further revision surgery because of loosening in four patients and amputation in two patients (due to infection in one and local tumor recurrence in the other). Mechanical failure was the cause in some of these cases. Initial implants were cast stems, but current stems are now forged, which is beneficial in preventing metal-fatigue fractures. The authors noted that function was only slightly lower after revision than after the primary procedure. The risk of failure was no greater for the revision than for the primary reconstruction.

Revision of a failed hinged prosthesis using a nonhinged implant may be considered in selected patients. Kim (45) reported good results at 2 to 6 years after revision of 14 failed Guepar or Walldius hinged implants to Total Condylar III prostheses (Johnson & Johnson, Raynham, MA). Twelve of the 14 knees, however, were stable preoperatively. Preoperative patellar subluxation was problematic, and all patients required a lateral release for patellar realignment. Radiolucent lines were incomplete and less than 1 mm in 13 of the 14 patients. The author noted no failure but recommended further follow-up.

The ability to successfully revise a failed hinged prosthesis with a constrained but nonhinged implant may be dictated by the soft tissues. In five patients with failed hinged implants and severe distal femoral bone loss, Krackow and Mihalko (46) observed that the tibia would "fall away" from the femur in flexion (enlarged flexion gap) yet maintain a normal relationship to the femur in extension. They hypothesized that distraction of the tibia from the femur in flexion was due to loss of collateral ligaments and posterior capsule but that the intact posterior structures (gastrocnemius and hamstring muscles, fascial planes, skin, etc.) would prevent such distraction in extension. They investigated this further in a cadaveric study. With loss of the collateral ligaments, the flexion gap at 90 degrees was 17.2 mm, but the joint space in extension was preserved at 1.5 mm. With additional loss of the posterior capsule, the corresponding flexion gap was 26.2 mm, but the extension gap was only 3.4 mm. The authors concluded that severe distal femoral bone loss increased the flexion gap more than the extension gap.

INDICATIONS FOR HINGED KNEE ARTHROPLASTY

Fixed-Hinge Knee Arthroplasty

In the author's opinion, there are currently no indications for use of a fixed-hinge knee arthroplasty, with the exception of a fixed-hinge prosthesis permitting nonoperative lengthening (Repiphysis), which is used in young patients who have undergone bone sarcoma resection with a significant anticipated discrepancy in leg length.

Rotating-Hinge Knee Arthroplasty

Indications for use of a rotating-hinge prosthesis are varied. The reconstructive decision must be individualized to each patient, and multiple indications may be applicable to a given patient.

Reconstruction after Resection of the Distal Femur

Segmental modular rotating-hinge knee systems (megaprostheses) are particularly appropriate for patients who will receive post-

operative chemotherapy. Use of a structural allograft combined with a nonhinged constrained prosthesis still exposes the patient to some risk, albeit extremely low, of disease transmission associated with the allograft. Healing of the allograft to the host bone is necessary for long-term success of the reconstruction, and factors that would negatively influence bone healing (e.g., chemotherapy and radiation therapy) support use of a megaprosthesis. Although several clinical series report satisfactory early to intermediate results with use of large structural allografts combined with nonhinged prostheses in patients with severe bone loss about the knee (47–49), the concept of using a structural allograft to restore bone stock is limited. Only a small amount of remodeling of the allograft to living bone occurs over time (50), but resorption of the allograft can occur and result in weakening of the construct (51).

Reconstruction after Resection of the Proximal Tibia

Currently, effective soft tissue attachment to a megaprosthesis cannot always be achieved. Thus, after resections that are distal to the tibial tubercle, use of an allograft combined with a nonhinged implant may be considered. Use of an allograft-prosthesis composite may permit more effective healing of the host extensor mechanism to the proximal tibial reconstruction. In patients with risk factors that would negatively influence bone healing, however, a megaprosthesis should be considered, and specialized soft tissue procedures should be used to augment active knee extension. If solutions to the problem of tendon attachment to prostheses become available, megaprostheses may become the preferred method of reconstruction after proximal tibial resections.

Extensive Bone Loss

Extensive bone loss may result from trauma and failed arthroplasty. In such cases, metal augmentation on femoral and tibial components may be inadequate, and a choice must be made between a structural allograft combined with a standard prosthesis and a rotating-hinge implant or megaprosthesis.

Severe Varus or Valgus Ligamentous Instability

As the degree of constraint increased in many condylar-type prosthetic systems, the use of rotating-hinge prostheses for ligamentous instability decreased. Nonetheless, patients with severe ligamentous imbalance—particularly chronic, complete medial collateral ligament compromise—are potential candidates for a rotating-hinge implant (12,26,27,52). Intraoperative disruption of the medial collateral ligament during total knee arthroplasty can be treated successfully with repair or reattachment to bone (53). Complete absence of any lateralizing structure resulting in lateral rotatory instability may also be a factor favoring a hinged articulation (12).

Severe Malalignment

Severe malalignment is often associated with ligamentous imbalance, and correction of the deformity may require extensive soft tissue release and hence consideration of a rotating-hinge implant (Fig. 1) (28).

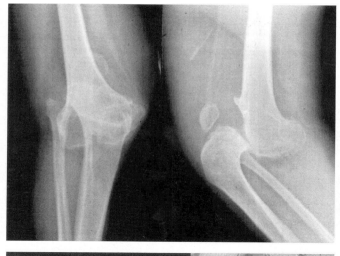

A,B

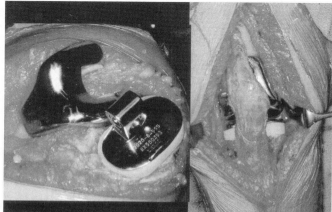

C,D

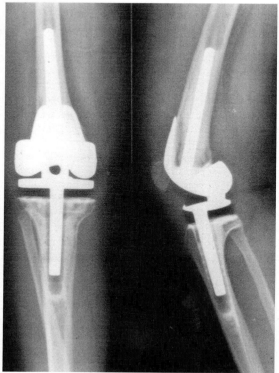

E,F

FIG. 1. Congenital knee dislocation in a 54-year-old woman with severe pain due to arthritic change. **A, B:** Anteroposterior and lateral radiographs before surgery. **C:** Intraoperative photograph of rotating-hinge arthroplasty before articulation of components and placement of axle pin and polyethylene (extensor) bumper. **D:** Intraoperative photograph of articulated rotating-hinge arthroplasty with centered extensor mechanism. **E, F:** Anteroposterior and lateral radiographs at 5-year follow-up. Patient had good clinical function. (**E** and **F** from Springer BD, Hanssen AD, Sim FH, et al. The Kinematic rotating hinge prosthesis for complex knee arthroplasty. *Clin Orthop* 2001;392:283–291, with permission.)

Extreme Imbalance of the Flexion-Extension Gap

Use of metal augmentation and a polyethylene insert of maximum thickness can compensate for a maximum flexion-extension gap of 4 cm (54). Flexion-extension imbalance beyond this requires use of a structural allograft or consideration of a rotating-hinge implant.

Absence of a Functional Extensor Mechanism

With loss of the extensor mechanism, the anteroposterior stability of the knee is markedly compromised and use of a hinged component should be considered (12).

Management of Certain Fractures

Periprosthetic fractures in elderly patients with osteoporotic bone, failed internal fixation of periprosthetic fractures in elderly patients, and acute pathologic fractures with significant neoplas-

tic bone destruction (particularly when goals of immediate weightbearing and range of motion are important) are all situations in which consideration of a rotating-hinge arthroplasty is appropriate (Fig. 2).

Revision of Previous Hinged Knee Arthroplasty

Patients with a failed hinged-knee arthroplasty typically require revision with another hinged prosthesis (28). Selected patients may be candidates for revision with a highly constrained nonhinged implant (45).

Neurologic Disorders

In patients with neurologic problems that result in stretched capsular and ligamentous tissues (e.g., poliomyelitis), resurfacing arthroplasties may fail because further compromise of these soft tissues may occur with time. In such cases, consideration of a rotating-hinge implant is appropriate (13).

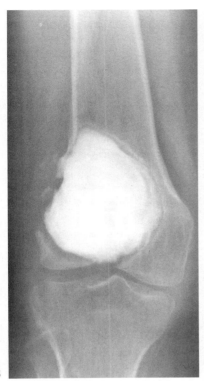
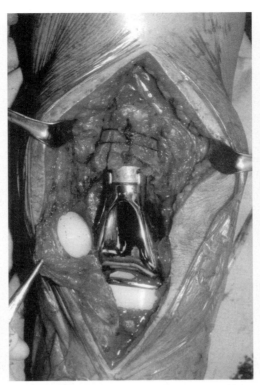
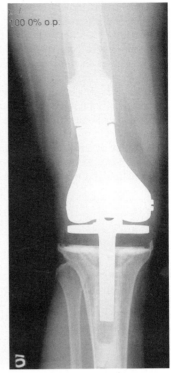

A,B

D

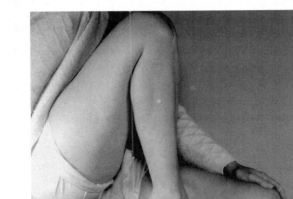

C

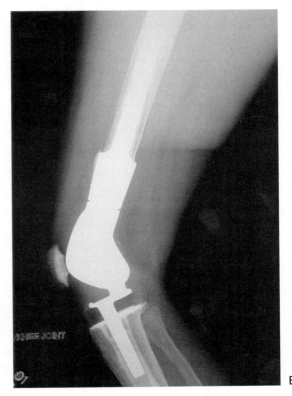

E

FIG. 2. The patient was a 54-year-old woman with an intercondy-lar fracture and a history of a giant cell tumor of the distal femur treated with cementation. **A:** Radiograph showing area of cementation and fracture. Severe loss of bone necessitated use of a distal femoral replacement implant. **B:** Intraoperative photograph showing distal femoral replacement implant. **C:** Clinical photograph of knee flexion 2 years after surgery. Anteroposterior **(D)** and lateral **(E)** radiographs of implant at 9-year follow-up. The patient continues to enjoy active range of motion of 0 to 140 degrees with no pain and no evidence of implant loosening or tumor recurrence. As instructed by her surgeon, she does use a cane for extended walking.

Technical Pearls

- There are currently very limited indications for use of a fixed-hinge knee implant.
- The decision to use a rotating-hinge prosthesis for reconstruction must be individualized to each patient.

- Indications for use of a rotating-hinge prosthesis include reconstruction after resection of the distal femur or proximal tibia, extensive bone loss, severe varus or valgus ligamentous instability, severe malalignment, extreme imbalance of the flexion-extension gap, absence of a functional extensor mechanism, management of certain fractures, revision of previous hinged-knee arthroplasty, and neurologic disorders that result in stretched capsular and ligamentous tissues.

- Particular attention should be directed to proper rotational positioning of components and balancing of the extension mechanism to minimize related postoperative complications.
- With use of a modular megaprosthesis, selection of a smaller distal femoral body component may assist with soft tissue closure and decrease the need for muscle flap coverage.
- With use of a megaprosthesis an attempt should be made to achieve extracortical bone bridging between the implant and host bone because this may improve implant survival.

CONCLUSION

Rotating-hinge knee arthroplasty still has a place in the armamentarium of the reconstructive knee surgeon. In some patients, a hinged implant may be the only alternative to arthrodesis or amputation. Satisfactory results may be achieved in these challenging cases.

REFERENCES

1. Walldius B. Arthroplasty of the knee using an endoprosthesis. Eight years' experience. *Acta Orthop Scand* 1960;30:137–140.
2. Shiers LGP. Arthroplasty of the knee: preliminary report of a new method. *J Bone Joint Surg Br* 1954;36:553–560.
3. Blauth W, Hassenpflug J. Are unconstrained components essential in total knee arthroplasty? Long-term results of the Blauth knee prosthesis. *Clin Orthop* 1990;258:86–94.
4. Lettin AW, Deliss LJ, Blackburne JS, et al. The Stanmore hinged knee arthroplasty. *J Bone Joint Surg Br* 1978;60:327–332.
5. Deburge A, GUEPAR. Guepar hinge prosthesis: complications and results with two years' follow-up. *Clin Orthop* 1976;120:47–53.
6. Hui FC, Fitzgerald RH Jr. Hinged total knee arthroplasty. *J Bone Joint Surg Am* 1980;62:513–519.
7. Hoikka V, Vankka E, Eskola A, et al. Results and complications after arthroplasty with a totally constrained total knee prosthesis (GUEPAR). *Ann Chir Gynaecol* 1989;78:94–96.
8. Knutson K, Lindstrand A, Lidgren L. Survival of knee arthroplasties. A nation-wide multicentre investigation of 8000 cases. *J Bone Joint Surg Br* 1986;68:795–803.
9. Jones EC, Insall JN, Inglis AE, et al. GUEPAR knee arthroplasty: results and late complications. *Clin Orthop* 1979;140:145–152.
10. Bargar WL, Cracchiolo A III, Amstutz HC. Results with the constrained total knee prosthesis in treating severely disabled patients and patients with failed total knee replacements. *J Bone Joint Surg Am* 1980;62:504–512.
11. Cracchiolo A III, Revell P. Metal concentration in synovial fluids of patients with prosthetic knee arthroplasty. *Clin Orthop* 1982;170:169–174.
12. Cameron HU, Hu C, Vyamont D. Hinge total knee replacement revisited. *Can J Surg* 1997;40:278–283.
13. Cameron HU, Jung YB. Hinged total knee replacement: indications and results. *Can J Surg* 1990;33:53–57.
14. Grimer RJ, Karpinski MR, Edwards AN. The long-term results of Stanmore total knee replacements. *J Bone Joint Surg Br* 1984;66:55–62.
15. Böhm P, Holy T. Is there a future for hinged prostheses in primary total knee arthroplasty? A 20-year survivorship analysis of the Blauth prosthesis. *J Bone Joint Surg Br* 1998;80:302–309.
16. Kaufer H, Matthews LS. Spherocentric knee arthroplasty. *Clin Orthop* 1979;145:110–116.
17. Sheehan JM. Arthroplasty of the knee. *J Bone Joint Surg Br* 1978;60:333–338.
18. Murray DG, Wilde AH, Werner F, et al. Herbert total knee prosthesis: combined laboratory and clinical assessment. *J Bone Joint Surg Am* 1977;59:1026–1032.
19. Accardo NJ, Noiles DG, Pena R. Noiles total knee replacement procedure. *Orthopedics* 1979;2:37–45.
20. Kester MA, Cook SD, Harding AF, et al. An evaluation of the mechanical failure modalities of a rotating hinge knee prosthesis. *Clin Orthop* 1988;228:156–163.
21. Shindell R, Neumann R, Connolly JF, et al. Evaluation of the Noiles hinged knee prosthesis. A five-year study of seventeen knees. *J Bone Joint Surg Am* 1986;68:579–585.
22. Walker PS, Emerson R, Potter T, et al. The Kinematic rotating hinge: biomechanics and clinical application. *Orthop Clin North Am* 1982;13:187–199.
23. Rand JA, Chao EY, Stauffer RN. Kinematic rotating-hinge total knee arthroplasty. *J Bone Joint Surg Am* 1987;69:489–497.
24. Shaw JA, Balcom W, Greer RB III. Total knee arthroplasty using the Kinematic rotating hinge prosthesis. *Orthopedics* 1989;12:647–654.
25. Springer BD, Hanssen AD, Sim FH, et al. The Kinematic rotating hinge prosthesis for complex knee arthroplasty. *Clin Orthop* 2001;392:283–291.
26. Lombardi AV Jr, Mallory TH, Eberle RW. Rotating hinge prosthesis in revision total knee arthroplasty: indications and results. *Surg Technol Int* 1997;6:379–382.
27. Barrack RL, Lyons TR, Ingraham RQ, et al. The use of a modular rotating hinge component in salvage revision total knee arthroplasty. *J Arthroplasty* 2000;15:858–866.
28. Jones RE, Skedros JG, Chan AJ, et al. Total knee arthroplasty using the S-ROM mobile-bearing hinge prosthesis. *J Arthroplasty* 2001;16:279–287.
29. Ward WG, Johnston KS, Dorey FJ, et al. Extramedullary porous coating to prevent diaphyseal osteolysis and radiolucent lines around proximal tibial replacements. A preliminary report. *J Bone Joint Surg Am* 1993;75:976–987.
30. Finn HA, Golden D, Kneisle JA, et al. The Finn knee: rotating hinge replacement of the knee. Preliminary report of a new design. In: Brown KLB, ed. *Complications of limb salvage: prevention, management and outcome.* Montreal: Isols, 1991:413–416.
31. Finn HA, Smith SR, Salob P, et al. The Finn knee: design, evolution and clinical use of a new hinge. *Orthop Trans* 1996;20:964 (abst).
32. Unwin PS, Cobb JP, Walker PS. Distal femoral arthroplasty using custom-made prostheses. The first 218 cases. *J Arthroplasty* 1993;8:259–268.
33. Choong PF, Sim FH, Pritchard DJ, et al. Megaprostheses after resection of distal femoral tumors. A rotating hinge design in 30 patients followed for 2–7 years. *Acta Orthop Scand* 1996;67:345–351.
34. Ward WG, Eckardt JJ, Johnston-Jones KS, et al. Five to ten year results of custom endoprosthetic replacement for tumors of the distal femur. In: Brown KLB, ed. *Complications of limb salvage: prevention, management and outcome.* Montreal: Isols, 1991:483–491.
35. Kawai A, Healey JH, Boland PJ, et al. A rotating-hinge knee replacement for malignant tumors of the femur and tibia. *J Arthroplasty* 1999;14:187–196.
36. Cobb JP, Grimer R, Unwin P, et al. Less is more in massive replacements about the knee. *J Bone Joint Surg Br* 1994;76:140(abst).
37. Draganich LF, Whitehurst JB, Chou LS, et al. The effects of the rotating-hinge total knee replacement on gait and stair stepping. *J Arthroplasty* 1999;14:743–755.
38. Kabo JM, Yang RS, Dorey FJ, et al. In vivo rotational stability of the Kinematic rotating hinge knee prosthesis. *Clin Orthop* 1997;336:166–176.
39. Karpinski MR, Grimer RJ. Hinged knee replacement in revision arthroplasty. *Clin Orthop* 1987;220:185–191.
40. Bell RS. Fixed hinge knee arthroplasty [editorial]. *Can J Surg* 1997;40:250.
41. Gold DA, Scott SC, Scott WN. Soft tissue expansion prior to arthroplasty in the multiply-operated knee. A new method of preventing catastrophic skin problems. *J Arthroplasty* 1996;11:512–521.
42. Inglis AE, Walker PS. Revision of failed knee replacements using fixed-axis hinges. *J Bone Joint Surg Br* 1991;73:757–761.
43. Shin DS, Weber KL, Chao EY, et al. Reoperation for failed prosthetic replacement used for limb salvage. *Clin Orthop* 1999;358:53–63.

44. Wirganowicz PZ, Eckardt JJ, Dorey FJ, et al. Etiology and results of tumor endoprosthesis revision surgery in 64 patients. *Clin Orthop* 1999;358:64–74.

45. Kim YH. Salvage of failed hinge knee arthroplasty with a Total Condylar III type prosthesis. *Clin Orthop* 1987;221:272–277.

46. Krackow KA, Mihalko WM. The effects of severe femoral bone loss on the flexion-extension joint space in revision total knee arthroplasty: a cadaveric analysis and clinical consequences. *Orthopedics* 2001;24:121–126.

47. Ghazavi MT, Stockley I, Yee G, et al. Reconstruction of massive bone defects with allograft in revision total knee arthroplasty. *J Bone Joint Surg Am* 1997;79:17–25.

48. Harris AI, Poddar S, Gitelis S, et al. Arthroplasty with a composite of an allograft and a prosthesis for knees with severe deficiency of bone. *J Bone Joint Surg Am* 1995;77:373–386.

49. Tsahakis PJ, Beaver WB, Brick GW. Technique and results of allograft reconstruction in revision total knee arthroplasty. *Clin Orthop* 1994;303:86–94.

50. Enneking WF, Mindell ER. Observations on massive retrieved human allografts. *J Bone Joint Surg Am* 1991;73:1123–1142.

51. Berrey BH Jr, Lord CF, Gebhardt MC, et al. Fractures of allografts. Frequency, treatment, and end-results. *J Bone Joint Surg Am* 1990;72:825–833.

52. Nelson TE. The use of modular revision knee systems. *Orthopedics* 1999;5(special edition):17–19.

53. Leopold SS, McStay C, Klafeta K, et al. Primary repair of intraoperative disruption of the medial collateral ligament during total knee arthroplasty. *J Bone Joint Surg Am* 2001;83:86–91.

54. Rorabeck CH, Smith PN. Results of revision total knee arthroplasty in the face of significant bone deficiency. *Orthop Clin North Am* 1998;29(2):361–371.

CHAPTER 105

Implant Removal in Revision Total Knee Arthroplasty

Thomas A. St. John, William J. Hozack, and Peter F. Sharkey

The removal of components during revision total knee arthroplasty can be a challenge to the joint surgeon. Knowledge of effective techniques that minimize bone loss can greatly facilitate knee reconstruction. As a procedure, it is practical to think of revision knee arthroplasty in three stages: exposure, removal of the components and cement, and reconstruction. These three stages are intimately linked in that the success of each stage depends on the satisfactory completion of the previous stage.

The goal of this chapter is to provide the revision knee surgeon with an organized and atraumatic technique for the removal of components. We begin with a discussion on exposure, and then focus on the specific tools and techniques for removal of the femoral, tibial, and patellar components. Emphasis is placed on cemented as well as cementless fixation.

EXPOSURE

An adequate exposure is a prerequisite for the timely and safe removal of components. There are many surgical approaches available to the knee surgeon, such as the V-Y quadricepsplasty, the quadriceps snip, and the tibial tubercle osteotomy, all of which can enhance the surgeon's access to the knee joint. Although it is important to be familiar with these techniques, they are not often necessary if one has performed a complete extensor mechanism tenolysis.

A wide exposure is usually accomplished by thoroughly mobilizing the extensor mechanism through resection of all scar tissue, with particular attention to the lateral gutter and the undersurfaces of the quadriceps and patellar tendons. The often thickened and fibrosed patellar tendon should be dissected free and mobilized (Fig. 1). Furthermore, the attachment to the tibia should be released down to the insertion on the tibial tubercle and clearly defined. This release should extend around the lateral aspect of the tibia, freeing the adhered extensor mechanism from the joint line. Placing a right-angle retractor under the tendon can facilitate visualization of this area (Fig. 2).

After mobilization of the patellar tendon, the lateral gutter should be addressed. The lateral gutter is often obliterated by adhesions, which can be resected with a large rongeur. Resection should proceed until the normal lateral gutter volume has been restored. Furthermore, the lateral border of the patella is usually overgrown with fibrotic tissue. Dissection and definition of the patellar lateral border improve eversion. Extensor mechanism tenolysis is completed by dissection of the quadriceps tendon, which is often adhered to the lateral border of the distal femur. These adhesions should be released from the lateral gutter proximally. Finally, the tendon itself should be thinned until normal tendinous fibers are identified.

In this fashion, the patella is usually readily everted (Fig. 3), which allows direct access to the component-bone interfaces, particularly on the harder to reach lateral side. This is important to minimize bone destruction during disruption of these interfaces.

TOOLS

There are a variety of specific tools that can be used for removal of components or cement or both. Several different

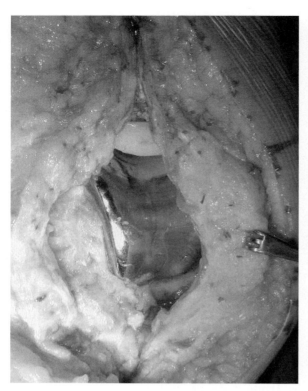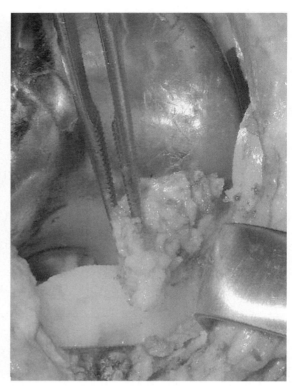

FIG. 1. Intraoperative photographs showing patellar tendon débridement.

instruments and techniques can be applied equally well for the same purpose. The revision surgeon should be familiar with a broad spectrum of these techniques, which can be used individually, depending on the situation, or in combination to achieve safe component extraction. Tools specifically designed for knee revisions are available in the Moreland Knee Revision Instrumentation set (Depuy, Warsaw, IN). There are a variety of osteotomes, chisels, and extractors that were designed to accommodate the special needs of the knee revision surgeon.

Component-Specific Tools

The majority of revision total knee arthroplasties can be performed successfully with the use of universal extraction devices, which are designed to be applied to a variety of different components. The availability of "universal" equipment reduces the number of instruments that must be on hand and that the surgeon must be familiar with. Certain knee designs, however, may be removed more easily with the use of manufacturer-specific extraction devices. Awareness of their availability can greatly

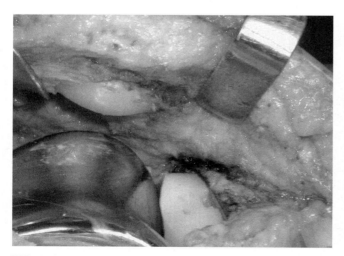

FIG. 2. Intraoperative photograph showing exposure of lateral gutter with a right-angled retractor in place.

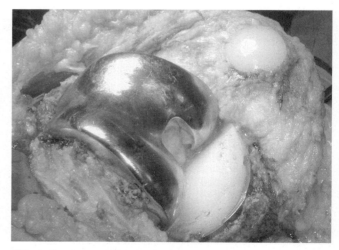

FIG. 3. Intraoperative photograph showing complete knee exposure and eversion of the patella.

reduce operative time and effort. Preoperative planning is essential to ensure that the proper instrumentation is available. Obtaining the operative note for the index procedure can be helpful in determining the implant manufacturer and design.

Hand and Power Tools

The instruments described in the following subsections should be available during all revision total knee arthroplasties. Their specific use is mentioned briefly in this section and is elaborated on in the sections dealing with femoral, tibial, and patellar component removal.

Osteotome

Osteotomes are one of the most effective and widely used instruments for component removal. Gently curved osteotomes, straight osteotomes, and angled osteotomes are available in a variety of widths. These are carefully inserted at the femoral and tibial component interfaces. One must use caution, however, to keep the osteotome against the component surface and counter the tendency for it to travel into the softer cancellous bone (1). Small curved osteotomes are particularly useful for removing tibial canal cement.

Power Saw

Power saws can be used in a fashion similar to osteotomes to disrupt the component interface. Thin saw blades are recommended; as with osteotomes, the blade should abut the component surface so that the least amount of bone is removed. In addition, power saws can be used to readily remove an all-polyethylene component, exposing the underlying cement.

Power Burr

A power burr with a very fine tip can be used to define the prosthesis-bone or prosthesis-cement interface. If it is used cautiously, the correct plane can be established adjacent to the component, and removal can then be completed with a saw or osteotome. Burrs are also useful for removal of residual cement and sclerotic bone once the implant has been removed.

Gigli Saw

For certain implant designs, a Gigli saw can be used to expediently remove well-fixed cemented and cementless femoral components (2). The Gigli saw is placed at the most proximal edge of the trochlear flange and directed distally and anteriorly. As with other instruments, the saw is kept against the component to minimize bone loss. If the maneuver is performed properly, the saw is in constant contact with the metal prosthesis, which often causes the saw wire to break. The surgeon should be aware of this possibility, and several wires should be available. The distal femoral component interface can be disrupted to a variable degree, depending on the presence of pegs or a metal intercondylar notch. The posterior condylar interface can be

partially disrupted in the following manner: a hole is made with a drill bit or Steinmann pin, adjacent to the component and directed toward the notch (2). One end of the Gigli saw is passed through the hole, and the saw is then applied in a distal direction. The remainder of the posterior interface can then be divided with the use of osteotomes.

High-Speed Instruments

High-speed cutting tools should be available during revision total knee arthroplasties for situations that require cutting the prosthesis to gain access to well-fixed distal stems. Diamond-tipped wheels are also very useful when removing well-fixed metal-backed patellar components. Several manufacturers (Midas Rex, Fort Worth, TX; Anspach, Lake Park, FL; Zimmer, Warsaw, IN) make high-speed tools with metal cutting tips (i.e., a diamond-edge circular saw blade). Specialty training courses are available for the proper use of these tools. Great care should be exercised when using these tools because of the rapidity with which they can remove bone. A wet surgical sponge should be placed on the surrounding tissue to prevent the spread of metal debris. Furthermore, continuous irrigation should be used if the saw blade is adjacent to any bone surface to prevent thermal necrosis.

Ultrasonic Tools

Ultrasonic powered tools have been developed in an attempt to mimic the function of hand tools without generating the impact they typically require for effectiveness. The ultrasonic device converts electrical energy to mechanical energy, which can be applied to a specially designed tip (3). Methylmethacrylate selectively absorbs this energy, which causes the cement to soften and facilitates its removal. The ultrasonic tip provides both tactile and auditory feedback when cortical bone is contacted instead of cement. Ultrasonic tools typically require considerably more force to penetrate cortical bone. Thus, one can safely and selectively remove cement with minimal damage to surrounding bone (4). Ultrasonic tools have proved invaluable in revision hip surgery due to the difficulty of visualizing the cement within the femoral canal. During knee arthroplasty revisions, however, the surgeon often has direct access to the cement. Therefore, the benefit of ultrasonic tools in knee revision surgery may not be as dramatic as it is for hip revisions.

REMOVAL OF COMPONENTS

The order in which components should be removed depends, in part, on the amount of exposure that one is able to obtain. If a wide exposure is achievable, whereby the patella can be everted and the knee can safely be dislocated, the tibial component should be removed first. When the femoral component is in place, the underlying bone is protected from damage when levering on the metal femur with a Homan retractor. It is not always possible to obtain this amount of exposure, however. In this circumstance, the femoral component can be removed first, which allows access to the underlying tibial component. Care should be taken not to damage the distal femur with a retractor

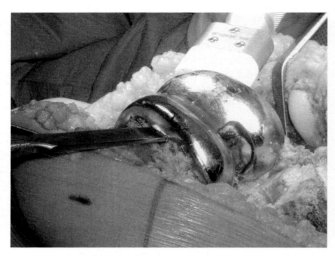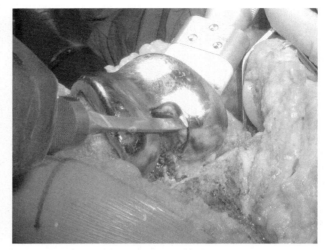

FIG. 4. Intraoperative photographs showing femoral component removal with an osteotome.

once the implant has been removed. If it is possible, early removal of the polyethylene tibial tray relaxes the soft tissues of the knee, which facilitates the exposure.

Femoral Component

Whether the femoral component is cemented or uncemented, the general principles of removal remain the same. Time must be spent to carefully disrupt the entire component interface (prosthesis-bone or prosthesis-cement) while causing minimal bone damage. Forcible extraction of a well-fixed component can lead to severe bone loss, which may compromise the successful reconstruction of the knee (1).

To accomplish the complete disruption of the component interface, one of several different techniques may be used. Careful dissection with a sharp curved osteotome can result in a successful bone-sparing extraction. The anterior, medial, and lateral margins of the component should be débrided of all soft tissue using a

Bovie. Once the interfaces are adequately visualized, an osteotome can be introduced into the appropriate space (Fig. 4). The hard prosthesis or cement has the tendency to drive instruments into the softer cancellous bone. Therefore, the osteotome should be carefully angled up against the metal prosthesis at all times. Using a gently curved osteotome with the curve angled toward the metal restricts the tendency to violate the bone. Wider osteotomes are useful for the trochlear flange; however, 0.25-in. osteotomes may be necessary to disrupt the anterior and posterior chamfers and posterior condylar interface.

A power saw equipped with a thin blade may be used in place of osteotomes with similar efficacy. As with the osteotome, the saw blade must be kept adjacent to the prosthesis at all times, and the operator must carefully resist the tendency for the thin blade to be pushed into the soft bone. Thin saw blades remove less bone; however, they tend to be more flexible and are thus more prone to follow a path of least resistance. The use of osteotomes may still be necessary for disruption of the distal femoral interface due to the presence of pegs that may interfere with a saw blade.

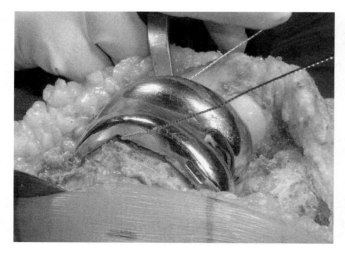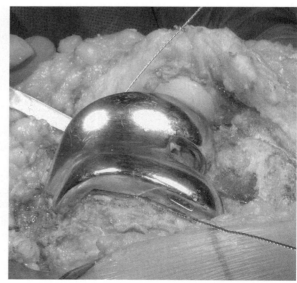

FIG. 5. Intraoperative photographs showing femoral component removal with a Gigli saw.

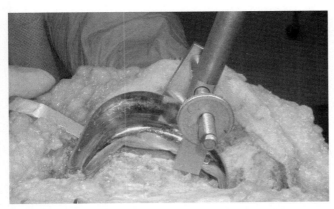

FIG. 6. Intraoperative photograph showing use of a femoral universal extractor.

Another technique for femoral component removal has been described using a Gigli saw (Fig. 5), as mentioned previously. When the Gigli saw is placed at the most proximal edge of the component and directed distally, the saw readily disrupts the anterior interface and a variable amount of the distal femoral interface (depending on the presence of a central stem or pegs) (2). Angling the saw anteriorly ensures contact with the prosthesis at all times, which minimizes the amount of bone resected. The posterior condylar interfaces are disrupted with a combination of the Gigli saw and osteotomes.

When all of the interfaces have been adequately disrupted, the femoral component is removed with either a universal or component-specific extractor (Fig. 6). If a cemented central stem is present, the stem often debonds from the cement, which allows extraction of the component and stem with minimal exertion. The remaining cement column can then be removed separately (1). Occasionally, however, the stem does not debond from the cement without excessive force, which risks a femoral fracture or severe bone damage. In this situation, the stem-cement or stem-bone interface must be accessed directly. This is best accomplished by cutting the prosthesis free from the stem with a metal-cutting high-speed saw (1). The majority of the femoral component with its disrupted interfaces can then easily be removed, with the well-fixed stem left behind. The stem can then be extracted by direct disruption of its interface with the use of a fine-tipped burr, ultrasonic tools, small osteotomes, or some combination of these. It should be noted that most stemmed knee components are modular and are sometimes connected with a screw, which is easily accessible in the notch. In this case, metal-cutting tools would be unnecessary. Disengaging this screw may require a component-specific screwdriver. With the stem disengaged, removal of the femoral component allows direct access to the stem interfaces.

The techniques described earlier may be applied equally well to both cemented and uncemented femoral components. The power saw, osteotomes, and Gigli saw can efficiently disrupt the trochlear and anterior chamfer interfaces, whether they are prosthesis-cement or prosthesis-bone. Similarly, the posterior interfaces are readily disrupted with osteotomes or Gigli saw or both, regardless of the type of fixation. Perhaps the greatest challenge of an uncemented femoral component arises when a porous-coated central stem is present and is well fixed. Nevertheless, this is treated in the same manner as the well-bonded cemented

stem. As mentioned, removal requires that the prosthesis be cut free from the stem with a metal-cutting high-speed instrument, which allows direct access to the bone–ingrown stem interface.

Tibial Component

Removal of well-fixed tibial components tends to be somewhat easier than removal of well-fixed femoral components due to the simpler geometry of the tibial tray. The principles, however, remain the same. An adequate exposure is required to gain access to the component interfaces. Subsequently, these interfaces must be disrupted before any attempt at removal. In this fashion, successful removal of the tibial component can be accomplished with minimal damage to bone.

As with the femoral component, the tibial interfaces can efficiently be disrupted using osteotomes or a power saw, or both. The periphery of the component interface should initially be defined as completely as the exposure allows and the proper plane established. The lateral interface may be difficult to visualize directly. An osteotome or power saw is then introduced into this plane, with caution used to maintain the instrument adjacent to the component to minimize the amount of bone resected. The osteotomes can be used in a medial to lateral direction to disrupt the harder-to-reach lateral interface, both anterior and posterior to the central stem. The patellar tendon must be protected at all times from damage by the osteotomes or saw.

The "stacked" osteotome technique is an efficient way to lift the prosthesis away from the bone surface (Fig. 7) (1). Multiple osteotomes are introduced into the interface on top of one another to gradually lift the implant. A broad osteotome should be used closest to bone to help distribute the forces over a larger surface area. The osteotomes should not be used to forcibly remove the prosthesis by levering against the tibial plateau. This may crush the underlying cancellous bone. Rather, stacking the osteotomes in all accessible areas of the component interface should sufficiently loosen the prosthesis to allow easy removal with a bone tamp (Fig. 8).

Cemented central stems on the tibial prostheses are designed to debond from the surrounding cement when a reasonable amount of force is applied. If the circumstance should arise in which the stem does not debond from the cement without excessive force, despite adequate disruption of the tibial plateau interface, then the stem should be cut free from the tibial tray with a high-speed cutting device, to allow direct access to the stem interface (1).

Uncemented tibial components often have additional fixation with screws. This should be noted on the preoperative radiographs, and component-specific screwdrivers should be available if necessary. Otherwise, the prosthesis-bone interface is disrupted in a fashion similar to that described earlier. Bone-ingrown tibial stems that cannot be removed with reasonable force should be approached in the same manner as well-fixed cemented stems, by cutting the stem free of the prosthesis and directly disrupting the stem interface.

Patellar Component

Removal of the patellar component can be deceptively difficult because of the thinness of the patella and the presence of anchoring pegs in the already vulnerable bone. Poor technique

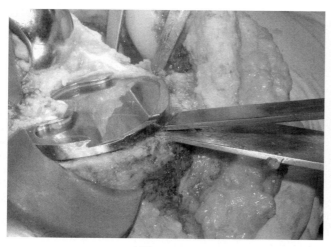 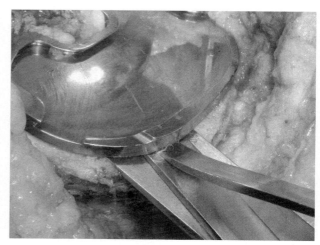

FIG. 7. Intraoperative photographs showing stacked osteotome technique.

risks removal of too much bone or fracture of the patella, or both, which compromises the extensor mechanism (1). If the component is well fixed and there is only cold-flow deformation of the polyethylene, then consideration should be given to leaving the patella in place. If removal is indicated, then a careful and meticulous technique as outlined for the femoral and tibial components should be used. Débridement of the peripatellar soft tissue is performed to gain access to the prosthetic interface. If the component is made entirely of polyethylene, removal can be readily accomplished by cutting across the polyethylene pegs and bone-cement interface with small osteotomes or a thin saw blade, or both. The pegs and remaining cement are then directly accessed and removed with a fine-tipped burr.

Metal-backed patellar components can be considerably more difficult to remove. The mode of failure of this design often involves polyethylene wear and subsequent dissociation from the underlying well-fixed metal plate (5). Conventional removal techniques with an osteotome are likely to be ineffective when the fixation pegs are ingrown with bone. Attempts to lever the patellar component free should be avoided because of the risk of fracture. A simple technique has been described in

which the pegs are cut free from the prosthetic plate using a metal-cutting wheel (6). After adequate peripatellar soft tissue débridement, the bone-prosthesis interface is defined with an osteotome, which provides a plane for a metal-cutting circular saw. The saw is introduced into this space and directed circumferentially around the patella, disrupting the bone-prosthesis interface as well as the peg-plate connection. After removal of the metal plate, the well-fixed pegs can be freed from the bone with a fine-tipped burr, or left in place, with new holes drilled. Placing a wet sponge with a hole cut in it is an effective way to isolate the debris from the remainder of the knee when working on the patella, particularly when a metal-cutting burr is used.

REMOVAL OF CEMENT

Cement that remains on the surfaces of the femur and tibia after component extraction can be removed using hand tools such as straight osteotomes or a rongeur, with minimal loss of underlying bone. If the cement-bone interface is not easily defined, use of a power burr to trim away any residual cement can be helpful. Well-fixed cement can also be left in place when it does not interfere with placement of the new component and the revision is not being performed for infection.

When cement is present in the canals (femoral or tibial), removal techniques that have been developed for total hip arthroplasty can be applied. A combination of splitter osteotomes, straight osteotomes, and gouges can be used to fragment the cement column. Ultrasonic tools are also very effective, particularly for removal of any well-fixed diaphyseal cement plugs. Care should be exercised to avoid perforation, particularly of the thin tibial cortices.

CONCLUSION

Proficiency in removing failed total knee components is a requirement for all total joint surgeons. The success of any revision is largely dependent on the ability to remove components without damaging the underlying bone. Proper exposure combined with meticulous extraction techniques expedites the

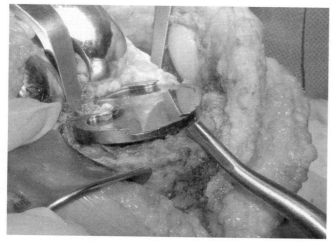

FIG. 8. Intraoperative photograph showing removal of tibial component with a bone tamp.

surgery, minimizes bone loss, and provides the optimal setting for a successful and durable reconstruction.

REFERENCES

1. Berry DJ. Component removal during revision total knee arthroplasty. In: Lotke PA, Garino JP, eds. *Revision total knee arthroplasty.* Philadelphia: Lippincott–Raven Publishers, 1999:187–196.
2. Firestone TP, Krackow KA. Removal of femoral components during revision knee arthroplasty. *J Bone Joint Surg Br* 1991;73(3):514.
3. Brooks AT, Nelson CL, et al. Effect of an ultrasonic device on temperatures generated in bone and on bone-cement structure. *J Arthroplasty* 1993;8(4):413–418.
4. Klapper RC, Caillouette JT, et al. Ultrasonic technology in revision joint arthroplasty. *Clin Orthop* 1992;285:147–154.
5. Bayley JC, Scott RD, et al. Failure of the metal-backed patellar component after total knee replacement. *J Bone Joint Surg Am* 1988;70:668.
6. Dennis DA. Removal of well-fixed cementless metal-backed patellar components. *J Arthroplasty* 1992;7(2):217–220.

CHAPTER 106

Use of Stems in Revision Total Knee Arthroplasty

Steven H. Weeden, Wayne G. Paprosky, and Todd D. Sekundiak

The goal in revision total knee arthroplasty is to re-create a stable joint that is positioned and oriented close to the normal anatomic axis in all planes. This becomes a more difficult task in the revision setting secondary to bone and soft tissue loss. The abnormalities present during revision surgery may result from a combination of different factors: primary disease deformity, infection, osteolysis, aseptic loosening, implant removal complications, and concomitant systemic disease. To anatomically re-create the knee joint, the surgeon may be required to use augments of a biologic or mechanical nature to compensate for the bone or soft tissue loss.

In the normal tibia, the cancellous and cortical bone of the proximal tibia buttresses and supports the overlying articular cartilage. The stiffness of the cancellous bone decreases distally as the stiffness of the cortical shell increases (1). The joint load is transmitted through the articular cartilage to the cancellous and cortical bone beneath. In the setting of primary knee arthroplasty, the combination of plastic, metal, and polymethylmethacrylate transmits the load directly to the underlying cancellous and cortical bone. In the revision setting, there is loss of the strongest supporting bone, and transmission of forces to the remaining subsurface could lead to early failure (2).

Revision total knee arthroplasty components are commonly stemmed to protect the limited autogenous bone stock that is remaining. This bone may be directly under the component or under the cement, metal augments, or structural bone graft. When one is using large volumes of morselized or structural grafts, one may want to protect the graft from significant load (3). Conclusively, revision components without stems can place abnormal stresses on the normal bone by their constrained design nature. Joint loads are several times body weight. A stemmed component can transfer these loads if it is composed of materials that can withstand the stresses imposed on them (4). If the stem fails to transfer the load, then the remaining cancellous bone experiences load beyond its ultimate strength, and this will lead to a loss in fixation (5).

A stem's purpose, therefore, is to transmit force away from the joint line and, in so doing, lessen the stresses placed on the joint (6,7). Stems perform this function by being rigid and by being attached to a solid femoral component or tibial base plate. Brooks et al. have shown that, in the varus deficient proximal tibia, the addition of a metal-backed component decreases stress and allows for a more uniform distribution of force across the proximal tibia (8). Because these components are more rigid than the remaining cancellous bone, force is transmitted through them and onto the stem or onto the remaining tibial cortical rim. Bartel and associates have shown by finite element analysis that stresses on the cancellous bone beneath prostheses of conventional design can be diminished if a metal tray and a central peg are used (9). Lewis et al. found that tibial post designs provided the lowest stresses on host bone (10). Once a stem (or post) length reaches 70 mm, the axial load at the joint line can be reduced by 23% to 39% (6–8). The bending moment carried by the stem can be variable, as fixation of the stem occurs distally (8). Addition of a central post and stem to the tray, however, increases the stiffness of the component and, in doing so, decreases the bending moment (7). The force is then returned to the bone at the metadiaphyseal or diaphyseal area, depending on the geometry, size, length, position, and composition of the stem. Bourne and Finlay demonstrated in a fresh cadaveric strain-gauge study that loss of proximal cortical tibial contact resulted in a 33% to 60% decrease in strain values (15). When stems up to 15 cm long are evaluated, marked stress shielding of the proximal tibial cortex and doubling of the strain located at the tip is noted.

Two traditional methods of stem insertion have been used. Use of a cemented stem results in transmission of load closer to the joint line, as the stems are shorter and the force is transmitted

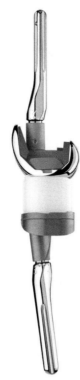

FIG. 1. Example of stemmed femoral and tibial components for press-fit use. Stems are fluted, which helps to engage endosteal bone. This allows control of rotational forces. Press-fitting of the stems also controls bending forces. The smooth surface allows subsidence to maintain compression forces at the joint line. The stems are offset to compensate for asymmetric joint surfaces. (Courtesy of Zimmer, Warsaw, IN.)

along the bone-cement interface. This should decrease severe stress shielding (11). Filling the intramedullary canal with cement can make future revisions more problematic, however, and may lead to further bone loss and destruction during cement removal (12). With cementless stems, forces are transmitted to the tip of the stem where cortical bone contact occurs (12–14). Researchers have raised concern regarding possible proximal stress shielding with cementless stems; however, this is, more often than not, technique dependent (15). Stress shielding may actually be less if the stem is not anchored in cement (13). Cementless stem insertion may actually weaken bone due to excessive reaming or may possibly promote early loosening if the stem is undersized (14,16). These arguments are technique related and should not be indications to avoid the use of cementless stems.

It is essential that the revision surgeon realize that stems are not a substitute for optimal component fit. They are simply an adjunct to relieve a portion of the excess stress seen by the components at the joint line. The type and size of stem are irrelevant if the juxtaarticular tissues are not adequately reconstructed. As stresses become greater or the soft tissues more compromised, the approach to stem fixation must be altered (16).

There are a multitude of different stem geometries available. Use of larger diameter stems leads to increased load transmissions, but this is usually negated by the fact that most systems have a set diameter fixation point at the stem-component junc-

tion (17). In addition, the bending moment of the base plate is determined at this junction (18). Longer stems in the knee result in more proximal bone shielding (7). This factor cannot be assessed in isolation, as shorter, wider stems impinge at their tips because of the conical shape of metaphyseal endosteum. The use of longer, thinner stems prevents tip impingement, as the stem can migrate in the sleeve of tubular diaphyseal endosteum. The contact area of the stem within the bone also determines how the load is transferred to the cortex. To complicate matters, the surface preparation of the stem may also alter fixation. Presently, most cementless stems are smooth or blasted without a porous coating. Flutes have been added to the stems to aid in fixation and decrease stem stiffness. Flutes or splines on the stem engage in endosteal bone and, it is hoped, function to decrease rotational stresses at the joint line. The flutes may also act to decrease the modulus of elasticity of the stems and thus decrease the severity of proximal stress shielding (Fig. 1).

PREOPERATIVE PLANNING

Preoperative planning is essential before knee revision arthroplasty. Full-length anteroposterior and lateral radiographs allow for complete assessment of the femur and tibia. Besides allowing determination of the position of the joint line, alignment of bony cuts, size and position of components, and need for augmentation, these radiographs permit assessment of the intramedullary canals to ensure that intramedullary alignment

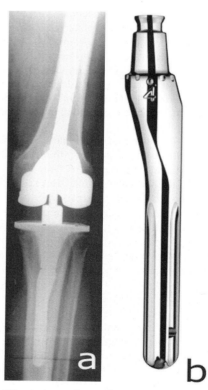

FIG. 2. a: Offset stem allows displacement of the tibial base plate in the desired direction to prevent component overhang and allow for optimal coverage. (Courtesy of Zimmer, Warsaw, IN.) **b:** Offset tibial stemmed component.

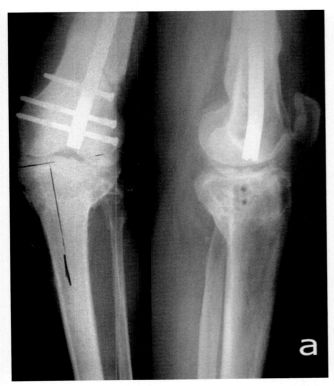
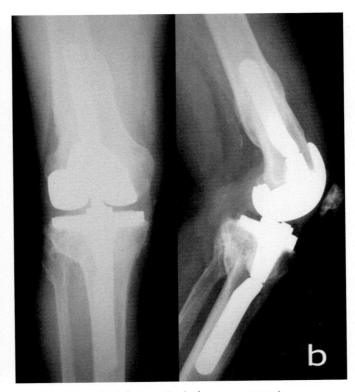

FIG. 3. Radiographs of the knee of a 77-year-old man who experienced a fall 9 months before assessment. Attempts at open reduction and internal fixation failed to achieve union. **a:** Anteroposterior and lateral radiographs of a supracondylar femur fracture with posttraumatic arthritis and failed internal fixation. **b:** Postoperative radiographs at 9 months.

conforms to the mechanical axis orientation. Eccentric joint surfaces may require the use of offset stems or tibial housings to ensure proper alignment of the component while optimizing tibial plateau coverage and preventing implant overhang (Figs. 1 and 2). Canal assessment ensures that straight-stemmed components may be inserted and possibly determines the need for an osteotomy secondary to severe deformity. Stem length and width are estimated to obtain adequate endosteal press-fit. Stem length must be estimated with the component to account for each component's respective housing. In general, longer stems are used to provide more rigid support, as their point of contact extends for a longer length along the endosteal diaphyseal surface. Length and degree of support cannot be assessed in isolation, as the extent of press-fit is a significant concomitant factor. Longer stems with tight diaphyseal endosteal cortical press-fit are chosen in cases of massive bony deficiencies (Fig. 3). Long stems may also be used to provide constrained component support when significant soft tissue imbalance or instability is present and more constrained implants are used (Fig. 4).

It is useful to template for at least two possible stem lengths with their corresponding different stem widths (Fig. 5). Commonly, a predetermined stem length may be too loose because of undersizing or the stem may impinge if it is oversized. Attempting to insert a stem of larger or smaller diameter, respectively, may then cause the reciprocal problem. Usually, the problem of impingement can be avoided by reaming away more endosteal bone. This helps lessen the impingement that occurs at the tip of the stem where the intramedullary canal begins to narrow. If the amount of bone removed is excessive, however, a

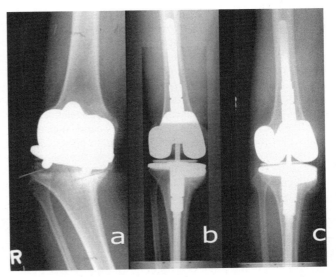

FIG. 4. Radiographs of a 55-year-old woman with primary uncemented total knee arthroplasty for degenerative osteoarthritis. Patient was complaining of significant medial knee and lower leg pain. **a:** Anteroposterior radiograph of an unstable uncemented total knee prosthesis. Two-month **(b)** and 2-year **(c)** postoperative anteroposterior radiographs of a cemented constrained total knee prosthesis with Press-Fit stems. Incompetency of the medial collateral ligamentous complex prevented balancing of the joint and therefore required the use of constrained polyethylene to compensate for ligamentous laxity.

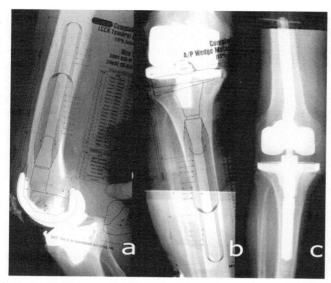

FIG. 5. Radiographs of the knee of a 65-year-old man with severe osteolysis secondary to excessive polyethylene wear. The patient had previously undergone removal of a metal-backed patella. Preoperative anteroposterior **(b)** and lateral **(a)** radiographs with overlying templates. With severe osteolysis, reconstitution of bone stock with bulk allografting or impaction grafting must be considered. **c:** Postoperative radiograph.

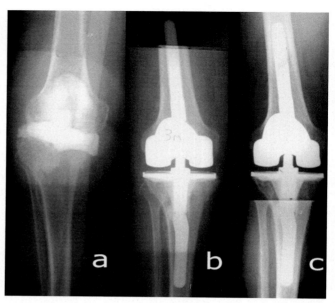

FIG. 6. Revision total knee arthroplasty requiring a tibial offset stem as the patient had previously undergone a high tibial osteotomy and was left with a deficient medial tibial plateau. The patient underwent a two-staged revision because of previous infection. **a:** Preoperative radiograph. **b:** Three-month postoperative radiograph. **c:** Two-year postoperative radiograph. The offset stem allowed for better lateral coverage of the tibial surface with no significant medical overhang of the component.

stress riser may be created at the tip of the stem, which can lead to stem tip pain or fracture. An alternative is to change to a stem of shorter or longer length with a different diameter. Templating helps ensure that the stem length chosen is sufficient so that structural bone will support the stem.

Most stems attach to a fixed point on the revision arthroplasty component. Estimation of component position in the coronal and sagittal planes is therefore essential. Commonly, the femoral component sizing in the coronal plane is decided by the knee anatomy, as the medial and lateral condyles have a relatively symmetric width in relation to the intramedullary canal. With straight stems, placement of the component in the sagittal plane is dictated by the stem and therefore predetermines the flexion gap. To increase or decrease the flexion gap during the use of straight stems, the only option is to upsize or downsize the femoral component, respectively (Fig. 5). Shifting of the component position or addition of posterior femoral augments cannot be used to alter the flexion gap, as component position has been predetermined by the straight intramedullary stem. If available, an offset stem or a component with a different housing junction point is another viable option. On the tibial side, stem positioning tends to be a greater problem in the coronal plane, as the medial and lateral tibial plateaus are commonly asymmetric (Fig. 6). Ultimately, position of the component must correlate with both the bone of the joint line and the intramedullary canal alignment to prevent significant overhang of the component.

Many newer revision knee systems have a swivel joint at the tibial component-stem junction or are equipped with an offset stem that allows for adjustment of component position (Figs. 1 and 2). Curved stems allow for longer support on the femoral side and attempt to lessen the possibility of endosteal impingement.

OPERATIVE TECHNIQUE

Before reconstruction of the knee joint, infection must be ruled out and the original components removed, with every attempt made to preserve the underlying host bone stock. The surrounding soft tissues must be adequately assessed and protected during the reconstruction.

In rare instances, a stemmed component may be considered during a primary arthroplasty because of severe deformity, significant bone loss, or severe ligamentous insufficiency. Conversion to a stemmed component cannot immediately proceed after implantation of a regular component if extramedullary alignment has been used. The possibility exists of mismatching the bone cuts to the intramedullary axes, which can cause impingement of the intramedullary stem on the endosteal surface. This can lead to malalignment of components, poor fit of components on the bone surfaces, or iatrogenic bone fractures from attempts to make the component fit with forceful impaction.

Preparation of the femoral and tibial bony surfaces is done with an intramedullary alignment guide. Rather than using the narrow intramedullary guide rods that attach to the cutting jigs of most systems, the authors prefer to use the intramedullary reamers from the cutting-jig guide rod. The initial step is to minimally ream and push the largest diameter reamer past the isthmus. The initial reamer produces an entry point in the juxtaarticular bone and is rotated to enlarge the entry site. This removes ectatic and sclerotic bone that can lever the reamers away from the true longitudinal axes of the bones. Reaming is then continued in millimeter increments until minimal endosteal cortical contact is felt or heard. As stated earlier, reaming is minimal, as the reamers are being used more as guide rods for cut alignment and stem position. Cutting blocks are then attached to this rod, and initial cuts are completed. By using the largest diameter rod in the canal and ensuring that the rod passes the isthmus, one can better assure that the bony cuts for the component optimally correlate with the stem orientation and prevent impingement or malpositioning of the component-stem construct. A full-length reamer or a reamer of equal width throughout its length provides for the best alignment, as there is minimal toggle along its shaft. Once the entry site has been cleared of sclerotic bone, the reamer should be gently pushed up the canal rather than forcibly reamed into the canal. The reamer is acting as a guide rod at this point.

Balancing of the joint in the flexion-extension and varus-valgus planes proceeds in a routine manner once the initial cuts have been made. The initial bone cuts required are the proximal tibial cut and the distal and posterior femoral cuts. Cuts should resect minimal bone and are performed before assessing the flexion and extension spaces. The use of premeasured spacer blocks or a measurable tensioning device is essential at this stage. Joint line positioning is decided by this assessment and by preoperative templating. The size of the femoral component, the amount of femoral distal buildup, and the amount of tibial thickness can then be determined arithmetically. The tibial component affects both the flexion and extension gaps. Its thickness is determined by an estimation of the position of the joint line. This measurement can be subtracted from the spacer block measurements of the flexion and extension gaps to determine the size of the femoral component required for flexion gap balance and the amount of distal femoral augment for extension gap balance.

It is essential to reiterate that the position of the femoral and tibial components is dictated by the position of the press-fit stem. The size of the tibial base plate determines the amount of coverage but also the amount of overhang on the tibia in the coronal plane. If the canal is eccentric or the tibial plateaus deficient, then a base plate with an offset housing or offset stem must be considered to correct this problem. A similar but less common problem occurs in the sagittal plane.

With the femoral component, there is an additional concern of altering the thickness in the sagittal plane. Changing the femoral sizing alters the flexion gap thickness by predetermined amounts and is the only way to alter the flexion gap when assessing the femoral component in isolation. The extent that a smaller-sized femoral component increases the flexion gap is system specific and must be known. Posterior femoral augments are used as a filler to ensure that the posterior aspect of the component is in bony contact and thus rotationally stable. Once the size of the femoral component is determined, chamfer cuts and housing resection can be completed. Final shaping for augments is also completed. All bone cuts should be performed in reference to an intramedullary alignment rod.

If bulk allograft is required, sizing, shaping, and fixation are now performed. Depending on defect size, grafting can be completed before gap assessment. Length estimates are performed with the calculations noted earlier if a complete structural allograft is required to replace the juxtaarticular bone. Completion of bony allograft resection is completed to accept the component and component housing. The cuts are performed on a satellite table with intramedullary alignment. The diameter of the intramedullary guide within the allograft is determined by the width of reaming required within the host bone. Appropriate graft size is required to ensure that excessive reaming of the graft does not occur and weaken the graft.

Femoral and tibial canals are then sequentially reamed to the appropriate length and width to accept the Press-Fit stem. A preoperative estimate along with the intraoperative assessment is required to determine the extent of press-fit required. With a wide variety of stems available, different permutations of stem length and width give adequate press-fit in most situations. For more severe defects, fewer stem choices exist, which emphasizes the need for preoperative templating to ensure appropriate stem availability. A greater degree of press-fit is required when there is greater structural bone loss or greater soft tissue imbalance or insufficiency. This translates to reaming to greater depths with removal of more endosteal bone to ensure that there is a sleeve of cortical endosteal bone supporting the stemmed component.

The width of reaming is templated preoperatively and correlates intraoperatively to the point at which cortical chatter is felt or heard with the reamer. Assessment of reamings is also of value in determining if endosteal cortical bone is being removed. Traditionally, the authors ream approximately 1 cm past the tip of the stem to ensure that there is no tip impingement with the possibility of cortical erosion. Remaining depth must include the stem length and the length of the component housing. A shorter stem of a wider variety is indicated if reaming past the tip of the stem will remove excess bone. For routine revisions, reaming should not be overly aggressive and does not need to proceed to the point of significant cortical chatter. Stem insertion and reaming proceeds line to line. If the revision requires more support from the stem, then reaming can be more aggressive. It is difficult to absolutely quantitate the extent of reaming for each situation; this must be done with clinical judgment as determined preoperatively and intraoperatively. It is important to compare the integrity of the bone and soft tissues to the primary arthroplasty setting and then determine the extent of extra support required. For structural bulk allografts, stem fixation along the endosteal bone should have cortical contact and should occur over a longer extent (Fig. 3). Reaming should therefore continue at least a millimeter or two wider beyond the point at which cortical chatter is felt and heard.

Trial reduction of the femoral and tibial components is performed with the required augments but without the stem extensions to assess the accuracy of the bony cuts. Before any recutting is attempted, it is important to retrial the components with the stems. Failure to seat components then can be assessed. Failure to seat the components without the stem indicates inaccurate bone cuts that require refinement. Easy seating of components without the stem but failure to easily seat with the stem either means that the stem has been incorrectly sized and endosteal impingement is occurring or that bony cuts have not correlated with the intramedullary positioning of the stem. If stem impingement is occurring, then rereaming of the canal or resizing of the stem is required. Cortication of the juxtaarticular bone occurs secondary to the osteolytic and loosening process in the revision setting. This bone can deflect the guide rod, reamer, stem, or component housing and lead to malpositioning. Ensuring adequate removal of bone for the component housing helps in alignment of the components. Failure to remove this bone or realize this problem leads to improper cut alignment and component malpositioning. At this stage, the only option is to replace the intramedullary guide rod and recut the femur.

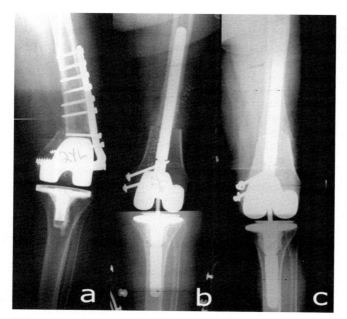

FIG. 7. Radiographs of the knee of a 69-year-old man who required bulk structural allograft for severe osteolysis and failed internal fixation. **a:** Preoperative radiograph. **b:** Immediately postoperative radiograph. The structural allograft was cut on a satellite table with an intramedullary rod of equal width to the reamer in the host endosteal canal. The component-graft composite was cemented, which ensured adequate stem for press-fit into host bone. Ideally, no cement should extend beyond or into the host-graft junction. **c:** Two-year follow-up radiograph.

Occasionally, when the relationship of the cut surfaces to the intramedullary alignment guide is reassessed, cuts are noted to be accurate; however, on upsizing reamers to accept a wider press-fit stem, cuts do not correlate with the stemmed component. This occurs because the bone is bowed or noncylindric, with the wider stem seating in a position, in that segment of bone, different from the longitudinal axis as determined by the intramedullary guide. The choice is then to recut the bone to correlate with the wider press-fit stem or to accept a narrower stem with or without increased length. The latter option better relates the bone cuts to the longitudinal axis of the bone and, in the majority of cases, the latter option is accepted, as the risk of malalignment is prevented. Once components are inserted, final assessment of flexion and extension gaps is performed.

In many revision situations, bulk allografting is not required for the contained cavitary defects that are present. Morselized autogenous or allogenic bone graft is useful in reconstituting bone stock in these situations. The trial stem, with or without the component, is inserted into the diaphysis but not fully seated. The stem acts as a mold for the actual component and a stopper to prevent graft from filling the intramedullary canal. Graft is placed around the stem and in the defects. The graft is then impacted, which gives it structure and more extensive contact with the host bone. The trial stem is then removed, with the graft maintaining its structural integrity.

Final components are then inserted in a routine manner. If components are cemented, cement should extend to but not include the stem-component junction. If cement extends to a point on the housing at which the taper of the component begins increasing in width, as in the junction of the component housing with a wider stem, removal of the component can be extremely difficult. The cement collar acts as an impediment to removal of the stem and can lead to fracturing at rerevision.

If complete juxtaarticular allografts are being used, attempts at trial reduction without the graft are performed to determine appropriate rotation of the component-allograft composite. Reduction of the joint should be possible, as the stemmed component will be stable in the host bone with the Press-Fit stem. Marking of the host bone and graft then allows for reproduction of the appropriate rotation and estimation of stem length. The graft-prosthesis composite is cemented, with the stem-graft junction kept void of cement. The composite is then impacted into the host, and final trimming of the junction is performed to ensure that host and graft cortical contact is maximized to minimize the stresses through the stem (Fig. 7).

RESULTS

The longest follow-up on revision total knee arthroplasties with stemmed components has occurred with cemented stems. Results have been very successful at a follow-up of 58.2 months. This presently is the gold standard to follow. Forty stemmed arthroplasty revisions were performed. Only one femoral component was radiographically determined to be loose, and three femurs and five tibias developed incomplete, progressive radiolucent lines (11).

Bertin et al. have reported early results of the use of uncemented stems in 53 patients (12). Stems were of limited sizes and, although uncemented, were not always press-fit. Excluding four knees that had serious postoperative complications, 91% of patients had relief of pain, 84% had more than 90 degrees of motion, and 80% were able to walk longer than 30 minutes. Eighty-eight percent of the stems were noted to have surrounding radiopaque lines, which were unrelated to degree of pain or failure rate.

The Insall group has performed follow-up on 76 knees at 42 months, with only three failures occurring from loosening and three from infection (14). Fluted diaphyseal stems were used in all patients. There was a 13% complication rate, with all complications being unrelated to the stems. Overall, 84% of patients had a good or excellent result according to the Hospital for Special Surgery rating scale. The procedure failed in six of the knees and another revision was required. In 67% of femoral rods and 69% of tibial rods, a 1- to 2-mm radiopaque line was noted to surround the stems completely or incompletely. These sclerotic lines usually appeared a few months after the procedure and had no correlation with outcome. In 4% of the femoral and 6% of the tibial rods, a progressive radiopaque line longer than 2 mm was present but again had no correlation to outcome (19). This appearance was markedly different from that of stems that fail (16).

Paprosky reported on a select group of patients in whom stemmed components were used with distal femoral allografts (20). This combination was used in cases of periprosthetic femoral fractures, fracture nonunion, and severe distal femoral bone loss. Distinctly absent from this patient population were patients with bone tumors. At an average follow-up of 32 months, seven of the nine patients had excellent or good results and the remaining two had fair results according to the Hospital for Special Surgery knee score. Complications were again unrelated to the stems. Soft tissue balancing was the greatest concern, with imbalance leading to patellar subluxation or genu recurvatum. Extreme emphasis was placed on protected weightbearing and bracing until union of the allograft site was evident. Results from the study of Mnaymneh et al. are similar, with union of allograft occurring in 86% of cases and motion averaging 92 degrees (21). Two patients experienced nonunion and fracture on the femoral side. These procedures were considered salvage procedures. Vince and Long reported on 44 revision knee arthroplasties using Press-Fit stems with 2 to 6 years of follow-up (16). Three patients developed clinical or radiographic evidence of loosening despite adequate canal fill. It was concluded that, even with adequate canal fill, fixation is inadequate in poor-quality bone using a Press-Fit stem, and consideration should be given to cementing the stem in position. Significant radiolucencies completely surrounded the stems of those components that failed. In addition to the endosteal radiolucencies, a cortical reaction was evident.

CONCLUSION

As time progresses, as with hip revision arthroplasty, the number of revision knee arthroplasties increases. As the numbers increase, so do the severity of the defects and the complexity of the reconstructions. Use of a Press-Fit stem on revision components can protect the juxtaarticular bone and transfer the load to stronger diaphyseal bone. The balance between overshielding the juxtaarticular bone and overloading it to failure still needs to be determined. Presently, these stems provide for excellent structural protection of the abnormal bone with no substantial evidence of stress shielding. The stems provide protection from shear, bending, and rotational forces while still allowing compression of the bone. This requires the presence of bone with enough structural integrity to support these remaining forces. Medium-term findings for procedures using these components have demonstrated results that have been unparalleled, so that these stems are an essential adjunct to the revision arthroplasty procedure. They are not, however, a substitute for ensuring solid juxtaarticular support for the components.

REFERENCES

1. Behrens JC, Walker PS, Shoji H. Variations in the strength and structure of cancellous bone at the knee. *J Biomechanics* 1974;7:201.
2. Albrektsson BEJ, Ryyd L, Carlsson LV, et al. The effect of a stem on the tibial component of knee arthroplasty: a roentgen stereophotogrammetric study of uncemented tibial components in the Freeman-Samuelson knee arthroplasty. *J Bone Joint Surg Br* 1990;72:252–258.
3. Dennis DA. Structural allografting in revision total knee arthroplasty. *Orthopaedics* 1994;17(9):849.
4. Bartel DL, Burstein AH, Santavicca EA, et al. Performance of the tibial component in total knee arthroplasty. *J Bone Joint Surg Am* 1982;64:1026–1033.
5. Wright T. Biomaterials and prosthesis design in total knee arthroplasty. *Orthopaedic knowledge update: hip and knee reconstruction.* Rosemont, IL: American Academy of Orthopaedic Surgeons, 1995.
6. Murase K, Crowingshield RD, Pedersen DR, et al. An analysis of tibial component design in total knee arthroplasty. *J Biomechanics* 1983;16:13.
7. Reilly D, Walker PS, Ben-Dov M, et al. Effects of tibial components on load transfer in the upper tibia. *Clin Orthop* 1982;170:131.
8. Brooks PJ, Walker PS, Scott RD. Tibial component fixation in deficient tibial bone stock. *Clin Orthop* 1984;184:302–308.
9. Bartel DL, Burstein AH, Santavicca EA, et al. Performance of the tibial component in total knee replacement: conventional and revision designs. *J Bone Joint Surg Am* 1982;64:1026–1033.
10. Lewis JL, Askew MJ, Jaycox DP. A comparative evaluation of tibial component designs of total knee prostheses. *J Bone Joint Surg Am* 1982;64:129–135.
11. Murray PB, Rand JA, Hanssen AD. Cemented long-stem revision knee arthroplasty. *Clin Orthop* 1994;309:116–123.
12. Bertin KC, Freeman MAR, Samuelson KM, et al. Stemmed revision arthroplasty for aseptic loosening of total knee replacement. *J Bone Joint Surg Br* 1985;67:242–248.
13. Elia EA, Lotke PA. Results of revision total knee arthroplasty associated with significant bone loss. *Clin Orthop* 1991;271:114–121.
14. Haas SB, Insall JN, Montgomery W, et al. Revision total knee arthroplasty with use of modular components with stems inserted without cement. *J Bone Joint Surg Am* 1995;77:1700–1777.
15. Bourne RB, Finlay JB. The influence of tibial component intramedullary stems and implant-cortex contact on the strain distribution of the proximal tibia following total knee arthroplasty: an in vitro study. *Clin Orthop* 1986;208:95–99.
16. Vince KG, Long W. Revision knee arthroplasty: the limits of press fit medullary fixation. *Clin Orthop* 1995;317:172–177.
17. Donaldson, WF, Sculco TP, Insall JN, et al. Total Condylar III knee prosthesis: long-term follow-up study. *Clin Orthop* 1988;226:22–28.
18. Askew MJ, Lewis JL, Jaycox DP, et al. Interface stresses in a prosthesis-tibia structure with varying bone properties. *Trans Orthop Res Soc* 1978;3:17.
19. Insall JN, Ranawat CS, Aglietti P, et al. A comparison of four models of total knee replacement prostheses. *J Bone Joint Surg Am* 1976;58:754–765.
20. Paprosky WG. Use of distal femoral allografts in revision total knee arthroplasty. In: Insall JN, Scott WN, Scuderi GR. *Current concepts in primary and revision total knee arthroplasty.* Lippincott–Raven Publishers, 1996:217–226.
21. Mnaymneh W, Emerson RH, Borja F, et al. Massive allografts in salvage revisions of failed total knee arthroplasties. *Clin Orthop* 1990;260:144–153.

CHAPTER 107

Implant Selection in Revision Total Knee Arthroplasty

Brian D. Haas and Douglas A. Dennis

PREOPERATIVE CLINICAL ASSESSMENT

An extensive preoperative patient evaluation is necessary to improve the outcome of revision total knee arthroplasty (TKA). This includes a thorough history taking and physical examination, laboratory assessment, and critical review of radiographs. A review of the patient's preoperative history is necessary to determine the cause of the failed TKA. Success rates of revision TKA procedures have clearly been unfavorable if the cause of failure is not identified preoperatively (1,2). Infection, Charcot arthropathy, neuromuscular disease, or significant preoperative medical conditions, which may contribute to adverse outcomes, should be addressed preoperatively.

Knowledge of previous surgical procedures and the prosthetic devices implanted is necessary. The previous surgical approach, soft tissue releases performed, and the size and type of prosthetic components implanted are critical information.

Clinical examination includes the assessment of range of motion, ligamentous stability, overall lower limb alignment, and patellofemoral tracking. Evaluation of the hip and ankle to assess for any factors contributing to overall limb alignment is mandatory. Other causes of limb pain, such as vascular insufficiency and radicular pain, should be evaluated and addressed before revision arthroplasty.

PREOPERATIVE ASSESSMENT OF THE EXISTING IMPLANT DESIGN

Preoperative assessment of the existing implant aids the surgeon in selecting the appropriate revision implant. The revision total knee surgeon will encounter patients implanted with a myriad of different prosthetic devices. A thorough knowledge of the implant type with available modularity and revision options for the implant in place is necessary. Some revision TKA procedures involve revising only a portion of the existing implant, and thorough knowledge of the implant system in place is necessary to prepare adequately for these cases. In addition, awareness of the specific implant design in place allows the surgeon to order implant-specific extraction devices, should these be indicated. If the previous arthroplasty was performed by another surgeon, the operative note and purchasing order should be obtained to verify implant type and size.

OPERATIVE APPROACH

The operative approach used in revision TKA depends on multiple factors. The most critical factors are maintenance of cutaneous circulation, protection of the extensor mechanism, and the ability of the surgeon to adequately gain exposure of the existing implants. Use of the previous skin incision is generally recommended. Although it is usually safe to ignore previous short medial or lateral peripatellar skin incisions, one should beware of wide scars with thin or absent subcutaneous tissue, as damage to the underlying dermal plexus is likely, which increases the risk of wound necrosis (3). If long parallel skin incisions exist, choice of the lateral-most skin incision is favorable to avoid a large lateral skin flap that has been previously compromised at the time of the initial lateral skin incision. In complex situations, such as in knees with multiple skin incisions or previously burned or irradiated skin, consideration of plastic surgical consultation is wise, both for the design of the upcoming skin incision as well as for consideration of preoperative muscle flap procedures or soft tissue expansion (4) if the risk of skin necrosis is substantial.

Avulsion of the patellar tendon remains a devastating complication (5) and must be avoided at all costs. Extensile exposures, such as the quadriceps snip (6) or tibial tubercle osteotomy (7), should be used before excessive tension is placed on the patellar tendon insertion. Adequate exposure to remove implants is essential to avoid further bone loss and to protect ligamentous structures.

BONE LOSS

The management of bone loss in TKA is dictated by the extent and location of bone deficiency. In revision TKA, significant bone loss is often encountered, and the extent is usually more than preoperative radiographs would indicate. Assessment of bone loss in revision TKA is best accomplished after removal of components. One should anticipate that the removal of well-fixed implants may accentuate the preoperative bone loss. Preliminary bone cuts should be made before determination of the method of bone defect management. A general principle is to remove only 1 to 2 mm of bone from the most prominent femoral or tibial condyle to provide a platform onto which cutting guides can be placed. Most literature classifies bone defects as contained (cavitary) or noncontained (segmental).

Bone cement is useful to fill smaller areas of bone deficiency, particularly in elderly patients. Its major indications are small bony defects up to 5 mm in depth, which are preferably contained. Bone cement fill of larger, noncontained defects is not recommended because of difficulty in pressurization and loss of support due to cement shrinkage during polymerization.

Autogenous bone graft is indicated for contained defects larger than 5 mm in depth. In cases in which bone resection provides adequate material, this is an excellent choice due to accelerated incorporation compared to allograft. Because the size and shape of available autogenous bone are limited, it is infrequently used in cases of larger noncontained defects.

Particulate allograft is often selected for large contained defects. This material is useful in cases in which autogenous bone graft is inadequate or the size of the defect is so large that autogenous bone grafting is impractical. Structural allograft bone grafting is reserved for large, noncontained bone defects. Allograft offers numerous advantages, including biocompatibility, bone stock restoration, and the potential for ligamentous reattachment, particularly if grafting is performed using bone block reattachment techniques (8–10). Disadvantages include expense and the potential for disease transmission (11) and biologic failure of the graft (9,11,12).

Modular metal augmentations have become a popular alternative to address bone loss (13–15). They are particularly useful for moderate-sized, peripheral bony defects. Disadvantages of use include a potential for increased fretting and their limited size and shapes, which often preclude use in repairing massive defects. They also do not restore bone stock, which is of particular concern in younger patients.

IMPLANT SELECTION CRITERIA

Although the principles of revision TKA are similar to those of primary arthroplasty, numerous additional difficulties are often encountered, including soft tissue scarring, bone loss, flexion-extension gap imbalance, ligamentous instability, and disturbance of the anatomic joint line. To deal with these difficulties, use of a revision implant system, which includes various levels of prosthetic constraint, augmentations, and diaphysis-engaging stems, is imperative. The surgeon's experience with the implant design system selected is paramount in ensuring the success of the revision arthroplasty.

In choosing a revision implant system, the surgeon must take into account multiple variables. The coronal and sagittal geometry of the implant must be appropriate to provide proper kinematic function. Prostheses with increasing levels of constraint, ranging from posterior cruciate retention to posterior cruciate substitution, varus-valgus constraint, and hinged designs, must be available. A vast array of implant designs is available, and these may have significant differences in eventual kinematic function. For example, cam-and-post mechanisms of posterior cruciate–substituting (PCS) designs vary widely in size, shape, and degree of flexion at which cam-post engagement occurs. These differences are reflected in variable levels of implant performance. The locking mechanism for polyethylene bearing fixation to the tibial tray should be evaluated. Research has indicated that back surface wear is a significant contributor to polyethylene debris production (16,17). A thorough knowledge of each implant type allows the surgeon to choose the appropriate implant for each individual patient. Because of the complexity of each procedure, no single implant type can be used for all cases.

Prosthetic components are selected based on intraoperative findings. Prosthetic constraint should be minimized to enhance the durability of fixation. In many cases, however, posterior cruciate ligament deficiency is common, and choice of a PCS device is wise. In most revisions, either large bone defects or weakened condylar bone is encountered, which necessitates use of either press-fit or cemented diaphysis-engaging stems for additional fixation and load distribution. The surgeon should evaluate the design, modular locking mechanism, and available lengths of the implant system selected.

POSTERIOR CRUCIATE–RETAINING REVISION TOTAL KNEE ARTHROPLASTY

The use of a posterior cruciate–retaining (PCR) prosthesis in revision TKA requires a surgeon skilled in appropriate balance of the posterior cruciate ligament. As previously stated, indications for revision TKA with PCR components are uncommon in our practice, and their use should be limited to cases with mini-

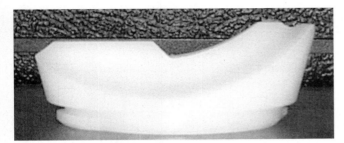

FIG. 1. Example of a tibial polyethylene insert designed with increased sagittal plane conformity.

mal deformity, instability, and bone loss. Preoperative assessment of both flexion and extension stability and the competence of the posterior cruciate ligament is essential to the use of this type of device.

Principles of posterior cruciate retention are the same in revision TKA as in primary TKA. If present, the posterior cruciate ligament may be retained if the operative surgeon can achieve flexion and extension balance with maintenance and competence of the posterior cruciate ligament and restoration of the anatomic joint line. Advantages of the use of PCR designs in revision knee arthroplasty are the preservation of bone stock and the theoretic advantages for retention of the posterior cruciate ligament found in primary TKA. The majority of cases in which this type of implant is used today are those in which polyethylene failure has led to wear and the need for revision. In these cases, the original primary implant remains well fixed and posterior cruciate ligament integrity is maintained.

Disadvantages of the use of PCR designs are the difficulty of balancing the posterior cruciate ligament, restoring the joint line to its anatomic position, and obtaining adequate flexion stability in revision cases in which the competency of the existing posterior cruciate ligament may be difficult to evaluate. Because of these factors, it is often wise to select a PCR design that provides enhanced sagittal plane conformity (Fig. 1) (18) to better control anteroposterior femorotibial translation in those cases in which integrity of the posterior cruciate ligament is questionable. Collateral ligament instability may necessitate further levels of constraint, which prohibits the retention of the posterior cruciate ligament. In the authors' experience, the use of these devices is limited because of the difficulties discussed earlier.

POSTERIOR CRUCIATE–SUBSTITUTING REVISION TOTAL KNEE ARTHROPLASTY

PCS devices remain the authors' implant choice for the majority of revision TKA cases. Advantages of the use of these designs include reliable substitution for an absent or incompetent posterior cruciate ligament, easier correction of deformity, increased flexion stability, and increased range of motion (19,20) secondary to forced posterior femoral rollback. This can be beneficial in those cases in which preoperative stiffness is problematic.

PCS TKA designs incorporate a cam-and-post mechanism to enhance flexion stability and posterior femoral rollback (Fig. 2). There are multiple types of cam-and-post mechanisms available that differ in post size (height and width), shape, and sagittal plane position. These design variances are reflected in differing patterns

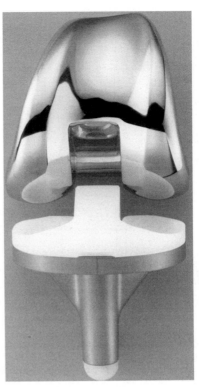

FIG. 2. Posterior cruciate–substituting design for total knee arthroplasty demonstrating the cam-and-post mechanism.

of kinematic function. The implanting surgeon must be aware of these differences and select a design that optimizes patient function while providing long-term durability. Historically, in the most commonly implanted (PCS) designs, the cam and post do not engage until approximately 70 degrees of knee flexion (21). Therefore, the cam and post are not engaged during lesser flexion activities such as walking. Other PCS TKA designs allow cam-and-post engagement as early as 30 degrees of knee flexion. Advocates of these designs report earlier posterior femoral rollback and enhanced quadriceps function due to an increased quadriceps lever arm (22). Polyethylene post wear in traditional PCS TKA designs has been limited. It is not yet known if post wear will become problematic in designs that permit earlier cam-post engagement.

Potential problems encountered with use of PCS TKA implants include posterior dislocation of the cam relative to the post (23,24), condylar fracture due to increased bone resection (25), and an increased incidence of patellar clunk syndrome (26–28). While mechanically enhancing flexion stability, the surgeon must still strictly adhere to the principle of obtaining flexion-extension gap balance to lessen the risk of dislocation. The risk of femoral condylar fracture is typically increased in the multiply revised TKA in which excessive distal femoral bone resection has previously been performed. The risk of condylar fracture is greatest medially because the medial metaphyseal contour transitions more abruptly to the diaphysis than the lateral contour. Because of this, the amount of bone remaining at the proximal margin of the intercondylar notch resection required for PCS TKA designs is less medially (Fig. 3).

Although the incidence of patellar clunk syndrome has been higher in PCS TKA (26–28), the incidence is clearly design

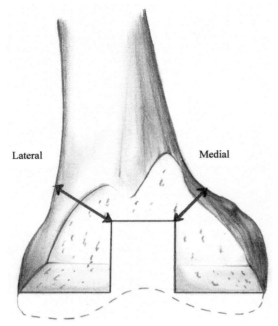

FIG. 3. Diagram showing reduced medial versus lateral bone mass (↕) present at the proximal margin of the intercondylar bone resection required for implantation of a posterior cruciate–substituting total knee prosthesis.

related. Designs with a more "boxy" (rectangular) sagittal geometry and those with a higher (more proximal) margin of the intercondylar box are at greater risk. Pollock et al. (29) reviewed the incidence of peripatellar synovial entrapment in three different PCS TKA designs (459 consecutively treated

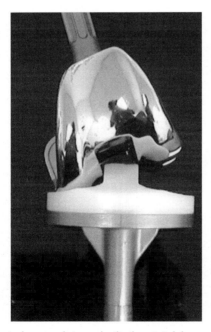

FIG. 4. Posterior cruciate–substituting total knee prosthesis demonstrating an absence of collateral stability provided by this implant design.

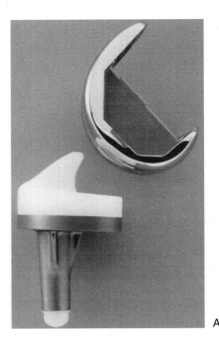

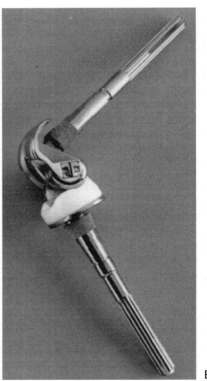

FIG. 5. Unlinked (**A**; PFC Sigma Total Condylar III) versus linked (**B**; S-ROM rotating hinge) constrained total knee arthroplasty designs.

cases). The incidence of symptomatic synovial entrapment varied based on implant type, with 12.8% (18 of 141) of patients implanted with a Congruency PCS (Depuy, Warsaw, IN), 4.2% (9 of 212) given an AMK PCS6, and 0% (none of 106) of those receiving a PFC Sigma PCS design experiencing synovial entrapment.

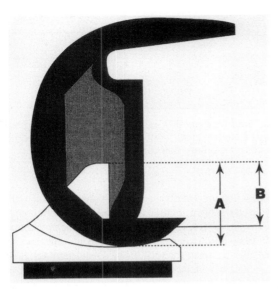

FIG. 6. Diagram of lateral view of generic varus-valgus constrained design. A, post height; B, subluxation height. (From Griffin WL, Fehring TK, Valadie A. Revision of the unstable total knee arthroplasty. In: Engh GA, Rorabeck CH, eds. *Revision total knee arthroplasty.* Baltimore: Williams & Wilkins, 1997:340–351, with permission.)

Last, one must realize that traditional PCS TKA designs do not provide stability in the presence of varus or valgus loads and therefore do not provide stability in cases of advanced collateral ligamentous laxity or loss (Fig. 4). Constrained TKA devices must be considered in these cases.

CONSTRAINED REVISION TOTAL KNEE ARTHROPLASTY

Constrained TKA implants provide stability in both the frontal and sagittal planes. Their use is indicated in cases with severe collateral ligamentous insufficiency or loss and in those with substantial flexion-extension gap imbalance in which flexion stability cannot be obtained using traditional ligament-balancing techniques and joint line restoration.

Constrained designs can be classified as unlinked or linked (Fig. 5). Unlinked constrained designs typically have a tibial polyethylene post that is enlarged (in height and width) and interlocks into a deepened femoral intercondylar box. Various unlinked constrained implants are available that differ in the degree of varus-valgus constraint, rotational constraint, and dislocation height (30) (Fig. 6, Table 1). Disadvantages of the use of unlinked constrained designs include premature tibial polyethylene post wear (31) and premature component loosening (32–34) due to increased load transmission to the fixation interface and implant dislocation.

With linked constrained devices, the femoral and tibial components are linked, typically via an intercondylar locking pin. In the authors' practice, the use of these devices is uncommon and limited to patients with total medial collateral ligament loss, severe flexion instability, uncontrolled hyperextension deformities, and massive bone loss from tumor resection or comminuted supracondylar femoral fractures.

Linked-hinge designs are often excessively constrained and have the same problems (premature polyethylene wear and prosthetic loosening) as unlinked constrained devices. Early linked-hinge implants allowed no rotational laxity and failed prematurely due to component loosening (35–37). Most modern hinged designs incorporate a mobile polyethylene bearing that permits rotation and lessens loads to both the polyethylene bearing and the fixation interface. These designs are favored in the rare situation that a constrained hinged TKA is required.

To maximize the longevity of constrained devices, surgeons must still concentrate on restoration of normal limb alignment, balancing the remaining soft tissue envelope, and not depending totally on implant constraint to provide knee stability.

CUSTOM PROSTHETIC DEVICES

The need for custom-designed TKA components has dramatically decreased since the evolution of modular TKA systems that allow the surgeon to build total knee components based on intraoperative findings. The most common indications for custom devices include the presence of marked angular deformities (congenital or acquired), massive bone loss when bone allograft is unavailable, and miniature bone anatomy such as in patients with juvenile rheumatoid arthritis or dwarfism.

Disadvantages of the use of custom components include difficulty in assessing bone loss preoperatively, which results in an inaccurate custom component design. In addition, these devices are costly and often are provided without custom-designed instruments to assist in accurate implantation.

TABLE 1. *Constraint level of various unlinked constrained total knee arthroplasty implants*

	Total Condylar III (Johnson & Johnson, Raynham, MA)	Maxim (Biomet, Warsaw, IN)	Zimmer constrained condylar knee (Zimmer, Warsaw, IN)	Coordinate (Depuy, Warsaw, IN)
Post height (mm)	24.6–27.22	24.2–24.4	22.7–29.5	17.1–26.7
Dislocation height (mm)	21.3–23.8	18.9–19.1	17.7–24.5	12.1–18.0
Varus-valgus constraint at 0 degrees	±2.2 degrees	±3.0 degrees	±1.25 degrees	±2.0 degrees
Rotational constraint at 0 degrees	±4.33 degrees	±4.0 degrees	±2.0 degrees	±1.3 degrees

From Griffin WL, Fehring TK, Valadie A. Revision of the unstable total knee arthroplasty. In: Engh GA, Rorabeck CH, eds. *Revision total knee arthroplasty.* Baltimore: Williams & Wilkins, 1997:340–351, with permission.

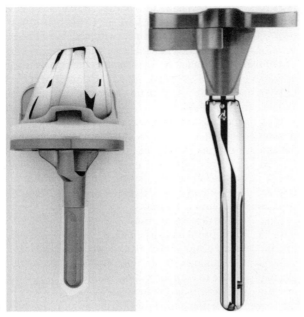

FIG. 7. Offset tibial tray **(A)** and offset tibial stem **(B)**, which are useful in cases of distortion of metaphyseal versus diaphyseal bone anatomy.

MODULAR STEMS AND AUGMENTATIONS

The use of diaphysis-engaging femoral and tibial stems has clearly improved the results of revision TKA (38–40). Stems enhance fixation of revision TKA components by dispersing load from weakened condylar bone.

Controversy exists as to whether the stem should be fully cemented or press-fit. Equivalent results have been reported using both techniques (38–40). Cementless stems should be canal filling and should provide rotational stability. Cemented stems should have rounded contours to facilitate removal if necessary. Modular locking mechanisms must be secure to prevent fretting or stem dissociation (41). The use of Press-Fit stems provides better remaining bone stock should future revision TKA be necessary. Due to the canal-filling nature of Press-Fit stems, the condylar position of the femoral or tibial component is determined by the stem position within the medullary canal. This fact may preclude their use in patients with angular deformity, particularly in the metaphyseal or diaphyseal regions. Use of offset tibial trays or offset intramedullary stems (Fig. 7) can be helpful in these situations, as long as angular deformity is limited. Cemented stems are favored in patients with anatomic deformity or severe osteopenia, and in cases in which rigid fixation cannot be obtained with a press-fit design.

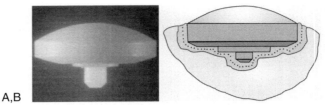

FIG. 9. Biconvex patellar component **(A)** and diagram of a biconvex patellar component implanted into a revision patella with a central cavitary defect **(B)**.

Modular femoral and tibial augmentations are useful to fill moderately sized (less than 2 cm) osseous defects. A common surgical error in revision TKA is failure to recognize the amount of distal femoral bone loss. Failure to do so results in joint line elevation and possibly an unsatisfactory result. Distal femoral augmentations are quite beneficial to assist in joint line restoration.

Modular tibial component augmentations are available in multiple shapes (angular vs. rectangular) and sizes (Fig. 8). Angular augmentations are often more bone preserving, whereas rectangular augmentations have been shown to be more stable biomechanically due to reduced shear forces (42).

When modular augmentations are required in revision TKA, condylar bone damage is common. Diaphysis-engaging Press-Fit or cemented stems used in conjunction with modular augmentation should be chosen to provide additional support and lessen condylar fixation stresses.

PATELLAR COMPONENT REVISION

Variable amounts of patellar bone loss may be encountered during patellar component revision. In the authors' experience, a minimum of 10 to 12 mm of remaining patellar bone stock is necessary if a new patellar component is to be implanted.

Designs with three peripheral lugs are often useful when revising central lug designs, in which bone loss is typically central. A circular, three-lug design is also often selected when revising a failed three-lug device. In this situation, rotation of the component from its original position often provides adequate bone for fixation of the new patellar component.

In cases with large, central cavitary bone loss, selection of a bioconvex, inset patellar component can facilitate patellar component fixation (Fig. 9) (43).

CONCLUSION

To successfully manage the myriad problems faced in revision TKA, a modular revision TKA system is favored. A pros-

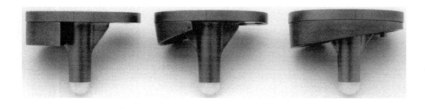

FIG. 8. Multiple shapes and sizes of modular tibial augmentation available to replace moderate-sized bone defects.

thetic system must provide multiple levels of prosthetic constraint, femoral and tibial augmentations, and diaphysis-engaging stems. Use of an implant system allows the surgeon to assemble the desired prosthetic components based on intraoperative findings. One must realize that long-term durability of prosthetic components is inversely proportional to prosthetic constraint. Selection of the least-constrained prosthetic components that provide satisfactory stability is recommended. Diaphysis-engaging stems are often used due to the weakened metaphyseal bone encountered in most cases of revision TKA.

REFERENCES

1. Dennis DA. Revision knee arthroplasty: how I do it. In: Insall JN, Scott WN, eds. *Surgery of the knee.* New York: Churchill Livingstone, 2001:1934–1941.
2. Mont MA, Serna FK, Krackow KA, et al. Exploration of radiographically normal total knee replacements for unexplained pain. *Clin Orthop* 1996;331:216–220.
3. Klein NE, Cox CV. Wound problems in total knee arthroplasty. In: Fu FH, Harner CD, Vince KG, et al. eds. *Knee surgery,* vol 2. Baltimore: Williams & Wilkins, 1994:1539–1552.
4. Gold DA, Scott SC, Scott WN, eds. Soft tissue expansion prior to arthroplasty in the multiply-operated knee: a new method of preventing catastrophic skin problems. *J Arthroplasty* 1996;11:512.
5. Rand JA, Morrey BF, Bryan RS. Patellar tendon rupture after total knee arthroplasty. *Clin Orthop* 1989;244:233–238.
6. Garvin KL, Scuderi G, Insall JN. Evolution of the quadriceps snip. *Clin Orthop* 1995;321:131–137.
7. Whiteside LA. Exposure in difficult total knee arthroplasty using tibial tubercle osteotomy. *Clin Orthop* 1995;321:32–35.
8. Mankin HJ, Doppelt S, Tomford W. Clinical experience with allograft implantation. The first ten years. *Clin Orthop* 1983;174:69–86.
9. Mnaymneh W, Emerson RH, Borja F, et al. Massive allografts in salvage revisions of failed total knee arthroplasties. *Clin Orthop* 1990;260:144–153.
10. Dennis DA. Structural allografting in revision total knee arthroplasty. *Orthopaedics* 1994;17:849–851.
11. Buck BE, Malinin TI, Brown MD. Bone transplantation and human immunodeficiency virus. An estimate of risk of acquired immunodeficiency syndrome (AIDS). *Clin Orthop* 1989;240:129–136.
12. Berrey BH Jr, Lord CF, Gebhardt MC, et al. Fractures of allografts. Frequency, treatment, and end-results. *J Bone Joint Surg Am* 1990;72:825–833.
13. Rand JA. Bone deficiency in total knee arthroplasty. *Clin Orthop* 1991;271:63–71.
14. Brand MG, Daley RJ, Ewald FC, et al. Tibial tray augmentation with modular metal wedges for tibial bone stock deficiency. *Clin Orthop* 1989;248:71–79.
15. Pagnano MW, Trousdale RT, Rand JA. Tibial wedge augmentation for bone deficiency in total knee arthroplasty. A follow-up study. *Clin Orthop* 1995;321:151–155.
16. Parks NL, Engh GA, Topoleski LD, et al. The Coventry Award. Modular tibial insert micromotion. A concern with contemporary knee implants. *Clin Orthop* 1998;356:10–15.
17. Wasielewski RC, Parks NL, Williams I, et al. The tibial insert undersurface as a contributing source of polyethylene wear debris. *Clin Orthop* 1997;345:53–59.
18. Laskin RS, Maruyama Y, Villanueva M, et al. Deep-dish congruent tibial component use knee arthroplasty. *Clin Orthop* 2000;380:36–44.
19. Dennis DA, Komistek RD, Stiehl JB, et al. Range of motion after total knee arthroplasty. *J Arthroplasty* 1998;13:748–752.
20. Hirsh HS, Lotke PA, Morrison LD. The posterior cruciate ligament in total knee surgery. *Clin Orthop* 1994;309:64.
21. Insall J, Lachiewicz P, Burstein A. The posterior stabilized condylar prosthesis: a modification of the total-condylar design; two- and four-year clinical experience. *J Bone Joint Surg Am* 1982;64:1317–1323.
22. Lombardi AV Jr, Metzger RG, Mallory TH, et al. Late versus early engagement of posterior stabilized prosthesis: effect on extensor moment arm and resultant extensor loads. Paper presented at: 68th Annual Meeting of the American Academy of Orthopaedic Surgeons; February 28–March 4, 2001; San Francisco, CA.
23. Lombardi AV Jr, Mallory TH, Vaughn BK, et al. Dislocation following primary posterior-stabilized total knee arthroplasty *J Arthroplasty* 1993;8(6):633–639.
24. Hossain S, Ayeko C, Anwar M, et al. Dislocation of Insall-Burstein II modified total knee arthroplasty. *J Arthroplasty* 2001;16:233–235.
25. Lombardi AV Jr, Mallory TH, Waterman RA, et al. Intercondylar distal femoral fracture. An unreported complication of posterior-stabilized total knee arthroplasty. *J Arthroplasty* 1995;10(5):643–650.
26. Hozack WJ, Rothman RH, Booth RE Jr, et al. The patellar clunk syndrome: a complication of posterior stabilized total knee arthroplasty. *Clin Orthop* 1989;241:203–208.
27. Beight JL, Yao B, Hozack WJ, et al. The patellar "clunk" syndrome after posterior stabilized total knee arthroplasty. *Clin Orthop* 1994;299:139–142.
28. Lucas TS, DeLuca PF, Nazarian DG, et al. Arthroscopic treatment of patellar clunk. *Clin Orthop* 1999;367:226–229.
29. Pollock DC, Engh GA, Ammeen DJ. Synovial entrapment: a complication of posterior stabilized total knee arthroplasty. Paper presented at: Knee Society Interim Meeting; September 14, 2000; Boston.
30. Griffin WL, Fehring TK, Valadie A. Revision of the unstable total knee arthroplasty. In: Engh GA, Rorabeck CH, eds. *Revision total knee arthroplasty.* Baltimore: Williams & Wilkins, 1997:340–351.
31. Puloski SK, McCalden RW, MacDonald SJ, et al. Tibial post wear in posterior stabilized total knee arthroplasty. An unrecognized source of polyethylene debris. *J Bone Joint Surg Am* 2001;83:390–394.
32. Rosenberg AG, Verner JJ, Galante JO. Clinical results of total knee revision using the Total Condylar III prosthesis. *Clin Orthop* 1991;273:83–90.
33. Donaldson WF, Sculco TP, Insall JN, et al. Total condylar III knee prosthesis. Long term follow-up study. *Clin Orthop* 1988;226:21–28.
34. Rand JA. Revision total knee arthroplasty using the total condylar III prosthesis. *J Arthroplasty* 1991;6:279.
35. DeBurge A, Guepar. Guepar hinge prosthesis: complications and results with 2 years followup. *Clin Orthop* 1976;120:47–53.
36. Bargar WL, Cracchiolo A III, Amstutz HC. Results with the constrained total knee prosthesis in treating severely disabled patients and patients with failed total knee replacements. *J Bone Joint Surg Am* 1980;62:504–512.
37. Hui FS, Fitzgerald RH Jr. Hinged total knee arthroplasty. *J Bone Joint Surg Am* 1980;62:513–519.
38. Murray PB, Rand JA, Hanssen AD. Cemented long-stem revision total knee arthroplasty. *Clin Orthop* 1994;309:116–123.
39. Haas SB, Insall JN, Montgomery W 3rd, et al. Revision total knee arthroplasty with use of modular components with stems inserted without cement. *J Bone Joint Surg Am* 1995;77(11):1700–1707.
40. Engh GA, Herzwurm PJ, Parks NL. Treatment of major defects of bone with bulk allografts and stemmed components during total knee arthroplasty. *J Bone Joint Surg Am* 1997;79:1030–1039.
41. Lim LA, Trousdale RT, Berry DJ, et al. Failure of the stem-condyle junction of a modular femoral stem in revision total knee arthroplasty. *J Arthroplasty* 2001;16:128–132.
42. Chen F, Krackow KA. Management of tibial defects in total knee arthroplasty. *Clin Orthop* 1994;305:249–257.
43. Kitsugi T, Gustilo RB, Bechtold JE. Results of nonmetal-backed, high-density polyethylene, biconvex patellar prostheses. A 5–7-year follow-up evaluation. *J Arthroplasty* 1994;9:151–162.

CHAPTER 108

Management of Bony Defects in Revision Total Knee Joint Replacement

Mark Clatworthy and Allan E. Gross

Surgeons treating patients who require revision arthroplasties may have to deal with osseous defects. The management of these defects depends on their size and location. Small defects may be amenable to repair with morselized allograft or augments and wedges that are an integral part of modern knee revision systems. In the face of massive bone loss, structural allografts or custom prostheses are a viable alternative.

In this chapter, we present the classification of bony defects in revision total knee arthroplasty, review the pathogenesis of bone destruction, appraise the treatment options for bony defects, outline the techniques for the treatment of bone loss, and review the results of these treatment options.

CLASSIFICATION

Bone defects encountered in revision total knee arthroplasty have been classified to enable the surgeon to categorize the extent of the bone loss preoperatively. This enables the surgeon to plan accurately for the revision procedure. The classification also allows comparison of the outcomes of revision procedures according to the degree of bone loss.

We use a simple classification: contained and noncontained defects.

Contained defects have an intact circumferential cortex. Contained defects are subdivided into

Type 1 defects, in which the metaphyseal bone is intact and no bone grafting or augmentation is required to restore a normal joint line. Small bone defects can be filled with cement, and a primary style prosthesis without stems can be used.
Type II defects, which have damaged metaphyseal bone requiring bone grafting, a cement fill, or augments to restore a normal joint line. These defects are best treated with stemmed revision prostheses with augments.

Uncontained defects have segmental bone loss with no remaining cortex.

These defects are subdivided as

Type III or noncircumferential defects requiring a partial distal femur, partial proximal tibia, or femoral head graft.
Type IV or circumferential defects requiring a segmental distal femur or proximal tibia.

PATHOGENESIS OF BONE DEFECTS IN TOTAL KNEE REPLACEMENT

The etiology of bony defects is multifactorial. In this section, we discuss mechanical bone loss, stress shielding, osteolysis, and infection.

Mechanical Bone Loss

Bone excision at the time of the primary knee replacement is the most obvious cause of bone loss. The early knee prostheses were hinged. They required significant bone resection and had large intramedullary stems that required a large amount of cancellous bone removal. Due to the excessive constraints, high rotational forces were distributed to the implant bone interface, which led to loosening of the implant. Gross loosening resulted in a windshield-wiper-like action, often with dramatic bone loss (1,2). The early 1980s saw a move to resurfacing-style prostheses requiring minimal bone resection and using very thin polyethylene inserts. Paradoxically, this resulted in increased polyethylene wear, which led to particulate-mediated osteolysis (3–6).

Significant bone loss can also occur at the revision of well-fixed components. The posterior femoral condyles are particularly at risk. Thus, great care must be taken to ensure that the bone-cement-implant interface is loosened adequately before implant removal.

Stress Shielding

The tibial component most commonly fails in total knee replacement. This is thought to be due to compressive failure of trabecular support (7). Stress shielding may be an important factor in this mechanism of failure. Use of a metal tibial tray and stem has been shown to reduce maximum compressive stresses in underlying bone by 16% to 39% (8).

The strength of the metaphyseal region of the distal femur is also reduced. In calculations using finite-element analysis, it has been shown that the rigid femoral component reduces stress to the anterior distal femur by a magnitude of 1 (9). Bone loss occurs primarily in the first year (10); however, one study has shown progressive bone loss with time (11). The effect of type of fixation on stress shielding is controversial. Mintzer et al. (10) showed that osteopenia was independent of implant design and fixation, whereas Seki et al. (12) demonstrated a 57% decrease in bone density with a cemented implant compared with 28% for a cementless implant of the same design. This stress shielding correlates with the clinically and radiographically observed area of osteopenia in the anterior distal femur.

Osteolysis

It has now been well shown that wear particle generation is a significant factor in stimulating periprosthetic inflammation and subsequent bone loss in total joint arthroplasty (13). Osteolysis is common in total knee arthroplasty and occurs in the femur, tibia, and patella. Osteolysis may result in catastrophic failure of the arthroplasty when the bone is unable to support the implant (14,15). Weakening of the bone by osteolysis may also lead to periprosthetic fractures (16,17).

The etiology of wear particle generation is multifactorial. Finite-element analysis has demonstrated much higher contact stresses in the nonconforming total knee arthroplasty than in the more conforming total hip arthroplasty (3,18,19). Clinically, this has been demonstrated from retrievals of tibial polyethylene inserts in less-conforming total knee arthroplasties (3,4,6,20). Contact stresses in knee arthroplasty can exceed the yield stress of polyethylene, particularly if the polyethylene is less than 6

mm. The nonarticulating surface of the polyethylene can also generate wear particles (21,22). This has been termed *backsided wear*. Studies by Engh et al. (21) demonstrate a wide variation in the degree of wear between implants. They have shown that wear characteristics of the inner tray surface and integrity of the tibial implant locking mechanism are important.

The number of wear particles increases with applied load and number of cycles. Thus, more osteolysis is expected in heavier and more active patients (19,23,24). Poor limb alignment can result in early failure. It has been suggested that this is due to increased contact stresses, which increase both wear and mechanical failure (25). The polyethylene patella button can also be a source of wear particles. The force across the patellofemoral joint can be in excess of 4,600 N. This can be over a small area, particularly if there is patella maltracking or tilt (26). Thus, the yield strength of polyethylene may be exceeded (20).

Materials-related causes of osteolysis include the use of poor-quality polyethylene (5,20), heat-pressed polyethylene (20,27), or gamma-irradiated polyethylene, which oxidizes (28); the use of titanium as a bearing surface (29–31); and screw fixation of tibial implants (32). Some reports suggest that osteolysis is more common with cementless implants (23,33). It is proposed that this is because the wear particles gain easier access where the bone-cement interface is not imperviously sealed. Extensive porous coating has been shown to decrease the incidence of osteolysis (34).

Infection

Infection causes an acute inflammatory reaction and the production of a purulent cytokine-rich inflammatory exudate. These osteolytic cytokines can result in rapid destructive bone loss. Infection with lower-virulence organisms such as *Staphylococcus epidermidis* can result in progressive periprosthetic radiolucencies without frank clinical signs of infection.

Further bone loss is associated with the treatment of an infection about a total knee prosthesis. There is bone loss at the time of implant removal. The two-stage revision is also likely to lead to further mechanical bone loss from compression and abrasion due to the use of antibiotic spacers. One study quantified the loss as an average of 12.8 mm for the femur and 6.2 mm for the tibia (35). No metal rods were inserted across the knee. The authors use Rush pins to bridge the knee to increase the strength of the construct and reduce bone loss.

TREATMENT

Options

Commonly accepted options for the treatment of bony defects in revision knee arthroplasty include bone cement, screw- or mesh-augmented cement, modular or custom implants, and autograft or allograft. The technique used depends on the degree of bone loss and the extent to which the defect is contained.

Bone Cement

Cement has a role in repair of contained defects in which the bone loss is minimal. The major advantage of bone cement is that it can be molded to fit an irregular defect. It is a nonphysiologic material, however, and it lacks biomechanical integrity in larger defects, even when used with screws. Thus, the use of cement alone is limited to cases in which the cement column is a maximum of 5 mm in height and the bone loss involves less than 50% of the tibial plateau (36).

Metal Augments

Modern revision total knee systems are able to address bone stock loss using metal augmentation on both the femoral and tibial sides. The maximum flexion-extension gap equates to approximately a 5-cm gap. Gaps larger than this require massive allograft reconstructions.

Tibial wedges have been shown to be biomechanically superior to cement alone or screw-augmented cement (37). Metal augments are also useful on the femoral side, as asymmetric bone loss is common. Medial and lateral augments are available for use distally and posteriorly. The use of distal augments is increasing as surgeons more accurately re-create the anatomic joint line, whereas posterior augments are helpful to correct rotational errors resulting from the primary procedure and asymmetric bone loss.

In a study performing a finite-element analysis of the metaphyseal stresses in the bone-deficient tibia, the use of a metal base plate and stem was found to significantly reduce stress (8). It has also been shown that, in the absence of a cancellous bed to support the component, the best solution is to transfer the load to the cortical rim. This work has been supported by Brooks et al. (38), who showed that a 70-mm tibial stem will bear approximately 30% of the total load, unloading the deficient tibia.

Megaprostheses

Another alternative to structural allograft is mega custom implants, which are used frequently in limb reconstruction for malignant tumors around the knee. Where there is loss of ligamentous integrity with bone loss, rotating hinge prostheses can be used. These megaprostheses require use of a cemented porous-coated stem, which makes revisions of these constructs difficult. In addition, the reattachment of ligaments and the patellar tendon is not biologic. This may necessitate the use of a rotating hinge for stability and a gastrocnemius flap for patellar tendon attachment. This approach is valuable in patients with tumors but is not necessary for revision cases.

Autograft

Autograft is the optimum material for grafting defects, as it is both osteoinductive and osteoconductive. Bony defects are often too large to be repaired solely with autograft; however, autograft is useful to augment and enhance morselized allograft in contained defects and its use is imperative at the host-allograft interface to ensure healing.

Allograft

Allograft is an appealing alternative to autograft. It is available in unlimited quantities, the graft can be tailored to match the geometry of the bony defect, and there is no donor site mor-

bidity. Allograft, however, is only osteoconductive not osteoinductive; thus, the incorporation of cancellous bone and the healing of cortical bone is slower than with autogenous grafts (39). Allograft incorporation varies with the clinical scenario. The most critical factor is the recipient host bed. Morselized allograft incorporation occurs through a combination of revascularization, osteoconduction, and remodeling. In contrast, a segmental allograft unites to the host at the host-allograft interface, but there is limited internal remodeling of the allograft (40).

Fresh allografts may be rejected by the host immune system. The initial response is inflammation followed by complete graft resorption (41). Because of this, allografts are processed. The most common techniques are freezing and freeze drying. This allows long-term preservation of the graft. Bone frozen at –70°C has a shelf life of 5 years (41). These techniques have been shown to decrease or eliminate the immunogenicity of allografts; however, they also decrease their biologic activity by killing live cells. The major histocompatibility complex class I and II antigens on specialized antigen-presenting cells are responsible for the immune response to allograft bone (41,42). Animal studies have shown a strong immune response if there are major histocompatibility differences; however, there is no difference in the biologic incorporation of the graft (43,44). Similarly, the effect of HLA matching in allografts has been evaluated. A multicenter study showed sensitization to HLA; however, no biologic or clinical effects were ascertained (45). Other studies have shown better radiographically demonstrated incorporation with HLA matching; however, this effect was not statistically significant (46,47). Thus, at present no major histocompatibility complex or HLA matching is performed in revision joint arthroplasty using allograft bone.

Techniques

In this chapter, we concentrate on the surgical technique for treatment of uncontained defects that are beyond the scope of implant supplements. Contained defects are easily treated with morselized allograft, whereas small uncontained defects are treated with modular implants. Excellent step-by-step treatment guides are provided by the implant companies.

Preoperative Planning

Radiographs must be evaluated for bone loss. Before surgery, an attempt is made to assess bone loss; however, often loss is more extensive than anticipated on the radiographs. The surgeon must have available an allograft that matches the anatomic site, which is a distal femur or proximal tibia. Sizing is important, and it is useful to compare radiographs of the operated and contralateral knee with radiographs of the proposed allograft. If a distal femur is required, it is essential to have a smaller allograft than the host's so that the allograft can be placed within the host cortical shell with its attached collateral ligaments. If there is concern about the extensor mechanism, a proximal tibia with an extensor mechanism attached should be made available.

It is also important to examine the knee to gain an indication of the sagittal and coronal instability so that an implant with appropriate constraint can be chosen. Maintaining the soft tissue envelope allows a less constraining implant to be used rather than a

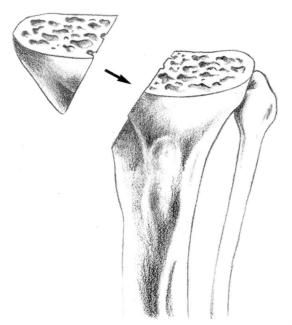

FIG. 1. A geometric defect is made in the noncircumferential defect to accept the allograft.

hinged prosthesis. We believe this decreases forces at the implant allograft and allograft-host interfaces, which should decrease the incidence of implant loosening and subsequent failure.

Allograft Procurement

The allograft is procured under sterile conditions according to the protocol of the American Association of Tissue Banks (48). The bone is deep-frozen at –70°C and treated with 25,000 Gy of radiation.

Surgical Technique

Noncircumferential Defects

For noncircumferential defects, a femoral head, partial distal femur, or proximal tibia is used. The bony defect is dissected out. A geometric cut is made where the host bone is structurally sound (Fig. 1). The structural allograft is then fashioned on the back table to fit the bony defect. The structural allograft is fixed to the bone with cancellous screws (Fig. 2), and additional fixation is obtained with long press-fit stems (Fig. 3). Care must be taken to ensure that the screws do not interfere with the press-fit stems. Two 6.5-mm AO screws are usually satisfactory. Morselized allograft is used to fill any contained bony defects. Cement is used to secure the allograft-implant and host-implant interfaces but is not used to enhance stem fixation in the diaphyseal region.

Circumferential Defects

For circumferential defects, the margins of the host bone are dissected out to reveal the extent of the bone loss. It is impera-

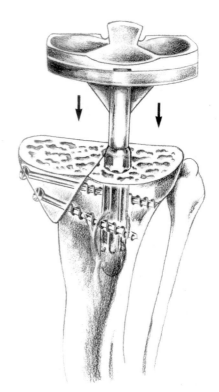

FIG. 2. The allograft is screwed to the host bone.

tive to retain as much residual host bone with soft tissue attachments as possible. The size and shape of the bony defect are evaluated, and a replacement construct is fashioned on the back table (Fig. 4). Appropriate cuts are made using revision total knee joint instrumentation. A step cut is made where the host

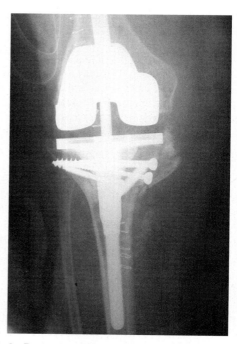

FIG. 3. Press-Fit stems are used to increase stability.

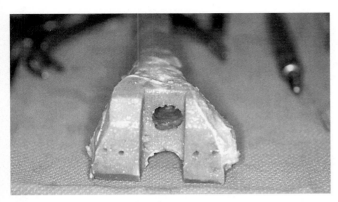

FIG. 4. The allograft is fashioned on the back table using revision instruments.

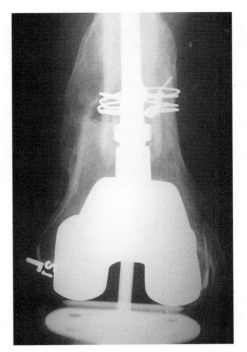

FIG. 6. Stems are used to enhance stability.

bone is structurally sound, and the allograft is fashioned to complement the step cut (Fig. 5). It is important to ensure that there is good approximation of bone at the allograft-host interface and that the allograft construct is satisfactorily externally rotated. A trial reduction is then performed. The level of the joint line must be carefully assessed, as there is a tendency to translate the joint line with allograft constructs. With a femoral allograft, the tendency is to depress the joint line, whereas a tibial allograft tends to elevate the joint line.

The most accurate method to measure the joint line is to measure the distance from the proximal tip of the fibula to the joint line on the normal contralateral knee radiograph. If the patient has undergone a joint replacement on the contralateral knee, guidelines for the joint line are the following: 1.5 cm proximal to the tip of the fibula, 2.5 cm distal to the medial epicondyle or the site of the residual meniscal rim scar. The surgeon must also ensure that the flexion and extension gaps are balanced, that the rotation of the components is correct, and that the alignment of the limb is acceptable. Rotational positioning of the implants is trialed with the epicondylar axis in the femur and the long axis of the tibia as a guide. It is important to ensure that the rotation is matched for the femoral and tibial components. We use patellar tracking as a guide to ensure that we have correct external rotation of the components.

Once the surgeon is satisfied that the aforementioned criteria for the allograft construct have been met, the components can be cemented to the allograft on the back table (Fig. 5). Cement is

used at the implant-allograft interface and the stem-allograft interface; however, care is taken to ensure that no cement is present at the proposed allograft-host interface or in the host canal. Stability of the construct is gained from the step cut and press-fit stems (Fig. 6). The stem is not cemented or porous coated, which makes the host canal available for further surgery. In the femur, the cortical shell of bone with the attached collateral ligaments is fixed with cerclage wires or screws to the construct to act as a vascularized graft at the host-allograft junction and to provide ligamentous support (Fig. 7). In the tibia, excellent stability is usually obtained with the step cut and press-fit stem; however, if there is any doubt, fixation can be augmented with cortical screws. Morselized autograft and allograft are laid around the allograft-host junction. We do not recommend plate fixation to enhance fixation of the allograft (49,50), as the multiple drill holes produce channels in the allograft that may facilitate revascularization and fracture of the graft (51). If there is concern regarding the stability

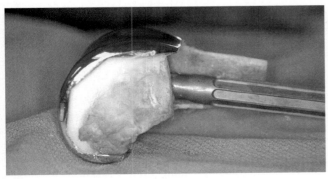

FIG. 5. A step cut is made in the allograft for stability. The allograft-implant interface is cemented only.

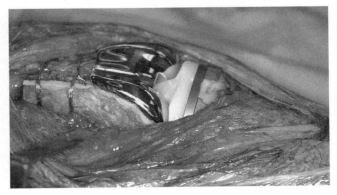

FIG. 7. The host-graft interface is stabilized with cerclage wire.

of the construct, cortical struts or plates may be used as a last resort. Plates and screws should be avoided in the proximal tibia due to concerns regarding soft tissue coverage.

Postoperative Management

Postoperative management varies according to the complexity of the surgery. Patients are encouraged to initiate range-of-motion exercises early in a hinged knee brace. The patient is kept touch weightbearing for 6 weeks and progresses to partial weightbearing until there is evidence of union at the allograft-host interface, which usually takes 3 months.

RESULTS OF TREATMENT

Cement

Two studies have evaluated the use of cement alone to fill a contained defect when long stems were used. Murray et al. (52) reported on a series of 40 revisions with an average follow-up of 58 months. Clinical results as measured by the Knee Society score were maintained at 83 points. Early radiolucent lines were seen; however, these were not progressive. Vince and Long (53) evaluated 31 patients with posterior stabilized implants and stems and 13 with constrained implants. Three of the 13 constrained implants failed; however, all these revisions were for infection. The investigators concluded that the press-fit technique with limited cement use may not provide adequate fixation for the constrained condylar implant, especially when bone quality is poor.

Ritter (54) evaluated 57 total knee arthroplasties in which defects in the tibial plateaus were filled with screw and cement; patients were followed for longer than 3 years. At 3 years, 15 of them had radiolucency between the cement and bone that was unchanged from that in the radiograph taken 2 months postoperatively. No radiolucency was noted about the stem bone-cement interface or between the screw and the bone. Ten of the 27 knees followed longer than 4 years showed similar findings. There were no loose tibial components in any of the 57 cases of total knee arthroplasty.

Metal Augments

The use of metal augments for tibial revisions was first reported by Brand et al. (37). Wedges were used to make up defects of approximately 2 cm. Twenty-two knees (20 patients) were followed for a minimum of 2 years with an average follow-up of 37 months. No failures of this technique or tibial component loosening was reported. The incidence of nonprogressive radiolucent lines was 27%. The investigators concluded that this technique is more appealing in the older age group with lower activity demands in whom restoration of bone stock is not so important. Pagnano et al. (55) followed 28 knees in 25 patients. Clinical results were excellent in 67%, good in 29%, and poor in 4%. Radiolucent lines at the cement-bone interface beneath the metal wedge were present in 13 knees. None was progressive. No deterioration of the wedge-prosthesis or wedge-cement-bone interface was seen at midterm follow-up.

Megaprostheses

To the best of our knowledge, there is no published series evaluating the outcome of mega modular prosthesis implantation in the revision total knee literature.

Three papers have reported on the use of the modular rotating-hinge prosthesis. Barrack et al. (56) evaluated 16 knees in 15 patients with a mean follow-up of 51 months. Clinical and radiographic results were reviewed and compared with those for 87 patients who underwent revision total knee arthroplasty with components of standard condylar revision design during the same period. Early results showed comparable postoperative knee scores and range of motion in the two groups despite the use of the rotating-hinge component in more complex revision cases. No patient exhibited radiographic evidence of definite component loosening. The investigators concluded that short-term clinical and radiographic results are encouraging and suggested that a second-generation modular rotating-hinge component can be used successfully in selected salvage revision cases. Westrich et al. (57) reviewed 24 knees in 21 patients who received a Finn rotating hinge device. The average follow-up was 33 months. There was a significant improvement in Knee Society clinical and functional scores. They concluded that the Finn total knee replacement appears to be an acceptable option for the treatment of the most severely affected knees with compromised bone and ligamentous instability. In contrast, Wang and Wang (58) documented that the polyethylene bushing in the rotating platform can fail as early as 5 months after implantation.

Morselized Allograft

The most comprehensive study on the use of morselized allograft was reported by Whiteside and Bicalho (59). They used morselized cancellous allograft to fill large contained femoral or tibial defects, or both, in 63 patients (63 knees). Firm seating of the components on a rim of viable bone and rigid fixation with a medullary stem were achieved in all cases. One patient was lost to follow-up; 62 patients had standard radiographic evaluation at 1 month, 3 months, and yearly intervals postoperatively. Fourteen patients required reoperation between 3 weeks and 37 months after revision; however, only two patients required revision surgery. A biopsy specimen was taken from the central portion of the allograft in each case. Evidence of healing, bone maturation, and formation of trabeculae was seen in all allografted areas visible on radiograph at 1 year after surgery. No sign of significant bone graft loss was seen in any case. Likewise, all biopsy specimens, including the 3-week specimen, showed evidence of active new bone formation in the allografted area. Active bone formation was found in and around the allograft pieces, and new osteoid formed directly on dead allograft trabeculae. Vascular stroma was present between the bone fragments deep in the allograft mass. Older biopsy specimens demonstrated progressive maturation, and evidence of active osteoclastic activity was absent by 18 months after surgery. All patients but one had significant improvement in their pain scores compared with their preoperative status. Although the complication rate was high (22%), all but one patient achieved lasting fixation to bone, adequate ligament balancing, good range of motion, and minimal to mild pain. Two patients required revision surgery. Both had greatly improved bone stock, so that new implants could be applied with minor additional grafting. The investigators concluded that this method of bone stock reconstitution appears to be reliable when used in conjunction with firm rim seating and rigid intramedullary stem fixation.

Structural Allograft

Clatworthy et al. (60) have reported the largest series with the longest follow-up. Fifty patients undergoing 52 revision knee replacements with 66 structural grafts were evaluated prospectively. This was a complex cohort of patients in whom 48 defects (73%) were circumferential. Thirty-one whole distal femurs and 17 whole proximal tibias were implanted.

Twenty-nine knees in 27 patients were independently reviewed at a mean of 96.9 months. Twelve knees were re-revised at a mean of 70.7 months. Two of these patients retained their allografts. Eleven patients died with their structural allografts and implants intact and were not awaiting revision at a mean of 93 months.

Failure was defined as an increase of less than 20 points in the modified Hospital for Special Surgery knee score at review or the need for an additional operation related to the allograft. Revisions of 13 knees were deemed failures, which indicates a 75% success rate. Graft resorption resulting in implant loosening occurred in five patients. Four revisions failed due to infection, and nonunion between the host bone and allograft was present in two. One patient undergoing two knee revisions failed to gain a 20-point improvement. Survival analysis showed a 92% survival at 5 years and 72% survival at 10 years. Clinically, the modified Hospital for Special Surgery score improved from a mean of 32.5 preoperatively to a mean of 75.6 at review.

There is concern that allografts resorb with time due to revascularization by creeping substitution. Allograft resorption was assessed using the following classification: Mild resorption is partial-thickness loss of less than 1 cm in length of one cortex. Moderate resorption is partial-thickness loss of 1 cm or more of one cortex. Major resorption is full-thickness loss of any length of one cortex. Radiographic analysis of the surviving grafts showed no severe resorption, one case of moderate resorption, and two cases of mild resorption.

Evaluation for loosening revealed that one patient had a loose tibial component, whereas three patients had nonprogressive tibial radiolucent lines. All four patients were asymptomatic. There is also concern with allograft implantation in the setting of previous infection. Six patients had an infected total knee replacement treated by a two-stage revision procedure with use of an antibiotic-impregnated spacer and a minimum of 6 weeks of intravenous antibiotics. Only one patient had ongoing infection. Nonvascularized allografts serve as an excellent nidus for the growth of organisms (61); hence, there is a concern for late allograft infection (62). The infection rate of 8% in this series is slightly higher than that in other revision knee series, in which a 0.0% to 4.5% infection rate is reported in patients not requiring allografts (63–65). The rate is comparable with that in other allograft procedures, however, in which the reported infection rate varies from 6% to 15% (50,61,66–70).

This study demonstrates encouraging medium-term survival of allografts used for revision knee replacement in a difficult population of patients with massive bone loss.

Others have also presented promising results in the short to medium term. Engh et al. (66) reviewed 35 patients at a mean of 50 months, of whom 83% received a femoral head graft. A good or excellent result was attained in 87%. Harris et al. (49) reported satisfactory clinical and radiographic results in 14 of 15 patients at a mean of 43 months. Mow et al. (71) demonstrated that 12 of 15 patients had no allograft-related complications at 47 months, whereas Mnaymneh et al. (50) reported a high complication rate in five of ten patients with massive bone loss who required whole distal femoral allografts or whole proximal tibial allografts, or both.

CONCLUSION

Revision total knee arthroplasty is becoming more frequent; thus, the need to treat significant bony defects is becoming more prevalent. Today's revision surgeon has a number of viable treatment options that yield good medium-term results.

The authors recommend cement use alone for a contained defect if the bone loss is minimal; however, we have a low threshold for packing the defect with morselized allograft, augmented with autograft where possible, to restore bone. With moderate or significant contained bone loss, morselized graft is used.

For an uncontained defect in which the bone loss is 2 cm or less in the femur or tibia, we recommend the use of modular augments and wedges. In the face of significant noncircumferential or circumferential bone loss, we favor structural allografts. In our minds, the golden rule of revision joint arthroplasty is to minimize bone resection and restore bone stock wherever possible.

REFERENCES

1. Grimer RJ, Karpinski MR, Edwards AN. The long-term results of Stanmore total knee replacements. *J Bone Joint Surg Br* 1984;66:55–62.
2. Rand JA, Chao EY, Stauffer RN. Kinematic rotating-hinge total knee arthroplasty. *J Bone Joint Surg Am* 1987;69:489–497.
3. Bartel DL, Bicknell VL, Wright TM. The effect of conformity, thickness, and material on stresses in ultra-high molecular weight components for total joint replacement. *J Bone Joint Surg Am* 1986;68:1041–1051.
4. Bartel DL, Rawlinson JJ, Burstein AH, et al. Stresses in polyethylene components of contemporary total knee replacements. *Clin Orthop* 1995;317:76–82.
5. Collier JP, Mayor MB, Surprenant VA, et al. The biomechanical problems of polyethylene as a bearing surface. *Clin Orthop* 1990;261:107–113.
6. Engh GA. Failure of the polyethylene bearing surface of a total knee replacement within four years. A case report. *J Bone Joint Surg Am* 1988;70:1093–1096.
7. Hvid I, Bentzen SM, Jorgensen J. Remodeling of the tibial plateau after knee replacement. CT bone densitometry. *Acta Orthop Scand* 1988;59:567–573.
8. Bartel DL, Burstein AH, Santavicca EA, et al. Performance of the tibial component in total knee replacement. *J Bone Joint Surg Am* 1982;64:1026–1033.
9. Angelides M, Shirazi-Adl A, Shrivastava SC, et al. A stress compatible finite element for implant/cement interface analyses. *J Biomech Eng* 1988;110:42–49.
10. Mintzer CM, Robertson DD, Rackemann S, et al. Bone loss in the distal anterior femur after total knee arthroplasty. *Clin Orthop* 1990;260:135–143.
11. Van Lenthe GH, Waal Malefijt MC, Huiskes R. Stress shielding after total knee replacement may cause bone resorption in the distal femur. *J Bone Joint Surg Br* 1997;79:117–122.

12. Seki T, Omori G, Koga Y, et al. Is bone density in the distal femur affected by use of cement and by femoral component design in total knee arthroplasty? *J Orthop Sci* 1999;4:180–186.

13. Goldring SR, Clark CR, Wright TM. The problem in total joint arthroplasty: aseptic loosening. *J Bone Joint Surg Am* 1993;75:799–801.

14. Hvid I, Bentzen SM, Jorgensen J. Remodeling of the tibial plateau after knee replacement. CT bone densitometry. *Acta Orthop Scand* 1988;59:567–573.

15. Robinson EJ, Mulliken BD, Bourne RB, et al. Catastrophic osteolysis in total knee replacement. A report of 17 cases. *Clin Orthop* 1995;321:98–105.

16. Morrey BF, Chao EY. Fracture of the porous-coated metal tray of a biologically fixed knee prosthesis. Report of a case. *Clin Orthop* 1988;228:182–189.

17. Scott RD, Ewald FC, Walker PS. Fracture of the metallic tibial tray following total knee replacement. Report of two cases. *J Bone Joint Surg Am* 1984;66:780–782.

18. Levitz CL, Lotke PA, Karp JS. Long-term changes in bone mineral density following total knee replacement. *Clin Orthop* 1995;321:68–72.

19. Wright TM, Bartel DL. The problem of surface damage in polyethylene total knee components. *Clin Orthop* 1986;205:67–74.

20. Collier JP, Mayor MB, McNamara JL, et al. Analysis of the failure of 122 polyethylene inserts from uncemented tibial knee components. *Clin Orthop* 1991;273:232–242.

21. Engh GA, Dwyer KA, Hanes CK. Polyethylene wear of metal-backed tibial components in total and unicompartmental knee prostheses. *J Bone Joint Surg Br* 1992;74:9–17.

22. Wasielewski RC, Parks N, Williams I, et al. Tibial insert undersurface as a contributing source of polyethylene wear debris. *Clin Orthop* 1997;345:53–59.

23. Cadambi A, Engh GA, Dwyer KA, et al. Osteolysis of the distal femur after total knee arthroplasty. *J Arthroplasty* 1994;9:579–594.

24. Hirakawa K, Bauer TW, Stulberg BN, et al. Characterization of debris adjacent to failed knee implants of 3 different designs. *Clin Orthop* 1996;331:151–158.

25. Lotke PA, Ecker ML. Influence of positioning of prosthesis in total knee replacement. *J Bone Joint Surg Am* 1977;59:77–79.

26. Leblanc JM. Patellar complications in total knee arthroplasty. A literature review. *Orthop Rev* 1989;18:296–304.

27. Bloebaum RD, Nelson K, Dorr LD, et al. Investigation of early surface delamination observed in retrieved heat-pressed tibial inserts. *Clin Orthop* 1991;269:120–127.

28. Sutula LC, Collier JP, Saum KA, et al. The Otto Aufranc Award. Impact of gamma sterilization on clinical performance of polyethylene in the hip. *Clin Orthop* 1995;319:28–40.

29. La Budde JK, Orosz JF, Bonfiglio TA, et al. Particulate titanium and cobalt-chrome metallic debris in failed total knee arthroplasty. A quantitative histologic analysis. *J Arthroplasty* 1994;9:291–304.

30. Milliano MT, Whiteside LA. Articular surface material effect on metal-backed patellar components. A microscopic evaluation. *Clin Orthop* 1991;273:204–214.

31. Milliano MT, Whiteside LA, Kaiser AD, et al. Evaluation of the effect of the femoral articular surface material on the wear of a metal-backed patellar component. *Clin Orthop* 1993;287:178–186.

32. Lewis PL, Rorabeck CH, Bourne RB. Screw osteolysis after cementless total knee replacement. *Clin Orthop* 1995;321:173–177.

33. Peters PC, Engh GA, Dwyer KA, et al. Osteolysis after total knee arthroplasty without cement. *J Bone Joint Surg Am* 1992;74:864–876.

34. Whiteside LA. Effect of porous-coating configuration on tibial osteolysis after total knee arthroplasty. *Clin Orthop* 1995;321:92–97.

35. Calton TF, Fehring TK, Griffin WL. Bone loss associated with the use of spacer blocks in infected total knee arthroplasty. *Clin Orthop* 1997;345:148–154.

36. Dorr LD, Ranawat CS, Sculco TA, et al. Bone graft for tibial defects in total knee arthroplasty. *Clin Orthop* 1986;205:153–165.

37. Brand MG, Daley RJ, Ewald FC, et al. Tibial tray augmentation with modular metal wedges for tibial bone stock deficiency. *Clin Orthop* 1989;248:71–79.

38. Brooks PJ, Walker PS, Scott RD. Tibial component fixation in deficient tibial bone stock. *Clin Orthop* 1984;184:302–308.

39. Goldberg VM, Stevenson S, Shaffer JW. Biology of autografts and allografts. In: Friedleander GE, Goldberg VM, eds. Bone and cartilage allografts: biology and clinical applications. Park Ridge, IL: American Academy of Orthopaedic Surgeons, 1991:3–13.

40. Enneking WF, Mindell ER. Observations on massive retrieved human allografts. *J Bone Joint Surg Am* 1991;73:1123–1142.

41. Czitrom A. Biology of bone grafting and principles of bone banking. In: Weinstein SL, ed. *The paediatric spine: principles and practice.* New York: Raven Press, 1994:1285–1298.

42. Stevenson S, Horowitz M. The response to bone allografts. *J Bone Joint Surg Am* 1992;74:939–950.

43. Bos GD, Goldberg VM, Zika JM, et al. Immune responses of rats to frozen bone allografts. *J Bone Joint Surg Am* 1983;65:239–246.

44. Stevenson S, Li XQ, Davy DT, et al. Critical biological determinants of incorporation of non-vascularized cortical bone grafts. Quantification of a complex process and structure. *J Bone Joint Surg Am* 1997;79:1–16.

45. Strong DM, Friedlaender GE, Tomford WW, et al. Immunologic responses in human recipients of osseous and osteochondral allografts. *Clin Orthop* 1996;326:107–114.

46. Muscolo DL, Ayerza MA, Calabrese ME, et al. Human leukocyte antigen matching, radiographic score, and histologic findings in massive frozen bone allografts. *Clin Orthop* 1996;326:115–126.

47. Muscolo DL, Caletti E, Schajowicz F, et al. Tissue-typing in human massive allografts of frozen bone. *J Bone Joint Surg Am* 1987;69:583–595.

48. Fawcett K, Barr AR. *Tissue banking.* Arlington, VA: American Association of Blood Banks, 1987:97–107.

49. Harris AI, Poddar S, Gitelis S, et al. Arthroplasty with a composite of an allograft and a prosthesis for knees with severe deficiency of bone. *J Bone Joint Surg Am* 1995;77:373–386.

50. Mnaymneh W, Emerson RH, Borja F, et al. Massive allografts in salvage revisions of failed total knee arthroplasties. *Clin Orthop* 1990;260:144–153.

51. Burchardt H. The biology of bone graft repair. *Clin Orthop* 1983;174:28–42.

52. Murray PB, Rand JA, Hanssen AD. Cemented long-stem revision total knee arthroplasty. *Clin Orthop* 1994;309:116–123.

53. Vince KG, Long W. Revision knee arthroplasty. The limits of press fit medullary fixation. *Clin Orthop* 1995;317:172–177.

54. Ritter MA. Screw and cement fixation of large defects in total knee arthroplasty. *J Arthroplasty* 1986;1:125–129.

55. Pagnano MW, Trousdale RT, Rand JA. Tibial wedge augmentation for bone deficiency in total knee arthroplasty. A followup study. *Clin Orthop* 1995;321:151–155.

56. Barrack RL, Lyons TR, Ingraham RQ, et al. The use of a modular rotating hinge component in salvage revision total knee arthroplasty. *J Arthroplasty* 2000;15:858–866.

57. Westrich GH, Mollano AV, Sculco TP, et al. Rotating hinge total knee arthroplasty in severely affected knees. *Clin Orthop* 2000;379:195–208.

58. Wang CJ, Wang HE. Early catastrophic failure of rotating hinge total knee prosthesis. *J Arthroplasty* 2000;15:387–391.

59. Whiteside LA, Bicalho PS. Radiologic and histologic analysis of morselized allograft in revision total knee replacement. *Clin Orthop* 1998;357:149–156.

60. Clatworthy MG, Ballance J, Brick GW, et al. The use of structural allograft for uncontained defects in revision total knee arthroplasty. A minimum five-year review. *J Bone Joint Surg Am* 2001;83:404–411.

61. Stockley I, McAuley JP, Gross AE. Allograft reconstruction in total knee arthroplasty. *J Bone Joint Surg Br* 1992;74:393–397.

62. Rorabeck CH, Smith PN. Results of revision total knee arthroplasty in the face of significant bone deficiency. *Orthop Clin North Am* 1998;29:361–371.

63. Friedman RJ, Hirst P, Poss R, et al. Results of revision total knee arthroplasty performed for aseptic loosening. *Clin Orthop* 1990;255:235–241.

64. Goldberg VM, Figgie MP, Figgie HE, et al. The results of revision total knee arthroplasty. *Clin Orthop* 1988;226:86–92.

65. Mow CS, Wiedel JD. Revision total knee arthroplasty using the porous-coated anatomic revision prosthesis: six- to twelve-year results. *J Arthroplasty* 1998;13:681–686.

66. Engh GA, Herzwurm PJ, Parks NL. Treatment of major defects of bone with bulk allografts and stemmed components during total knee arthroplasty. *J Bone Joint Surg Am* 1997;79:1030–1039.

67. Engh GA, Parks NL. The management of bone defects in revision total knee arthroplasty. *Instr Course Lect* 1997;46:227–236.

68. Ghazavi MT, Stockley I, Yee G, et al. Reconstruction of massive bone defects with allograft in revision total knee arthroplasty. *J Bone Joint Surg Am* 1997;79:17–25.

69. Lord CF, Gebhardt MC, Tomford WW, et al. Infection in bone allografts. Incidence, nature, and treatment. *J Bone Joint Surg Am* 1988;70:369–376.

70. van Loon CJ, Waal Malefijt MC, Buma P, et al. Femoral bone loss in total knee arthroplasty. A review. *Acta Orthop Belg* 1999;65:154–163.

71. Mow CS, Wiedel JD. Structural allografting in revision total knee arthroplasty. *J Arthroplasty* 1996;11:235–241.

CHAPTER 109

Cementless Revision Total Knee Arthroplasty

Leo A. Whiteside

Implant fixation, bone reconstruction, and ligament balancing are the three primary goals of revision total knee arthroplasty (Fig. 1). Fixation often is difficult to achieve because the cancellous bone has been depleted, so it is tempting to cement the implant to diaphyseal cortical bone. Cemented fixation usually is tenuous when the cancellous bone has been depleted, however, and revision with cement ultimately destroys more bone stock. A more reliable and durable technique uses an uncemented stem to engage the isthmus and rim contact on metaphyseal cortical bone. This creates a stable construct around which the bone can be rebuilt (1–3). In almost all cases of revision, the implant can be fixed to available bone stock, which obviates the need for massive allografts that do not reconstitute the lost bone stock and often fail due to late collapse and infection (4). Two major concerns with massive bone grafting—vascularization and incorporation—remain significant issues in the knee (4), and bone grafting with allograft still raises the questions of immunocompatibility. Bone tissue itself is not highly immunogenic, but the marrow cells incite a vigorous immune response (5) and can create an inflammatory process that blocks ossification and incorporation of the graft (6).

An effort has been made since 1984 to reconstruct bone defects with morselized allograft bone and to fix the implants to the patient's remaining bone structure without cement. Durability of the construct and reliability of fixation of the implants have been very good, and repeated revision due to mechanical failure has been rare (1–3,7,8).

In cases of infection about a total knee prosthesis, the standard treatment has been to remove the implants, treat with antibiotics for 6 weeks, and finally perform revision arthroplasty with antibiotic-impregnated cement (9–12). Cementless reconstruction, however, is attractive for these revision cases because further bone destruction is avoided and bone stock also can be restored (1,2,13,14). Since 1984, a regimen of cementless reconstruction has been used in cases of infection. The implants

are removed and the knee is thoroughly débrided, then the patient is treated with parenteral antibiotics for 6 weeks. Three months after the final débridement, the joint is reconstructed using stemmed implants and morselized allograft.

GRAFTING TECHNIQUE

Block allografts traditionally have been used for massive bone deficiency, but complication rates with their use are high, and the destructive effects of allograft rejection can limit their long-term success (6,15). Because marrow is immunogenic, rejection can be a major problem with allograft (6,15). Marrow elements, however, can be thoroughly removed from morselized allograft to minimize the inflammatory response and loss of graft and to capitalize on the osteoconductive potential of the allograft. Washing and soaking the components in an antibiotic solution have the added benefit of making available a reservoir of antibiotic that is released slowly during the postoperative period (16). Large segments of allograft also heal slowly, are never replaced by new bone, and weaken as the ossification and vascularization front proceeds (17,18). In contrast, morselized allograft, if protected initially by stem and rim fixation of the implants, has proven reliable both for small and large defects while supporting new bone formation (19,20). Morsels that are 1 cm in diameter maintain their integrity long enough to act as a substrate for new bone formation. Morsels that are much less than 0.5 to 1.0 cm in diameter tend to be resorbed, whereas those larger than 1 cm incorporate slowly, if ever, and tend to collapse under weightbearing stress.

The allograft is not osteoinductive but acts as scaffolding for new bone growth. Demineralized bone, which is mildly osteoinductive, can be added to the allograft to enhance bone formation. The surrounding bone structure supplies most of the osteoinductive activity because metaphyseal bone has a rich

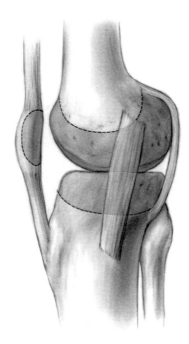

FIG. 1. Bone loss from the femur, tibia, and patella may be extensive in failed total knee arthroplasty, but the ligaments and capsule usually are competent. Cancellous bone stock rarely is intact. The shaded area represents loss of cortical wall and cancellous structure. (From Whiteside LA. Results: cementless. In: Rorabeck CH, Engh GA, eds. *Revision total knee arthroplasty.* Baltimore: Williams & Wilkins, 1997, with permission.)

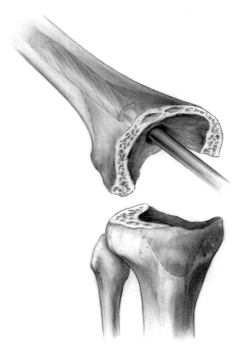

FIG. 2. Intramedullary alignment provides the only reliable landmark for minimal resection. Recognizing that severe bone loss has occurred, the surgeon should resect only a small amount of bone to allow firm footing for the implant. (From Whiteside LA. Results: cementless. In: Rorabeck CH, Engh GA, eds. *Revision total knee arthroplasty.* Baltimore: Williams & Wilkins, 1997, with permission.)

blood supply and maintains the capacity to heal even after repeated failure of arthroplasty.

BONE PREPARATION TECHNIQUE

Because bone loss is one of the major problems in failed total knee arthroplasty, minimal bone should be resected during preparation (Fig. 2). Bone erosion already present makes complete seating of the component nearly impossible, but side-to-side and front-to-back toggle of the implants can be eliminated by placing a stem rigidly in the medullary canal. The implant seats on the remaining rim of metaphyseal bone. Seating the implant on the patient's own bone stock controls axial migration, and the stem prevents the implant from tilting into the defect. Screw and peg fixation may be used to add stability to the construct. This technique results in substantial uncontained cavitary defects that may be filled with morselized bone. This bone-grafting technique promotes rapid healing and reconstitution of bone stock without the technical difficulty and late collapse associated with massive allograft replacement.

Tibial Preparation

Reconstruction of massive tibial defects relies on rim support for axial loading and stem fixation for toggle control. The use of screws can be effective in the tibial component to augment fixation, combined with the use of nonstructural allograft to fill central and peripheral defects. Massive block allografting also may be used for these defects; however, with long-stem and augmented fixation, morselized cancellous allografting can reconstruct the proximal tibial bone with low failure and complication rates (3).

The lateral tibial cortex usually is relatively well preserved. The fibular head almost always is present and can be used for proximal seating of the tibial component if the rest of the tibial architecture is destroyed (Fig. 3). In the worst cases, all cancellous bone is gone, which leaves a large cavitary defect and substantial deficiency of the tibial rim. Long-stem fixation is advised in these cases regardless of whether block or morselized allograft is used. When morselized graft is used, the tibial tray should seat on the intact portion of the tibial rim, and the stem should engage the isthmus of the tibia. As with the femoral component, the tightly fit diaphyseal stem maintains stability and prevents tilting of the component, so that massive defects may be filled with allograft and protected until healing and bone formation occur in the grafted area (Fig. 4).

Femoral Preparation

When bone destruction is assessed, the medial and lateral condyles usually are found to be at least partially intact. With intramedullary instrumentation as a guide, the distal surface of the femur should be resected just enough to achieve firm seating of the femoral component on one side of the bone. Both sides may be engaged by the implant in some cases, but often only

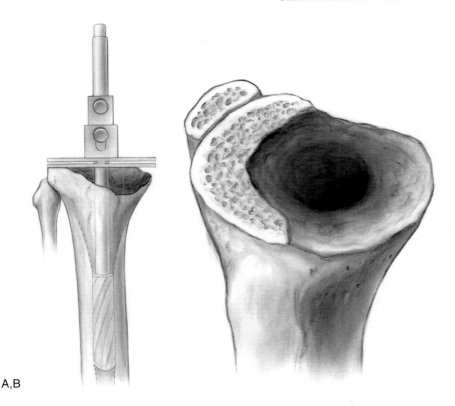

A,B

FIG. 3. A: Intramedullary instruments allow accurate alignment. Here, a tibial cutting guide is used to trim the upper tibial rim. Minimal resection should be done, which may leave large rim defects. **B:** With long-stem support of the tibial component, one-fourth of the rim of the proximal tibia can be used to support the implant. The fibular head also may be used for tibial support. (From Whiteside LA. Results: cementless. In: Rorabeck CH, Engh GA, eds. *Revision total knee arthroplasty.* Baltimore: Williams & Wilkins, 1997, with permission.)

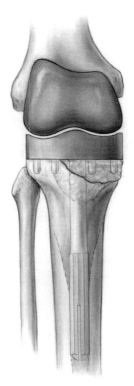

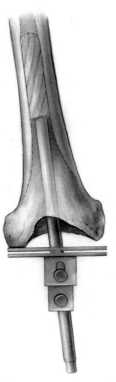

FIG. 4. Fixation of the tibial component with rim contact on viable bone, screw fixation into the cortical shell, peg fixation into intact bone structure, and stem fixation into the diaphysis allows adequate stabilization until the grafted area can be incorporated. (From Whiteside LA. Results: cementless. In: Rorabeck CH, Engh GA, eds. *Revision total knee arthroplasty.* Baltimore: Williams & Wilkins, 1997, with permission.)

FIG. 5. An intramedullary reamer is used to align the femoral cutting guide. The guide is set at 5 degrees of valgus alignment and positioned to resect minimal bone from the most prominent distal surface of the femur. (From Whiteside LA. Results: cementless. In: Rorabeck CH, Engh GA, eds. *Revision total knee arthroplasty.* Baltimore: Williams & Wilkins, 1997, with permission.)

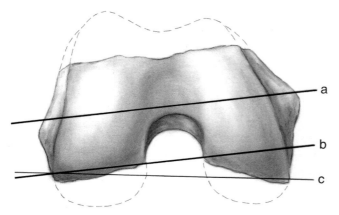

FIG. 6. A straight line through the medial and lateral femoral epicondyles provides correct rotational alignment. The dotted lines represent the original contours of the distal femur before total knee failure. Line a passes through the epicondyles. Line b represents the proper resection line for the posterior femoral condyles. If line c is followed, severe internal rotation of the femoral component will occur. (From Whiteside LA. Results: cementless. In: Rorabeck CH, Engh GA, eds. *Revision total knee arthroplasty.* Baltimore: Williams & Wilkins, 1997, with permission.)

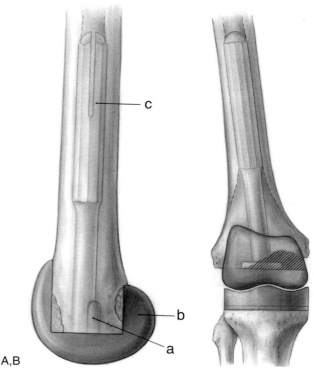

A,B

FIG. 7. A: Fixation of the femoral component into viable bone is achieved by means of a posterior stabilizing housing, a peg driven into the distal femoral surface (a), a thickened posterior surface (b), and a long stem (c), which allows soft bone graft to be used. **B:** Tight fixation of the stem in the diaphysis in combination with rim seating prevents the implant from migrating proximally and tilting into the defect. (From Whiteside LA. Results: cementless. In: Rorabeck CH, Engh GA, eds. *Revision total knee arthroplasty.* Baltimore: Williams & Wilkins, 1997, with permission.)

one of the two condyles can afford firm seating for the femoral component without excessive resection of the distal femur (Fig. 5). Adequate fixation of the femoral component requires posterior seating to prevent anteroposterior translation of the component in flexion and to augment torsional fixation. The posterior surfaces also are minimally resected, with as much bone stock as possible left on which to seat the surfaces of the femoral component. In many cases, the posterior bone erosion leaves little or nothing of the posterior femoral condyles, and the posterior femoral cuts are flush with the posterior cortex of the femur (Figs. 6 and 7). These posterior femoral surfaces are aligned with the epicondylar axis of the femur to achieve correct varus-valgus alignment of the femoral implant in flexion. Trial components then are inserted, and buildups are chosen to achieve adequate purchase on the distal and posterior surfaces of the femur and upper surface of the tibia, while at the same time placing the joint line correctly both in flexion and extension. After the implant has been fully seated, more bone graft can be packed into the distal and posterior cavitary defects (Fig. 7). Prolonged protection from weightbearing usually is not necessary because the implants are supported well on viable bone.

Graft Preparation and Placement

Fresh frozen cancellous allograft in morsels measuring 0.5 to 1.0 cm in diameter is soaked for 5 to 10 minutes in normal saline solution that contains polymyxin B sulfate 500,000 U, bacitracin zinc 50,000 U, and cephazolin 1 g per L. The fluid is removed and 10 cm^3 of powdered demineralized cancellous bone is added to each 30 cm^3 of the cancellous morsels. To improve the osteoinductive potential, autogenous bone fragments and diaphyseal reamings are added. This mixture is packed loosely into the bone defects, and then the implants are

impacted so as to seat on the remnant of viable bone while compacting the morselized bone graft. Remaining cavitary defects are filled with bone graft, but the bone is not compacted so that early vascularization and healing will not be impeded.

CLINICAL EXPERIENCE

Since 1984, a cementless fixation technique has been used at the author's institution in aseptic and infected cases of revision total knee arthroplasty (2,3,7,8,14). Clean revision cases followed for 2 to 10 years had a failure rate of 3% due to loosening (14). The remainder had radiographic evidence of stable fixation. Biopsy results for 17 knees showed early, vigorous bone formation and late maturation throughout the grafts (Figs. 8 through 11). Thirty-three infected knees underwent revision using this technique 6 to 12 weeks after débridement (7). Four knees required repeated débridement and revision due to recurrent infection, but currently are functioning well. One had repeated infection that required amputation.

Clinical experience has shown that migration of the tibial component after reconstruction with morselized allograft is rare during the first 2 to 5 years after surgery (4). These results are

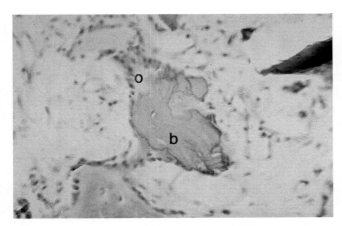

FIG. 8. Histologic section from the 3-week biopsy specimen. Granules of demineralized bone (b) are visible and are surrounded by plump osteoblasts (o) and new osteoid. Vascular stroma is present throughout the allografted area. There is no histologic evidence of bone resorption. (From Whiteside LA. Results: cementless. In: Rorabeck CH, Engh GA, eds. *Revision total knee arthroplasty.* Baltimore: Williams & Wilkins, 1997, with permission.)

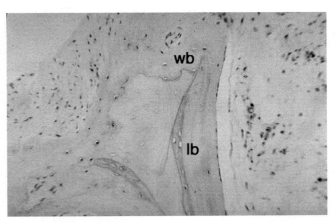

FIG. 10. Histologic section from the 21-month biopsy specimen. Mature lamellar bone (lb) and disorganized woven bone (wb) surround the allograft. The bone remodeling rate in the allografted area has decreased significantly. Trabeculae now are completely entombed by mature or woven bone. Bone remodeling has decreased, and osteoblastic or osteoclastic activity is directed toward new bone, not toward allograft. (From Whiteside LA. Results: cementless. In: Rorabeck CH, Engh GA, eds. *Revision total knee arthroplasty.* Baltimore: Williams & Wilkins, 1997, with permission.)

surprising in light of reported experience with structural allograft in the acetabulum. Jasty and Harris (20) reported loosening of acetabular components after 4 years in 32% of their cases. The biologic behavior of morselized allograft differs from that of block allograft, however. Vascularization and ossification are rapid, and a permanent, competent load-bearing structure is achieved by filling large deficient areas (1,2) (Figs. 12 through 15). The biologic response obtained with the correct technique appears to be early and vigorous. It does not seem

likely that progressive collapse will occur after remodeling and healing have been established.

Bone graft handling is probably crucial to the success of grafting the knee. Antibiotic soaking and washing, removal of bone marrow, and adequate support of the implants are all necessary for consistent success with this technique. The results of this salvage procedure have been encouraging. The grafting technique appears to provide long-term support for the implant, so that repeat revision likely will be uncommon.

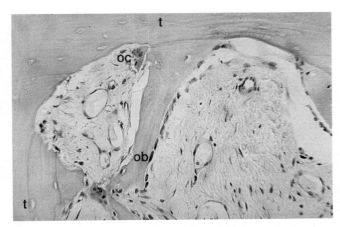

FIG. 9. Histologic section from the 3-month biopsy specimen. Dead trabeculae (t) are still abundant. Osteoclasts (oc) and new osteoid with osteoblasts (ob) are evident adjacent to the allograft. The allografted area contains multiple sites of bone resorption. New osteoid is often found on one surface of a trabecula and osteoclastic resorption on the opposite surface. Osteoblasts at this time are flatter and less numerous than in the 3-week biopsy specimen. (From Whiteside LA. Results: cementless. In: Rorabeck CH, Engh GA, eds. *Revision total knee arthroplasty.* Baltimore: Williams & Wilkins, 1997, with permission.)

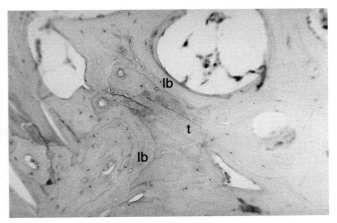

FIG. 11. Histologic section from the 37-month biopsy specimen. Entombed trabeculae (t) are present throughout the biopsied allograft. The visible allograft is completely encased by mature lamellar bone (lb). Bone remodeling continues at normal levels; few osteoclasts are found, and there is minimal evidence of osteoblastic activity. (From Whiteside LA. Results: cementless. In: Rorabeck CH, Engh GA, eds. *Revision total knee arthroplasty.* Baltimore: Williams & Wilkins, 1997, with permission.)

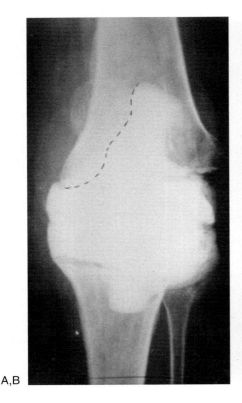
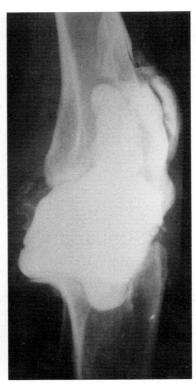

A,B

FIG. 12. A: Preoperative anteroposterior radiograph of the knee of a patient who had undergone a total knee replacement with a history of two previous infections. The dotted line indicates the interface between the cement spacer and bone. The medial and lateral femoral condyles are severely deficient; the medial and lateral tibial plateaus, the upper half of the fibular head, and the tibiofibular joint have been destroyed. B: Preoperative lateral radiograph of the same case as in A. The anterior femoral bone stock and posterior femoral condyles have been destroyed.

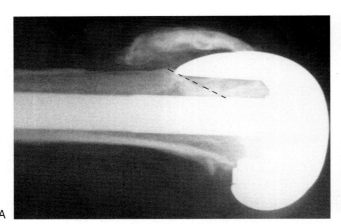

A

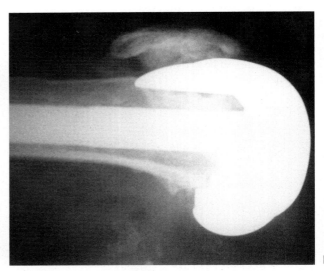

B

FIG. 13. A: Postoperative lateral view of the same knee as in Figure 12A 1 month after surgery. The dotted line indicates the distal extent of the patient's own anterior femoral bone stock. The material under the femoral flange is morselized cancellous allograft and demineralized allograft bone. The posterior surfaces of the femoral component are seated against the remaining portion of the femoral diaphysis. B: Postoperative lateral radiograph of the same knee 2 years after surgery. The bone graft has consolidated.

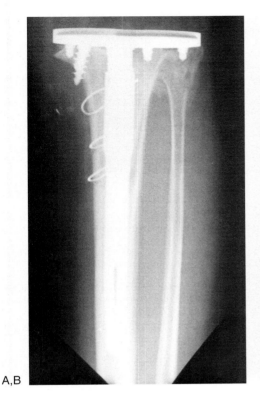
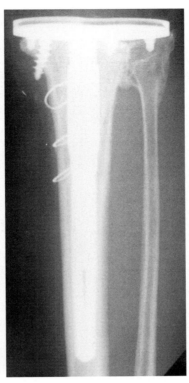

A,B

FIG. 14. A: Anteroposterior radiograph of the tibia of the same knee as in Figure 12A 1 month after surgery. The long stem engages the diaphysis of the tibia, and the distal slot is closed. Fresh graft is visible in the tibiofibular joint. The medial edge of the tibia and upper surfaces of the fibular head support the tibial component until healing is complete. **B:** Anteroposterior radiograph of the tibia of the same knee, taken 2 years after surgery. The slot in the stem is still closed, and the tibiofibular joint appears to be solidly healed.

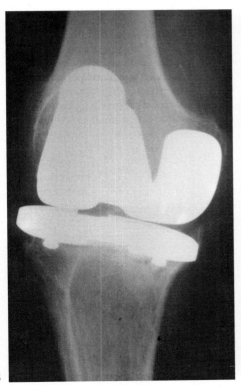
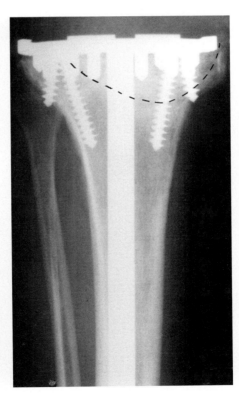

A,B

FIG. 15. A: Anteroposterior radiograph of a cemented total knee replacement 5 years after surgery. The tibial component has loosened and migrated into a varus position, destroying much of the medial tibial plateau. **B:** Anteroposterior radiograph of the same knee as in **A** 1 year after surgery. The dotted line indicates the previous bony defect. The lateral rim and diaphyseal stem have supported the tibial component as bone grew and healed under the medial side of the tibial component. The bone graft has healed, producing supporting bone stock for the medial side of the tibial component.

REFERENCES

1. Samuelson K. Bone grafting and noncemented revision arthroplasty of the knee. *Clin Orthop* 1988;226:93–101.
2. Whiteside L. Cementless reconstruction of massive tibial bone loss in revision total knee arthroplasty. *Clin Orthop* 1989;248:80–86.
3. Whiteside L, Ohl M. Tibial tubercle osteotomy for exposure of the difficult knee arthroplasty. *Clin Orthop* 1990;260:6–9.
4. Wilde A, Schickendantz M, Stulberg B, et al. The incorporation of tibial allografts in total knee arthroplasty. *J Bone Joint Surg Am* 1990;72:815–824.
5. Goldberg V, Powell A, Shaffer J, et al. Bone grafting: role of histocompatibility in transplantation. *J Orthop Res* 1985;3:389–404.
6. Muscolo D, Caletti E, Schajowicz F, et al. Tissue-typing in human massive allografts of frozen bone. *J Bone Joint Surg Am* 1987;69:583–595.
7. Whiteside L. Treatment of infected total knee arthroplasty. *Clin Orthop* 1994;299:169–172.
8. Whiteside L, Bicalho PS. Radiologic and histologic analysis of morselized allograft in revision total knee replacement. *Clin Orthop* 1998;357:149–156.
9. Booth R Jr, Lotke P. The results of spacer block technique in revision of infected total knee arthroplasty. *Clin Orthop* 1989;248:57–60.
10. Freeman M, Sudlow R, Casewell M, et al. The management of infected total knee replacements. *J Bone Joint Surg Br* 1985;67:764–768.
11. Jacobs M, Hungerford D, Krackow K, et al. Revision of septic total knee replacement. *Clin Orthop* 1989;238:159–166.
12. Windsor R, Miller D, Insall J, et al. Two-stage reimplantation for the salvage of total knee arthroplasty complicated by infection. *J Bone Joint Surg Am* 1990;72:272–278.
13. Whiteside L. Bone grafting in revision cementless total knee arthroplasty. *Tech Orthop* 1992;7:39–46.
14. Whiteside L. Cementless revision total knee arthroplasty. *Clin Orthop* 1993;286:160–167.
15. Friedlaender G. Current concepts review: bone grafts. *J Bone Joint Surg Am* 1987;69:786–790.
16. McLaren A. Antibiotic bone graft: early clinical results. Paper presented at: 57th Annual Meeting of the American Academy of Orthopaedics Surgeons; February 8–13, 1990; New Orleans.
17. Gitelis S, Helgimen D, Quill G, et al. The use of large allografts for tumor reconstruction and salvage of the failed total hip arthroplasty. *Clin Orthop* 1988;231:62–70.
18. Head W, Malinn T, Berklacich F. Freeze-dried proximal femur allografts in revision total hip arthroplasty. *Clin Orthop* 1987;215:109–120.
19. Gerber S, Harris W. Femoral head autografting to augment acetabular deficiency in patients requiring total hip replacement. *J Bone Joint Surg Am* 1986;68:1241–1248.
20. Jasty M, Harris WH. Salvage total hip reconstruction in patients with major acetabular bone deficiency using structural femoral head allografts. *J Bone Joint Surg Br* 1990;72:63–67.

CHAPTER 110

Managing the Patella in Revision Total Knee Arthroplasty

Robert L. Barrack

When performing a revision total knee arthroplasty (TKA), the patella is usually the last issue addressed. As Rand stated, "[T]he patella has too often been neglected in discussions of total knee arthroplasty revision" (1). Many studies on revision TKA, in fact, do not even specify the method of patellar treatment. There are a number of potential treatment options for the patella. In a study of 79 revision TKAs reported by Haas et al., in 38 knees a well-fixed component was left in place, in 28 the patellar component was revised to a new component, in 10 knees the component was resected and left unresurfaced, and in three cases a patellectomy had been performed (2). In a multicenter study of 242 revision total knees reported by Coon et al. (3), a similar distribution of patellar treatment options was reported (Table 1). The study by Coon et al. concluded that the method of patellar treatment significantly impacted the clinical result. Patients who had a revision total knee with prior patellectomy or with patellar resection arthroplasty had significantly worse results compared with the other groups. In recent years a number of novel new techniques have been described for dealing with these difficult patellar problems encountered during revision knee arthroplasty. The purpose of this chapter is to review the general surgical principles in approaching the patella during revision knee arthroplasty, discuss the options available for patellar management, review the previously documented results of these traditional options, and finally describe new techniques for patellar treatment during revision TKA.

SURGICAL CONSIDERATIONS

The first priority in the treatment of the patella in revision TKA is to avoid extensor mechanism disruption in the form of either a patellar tendon avulsion or patella fracture. This begins with the surgical approach to the knee at the outset of the case. Eversion of the patella is necessary to assess the status of the patellar component and to proceed with definitive treatment. This should be accomplished in a careful sequential manner. The patella should not be immediately everted while flexing the knee past 90 degrees, as is often possible in a primary knee replacement. The gutters should be cleared of adhesions, particularly on the lateral side. The patella should be placed under tension with a laterally directed retractor while adhesions are released starting with the patellofemoral ligament. Before flexing the knee, Laskin has recommended placing a Steinmann pin through the patellar tendon just proximal to the tibial tubercle to act as a stress reliever and minimize the risk of avulsion (4). This also focuses attention on the patellar tendon insertion so that inadvertent avulsion is less likely. When complete release of adhesions has been carried down to the periphery of the lateral tibial plateau and the adhesions have been released between the proximal tibia and the patellar tendon down to the level of the insertion on the tibial tubercle, an attempt can be made to evert the patella while gently flexing the knee. If undue tension on the patellar tendon insertion is still apparent with attempted patellar eversion, an alternative surgical approach can be considered (5). The options include rectus snip with or without lateral release, partial or complete V-Y quadricepsplasty, or tibial tubercle osteotomy.

After patellar eversion has been accomplished, it is necessary to expose the interface between the patellar component and underlying bone. Frequently this interface is obscured by overlying fibrous tissue, the so-called patellar meniscus (6). This should be circumferentially removed and the interface examined. An osteotome can be placed under the patellar com-

TABLE 1. *Methods of patellar treatment in two series of revision total knee arthroplasty*

	Haas et al. (2)		Coon et al. (3)	
	Number	%	Number	%
Well-fixed component retained	38	48.1	83	34.3
Component revised	28	35.4	78	32.2
Component resected	10	12.7	36	14.9
Resurfaced, originally intact	0	0	33	13.6
Prior patellectomy	3	3.8	12	5
Total	79	100	242	100

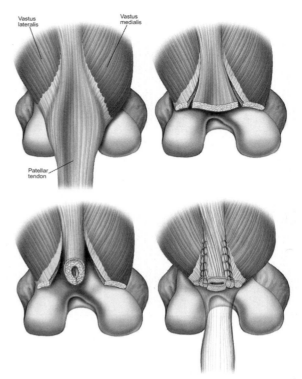

FIG. 1. "Tubularization" attempts to improve the cosmetic appearance as well as the mechanical lever arm of the extensor mechanism after patellectomy. (From Brown TE, Diduch DR. Fractures of the patella. In: Insall JN, Scott WN, eds. *Surgery of the knee*, 3rd ed. New York: Churchill Livingstone, 2001, with permission.)

ponent to determine if it can be levered out. Occasionally a component that appears well fixed radiographically will prove to be loose when tested in this manner. If the patella is not loose, radiographically or at intraoperative testing, a decision must be made as to whether there are other indications for removal of the component.

After a definitive method of patellar treatment has been elected, the final surgical consideration is ensuring optimal tracking of the extensor mechanism. This is equally important regardless of the method of patellar treatment elected. The major methods of optimizing tracking include attaining appropriate prosthetic rotation, especially an appropriate degree of femoral component external rotation. This is most reliably obtained in the revision situation by aligning the femoral component with the epicondyles. Tibial component internal rotation should be avoided and generally alignment of the mid-portion of the tibial component just medial to the midpoint of the tibial tubercle will position the tibial component appropriately. If the extensor mechanism does not track centrally, the femoral and tibial component rotation should be carefully reassessed with these landmarks in mind.

Certain component positioning parameters can place undue stress on the extensor mechanism. If the anterior flange of the femoral component is displaced anteriorly so that the flange is not flush with the femoral cortex, this will increase the forces on the extensor mechanism during knee flexion. Elevation of the joint line will have the same effect. If a very thick polyethylene tibial insert is used and there is undue stress on the extensor mechanism with flexion, the position of the patella relative to the joint line should be carefully assessed. The joint line is normally approximately 1 cm above the fibular head and in extension the inferior pole of the patella should be approximately 1 cm proximal to the surface of the tibial insert. If a thick tibial insert is necessary to obtain stability in extension and this results in a relative patellar baja, consideration should be given to using distal femoral augments and a thinner tibial insert to effectively lower the joint line.

Once the patellar component has been adequately exposed and its fixation status has been assessed, a decision must be made regarding the optimal method of treatment for the patella. If removal of the patellar component is elected, there are certain surgical technique considerations. The patellar component should be stabilized, usually with towel clips through the quadriceps tendon and the patella tendon. If the remaining patellar component bone is overly thick (more than

15 mm), it may be possible to simply take a saw and undercut the pegs of the component. This is not frequently possible. A well-fixed all-polyethylene component, however, can still be removed by placing a saw blade right at the implant–bone interface and sawing off the polyethylene from the pegs. The cement can then be removed with narrow sharp osteotomes, with care being taken not to fragment the residual patellar bone. Well-fixed polyethylene pegs can be efficiently removed by drilling the center of the peg with a sharp drill bit. This will remove the polyethylene from the cement and the cement can then be removed with sharp curettes and small osteotomes, again with care being taken not to fragment the bone. When a metal-backed component is removed it is usually easier to first remove the polyethylene from the metal. Cemented metal-backed components are carefully removed with osteotomes around the periphery. The most difficult component to remove is the bone-ingrown metal-backed component. In this situation, sectioning of the metal baseplate has been suggested as a method of minimizing the risk of patellar fracture during component removal (4).

The most commonly elected options for patellar treatment are either to leave a well-fixed patellar component in place or to revise the patellar component to one that is specific for the revision component being implanted. After patellar component removal, there may not be enough residual bone to implant a standard three-peg patellar component. In this scenario, a number of options exist, including using a special

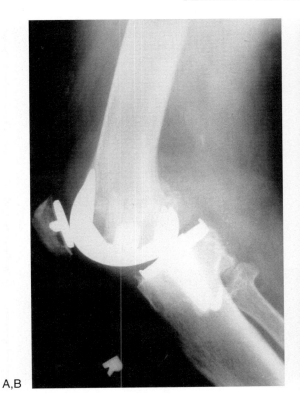
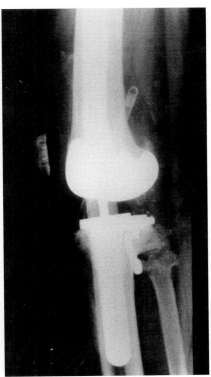

A,B

FIG. 2. Lateral radiograph of a metal-backed patellar component with evidence of osteolysis and loosening **(A)**. Revision to an all-polyethylene cemented component was performed **(B)**.

biconvex revision component, leaving the residual bone unresurfaced, impaction grafting, using a "crossed K-wire" technique, and using the so-called gull wing osteotomy. Another clinical scenario occasionally encountered is a patient with a prior patellectomy. This group of patients has traditionally had the least optimal results. Attempts to reestablish some of the mechanical advantages of the patella in this scenario include tubularization of the residual extensor mechanism (Fig. 1) (7), iliac crest bone grafting, or attaching a patellar component to the soft tissue of the residual extensor mechanism. These treat-

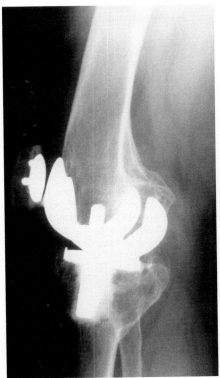
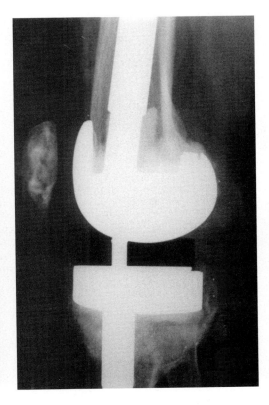

A,B

FIG. 3. Lateral radiograph demonstrating a well-fixed metal-backed patellar component in the presence of adequate bone to support a revision component **(A)**. Because of the poor track record of metal-backed components and the presence of more than 12 mm of residual bone, revision to a cemented all-polyethylene component was performed **(B)**.

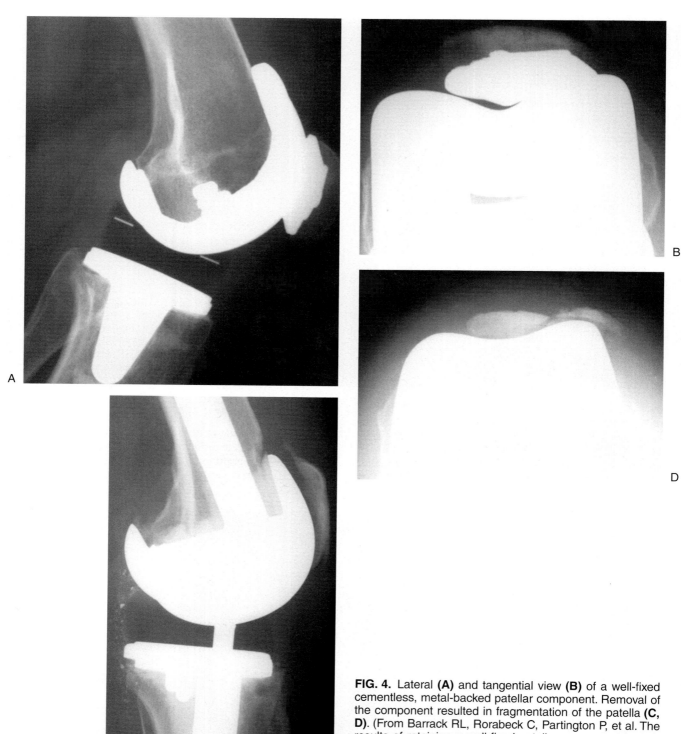

FIG. 4. Lateral **(A)** and tangential view **(B)** of a well-fixed cementless, metal-backed patellar component. Removal of the component resulted in fragmentation of the patella **(C, D)**. (From Barrack RL, Rorabeck C, Partington P, et al. The results of retaining a well-fixed patellar component in revision total knee arthroplasty. *J Arthroplasty* 2000;15:590–596, with permission.)

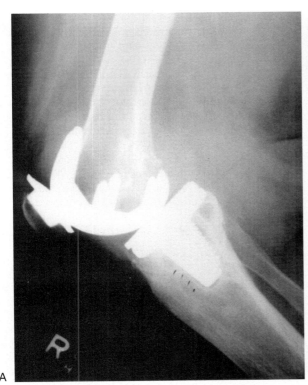
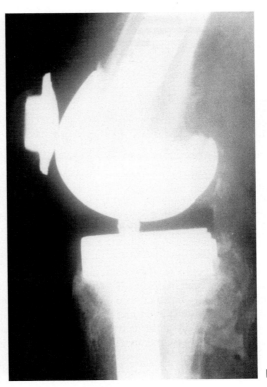

FIG. 5. A well-fixed uncemented, metal-backed patellar component with a thin residual patellar bone is present in this failed cementless total knee **(A)**. The well-fixed component was retained in spite of being metal backed and was well functioning years later **(B)**.

ment options and the clinical results that have been described to date are discussed.

RETAINING A WELL-FIXED PATELLAR COMPONENT

Retaining a patellar component that is not loose has a number of distinct advantages, including eliminating the risk of patellar fracture during component removal, retaining the maximal patellar bone stock and thus minimizing the risk of subsequent patella fracture, decreased operative time, and elimination of the additional component expense. There are a number of prerequisites to retain a well-fixed component. First, the fixation must be ensured both on preoperative radiographs as well as at the time of intraoperative testing. Any component with evidence of loosening or significant osteolysis should be removed (Fig. 2). Obviously in the presence of infection the component and underlying cement should be removed. If the component has gross evidence of surface damage it should also be revised. If the patellar component is well fixed, is minimally damaged, and tracks well, it still must be geometrically compatible with the femoral component in place. Most patellar components are domes that are symmetric in geometry and compatible with the trochlear flange of the vast majority of femoral components.

Controversy exists on the subject of retaining a well-fixed metal-backed patellar component. Most metal-backed patellar components have had a relatively high failure (8–10). For this reason alone some authors have recommended revision of all metal-backed patellar components at the revision knee arthro-

plasty (4). If there is adequate thickness of residual bone so that 12 mm or more of bone will remain after removal of a metal-backed component, then certainly revision to a cemented all-polyethylene component is preferable (Fig. 3). If, however, the metal-backed component is well fixed and the residual bone is already less than 12 mm in thickness and there has not been substantial wear, removal of such a metal-backed patellar component is probably not advisable (Fig. 4).

Barrack et al. reported on the results of retaining a well-fixed patellar component in revision TKA (11). A series of 34 cases in which a well-fixed component was retained was compared with 39 cases in which the patellar component was revised to a cemented all-polyethylene component at the time of revision TKA. The groups were compared with knee scores, a satisfaction survey, and response to patellofemoral questions. Twelve of the 34 well-fixed retained patellar components were metal-backed and none had shown any signs of loosening in an average of 3 years (11). At further follow-up beyond 5 years, none of the retained components showed clinical radiographic signs of loosening. This seems to support retaining a well-fixed metal-backed patellar component when the residual bone is thin and prone to fracture with component removal (Fig. 5). The fact that these components were not worn at the time of revision indicates that the extensor mechanism was probably reasonably well balanced and this probably also explains why they continue to do well when retained subsequent to the revision procedure.

If revision to another component is performed, there must be adequate bone for interdigitation of cement so that early loosening does not occur. Attempts should also be made to ensure symmetric thickness of the resurfaced patella, and it has been

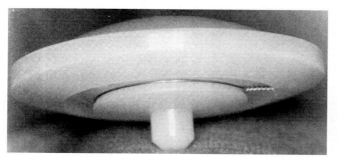

FIG. 6. A biconvex patellar component particularly suited for large central defects. (From Kolessar DJ, Rand JA. Extensor mechanism problems following total knee arthroplasty. In: Morrey BF, ed. *Reconstructive surgery of the joints*, 2nd ed. New York: Churchill Livingstone, 1996, with permission.)

suggested that a caliper be used to ensure that the thickness of the patella is within 2 mm in medial, lateral, proximal, and distal measurements (1). In many cases the residual patellar bone is deficient and is not amenable to implantation of a standard three-peg patellar component. In such instances, one of a number of options of dealing with deficient patellar bone must be selected.

TREATING THE DEFICIENT PATELLA

A certain amount of residual patellar bone is necessary to provide adequate support for implantation of a patellar component. There is a general agreement that the remaining thickness of bone in the range of 10 mm is necessary to provide adequate

support for fixation (1). If the patella is more than 10 mm in thickness but has a large central concavity, a special component such as biconvex patellar implant may be preferable to a standard three-peg component (Fig. 6) (4,12). Laskin reported on 85 total knees with use of such a domed-inset patellar implant (4). There was only one intraoperative fracture during reaming and no cases of postoperative fracture. A biconvex reamer is used to implant such a component and it is recommended that any remaining fibrous tissue be removed with the reamer in addition to 1 to 2 mm of underlying bone (4,12). This type of component requires that some degree of cancellous bone be present to allow interdigitation of bone cement (Fig. 7). When only a cortical shell is present with or without fracture, simple component removal without reinsertion of another component is a treatment option (Fig. 8).

PATELLOPLASTY

There is substantial dispute in the literature regarding the results of resection arthroplasty of the patella. The dispute begins with what the appropriate label for this procedure is. It has been variously called *patellar resection arthroplasty* (13), *patellar component resection* (14), and *patellar bony shell* (Fig. 8) (15). Drakeford et al. first reported on nine revision cases in which there was insufficient patellar bone stock for implantation of another component (13). A good to excellent Hospital for Special Surgery Knee score was reported in seven of the nine patients, with fair results in the other two. There were no cases of quadriceps lag, extension weakness, or anterior knee pain in this patient group, which caused the authors to recommend this as an acceptable alternative in revision knee replacement when there is inadequate patellar bone stock. Seel et al. reported on a larger group

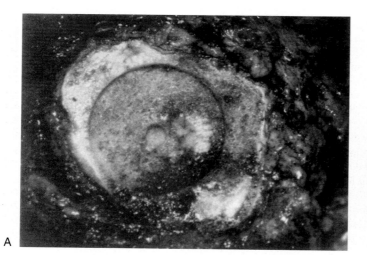

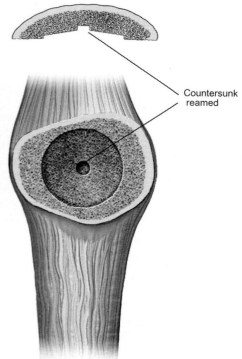

Countersunk reamed

FIG. 7. Technique of implanting a biconvex patella involves a reamer and requires the presence of some residual cancellous bone. **A:** Schematic of patella after reaming from the lateral and anteroposterior views **(B)**. (From Rand JA. Revision total knee arthroplasty: techniques and results. In: Morrey BF, ed. *Reconstructive surgery of the joints*, 2nd ed. New York: Churchill Livingstone, 1996, with permission.)

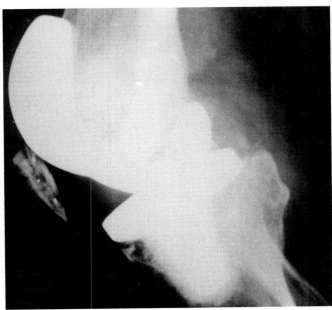

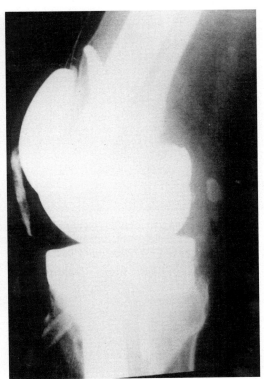

FIG. 8. Lateral radiograph demonstrates loosening of the cemented all-polyethylene patellar component with a very thin, sclerotic-appearing residual patellar bone fragment **(A)**. A simple patellar component resection was performed because of the sclerotic shell of remaining bone **(B)**.

of 18 patients with severely compromised patellar bone stock during revision TKA (16). This series was somewhat different in that a patella fracture was present in 10 of the 18 knees. Generalized knee pain was present in 10 of 18 knees (56%) and was classified as moderate or severe in four of the 18 (22%). The authors concluded that this provided an acceptable management option with a relatively low complication rate (one of 18, 6% fractured at 24 months) and was preferable to patellectomy or patellar component revision in patients with serious bone loss. Pagnano et al. reported on 34 knees in 31 patients at 3.5-year follow-up (range of 2 to 14 years) that had undergone revision TKA in which a patellar component could not be reinserted (14). Ten of 31 patients (32%) had persistent patellofemoral symptoms, seven of which (23%) were rated moderate or severe. Once again the authors concluded that patellar component resection without reimplantation was a reasonable approach for patients with markedly compromised patella bone stock; however, persistent anterior knee pain could be expected approximately one-third of the time. Barrack et al. reported on 21 knees that had a shell of bone left during revision TKA because of inadequate residual patellar bone (15). This study was unique in that it compared this series of 21 knees with 92 knees that had a patellar component in place after revision TKA. Among patients with a patellar bony shell, there was a significantly higher percentage of patients who had difficulty with stairs, a higher percentage of patients who were not satisfied with their surgery, and a higher percentage of patients who rated their surgeries unsuccessful in returning them to normal daily activities (15). Although the consensus of recent studies of patellar resection arthroplasty is that this is an "acceptable alternative," the relatively high incidence of persistent symptoms appears suboptimal and has led others to seek alternative approaches to the patient with patellar bone loss during revision TKA.

OPTIONS FOR THE DEFICIENT PATELLA

Hanssen recently described the technique and results of impaction grafting for severe patellar bone loss during revision TKA (17). Cancellous bone graft is tightly impacted into the patellar defect, which is then covered with a tissue flap created from peripatellar fibrotic tissue or free tissue obtained from the suprapatellar pouch (Fig. 9). This procedure was performed in nine knees in eight patients, with an average follow-up of 26.8 months (range of 15 to 43). The average arc of motion postoperatively was 1 to 98.9 degrees. There was dramatic improvement in pain and function scores from 39.1 to 91 points and 40 to 84 points, respectively. Radiographic analysis showed that the mean patella height on Merchant views averaged 19.7 mm (range of 17 to 22.5). The short-term results of this procedure represented an improvement over previous series of resection arthroplasty of the patella in terms of pain relief and knee score.

Fisher (18) described a technique of using crossed K-wires to provide support for cementing a patellar component in place when a cortical shell of bone is encountered during revision TKA (Fig. 10). This technique has been used in six knees that have been followed for 2 to 5 years, with good clinical results and no loosening reported to date (18).

Vince et al. described a treatment option when a shell of patellar bone is encountered that is scaphoid in shape, as might be seen in a case with extensive patellar osteolysis (19). Such cases tend to sublux laterally and articulate with the lateral femoral condyle. Four patients were treated with a gull wing sagittal osteotomy of the patella. The dorsal surface of the osteotomy is bone-grafted and the reshaped patella remnant is centralized over the patella groove (Fig. 11). Short-term follow-up on these patients revealed that the patients had a centrally tracking patella on physical examination and on Merchant view postop-

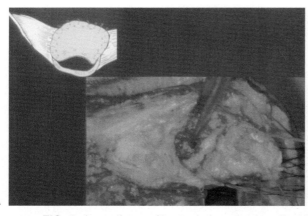

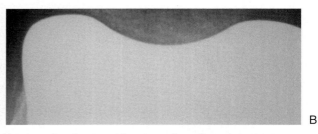

A

B

FIG. 9. Impaction grafting technique as described by Hanssen involves packing cancellous bone into the deficient patellar shell, which is then covered by a flap of locally obtained tissue **(A)**. The mean patellar height measured radiographically was approximately 20 mm **(B)**. (From Hanssen AD. Bone-grafting for severe patellar bone loss during revision total knee arthroplasty. *J Bone Joint Surg Am* 2001;83:171–176, with permission.)

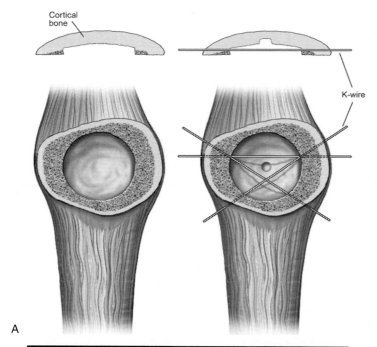

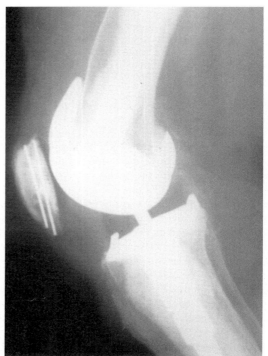

A

B

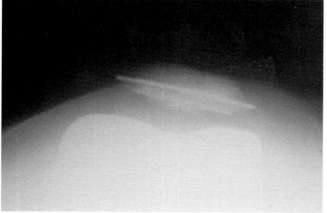

C

FIG. 10. The crossed K-wire technique as described by Fisher **(A)**. Follow-up lateral radiographic **(B)** and tangential view **(C)** demonstrating 2-year results of this technique. (Reprinted courtesy of David A. Fisher, MD, Indianapolis.)

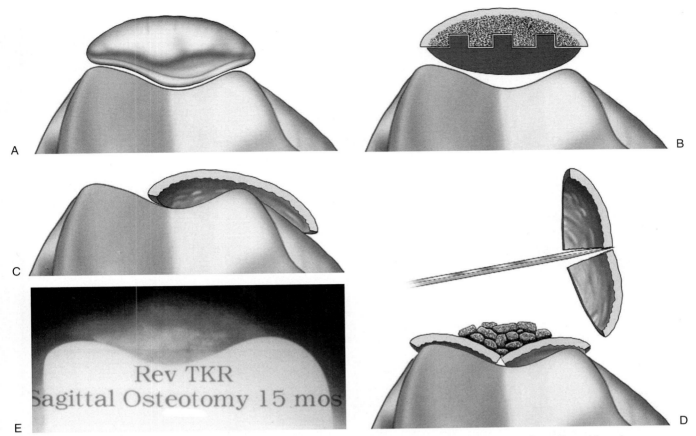

FIG. 11. Gull wing osteotomy technique as described by Vince is applicable to a laterally subluxed scaphoid-shaped shell of bone **(A–D)**. At short-term follow-up, more normal anatomy is demonstrated, with a patellar component remaining centrally located **(E)**. Rev TKR, revision total knee arthroplasty. (Reprinted courtesy of Kelly Vince, MD, Los Angeles.)

eratively. The Hospital for Special Surgery Knee score improved from an average of 32 to 75 points and the patients specifically denied anterior knee pain. The authors recommended this technique in dealing with a large, thin patellar remnant, in which case the shape of the fragment would prevent central tracking.

Another technique for dealing with the patellar remnant uses iliac crest bone graft that is shaped to the patellar remnant and fixed with four 1.5-mm cortical screws (20). A patellar button is then cemented in place. Two cases were described, with a 5-year follow-up with a satisfactory clinical result.

POSTPATELLECTOMY OPTIONS

The most difficult patellar situation to address is absence of the patella. This subgroup of patients had the lowest knee scores and the most functional disability compared with all other patellar treatment groups reported in the study by Coon et al. (3). Patients with a patellectomy typically experience extensor weakness, extension lag, and difficulty with patellofemoral activities such as stairs in a high percentage of cases (4). Buechel described a technique for restoring the patellar moment arm in an attempt to minimize the functional disability after TKA in cases with prior patellectomy (21). A 2.5-cm × 1-cm-thick iliac crest bone graft is sewn into a subsynovial pouch in the previous anatomic position of the patella (Fig. 12). Seven knees in six patients were treated with such an autografting technique and followed for a mean of 75.4 months (range of 24 to 125). Good or excellent results were reported in six of seven knees. All but one achieved painless active extension.

Another option in a patient who has had a prior patellectomy is to attempt attachment of a component to the soft tissue of the extensor mechanism. Simply sewing an all-polyethylene component to the undersurface of the extensor mechanism has resulted in generally unsatisfactory results (22). This approach was modified recently by Stulberg, who has sutured a metal porous tantalum baseplate into position at the desired location of the patella in the quadriceps tendon (23). Prior studies have documented that extensive fibrous tissue ingrowth can occur to attach the porous tantalum device via soft tissue fixation (24). An all-polyethylene component is then cemented onto the metal baseplate. Three patients were treated in this manner and followed for 1 year, at which time the implant appeared to be well fixed and functioning like a normal total knee patella (Fig. 13). Range of motion averaged 2 to 110 degrees.

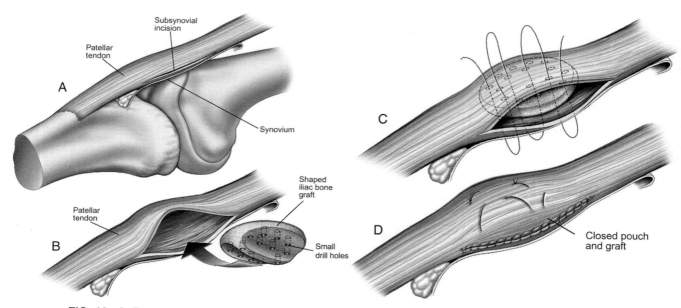

FIG. 12. A–D: Iliac crest bone-grafting technique with patients with prior patellectomy as described by Buechel. (From Buechel FF. Patellar tendon bone grafting for patellectomized patients having total knee arthroplasty. *Clin Orthop* 1991;271:72–78, with permission.)

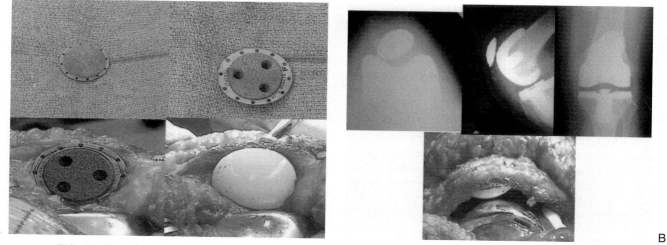

FIG. 13. Porous tantalum metal baseplate is sewn into the extensor mechanism in the appropriate position, after which an all-polyethylene component is cemented into the baseplate **(A)**. Clinical intraoperative photograph along with multiple postoperative views of the porous tantalum device used in knee replacement in a patient with prior patellectomy **(B)**. (Reprinted courtesy of David Stulberg, MD, Chicago.)

CONCLUSION

The method of patellar treatment significantly impacts the expected result after revision TKA. The most common procedures performed are revision to an all-polyethylene component designed for the revision total knee component used or retention of a well-fixed component. Both options appear to be equally satisfactory. For mild degrees of bone loss with some residual cancellous bone, a special revision component such as biconvex component can give consistently satisfactory results. Two patellar problem scenarios exist during revision TKA: the patient with a deficient patellar bone fragment and the patient who has had a patellectomy. For the patient with a deficient cortical shell of bone, recently described options include impaction grafting, a crossed K-wire technique, iliac crest bone grafting, and the gull wing osteotomy. For the patient with a patellectomy, options include iliac crest autograft into a subsynovial pouch and sewing in a porous metal baseplate designed for fibrous tissue attachment combined with a cemented all-polyethylene component. All of these options have shown promising results; however, the series to date have involved a small number of patients and the clinical follow-up has been relatively short.

Longer-term follow-up from a larger number of centers will be necessary to determine whether these patellar options in revision TKA prove to reliably improve on the results of these "patellar-problem patients" in revision TKA.

REFERENCES

1. Rand JA. Revision total knee arthroplasty: techniques and results. In: Morrey BF, ed. *Reconstructive surgery of the joints*, 2nd ed. New York: Churchill Livingstone, 1996.
2. Haas SB, Insall NJ, Montgomery W, et al. Revision total knee arthroplasty with use of modular components with stems inserted without cement. *J Bone Joint Surg Am* 1995;77:1700–1707.
3. Coon T, Drouillard P, Benjamin J, et al. *Patella management in revision total knee arthroplasty—a prospective study*. Presented at the 68th annual meeting of the American Academy of Orthopaedic Surgeons; February 2001; San Francisco.
4. Laskin RS. Management of the patella during revision total knee replacement arthroplasty. *Orthop Clin North Am* 1998;29:355–360.
5. Barrack RL. Specialized surgical exposure for revision total knee arthroplasty: quadriceps snip and patellar turndown. *Instr Course Lect* 1999;48:149–152.
6. Cameron HU, Cameron GM. The patellar meniscus in total knee replacement. *Orthop Rev* 1987;16:75–77.
7. Brown TE, Diduch DR. Fractures of the patella. In: Insall JN, Scott, WN, eds. *Surgery of the knee*, 3rd ed. New York: Churchill Livingstone, 2001.
8. Bayley JC, Scott RD. Further observations on metal-backed patellar component failure. *Clin Orthop* 1988;236:82–87.
9. Bayley JC, Scott RD, Ewald FC, et al. Failure of the metal-backed patellar component after total knee replacement. *J Bone Joint Surg Am* 1988;70:66–74.
10. Lombardi AV Jr, Engh GA, Volz RG, et al. Fracture/dislocation of the polyethylene in metal-backed patellar components in total knee arthroplasty. *J Bone Joint Surg Am* 1988;70:675–679.
11. Barrack RL, Rorabeck C, Partington P, et al. The results of retaining a well-fixed patellar component in revision total knee arthroplasty. *J Arthroplasty* 2000;15:590–596.
12. Kolessar DJ, Rand JA. Extensor mechanism problems following total knee arthroplasty. In: Morrey BF, ed. *Reconstructive surgery of the joints*, 2nd ed. New York: Churchill Livingstone, 1996.
13. Drakeford MK, Tsao AK, Lavernia C, et al. Resection arthroplasty for failed patellar components. *Ortho Trans* 1993–1994;17:992.
14. Pagnano MW, Scuderi GR, Insall JN. Patellar component resection in revision and reimplantation total knee arthroplasty. *Clin Orthop* 1998;356:134–138.
15. Barrack RL, Ingraham R, Matzkin E, et al. Revision knee arthroplasty with patella replacement versus bony shell. *Clin Orthop* 1998;356:139–143.
16. Seel MJ, Hanssen AD, Berry DJ, et al. Patellar component resection arthroplasty for the severely compromised patella during revision total knee arthroplasty. *Ortho Trans* 1995;19:338–339.
17. Hanssen AD. Bone-grafting for severe patellar bone loss during revision total knee arthroplasty. *J Bone Joint Surg Am* 2001;83:171–176.
18. Fisher DA. *The salvage knee*. Presented at the Issues in Orthopaedics: Clinical Results and Economic Outcomes; March 1997; Olympic Valley, CA.
19. Vince KG, Blackburn DC, Ortaaslan SG, et al. "Gull wing" osteotomy of the patella in total knee arthroplasty. *J Arthroplasty* 2000;15:254.
20. Tabutin J. Reconstruction osseuse de la patella par autogreffe vissee au cours des reprises des prostheses du genou. *Rev Chir Orthop Reparatrice Appar Mot* 1998;84:363–367.
21. Buechel FF. Patellar tendon bone grafting for patellectomized patients having total knee arthroplasty. *Clin Orthop* 1991;271:72–78.
22. Cameron HU, Fedorokow DM. The patella in total knee arthroplasty. *Clin Orthop* 1982;165:197–199.
23. Stulberg SD. *Treatment of the deficient patella in TKR surgery: rationale, surgical technique and initial clinical experience with the hedrocel revision patella*. Presented at the Interim Meeting of the Knee Society; September 2000; Boston.
24. Hacking SA, Bobyn JD, Toh KK, et al. Fibrous tissue ingrowth and attachment to porous tantalum. *J Biomed Mater Res* 2000;52:631–638.

CHAPTER 111

Diagnosis of Infection after Total Knee Arthroplasty

Kyle C. Swanson and Russell E. Windsor

The diagnosis of infection should always be considered when evaluating the patient with a painful total knee arthroplasty. Analysis of 18,749 total knee arthroplasties at the Mayo Clinic between 1969 and 1996 revealed the overall prevalence of infection 2.5%. Of 16,035 primary total knee arthroplasties, the incidence of infection was 2.0%. Of 2,714 revision total knee arthroplasties, the infection rate was 5.6% (1). The Hospital for Special Surgery reviewed 6,489 total knee replacements in 6,120 patients done between 1993 and 1999. Laminar airflow, hoods, panels, and perioperative antibiotics were used for these procedures. One hundred sixteen patients became infected, with 113 available for follow-up. Sixteen patients (14%) had superficial wound infections not in communication with the knee joint. These infections were all identified within the first 3 months after surgery. Ninety-seven cases (86%) developed deep periprosthetic infections. The overall infection rate for patients undergoing a primary total knee replacement was 0.39%. The overall infection rate for revision total knee arthroplasty was 0.97%. The time from implantation to the time of diagnosis ranged from 1 week to 156 months (2).

The diagnosis of infection after total knee arthroplasty is often challenging, with no single test being diagnostic in all patients. Instead, a careful history, with attention to host risk factors; physical examination; and selective microbacteriology, serum, and radiographic analyses, allows a reasonable prediction of infection. Although no individual test is 100% accurate, sensitive, and specific for establishing the presence of infection, the clinician must use every test result and clinical observation to make the diagnosis of infection.

EVALUATION OF HOST RISK FACTORS

Analysis of the painful total knee arthroplasty should prompt the evaluation and exclusion of infection. At times the diagnosis of infection is obvious in the setting of fever, acute swelling, and drainage. More often, the diagnosis is subtle and diagnostically challenging. A number of factors have been identified with an increased risk of infection after total knee arthroplasty.

The immune system of the host plays a critical role in the prevalence of infection. Patients on immunosuppressive medications have been shown to have an increased rate of postoperative infections (8). Although there is an array of direct and indirect laboratory studies for the surgeon to use to assess a patient's immune status, currently there is no accepted standard for delaying elective joint arthroplasty based on laboratory values that indicate compromised host immune function. Total lymphocyte count of less than 1,500 cells per μL and CD4 count of less than 100 obtained preoperatively have been shown to be significant risk factors in the development of postoperative infection (8–11).

The immune system is significantly dependent on a patient's nutritional status. Serum albumin and transferrin levels are well-recognized biologic markers of the patient's nutritional status, with serum transferrin levels having been shown to be more sensitive than both lymphocyte counts and albumin levels in predicting postoperative infection rates (8–11). Patients with these and other indicators that support a compromised immunity should raise the index of suspicion for infection.

The patient with diabetes mellitus is at increased risk for joint sepsis after total knee arthroplasty. England et al. (3) reviewed the results of 59 total knee arthroplasties in 40 patients diagnosed with diabetes mellitus. At 4.3 years average follow-up, the overall infection rate was 7%, a statistically higher rate of deep joint infection than the reported incidence of sepsis in nondiabetic patients. In another study of 60 patients with type II (adult-onset) diabetes mellitus matched with a nondiabetic control group, the incidence of postoperative medical and orthopedic complications was higher in diabetic patients. There were six early medical complications (12% versus 2% of the matched control group) and 21 orthopedic complications (31% versus 3% of the matched control group). Wound drainage, hematoma, or dehiscence occurred in 3 of 21 knees (4.4%). Superficial infection occurred in 1 of 21 knees (1.5%), and deep infection occurred in 1 of 21 knees (1.5%) with mean follow-up of 8 years (4). Yang et al. reviewed the outcome of 109 consecutive total knee arthroplasties in 86 diabetic patients. With a mean age of 69 years (range of 56 to 84 years) and mean follow-up of 42 months (range of 36 to 60 months), six knees (5.5%) subsequently developed deep joint infections (13).

Rheumatoid arthritis is a risk factor for the development of infection after total knee arthroplasty. Comparing osteoarthritis with rheumatoid arthritis in more than 2,000 total knee arthroplasties, the rate of infection was 2.4 times greater in patients with rheumatoid arthritis with metal-on-plastic designs and 2.5 times greater for hinged total knee designs. Although most infections were discovered within 2 years of surgery, all patients presenting with deep infection more than 3 years after operation had rheumatoid arthritis (5). Wilson et al. reviewed 4,171 total knee arthroplasties performed between 1973 and 1987 (6). Sixty-seven (1.6%) were followed by infection. The incidence of infection was significantly higher for knees affected by rheumatoid arthritis [45 (2.2%) of 2,076] than those affected by osteoarthritis [16 (1%) of 1,857]. Additionally, in the rheumatoid arthritis group, the incidence of infection was significantly higher in men [17 (4%) of 425 knees] than women [28 (1.7%) of 1,651].

Patients with psoriatic arthritis have an increased infection rate after total knee arthroplasty. Twenty-four arthroplasties performed in 16 patients with established long-standing psoriatic arthritis were reviewed. Four (17%) subsequently developed a deep infection. Two of the infections occurred at 1 and 6 months postoperatively; the other two occurred 3 and 5 years postoperatively (7).

Obesity has been evaluated as a risk factor for the development of infection after total knee arthroplasty. Winiarsky et al. found morbidly obese patients to have a statistically significant increase in the incidence of wound problems and development of deep periprosthetic infections in the perioperative period (12).

A history of old sepsis before total knee arthroplasty has demonstrated an increased susceptibility to the development of deep infection after total knee arthroplasty. In a review of 65 cemented total knee arthroplasties with a history of infection before total knee arthroplasty, deep infection occurred in five (7.7%) overall. In 20 of these 65 patients who demonstrated prior history of both bone and joint infection, three (15%) developed deep infection. In the other 45 patients who had a prior history of only joint sepsis, two (4%) developed deep infection (14).

Hemophilia also is a risk factor for the development of infection. Thomason et al. (15) reported the results of knee arthroplasty in hemophilic arthropathy. Twenty-three total knee arthroplasties were performed in 15 patients with severe hemophilia. Average follow-up was 7.5 years (range of 1 to 17 years), with a minimum of 4 years for the eight patients alive at the time of review. Thirteen patients were followed for at least 5 years and eight patients were followed for at least 10 years. There were two early infections, both in patients with human immunodeficiency virus. Two patients developed late infections, one at 18 months after implantation, and one at 4 years after implantation (15). Similarly, 29 arthroplasties performed in 21 disabled patients with severe hemophilia were evaluated from 1986 to 1995. With average follow-up of 4.8 years, 6 of 29 arthroplasties developed postoperative infections. Five were in patients with human immunodeficiency (16).

Numerous additional endogenous or host risk factors have been identified that may predispose certain patients to postoperative septic complications. These include alcohol abuse, chronic renal failure, infection at a remote site from total knee arthroplasty, malignancy, oral steroid use, multiple intraarticular injections before index arthroplasty, and development of postoperative hematoma (2,5,17–20).

HISTORY AND PHYSICAL EXAMINATION

A thorough history will elicit important host risk factors that may heighten the index of suspicion and aid in the diagnosis of infection. An investigation into the initiation and duration of pain is an important element of a thorough history. Unremitting pain with or without swelling and fever in the acute (within 3 months) postoperative period is uncommon and it should suggest the possibility of deep infection. Similarly, new-onset pain with or without swelling and fever, preceded by a quiescent period, is suggestive of late hematogenous infection. In both cases, indiscriminate administration of antibiotics may serve to mask certain physical findings such as swelling, erythema, and localized color; fever; and pain. Unfortunately, the end result is often an indolent subclinical infection and a painful prosthesis. Attempts should be made to isolate the organism if possible before antibiotic treatment commences.

Subclinical infections, with no overt physical findings of inflammation, swelling, or drainage, are more diagnostically challenging. Host factors, the infecting organism, or previous administration of antibiotics may contribute to the maintenance of a subclinical infection. Although certain mechanical factors may be excluded by physical examination, pain may be the only consistent finding in the presence of deep joint infection. In a study of 52 patients with infection after total knee replacement, pain was present in 100% of the patients (21). Seventy-seven percent had swelling of the knee, whereas 27% had active drainage.

Inquisition regarding prolonged drainage or delayed wound healing may aid in the diagnosis of infection. In the acute postoperative period, a small amount of drainage is not uncommon. However, prolonged wound drainage can effectively serve as a conduit through which bacteria can enter the wound. This is a recognized risk factor for the development of deep periprosthetic infection (23). Drainage occurs in approximately 25% of knee arthroplasty cases and may be further classified culture-negative or culture-positive (22). Cultures taken from wound drainage are generally unreliable and it is not recommended to base antibiotic treatment solely on this result. The onset of newly observable drainage in a healed wound after total knee arthroplasty is diagnostic of infection.

PLAIN RADIOGRAPHY

New radiographs should be obtained and when possible compared with old radiographs during an evaluation of the painful

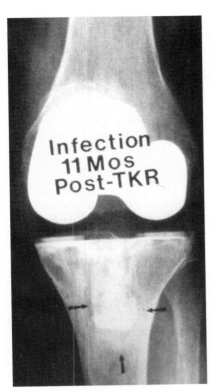

FIG. 1. Anteroposterior radiograph demonstrating progressive radiolucency (*arrows*) around the tibial component 11 months after Insall-Burstein II total knee arthroplasty.

total knee arthroplasty. Also, proper identification of the implants can aid in diagnosis, as the previous type of reconstruction has been shown to influence the subsequent risk of deep infection. Whereas surface replacements have an overall infection rate of less than 1%, metal-on-metal, constrained hinged total knee designs have a reported infection rate that approaches 14% (5,24,25). Many of these infections occur late, sometimes several years after implantation. The reason for this high incidence is not altogether clear but is probably related to the presence of metallic debris, which in turn causes the formation of a membranous sac containing fluid and debris around the prosthesis (26,27). Impregnation of the bone and soft tissues with metallic fragments and the large bone–cement interface may become factors, especially if the implant is loose. Constrained prostheses with metal-on-plastic bearing surfaces also demonstrate a higher infection rate. For example, the Stabilocondylar prosthesis (Howmedica, Rutherford, NJ) had an 8.3% infection rate in a small series of 36 cases. Rand et al. reported an infection rate of 16% in 50 kinematic rotating-hinge prostheses implanted between 1979 and 1981 (24). Cameron and Hunter reported similar results between the rotating-hinge and nonrotating-hinge prostheses (29). More recently, Wang and Wang reported on early catastrophic failure of two rotating-hinge total knee prostheses, illustrating that to date there are difficulties in the acute and long-term results with this type of prosthesis (30).

In the acute phase of deep periprosthetic infection, x-rays are often unremarkable, demonstrating a well-seated implant with no clear signs of premature loosening. Late findings of chronic infection may include progressive radiolucencies, focal osteopenia or

osteolysis of subchondral bone, and periosteal new bone formation, all suggestive of infection (28). Progressive prosthetic loosening is the most consistent radiographic finding associated with deep periprosthetic infection (Fig. 1) (1).

RADIOACTIVE ISOTOPE SCANNING (SCINTIGRAPHY)

No scintigraphic technique directly detects the presence of infection. Instead, all techniques reflect the inflammatory changes or localized bone reaction that may be associated with infection (65). With many causes of inflammation and accelerated bone turnover, scintigraphy often possesses less than optimal sensitivity and specificity. Additionally, increased uptake of radiopharmaceuticals may be seen in normal prostheses for up to 1 year after surgery, reflecting induced marginal osteoblastic activity (37). Despite their limitations, radioisotope scans may be used to facilitate the diagnosis of deep periprosthetic infection. Currently used radioisotopic tests include technetium-99m methylene diphosphonate, gallium-67 citrate, and indium-111–labeled leukocytes.

Prior reports of technetium-99m bone scanning have shown that this may be a useful screening tool in the evaluation of a painful implant. However, this procedure alone does not differentiate between infection and loosening (38,41). Technetium-99m scanning is performed in three phases. The first phase is a radionuclide angiogram, obtaining scans every 3 to 6 seconds for 1 minute after a bolus injection of the radionuclide. This demonstrates blood flow in the major vessels around the knee. The second phase includes a blood pool scan, for which a static image is obtained immediately after the flow study. This demonstrates radionuclide in the extravascular space. The first and second phases are the early phases and are a reflection of vascularity. The third, or late, phase consists of static images obtained 2 to 4 hours after injection. They demonstrate uptake of radionuclide by the bone and are a reflection of osteoblastic activity and bone blood flow (40). Technetium-99m scanning alone has a reported sensitivity of as high as 95% in detecting infection after total knee arthroplasty; its specificity, however, is only 20% (Fig. 2) (39).

Gallium-67 is taken up in white blood cells that subsequently migrate to areas of infection. It will also accumulate to a mild degree in the bone similar to a routine technetium-99m scan. Its independent use has a reported low specificity. Differential scanning comparing technetium-99m and gallium-67 was developed to increase the specificity for diagnosis of infection. A study is considered positive for infection if there is an area of high uptake on the bone scan as well as the gallium-67 scan. Also suggestive for infection is an area of uptake on the gallium-67 scan not matched on the bone scan. A study is considered negative for infection if there is no uptake on the gallium-67 scan or only a mild matched uptake. The study is indeterminate if there is moderate matched uptake (40). The clinical presentation of a technetium-99m scan that shows increased uptake but a gallium scan that is negative strongly suggests against the presence of infection. Many of the differential technetium-99m and gallium-67 scans, however, are indeterminate, showing only moderate matched increased uptake, which prevents a definitive diagnosis from being made (40). In fact, several authors have noted the limitations of sequential technetium-99m and

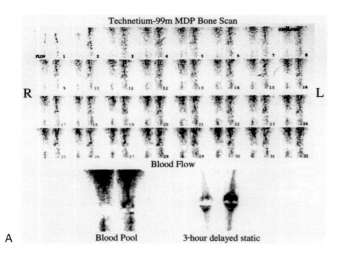

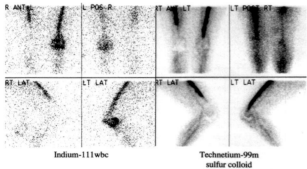

FIG. 2. A: Three-phase technetium-99m methylene diphos-phonate (MDP) bone scan shows increased vascularity on the blood flow and blood pool scans. The 3-hour delayed static images showed diffuse increased uptake around the left total knee prosthesis. **B:** A simultaneous indium-111 white blood cell scan and technetium-99m sulfur colloid bone marrow scan show increased uptake of the white blood cells around the left total knee prostheses that is not matched on the bone marrow scan. There is normal uptake in the marrow of diaphyses of the femurs. wbc, white blood cell.

gallium-67 bone scans, finding them inconsistent and unreliable in distinguishing infection from aseptic component loosening (44,46–48). LaManna et al. reported an accuracy of only 57% when using sequential technetium-99m and gallium-67 imaging in 60 patients with painful total joint arthroplasties (47).

Scanning with indium-111–labeled polymorphonuclear cells appears to be a sensitive and more specific test used in the diagnosis of infection (42). Reported values of sensitivity and specificity, however, have ranged from 50% to 100% (49). Variability in reported results may reflect inconsistent uptake around infected and uninfected arthroplasties. Although leukocytes may accumulate in bone marrow, there is considerable variation in marrow distribution. Prosthesis implantation adds variability, making interpretation of periprosthetic activity with indium-111 leukocyte scanning alone difficult (50). In 43 patients, indium-111–labeled white blood cell scanning used alone produced a sensitivity of 60% and a specificity of 73% (53). Using a canine model, Merkel et al. found that scintigraphy with indium-111–labeled autologous neutrophils was able to distinguish between septic and

aseptic loosening and a well-fixed prosthesis in 93% (14 of 15) of the study population (44). Rand et al. reviewed the value of indium-111 leukocyte scanning in the evaluation of painful and infected total knee arthroplasties. The series comprised 38 knees in 38 patients. All patients had surgical confirmation of the presence or absence of infection. Twenty patients were not infected and 18 patients had deep infection. The accuracy of the indium-111 leukocyte scan was 84%, the sensitivity was 83%, and the specificity was 85%. The three false-positive scans were obtained 1, 2, and 245 days before surgical exploration. The three false-negative scans were obtained 2, 3, and 2 days before surgical exploration, respectively (43).

To improve on the limitations regarding specificity, sequential imaging with complementary techniques has been advocated to provide the most accurate and reliable information to assist in the diagnosis of infection. Wukich et al. reported an 85% sensitivity and specificity using sequential technetium-99m and indium-111 in a retrospective examination of 24 patients with osteomyelitis or infection around a total joint prosthesis (64). Johnson et al. reported a sensitivity of 88% and a specificity of 95% using sequential technetium-99m and indium-111 leukocyte imaging (51). The study included 28 patients, nine of whom had a surgically confirmed infection. Palestro et al. reported a sensitivity of 67% and a specificity of 78% in 41 patients, with nine surgically confirmed infections using sequential technetium-99m and indium 111 scans (45). In a large study of 166 cases with 22 infected hip and knee arthroplasties, sequential use of technetium-99m and indium-111 leukocyte imaging was 64% sensitive and 78% specific (49).

Using available scintigraphic methods, other authors have advocated the use of sequential technetium-99m sulfur colloid and indium-111. If increased uptake is seen on the indium-111–labeled leukocyte scan, then further evaluation should be performed with a marrow-imaging agent such as technetium-99m–labeled sulfur colloid. If periprosthetic uptake of the leukocytes is more extensive than that of the sulfur colloid marrow agent, infection is likely. The use of the indium-111–labeled leukocyte scan with the technetium-99m–labeled sulfur colloid scan was the best combination of studies, with an 80% sensitivity and 100% specificity to evaluate infection after total knee arthroplasty (45).

New techniques such as indium-111–labeled immunoglobulin G and technetium-99m monoclonal antibody continue to be developed in an effort to improve on the diagnostic accuracy of infection.

LABORATORY STUDIES

Traditionally used hematologic tests in the diagnostic workup of infection include the white blood cell count, the erythrocyte sedimentation rate, and the C-reactive protein. These tests are dependent on the systemic response to the local infection. As is often the case with indolent periprosthetic infections, patients may generate normal laboratory results despite the presence of a deep infection.

The white blood cell count is rarely elevated and has been shown to have little or no value in predicting deep prosthetic infection (21,31–34). Grogan et al. identified 14 deep knee infections over a 10-year period (31). Although the peripheral leukocyte count ranged from 5,100 to 41,600 per mL at the time of diagnosis of the sepsis, the white blood cell count was greater than 10,000 per mL on only four occasions. Hanssen et al. reviewed 86 patients with 89 infected total knee arthroplasties (34). The leukocyte count averaged 8,440 (range of 3,800 to 19,200) and was elevated higher than 9,500 in only 17 patients.

The erythrocyte sedimentation rate and C-reactive protein are acute-phase reactants that can be an important adjunct to the diagnosis of deep periprosthetic infection. They are sensitive for an inflammatory process but lack specificity for infection. Furthermore, their value alone is limited in patients with systemic diseases that cause a baseline elevation of these markers such as rheumatoid arthritis and malignancy.

Postoperatively, both the erythrocyte sedimentation rate and the C-reactive protein levels are elevated. They generally return to normal as the inflammatory process abates. Variable sensitivities of the erythrocyte sedimentation rate and C-reactive protein have been reported in the literature depending on the level set for normal versus abnormal. Barrack et al. found a sensitivity of 100% when the abnormal erythrocyte sedimentation rate was set at more than 10 mm per hour and an 80% rate when an abnormal value was set at greater than 30 mm per hour (33). However, the specificity was only 25% and 62.5%, respectively. Levitsky et al. (35) found the sensitivity of the erythrocyte sedimentation rate to be 60% with a specificity of 65% when the abnormal rate was set at more than 30 mm per hour. This resulted in a positive predictive value of 25% and a negative predictive value of 89.5%. Other investigators have found the C-reactive protein to be more useful than the erythrocyte sedimentation rate, for it normalizes to presurgical levels in 2 to 3 weeks versus the 1 year it often takes for the sedimentation rate to normalize (36). Studies with the C-reactive protein have found that, like the sedimentation rate, it has a high sensitivity when the normal level is set less than 10 mg per L, but unfortunately it possesses a poor specificity. Analysis of obtaining C-reactive protein levels for this indication reveals an 85% sensitivity and specificity in detecting both acute postoperative infection and late hematogenous infections.

POLYMERASE CHAIN REACTION

Polymerase chain reaction is another method that has recently been used to ascertain evidence of infection. There are messenger DNA strands that can identify particular species of bacteria, allowing for the precise identification of the organism present in the joint. However, the polymerase chain reaction technique is expensive and has an approximately 2-hour turnaround time, which may be prohibitively long for practical use in the operating room setting. Additionally, observations of false-positive results have been reported recently (52). Polymerase chain reaction technology is still developing. In the future, this technique may become an extremely powerful tool in aiding the surgeon in both evaluation of infection and exact identification of the offending organism.

ASPIRATION

Arthrocentesis should be considered an essential element in the evaluation of the painful total knee arthroplasty. Obtaining a sample of synovial fluid for microscopic analysis and culture may establish an immediate diagnosis. Furthermore, isolation and identification of a bacterial species can help focus subsequent treatment, avoiding unnecessary cost and delay.

A synovial fluid white blood cell count of more than 25,000 per µL with more than 75% polymorphonuclear cells is highly suggestive of deep infection (54). In the presence of infection, fluid analysis may also reveal an increased protein level, a decreased glucose level, and poor mucin clot formation (55). Reported sensitivity of knee aspiration done under aseptic technique varies widely from 45% to 100% (32,35,53,56,57). This variation undoubtedly relates to the fact that administration of antibiotics before aspiration often leads to false-negative results.

If a patient is receiving antibiotics before isolation of a bacterial source, antibiotics should be discontinued. A period of 2 to 3 weeks should elapse before aspiration.

If the suspicion of infection remains high and the first aspiration is negative, repeat aspiration for 3 to 4 weeks is advised (1). Barrack et al. (33) evaluated 69 knees in 67 patients and found an overall sensitivity of 75%, specificity of 96%, and accuracy of 90%. Barrack et al. found the sensitivity of the knee aspiration to improve with multiple knee aspirations specifically if the patient had stopped the antibiotics (33). Multiple aspirations are prudent for two reasons: (a) Repeat aspirations may eventually yield an organism when no organisms were obtained from earlier aspirations, and (b) subsequent aspirations may be confirmatory if the original aspiration yielded growth of an organism and a contaminant or false-positive result is suspected. If an organism can be cultured, the surgeon will be more confident in obtaining a positive culture from the wound during surgery that accurately reflects the organism involved. Isolation of the organism(s) will facilitate the choice of postoperative antibiotic therapy and provide the actual infecting agents on culture media against which the bacteriocidal levels can be measured.

Procrastination of diagnosis and the prolonged use of oral antibiotics should be condemned, particularly when infection is suspected but not confirmed by proper bacteriologic evidence. The end result is likely to be an indolent subclinical infection and a painful prosthesis. Additionally, it may make subsequent culture of the organism very difficult, even after the components have been removed. Choosing appropriate antibiotic therapy may be nearly impossible, making successful salvage and reimplantation much less likely.

INTRAOPERATIVE ANALYSIS

Despite multiple attempts at aspiration, even in the absence of antibiotics, cultures may fail to yield an offending organism. False-positive cultures secondary to contamination from skin flora occasionally complicate the diagnosis. For this reason, many surgeons reserve the final diagnosis of infection until after intraoperative histopathologic analysis and tissue culture results.

The intraoperative use of Gram's staining alone is inadequate for excluding the diagnosis of infection. Della Valle et al. (58) reviewed the results of 413 intraoperative Gram's stains compared with the results of operative cultures, permanent histology, and the surgeon's intraoperative assessment to determine the ability of Gram's stains to identify periprosthetic infection. They found Gram's staining correctly identified the presence of infection in only 10 of the 68 cases that met the study criteria for infection (sensitivity of 14.7%). They concluded that Gram's

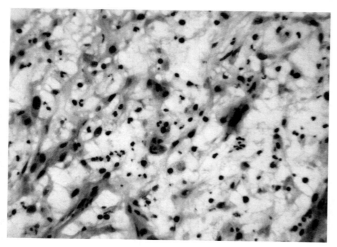

FIG. 3. High-power photomicrograph of an infected implant interface shows numerous neutrophils scattered throughout an edematous, slightly fibrotic, and moderately vascular stroma. Fibroblast and vascular endothelial elements show inflammatory atypia (hematoxylin and eosin stain, ×40).

stains alone do not have adequate sensitivity to be helpful in identifying periprosthetic infection and should not be performed on a routine basis. They may provide assistance in the case in which gross purulence is encountered to assist in the selection of initial antibiotic therapy.

Previous studies have demonstrated intraoperative frozen sections to be a reliable and accurate means of differentiating infection from a loose total joint prosthesis (Fig. 3) (59–61). Feldman et al. performed a retrospective analysis of thirty-three consecutive total hip and knee revision arthroplasties (62). To assess the usefulness of intraoperative frozen sections, they compared (a) the results of analyses of frozen sections with those of analyses of permanent histologic section; (b) the results of analyses of frozen sections with those of intraoperative cultures; (c) the results of clinical and radiographic follow-up with the final diagnosis; (d) the surgeon's operative impression regarding infection with the final pathologic result; and (e) the findings on preoperative radiographs, nuclear scans, laboratory studies, and intraoperative Gram's staining with the final pathologic result. Frozen sections were considered positive for infection if there were more than five polymorphonuclear leukocytes per high-power field in at least five distinct fields. Comparing the results of frozen sections (both positive and negative) with those of permanent sections of similar tissue was 100% sensitive, 100% specific, and 100% accurate. In patients with positive intraoperative cultures, all had positive frozen sections. Of the 24 patients who had negative intraoperative cultures, 23 had negative frozen sections (specificity, 96%). Of the nine positive intraoperative cultures, only two were found to have infection on intraoperative Gram's staining. The surgeon's operative assessment regarding the presence of infection compared with the final pathologic diagnosis demonstrated a sensitivity of 70%, a specificity of 87%, and an accuracy of 82% (62). In a follow-up study, Lonner et al. performed a prospective study of 175 consecutive revision joint surgeries and found that frozen sections have a sensitivity of 84% and a specificity of 96% for correctly distinguishing between infection and aseptic loosening when

the index five polymorphonuclear leukocytes per high-power field was used (63). The positive predictive value of the frozen sections increased significantly from 70% to 89% when the index increased from five to ten polymorphonuclear leukocytes per high-power field (63).

CONCLUSION

The diagnosis of infection is made by using the above observations derived from the clinical history, physical examination, and laboratory tests. Aspiration and x-ray evaluation contribute to the overall assessment of infection. If the presence of infection is confirmed, the surgeon should rapidly initiate definitive treatment using a variety of available options. Antibiotic suppression alone, surgical débridement with retention of the components plus antibiotic suppression, and one- or two-stage exchange of the total knee replacement should be done depending on the clinical situation. Salvage procedures such as arthrodesis, excision arthroplasty, and amputation should be considered only in the most difficult and extenuating circumstances.

REFERENCES

1. Hanssen AD, Rand JA. Evaluation and treatment of infection at the site of a total hip and knee arthroplasty. *Instr Course Lect* 1999;48:111–122.
2. Peersman G, Laskin RS, Davis J, et al. Infection in total knee replacement: a retrospective review of 6,489 total knee replacements. *Clin Orthop* 2001;392:15–23.
3. England SP, Stern SH, Insall JN, et al. Total knee arthroplasty in diabetes mellitus. *Clin Orthop* 1990;260:130–134.
4. Papagelopoulos PJ, Idusuyi OB, Wallrichs SL, et al. Long term outcome and survivorship analysis of primary total knee arthroplasty in patients with diabetes mellitus. *Clin Orthop* 1996;330:124–132.
5. Poss R, Thornhill TS, Ewald FC, et al. Factors influencing the incidence and outcome of infection following total joint arthroplasty. *Clin Orthop* 1984;182:117–126.
6. Wilson MG, Kelly K, Thornhill TS. Infection as a complication of total knee-replacement arthroplasty. Risk factors and treatment in 67 cases. *J Bone Joint Surg Am* 1990;72:878–883.
7. Stern SH, Insall JN, Windsor RE, et al. Total knee arthroplasty in patients with psoriasis. *Clin Orthop* 1989;248:108–111.
8. Greene KA, Wilde AH, Stulberg BN. Preoperative nutritional status of total joint patients. Relationship to postoperative wound complications. *J Arthroplasty* 1991;6:321–325.
9. Dreblow DM, Anderson CF, Moxness K. Nutritional assessment of orthopaedic patients. *Mayo Clin Proc* 2001;56:51–54.
10. Smith TK. Nutrition: its relationship to orthopaedic infections. *Orthop Clin* 1991;22:373–377.
11. Jensen JE, Jensen TG, Smith TK, et al. Nutrition in orthopaedic surgery. *J Bone Joint Surg Am* 1982;64:1263–1272.
12. Winiarsky R, Bath P, Lotto P. Total knee arthroplasty in the morbidly obese patient. *J Bone Joint Surg Am* 1998;80:1770–1774.
13. Yang K, Yeo SJ, Lee BP, et al. Total knee arthroplasty in diabetic patients: a study of 109 consecutive cases. *J Arthroplasty* 2001;16:102–106.
14. Jerry GJ, Rand JA, Ilstrup D. Old sepsis prior to total knee arthroplasty. *Clin Orthop* 1988;236:135–140.
15. Thomason HC, Wilson FC, Lachiewicz PF, et al. Knee arthroplasty in hemophilic arthropathy. *Clin Orthop* 1999;360:169–173.
16. Vastel L, Courpied JP, Sultan Y, et al. Knee replacement arthroplasty in hemophilia: results, complications and predictive elements of their occurrence. *Rev Chir Orthop Reparatrice Appar Mot* 1999;85:458–465.
17. D'Ambrosia RD, Shoji H, Heater R. Secondarily infected total joint replacements by hematogenous spread. *J Bone Joint Surg Am* 1976;58:450–453.

18. Hall AJ. Late infections about a total knee prosthesis. *J Bone Joint Surg Br* 1974;56:144–147.
19. Stinchfield FE, Bigliani LV, Nere HC, et al. Late hematogenous infections of total joint replacements. *J Bone Joint Surg Am* 1980;62:1345–1350.
20. Thomas BJ, Moreland JR, Amstutz HC. Infection after total joint arthroplasty from distal extremity sepsis. *Clin Orthop* 1983;181:121–125.
21. Windsor RE, Insall JN, Urs WK, et al. Two-stage reimplantation for the salvage of total knee arthroplasty complicated by infection. *J Bone Joint Surg Am* 1990;72:272–278.
22. Hanssen AD, Rand JA. Evaluation and treatment of infection at the site of a total hip or knee arthroplasty. *J Bone Joint Surg Am* 1998;80:910–922.
23. Weiss AP, Krackow KA. Persistent wound drainage after primary total knee arthroplasty. *J Arthroplasty* 1993;8:285–289.
24. Rand, JA, Cho, EY, Stouffer RN. Kinematic rotating-hinge total knee arthroplasty. *J Bone Joint Surg Am* 1987;69:489–497.
25. Deburge A, GUEPAR Group. Guepar hinge prosthesis: complications and results with two years follow-up. *Clin Orthop* 1976;120:47–53.
26. Rae T. A study on the effects of particulate metals of orthopaedic interest on murine macrophages in vitro. *J Bone Joint Surg Br* 1975;57:444–450.
27. Schurman DJ, Johnson BL Jr, Amstutz HC. Knee joint infections with *Staphylococcus aureus* and *Micrococcus* species: influence of antibiotics, metal debris, bacteremia, blood, and steroids in a rabbit model. *J Bone Joint Surg Am* 1975;57:40–49.
28. Rand JA, Bryan RS, Morrey BF, et al. Management of infected total knee arthroplasty. *Clin Orthop* 1986;205:75.
29. Cameron HU, Hunter GA. Failure in total knee arthroplasty: mechanisms, revisions, and results. *Clin Orthop* 1982;170:141–146.
30. Wang C, Wang HE. Early catastrophic failure of rotating hinge total knee prosthesis. *J Arthroplasty* 2000;15:387–391.
31. Grogan TJ, Dorey F, Rollins J, et al. Deep sepsis following total knee arthroplasty. *J Bone Joint Surg Am* 1987;69:489–497.
32. Windsor RE, Insall JN. Management of the infected total knee arthroplasty. In: Insall JN, ed. *Surgery of the knee*, 2nd ed. New York: Churchill Livingstone, 1993:959–974.
33. Barrack RL, Jennings RW, Wolfe MW, et al. The value of preoperative aspiration before total knee revision. *Clin Orthop* 1997;345:8–16.
34. Hanssen AD, Rand JA, Osmon DR. Treatment of the infected total knee arthroplasty with insertion of another prosthesis: the effect of antibiotic-impregnated bone cement. *Clin Orthop* 1994;309:44–54.
35. Levitsky KA, Hozak WJ, Balderson RA, et al. Evaluation of the painful prosthetic joint: relative value of bone scan, sedimentation rate, and joint aspiration. *J Arthroplasty* 1991;6:237–244.
36. Shih LY, Wu JJ, Yang DJ. Erythrocyte sedimentation rate and C-reactive protein values in patients with total hip arthroplasties. *Clin Orthop* 1987;225:238–246.
37. Eustace S, Shah Binod, Mason M. Imaging orthopedic hardware with an emphasis on hip prostheses. *Orthop Clin* 1998;29:67–84.
38. Reing CM, Richin PF, Kenmore PI. Differential bone-scanning in the evaluation of a painful total joint replacement. *J Bone Joint Surg Am* 1979;61:933–936.
39. Davis LP. Nuclear imaging in the diagnosis of the infected total joint arthroplasty. *Semin Arthroplasty* 1994;5:147–152.
40. Schneider R, Soudry M. Radiographic and scintigraphic evaluation of total knee arthroplasty. *Clin Orthop* 1985;205:108–120.
41. Al-Sheikh W, Sfakianakis GN, Mnaymneh W, et al. Subacute and chronic bone infections: diagnosis using In-111, Ga-67 and Tc-99m MDP bone scintigraphy, and radiography. *Radiology* 1985;155:501.
42. Propst-Proctor SL, Dillingham MF, McDougall IR, et al. The white blood cell scan in orthopaedics. *Clin Orthop* 1982;168:157.
43. Rand JA, Brown ML. The value of indium-111 leukocyte scanning in the evaluation of painful or infected total knee arthroplasties. *Clin Orthop* 1989;259:179–182.
44. Merkel KD, Brown ML, Dewanjee MK, et al. Comparison of indium-labeled imaging with sequential technetium-gallium scanning in the diagnosis of low-grade musculoskeletal sepsis. *J Bone Joint Surg Am* 1985;67:465–476.
45. Palestro CJ, Swyer AJ, Kim CK et al. Infected knee prosthesis: diagnosis with In-111-leukocyte, Tc-99m sulfur colloid, and Tc-99m MDP imaging. *Radiology* 1991;179:645–648.
46. Hattner RS, Chafetz N, Ruarke WC, et al. Clinical utility of Tc-99m-MDP/Ga-67 digital subtraction imaging in evaluating prosthetic joints. *J Nucl Med* 1982;23:29–36.
47. LaManna MM, Garbarino JL, Berman AT, et al. An assessment of technetium and gallium scanning in the patient with painful total joint arthroplasty. *Orthopedics* 1983;6:580–586.
48. Merkel KD, Brown ML, Fitzgerald RH. Sequential technetium-99m HDP-gallium-67 citrate imaging for the evaluation of infection in the painful prosthesis. *J Nucl Med* 1986;27:1413–1417.
49. Teller RE, Christie MJ, Martin W, et al. Sequential indium-labeled leukocyte and bone scans to diagnose prosthetic joint infection. *Clin Orthop* 2000;373:241–247.
50. Palestro CJ, Kim CK, Swyer AJ, et al. Total-hip arthroplasty: periprosthetic indium-111 labeled leukocyte activity and complementary technetium-99m-sulfur colloid imaging in suspected infection. *J Nucl Med* 1990;31:1950–1955.
51. Johnson JA, Christie MJ, Sandler MP, et al. Detection of occult infection following total joint arthroplasty using sequential technetium-99m HDP bone scintigraphy and indium-111 WBC imaging. *J Nucl Med* 1988;29:1347–1353.
52. Mariani BD, Martin DS, Levine MJ, et al. Polymerase chain reaction detection of bacterial infection in total knee arthroplasty. *Clin Orthop* 1996;331:11–22.
53. Cuckler JM, Star AM, Alavi A, et al. Diagnosis and management of the infected total joint arthroplasty. *Ortho Clin* 1991;22:523–530.
54. Insall JN. Infection of total knee arthroplasty. *Instr Course Lect* 1986;35:319–324.
55. Brause BD. Infected total knee arthroplasty. *Orthop Clin* 1982;13:245–249.
56. Morrey BF, Westholm F, Schoifet S, et al. Long-term results of various treatment options for infected total knee arthroplasty. *Clin Orthop* 1989;248:120–128.
57. Duff GP, Lachiewicz PF, Kelley SS. Aspiration of the knee joint before revision arthroplasty. *Clin Orthop* 1996;331:132–139.
58. Della Valle CJ, Scher DM, Yong YH, et al. The role of intraoperative Gram stain in revision total joint arthroplasty. *J Arthroplasty* 1999;14:500–504.
59. Bullough PG. Tissue reaction to wear debris generated from total hip replacements. In: *The hip. Proceedings of the first open scientific meeting of The Hip Society.* St. Louis: Mosby, 1973:80–91.
60. Charosky CB, Bullough PG, Wilson PD Jr. Total hip replacement failures. A histological evaluation. *J Bone Joint Surg Am* 1973;55:49–58.
61. Mirra JM, Amstutz HC, Matos M, et al. The pathology of the joint tissues and its clinical relevance in prosthesis failure. *Clin Orthop* 1976;117:221–240.
62. Feldman DS, Lonner JH, Desai P, et al. The role of intraoperative frozen sections in revision total joint arthroplasty. *J Bone Joint Surg Am* 1995;77:1807–1813.
63. Lonner JH, Desai P, DiCesare PE, et al. The reliability of analysis of intraoperative frozen sections for identifying active infection during revision hip or knee arthroplasty. *J Bone Joint Surg Am* 1996;78:1553–1558.
64. Wukich DK, Abren SH, Callaghan JJ, et al. Diagnosis of infection by preoperative scintigraphy with indium-labeled white blood cells. *J Bone Joint Surg Am* 1987;69:1353–1360.
65. Wegener WA, Alavi A. Diagnostic imaging of musculoskeletal infection. *Orthop Clin* 1991;22:401–418.

CHAPTER 112

Microbes and Antibiotics

Barry D. Brause

Total knee arthroplasty has become commonplace because of its magnificent success in restoring function to disabled arthritic individuals. However, 1% to 5% of indwelling joint prostheses develop infection, associated with significant morbidity and occasionally death. This chapter discusses the pathogenesis of these infections as it relates to the current spectrum of pathogens, the difficulties encountered in designing effective antimicrobial therapy in the present era of emerging multidrug resistance, and specific approaches to sepsis prevention.

MICROBIOLOGY OF PROSTHETIC KNEE INFECTION

Infection of prosthetic joints occurs by either the introduced-contiguous or hematogenous route. On the basis of observations at the Hospital for Special Surgery, approximately one-half of joint implants become infected by the introduced-contiguous route and one-third are blood-borne, with the remainder being of uncertain mode of origin (Table 1) (1).

The introduced-contiguous form of joint sepsis results from wound infection overlying the prosthesis or operative contamination. Any factor or event that delays wound healing increases the risk of infection. Ischemic necrosis, infected wound hematomas, superficial wound infection, and suture abscesses are common events preceding joint replacement sepsis. During the early postoperative period when these infections develop, the fascial tissue layers are not yet healed and the deep, periprosthesis tissue is unprotected by the usual physical barriers. Rarely, latent foci of chronic, quiescent osteomyelitis are reactivated by the disruption of tissue that accompanies implantation surgery. Although operative cultures at the time of joint replacement are sterile, *Staphylococcus aureus* and *Mycobacterium tuberculosis* infections have recrudesced in this setting.

Introduced-contiguous–type infections are usually caused by a single pathogen, but polymicrobial sepsis with as many as three to five different organisms is seen in as many as one-fourth of patients with this form of prosthesis infection (Table 2) (1). Two-thirds of introduced-contiguous infections are caused by gram-positive aerobes. Coagulase-negative staphylococci (*Staphylococcus epidermidis* and other species), the principal constituents of skin microflora, are the predominant etiologic agents, isolated in 37% of cases, followed by *S. aureus* in 16% and group D streptococci (enterococcal and nonenterococcal) in 10%. Gram-negative aerobes are found in 22% and anaerobes in 10% of patients.

Any bacteremia can cause infection of a total joint replacement by the hematogenous route. Sepsis usually becomes established at the interface of the bone with the foreign body (cement or prosthesis), and the pathogens reflect the resident microflora at the source of the bacteremia. Table 3 describes the attributed pathogenetic events in 36 patients with hematogenous prosthetic joint infections evaluated at the Hospital for Special Surgery (1). Dentogingival infections and manipulations are known causes of viridans streptococcal and anaerobic (*Peptococcus* and *Peptostreptococcus*) infections around prostheses (2,3). Pyogenic skin processes can cause staphylococcal (*S. aureus* and *S. epidermidis*) and streptococcal (groups A, B, C, and G streptococci) infections of prosthetic joint arthroplasties. Genitourinary and gastrointestinal tract procedures and infections are associated with gram-negative bacillary, enterococcal, and anaerobic infections of total joint replacements (4,5).

A general view of the microbial spectrum observed among joint implants infected by all routes is described in Table 4 (1). Staphylococci are the principal causative agents (44%), evenly

TABLE 1. *Routes of infection for joint prostheses: the Hospital for Special Surgery experience*

Route	Patients	Percent
Introduced-contiguous	(54/105)	51
Hematogenous	(36/105)	34
Unknown	(15/105)	14

divided between *S. epidermidis* and *S. aureus* in frequency. Aerobic streptococci are responsible for more than 20% of infections. Gram-negative aerobic bacilli are identified in 25% of patients, and anaerobes represent 10% of culture-proven pathogens. Anaerobes may not be isolated by routine culture techniques because of their fastidious growth requirements and their rapid demise on exposure to air. Therefore, the frequency of anaerobic involvement in prosthetic joint infections is likely understated and several studies report no incidence of anaerobic organisms (6). Recovery of anaerobes from infected tissues and fluids can be substantially increased by placing the specimen directly and immediately into a prereduced incubation medium, such as thioglycollate broth. Supplies of this inexpensive medium can be made available in the operating room and at the bedside to encourage its use. The frequency of culture-negative cases should be reduced with this approach to delineating the microbiologic diagnosis. In those difficult clinical situations in which antibiotic therapy is designed empirically, because of a high suspicion of infection in the absence of positive cultures, strong consideration should be given to include an antianaerobic agent in the therapeutic regimen.

FUNGAL INFECTIONS

Although these pathogens have been isolated in less than 1% of infected total joint arthroplasties, they represent significant

TABLE 2. *Introduced-contiguous–type prosthetic joint infection bacteriology (Hospital for Special Surgery)*

Pathogen	Percent
Gram-positive aerobes (67%)	
Staphylococcus epidermidis	37
Staphylococcus aureus	16
Group D streptococci	10
Group B streptococci	1
Corynebacteria	3
Gram-negative aerobes (22%)	
Proteus	6
Enterobacter	6
Pseudomonas aeruginosa	4
Serratia	4
Escherichia coli	1
Klebsiella	1
Anaerobes (10%)	
Propionibacteria	3
Clostridia	3
Peptococcus	1
Peptostreptococcus	1
Bacteroides	1
Arachnia	1
Polymicrobial infections (24%)	

TABLE 3. *Pathogenesis of hematogenous prosthetic joint infection*

Clinical Event	Organisms
Dental	
Manipulation with extensive gingival bleeding, abscesses, root canal	Viridans streptococci (4)
Infected wisdom tooth	*Peptostreptococcus* (1)
Capping	*Peptococcus* (1)
Urinary tract	
Infection	*Proteus mirabilis* (6)
	Escherichia coli (4)
Skin	
Abscesses, infected cyst, infected dermatitis, cellulitis, infected intravenous site	*Staphylococcus aureus* (9)
Cellulitis	Group G streptococci (2)
Desquamative dermatitis	*Staphylococcus epidermidis* (1)
Bowel	
Tumor, radiation colitis, diverticulitis, multiple enemas for obstipation	Viridans streptococci (4)
Proctitis	*Peptococcus* (1)
Diverticulitis	*E. coli* (1)
Enteritis	*Salmonella* (1)
Genital tract	
Cervical polypectomy	*Lactobacillus* (1)

problems for both diagnosis and treatment. All four principal species of *Candida* (*Candida albicans*, *Candida parapsilosis*, *Candida tropicalis*, and *Candida glabrata*) are capable of infecting joint prostheses (7–11). Because of the rarity of mycotic infection in this setting, initial cultures revealing *Candida* species may be interpreted as contaminants, thereby delaying appropriate therapy. Usually, fungal infections are found in patients with underlying conditions, including immunosuppression, prolonged antibiotic therapy, or intravenous drug abuse, but this is not true for patients with *Candida* infection of prosthetic articulations. The majority of patients described have had no identifiable predisposing conditions, have not had *Candida* infections elsewhere in their body, and have not had evidence of

TABLE 4. *Microbiology of prosthetic joint infection (all routes)*

Pathogens	Frequency (%)
Staphylococci	**44**
Staphylococcus aureus	22
Staphylococcus epidermidis	22
Streptococci	**21**
Viridans streptococci	9
Groups A, B, G	5
Group D (enterococci)	7
Gram-negative aerobic bacilli	**25**
Anaerobes	**10**
Fungi	**<1**
Mycobacteria	**<1**

disseminated candidiasis. These infections typically present within 5 years of joint replacement, and symptom evolution follows an indolent course, with an average of 10 months (range of 2 weeks to 4 years) between the onset of joint pain and diagnosis. Clinical presentations are the same as seen in bacterial infections of prosthetic joints. The periarticular fluid and tissues examined reveal purulent material with polymorphonuclear leukocytes. The individualized therapeutic approaches have varied from resection arthroplasties with intravenous amphotericin B to implant retention with suppressive oral therapy with an imidazole (12).

TUBERCULOUS INFECTIONS

Bacillemia during the earliest stage of tuberculous infection (with *M. tuberculosis*) can seed osseous tissue without causing systemic or local symptoms. Then, many years later, these foci of old, quiescent tuberculosis can reactivate in bones receiving prosthesis implantation (13–18). The risk of recrudescent infection is very low (approximating 1%) in patients with inactive tuberculosis for more than 10 years but can be as high as 43% in patients with active tuberculosis within the previous 10 years (19). It appears that perioperative antituberculous therapy is an appropriate consideration, especially if the initial tuberculous infection had been inadequately treated and if the patient is likely to tolerate antituberculous medication (20). The possibility of a mycobacterial infection should be considered in patients with otherwise unexplained recurrent joint prosthesis failure.

Optimally, patients with active tuberculosis should be treated before undertaking prosthesis implantation. Occasionally, *M. tuberculosis* infection is discovered at the time of joint replacement arthroplasty on the basis of subsequently available histopathology or culture results. In this clinical situation, successful treatment can be accomplished with triple-drug antituberculous chemotherapy given for 18 months postoperatively (21). It is noteworthy that almost all of these tuberculous infections were effectively controlled by antimicrobial therapy without removal of the prosthesis. However, the recent emergence of multidrug-resistant tuberculosis makes the efficacy of future treatments uncertain (22).

ESTABLISHING THE DEFINITIVE MICROBIOLOGIC DIAGNOSIS

The diagnosis of joint replacement infection is dependent, in large part, on isolation of the pathogen. Usually, the clinical history, physical examination, x-rays, and radioisotopic scans have inadequate specificity. Therefore, the single observation that delineates the presence of implant infection is isolation of the pathogen by arthrocentesis or surgical débridement. Moreover, microbiologic evaluations (e.g., susceptibility studies) of the etiologic microorganism are essential to design optimal antibiotic therapy.

Prosthetic joint fluid aspirates demonstrate the pathogen in 85% to 98% of cases (23,24).

When difficulty is encountered in obtaining intraarticular fluid, irrigation with sterile normal saline (without antiseptic preservative additives) can be used to provide fluid for culture. If initial cultures reveal a relatively avirulent organism (coagulase-negative staphylococci, corynebacteria, propionibacteria,

or *Bacillus* species), a second aspirate should be considered to confirm that the isolate is the pathogen and not a contaminant artifact.

Early isolation of the infecting organism is important in establishing the correct cause of the patient's painful prosthesis and is essential for optimal selection of the surgical and medicinal therapeutic approaches. Availability of antibiotic susceptibility studies preoperatively permits proper selection of the appropriate antimicrobial agent for incorporation into the antibiotic-loaded cement spacer. Preoperative knowledge of the pathogen's quantitative sensitivity (minimum bactericidal concentration) can be extremely valuable in determining whether a single-stage or a two-stage (prosthesis removal and reimplantation) procedure is the best alternative in individual cases. Because the success of the single-stage exchange procedure is largely dependent on the efficacy of the antibiotic selected for mixing with cement during reimplantation, the choice of this antimicrobial agent should be based on the quantitative susceptibility of the specific pathogen being treated. Most often tobramycin or gentamicin is used in the antibiotic–cement admixture because it is known that these agents leach from polymethylmethacrylate cement in predictably therapeutic concentrations (25). With the recent emergence of aminoglycoside (tobramycin, gentamicin) resistant staphylococci and streptococci, a successful clinical outcome may be related to how sensitive the pathogen is to these drugs. Most of these resistant gram-positive cocci remain sensitive to vancomycin; however, vancomycin leaches from cement in only very low concentrations (26). Recent studies have demonstrated significantly higher release of vancomycin when it is combined with tobramycin in the cement admixture and that the vancomycin/tobramycin combination releases substantial amounts of bioavailable bactericidal activity into joint fluids (27,28). Anaerobes are not susceptible to aminoglycosides but are usually sensitive to clindamycin. As more information is obtained regarding the usefulness (pharmacokinetics and patient tolerance) of clindamycin-cement admixtures, clindamycin may become the agent of choice for local depot therapy of anaerobic prosthesis infections.

Operative cultures are definitively diagnostic. Therefore, in the absence of acute illness, the patient should not receive any antibiotic therapy for several weeks before the procedure. Preoperative antibiotics should *not* be administered routinely. However, if individual patients need preoperative prophylactic antibiotics (because of the presence of other indwelling joint prostheses or abnormal cardiac valves, etc.), then a tourniquet, placed proximal to the infected knee implant, should be inflated before antimicrobial administration. Multiple specimens (five to seven) of tissue and fluid should be submitted for culture. Samples of purulence, abnormal tissue, and fluid are preferable to swabs for cultivation. Specific cultures for anaerobes using pre-reduced medium (e.g., thioglycollate broth) should be inoculated in the operating room if possible. Fungal and mycobacterial cultures should be arranged if appropriate. After culturing has been completed, intraoperative antibiotic therapy can be commenced. If a cement spacer is inserted, it should be loaded with antibiotics (tobramycin or gentamicin, with or without vancomycin) appropriate for the microbe anticipated. If the infecting pathogen is not sufficiently susceptible to these leaching antibiotics, consider not inserting a spacer. A cement spacer that is not releasing antibiotics effective against the microorganisms present at the infected site may allow organisms to persist on its surface and result in a failure to eradicate the infection.

Once the specific microbiologic diagnosis has been delineated, quantitative sensitivity studies (optimally, minimum bactericidal concentrations) can be used to design the best antimicrobial regimen for each individual patient. Selection of specific antibiotic agents and their route of administration (intravenous or oral) is facilitated by the availability of these data. Decisions regarding the usefulness of combinations of antibiotics to provide additive or synergistic activity can also be made more easily with these studies. The isolated pathogen can then be used to determine the potency of the therapeutic regimen by incubating it with a sample of the patient's blood in the serum bactericidal test. This test has been very useful for confirming the efficacy of antibiotic therapy for prosthetic joint infection when the two-stage (removal/reimplantation) approach is used. For this purpose, the blood for the serum bactericidal test is drawn at the postpeak period, 25% into the interval between doses. When this postpeak serum bactericidal test titer is equal to or greater than 1:8, cure rates are 90% to 95% for prosthetic hip arthroplasties and 97% for prosthetic knee arthroplasties (29–31). For all of the above reasons it is essential to isolate the pathogen in total joint replacement infections. However, there will always be clinical situations in which the etiologic microorganism is not isolated. In these uncommon circumstances, empiric antibiotic therapy should be designed on the basis of the likely pathogen(s), with special attention to the possible involvement of anaerobes in the infection.

ANTIMICROBIAL RESISTANCE

In the presence of prosthetic devices, many bacteria (especially strains of staphylococci and *Pseudomonas*) elaborate a fibrous exopolysaccharide material often termed "glycocalyx" or "slime." Organisms can grow within this matrix, forming thick biofilms. The glycocalyx modifies the local tissue environment in favor of the pathogen by concentrating microbial nutrients and by protecting the organism from surfactants, opsonic antibodies, phagocytes, and antimicrobial agents. These conditions increase the density of colonization on the surface of foreign materials *in vivo* and may predispose toward tissue invasion (20,32,33). These protective biofilms may also result in persistence of infection despite treatment with systemic antibiotic therapy (especially in the absence of extensive and meticulous débridement). Infections associated with biofilms and biomaterials may require special studies to determine the efficacy of specific antimicrobial agents (34–36). The routine tests for minimum inhibitory and minimum bactericidal concentrations are performed on suspensions of microorganisms in the logarithmic phase of growth. When the same bacteria are studied while they are adherent to foreign body substrates or in the stationary phase of growth, their resistance to antibiotics increases markedly (37). By this mechanism, all microorganisms that induce biofilms, in association with prosthetic device infection, are more resistant to the effects of antimicrobial agents. Rifampin is an antibiotic with superior tissue biofilm penetration characteristics and appears to have potency against pathogens even when the microbe is adherent to foreign materials. This capacity of rifampin may explain the observed apparent cures of infected prostheses after treatment with rifampin-containing antibiotic combinations even when the implant has been retained (38). Rifampin cannot be used as a single agent

due to the rapid development of rifampin-resistant strains when it is the sole therapeutic drug. Except for these scant published cases, approaches to treatment of infected retained total joint arthroplasties have been disappointing (39). When prolonged suppressive antibiotic therapy has been used to treat indwelling knee prostheses, joint function is maintained in only 26% (40). It should be anticipated that with greater understanding of the interaction between antimicrobial agents and substrate-adherent microorganisms, this success rate should improve.

Resistance of bacteria in general to specific antibiotics continues to increase as a consequence of microbial genetic responses to antimicrobial agents. Certain microorganisms important in prosthetic joint infections have developed particularly troublesome patterns of resistance. Methicillin-resistant *S. aureus* and methicillin-resistant *S. epidermidis* have become common nosocomial pathogens often requiring multidrug, substantially toxic antibiotic regimens for effective treatment (41). Vancomycin, associated with frequent chemical phlebitis and potential nephrotoxicity, is usually the drug of choice in combating these pathogens. Recently, vancomycin-resistant strains of *Enterococcus faecalis* and *Enterococcus faecium* have been isolated in hospital settings, representing potentially untreatable microorganisms (42,43). These vancomycin-resistant organisms are able to transfer vancomycin resistance to staphylococci *in vitro*, thereby producing methicillin-resistant *S. aureus* (and potentially methicillin-resistant *S. epidermidis*) strains that could also be untreatable with presently available antimicrobial agents. *S. aureus* strains have also developed intermediate resistance to vancomycin in hospitals and in patients using extensive amounts of vancomycin. Because staphylococci together with enterococci account for 63% of introduced-type prosthetic joint infection, the potential emergence of this degree of antibiotic-resistance would be a clinical problem of immense proportions. Aminoglycoside (gentamicin, tobramycin, amikacin, streptomycin) resistance is also being observed with staphylococci and streptococci (44). This eliminates our ability to use these antibiotics in combination with cell wall–active agents in synergistic, multidrug, systemic therapeutic regimens. Even more important, the emergence of this resistance will substantially interfere with the efficacy of antibiotic-impregnated cement for local therapy because tobramycin and gentamicin are the most commonly used antibiotics in these admixtures worldwide.

Antibiotic resistance among Gram-negative bacilli continues to outpace the development of new antibiotics. Treatment of these bacteria has been problematic and often ineffective. As a result of this experience, patients with Gram-negative infections of their joint prostheses have often been refused reimplantation, or reimplantation has been delayed for many months because insufficient confidence could be established regarding the eradication of this type of infection. Because this resistance pattern is strain-specific, decisions concerning therapeutic approaches, including the timing of reimplantation, should be made on the basis of the quantitative sensitivity (minimum inhibitory concentration, minimum bactericidal concentration, and serum bactericidal testing) of the particular microbe isolated (1,30,31). Treatment choices should not be based on the Gram stain characteristics of the organism or the genus and species involved. Instead, each cultured strain should be evaluated for our ability to eradicate it from the infected tissue with currently available antimicrobial strategies (including the variety of systemic agents as well as local therapy with antibiotic-loaded polymeric cement). At the present time, we encounter Gram-negative

TABLE 5. *Highlight points and technical pearls*

Microbiology of prosthetic knee infection
Introduced-contiguous form (51%)
    Any factor or event that delays wound healing increases
      the risk of infection
    Coagulase-negative staphylococci (including
      Staphylococcus epidermidis) (37%)
    Staphylococcus aureus (16%)
    Group D streptococci (including enterococci) (10%)
    Gram-negative aerobes (22%)
    Anaerobes (10%)
Hematogenous form (34%)
    Any bacteremia
    Dentogingival infections
    Pyogenic skin processes
    Genitourinary and gastrointestinal tract procedures and
      infections
Frequency of various pathogens
    Staphylococci (44%)
    Streptococci (21%)
    Gram-negative aerobic bacilli (25%)
    Anaerobes (10%)
    Fungal infections (<1%)
    Tuberculous infections (<1%)
Prophylactic use of antibiotics
Perioperative antibiotic prophylaxis
Postoperative considerations
    Prompt treatment of infections at remote sites
    Prophylactic antibiotic administration in anticipation of
      bacteremic events
      Dental procedures with significant bleeding
      American Dental Association and American Academy of
        Orthopaedic Surgeon recommendations

Establishing the definitive microbiologic diagnosis
History, physical examination, x-rays, radioisotopic scans
    Inadequate specificity
Isolation of the pathogen
    Joint aspirates (85–98% positivity)
    Operative cultures are definitively diagnostic
      No antibiotics for several weeks before surgery
      Multiple specimens (five to seven) of tissues and fluid
    Early isolation of the pathogen is important
      Allows for proper selection of antibiotics for spacer and
        for systemic use
      Helps determine the value of single-stage or two-stage
        approach to therapy
      Allows for quantitative antibiotic susceptibility studies
      Allows decision making regarding the use of antibiotic
        combinations
      Allows for the subsequent performance of serum
        bactericidal tests
Antimicrobial resistance
Bacterial exopolysaccharide (glycocalyx, slime)
    Protective biofilms may result in persistence of infection
Microbial genetic responses to antimicrobial agents
    Methicillin-resistant *S. aureus*, methicillin-resistant *S.
      epidermidis*, vancomycin-resistant strains of *Enterococcus
      faecalis*
    Vancomycin-intermediate-resistant *S. aureus*
    Aminoglycoside-resistant staphylococci and streptococci can
      interfere with the efficacy of antibiotic-loaded cements
    Gram-negative bacillary *strain-specific* antibiotic resistance

Technical pearls
1. Any factor or event that delays wound healing increases the risk of infection. Ischemic necrosis, infected wound hematomas, superficial wound infections, and suture abscesses are common events preceding joint replacement sepsis.
2. Anaerobes represent 10% of culture-proven pathogens in prosthetic joint infection. The frequency of anaerobic involvement is likely understated due to anaerobes' fastidious growth requirements. Recovery of anaerobes from infected tissues can be substantially increased by placing the specimen directly and immediately into a prereduced incubation medium such as thioglycollate broth.
3. In those difficult clinical situations in which antibiotic therapy is designed empirically, because of a high suspicion of prosthetic joint infection in the absence of positive cultures, strong consideration should be given to include an antianaerobic agent in the therapeutic regimen.
4. Usually, the clinical history, physical examination, x-rays, and radioisotopic scans have inadequate specificity. Therefore, the single observation that delineates the presence of implant infection is isolation of the pathogen by arthrocentesis or surgical débridement.
5. If initial cultures of prosthetic joint fluid reveal a relatively avirulent organism (coagulase-negative staphylococci, corynebacteria, propionibacteria, or *Bacillus* species), a second aspirate should be considered to confirm that the isolate is the pathogen and not a contaminant artifact.
6. Operative cultures are usually definitively diagnostic of prosthetic joint infection. Multiple specimens (five to seven) of tissue and fluids should be submitted for culture. Samples of purulence, abnormal tissue, and fluid are preferable to swabs for cultivation.
7. In designing therapy for an infected knee prosthesis, consider *not inserting a spacer* if the pathogen is not sufficiently susceptible to the antibiotics that leach adequately from polymethylmethacrylate spacers (tobramycin, gentamicin, or vancomycin combined with tobramycin or gentamicin). A cement spacer that is not releasing antibiotics effective against the microorganisms present at the infected site may allow organisms to persist on its surface and result in a failure to eradicate the infection.

bacilli that are far more readily eradicated than specific strains of Gram-positive cocci (e.g., methicillin-resistant *S. aureus*, methicillin-resistant *S. epidermidis*, and vancomycin-resistant strains of *E. faecalis*).

Our ability to control and eliminate specific pathogens is uncertain as antibiotic resistance continues to increase. The present problems we encounter with routine and nosocomial

bacteria may be dwarfed by the recent reemergence of multi-drug-resistant *M. tuberculosis* (22). Infection has often plagued the development of novel biotechnologic advances, including total joint arthroplasty. Innovative solutions to these clinical problems will require continued collaboration among clinicians and researchers from the different disciplines of orthopedics, bioengineering, and infectious disease.

PROPHYLACTIC USE OF ANTIBIOTICS

Perioperative antibiotic prophylaxis has been shown to reduce deep wound infection effectively in total joint replacement surgery (Table 5) (45). Oxacillin and cefazolin are commonly administered as antistaphylococcal agents immediately before implantation and for 24 hours thereafter. Vancomycin is an appropriate antimicrobial in those patients allergic to penicillins and cephalosporins. The duration of prophylactic antibiotic administration postoperatively has steadily decreased over the past two decades. Presently, prophylaxis is justifiable for 24 hours after surgery, but as more data accumulate in this regard, even shorter courses may become standard (46,47).

In patients with indwelling joint prostheses, early recognition and treatment of infection in any location are critical to decrease the risk of seeding the implant hematogenously. Circumstances likely to cause bacteremia should be avoided. Prophylactic antibiotic administration in anticipation of bacteremic events (e.g., dental surgery, cystoscopy, surgical procedures on infected or contaminated tissues) has been suggested on the same empiric basis on which endocarditis prophylaxis is recommended (3,20,48–50). This approach to prevention is controversial at the present time, and no data are available with which to determine the adequacy or cost-effectiveness of such measures. The American Dental Association and the American Academy of Orthopaedic Surgeons have jointly advised that a single dose of prophylactic antibiotic be given to selected patients undergoing dental procedures associated with significant bleeding (including periodontal scaling) (51). The selected populations include patients with inflammatory arthropathies, immunosuppression, diabetes mellitus, malnutrition, hemophilia, or previous prosthetic joint infection and all others undergoing these dental procedures within 2 years after joint implantation.

Prophylactic antibiotics may be advisable for other events (e.g., certain gastrointestinal or genitourinary tract procedures, surgery in an infected area) with a high risk of bacteremia and possibly in selected patients at high risk for infection (52). Clinical decisions regarding prophylactic antibiotics for expected bacteremias in patients with prosthetic joints should be made on an individual basis.

REFERENCES

1. Brause BD. Infected orthopedic prostheses. In: Bisno AL, Waldvogel FA, eds. *Infections associated with indwelling medical devices.* Washington, DC: American Society for Microbiology, 1989:111–127.
2. Lindqvist C, Slatis P. Dental bacteremia—a neglected cause of arthroplasty infections? *Acta Orthop Scand* 1985;56:506–508.
3. Maderazo EG, Judson S, Pasternak H. Late infections of total joint prostheses: a review and recommendations for prevention. *Clin Orthop* 1988;229:131–142.
4. Ahlberg A, Carlsson AS, Lindberg L. Hematogenous infection in total joint replacement. *Clin Orthop* 1978;137:69–75.
5. Inman JN, Gallegos KV, Brause BD, et al. Clinical and microbial features of prosthetic joint infection. *Am J Med* 1984;77:47–53.
6. Davies IM, Leak AM, Dave J. Infection of a prosthetic knee joint with Peptococcus magnus. *Ann Rheum Dis* 1988;47:866–868.
7. Darouiche RO, Hamill RJ, Musher DM, et al. Periprosthetic candidal infections following arthroplasty. *Rev Infect Dis* 1989;11:89–96.
8. Evans RP, Nelson CL. Staged reimplantation of a total hip prosthesis after infection with Candida albicans: a report of two cases. *J Bone Joint Surg Am* 1990;72:1551–1553.
9. Koch AE. *Candida albicans* infection of a prosthetic knee replacement. *J Rheumatol* 1988;15:362–365.
10. Lambertus M, Throdarson D, Goetz MB. Fungal prosthetic arthritis: presentation of two cases and review of the literature. *Rev Infect Dis* 1988;10:1038–1043.
11. Levine M, Rehm SJ, Wilde AH. Infection with *Candida albicans* of a total knee arthroplasty: a case report and review of the literature. *Clin Orthop* 1988;226:235–239.
12. Simonian PT, Brause BD, Wickiewicz TL. *Candida* infection after total knee arthroplasty. Management without resection or amphotericin B. *J Arthroplasty* 1997;12:825–829.
13. Baldini N, Toni A, Gregg I, Giunta A. Deep sepsis from *Mycobacterium tuberculosis* after total hip replacement. *Arch Orthop Trauma Surg* 1988;107:186–188.
14. Eskola A, Santavirta S, Konttinen YT, et al. Cementless total replacement for old tuberculosis of the hip. *J Bone Joint Surg Br* 1988;70:603–606.
15. Eskola A, Santavirta S, Konttinen YT, et al. Arthroplasty for old tuberculosis of the knee. *J Bone Joint Surg Br* 1988;70:767–769.
16. Kim YY, Ko CU, Ahn JY, et al. Charnley low friction arthroplasty in tuberculosis of the hip—an 8 year to 13 year follow-up. *J Bone Joint Surg Br* 1988;70:756–760.
17. Laforgia R, Murphy JCM, Redfern TR. Low friction arthroplasty for old quiescent (Tb) infection of the hip. *J Bone Joint Surg Br* 1988;70:373–376.
18. Santavirta S, Eskola A, Konttinen YT, et al. Total hip replacement in old tuberculosis: a report of 14 cases. *Acta Orthop Scand* 1988;59:391–395.
19. Kim YH, Han DY, Park BM. Total hip arthroplasty for tuberculous coxarthrosis. *J Bone Joint Surg Am* 1987;69:718–727.
20. Brause BD. Prosthetic joint infections. *Curr Opin Rheumatol* 1989;1:194–198.
21. Kim YH. Total knee arthroplasty for tuberculous arthritis. *J Bone Joint Surg Am* 1988;70:1322–1330.
22. Barnes PF, Barrows SA. Tuberculosis in the 1990s. *Ann Intern Med* 1993;119:400–410.
23. Eftehar NS. Wound infection complicating total hip joint arthroplasty. *Orthop Rev* 1979;8:49–64.
24. O'Neill DA, Harris WH. Failed total hip replacement: assessment by plain radiographs, arthrograms and aspiration of the hip joint. *J Bone Joint Surg Am* 1984;66:540–546.
25. Trippel SB. Antibiotic impregnated cement in total joint arthroplasty. *J Bone Joint Surg Am* 1986;68:1297–1302.
26. Brien WW, Salvati EA, Klein R, et al. Antibiotic impregnated bone cement in total hip arthroplasty, an in vivo comparison of the elution properties of tobramycin and vancomycin. *Clin Orthop* 1993;296:242–248.
27. Masri BA, Duncan CP, Beauchamp CP. Long-term elution of antibiotics from bone cement: an in vivo study using the prosthesis of antibiotic-loaded acrylic cement (PROSTALAC) system. *J Arthroplasty* 1998;13:331–338.
28. Gonzalez Della Valle AG, Bostrom M, Brause B, et al. Effective bactericidal activity of tobramycin and vancomycin eluted from acrylic bone cement. *Acta Orthop Scand* 2001;72:237–240.
29. Callaghan JJ, Salvati EA, Brause BD, et al. Reimplantation for salvage of the infected hip: rationale for the use of gentamicin-impregnated cement and beads. In: *The hip: proceedings of the 13th open scientific meetings of The Hip Society.* St. Louis: CV Mosby, 1986:65–94.
30. Salvati EA, Chekofsky KM, Brause BD, et al. Reimplantation in infection: a 12 year experience. *Clin Orthop* 1982;170:62–75.
31. Windsor RE, Insall JN, Urs WK, et al. Two-stage reimplantation for the salvage of total knee arthroplasty complicated by infection. *J Bone Joint Surg Am* 1990;72:272–278.
32. Costerton JW, Irvin RT, Cheng K-J. The bacterial glycocalyx in nature and disease. *Annu Rev Microbiol* 1981;35:299–324.
33. Gristina AG, Kolkin J. Total joint replacement and sepsis. *J Bone Joint Surg Am* 1983;65:128–134.
34. Dix BA, Cohen PS, Laux DC, et al. Radiochemical method for evaluating the effect of antibiotics on *Escherichia coli* biofilms. *Antimicrob Agents Chemother* 1988;32:770–772.
35. Farber BF, Kaplan MH, Clogston AG. *Staphylococcus epidermidis* extracted slime inhibits the antimicrobial action of glycopeptide antibiotics. *J Infect Dis* 1990;161:37–40.

36. Prosser BL, Taylor D, Dix BA, et al. Method of evaluating effects of antibiotics on bacterial biofilm. *Antimicrob Agents Chemother* 1987;31:1502–1506.

37. Gristina AG, Jennings RA, Naylor PT, et al. Comparative in vitro antibiotic resistance of surface-colonizing coagulase-negative staphylococci. *Antimicrob Agents Chemother* 1989;33:813–816.

38. Zimmerli W, Widmer AF, Blatter M, et al. Role of rifampin for treatment of orthopedic implant-related staphylococcal infections. *JAMA* 1998;279:1537–1541.

39. Brandt CM, Sistrunk WW, Duffy MC, et al. *Staphylococcus aureus* prosthetic joint infection treated with debridement and prosthesis retention. *Clin Infect Dis* 1997;24:914–919.

40. Ayers DC, Dennis DA, Johanson NA, et al. Common complications of total knee arthroplasty. *J Bone Joint Surg Am* 1997;79:278–311.

41. Goetz MB, Mulligan ME, Kwok R, et al. Management and epidemiologic analyses of an outbreak due to methicillin-resistant *Staphylococcus aureus*. *Am J Med* 1992;92:607–614.

42. Shales DM, Bouvet A, Shales JH, et al. Inducible, transferable resistance to vancomycin in *Enterococcus faecalis* A256. *Antimicrob Agents Chemother* 1989;33:198–203.

43. Whitman MS, Pitsakis PG, Zausner A, et al. Antibiotic treatment of experimental endocarditis due to vancomycin- and ampicillin-resistant *Enterococcus faecium*. *Antimicrob Agents Chemother* 1993;37:2069–2073.

44. Montecalvo MA, Horowitz H, Gedris C, et al. Outbreak of vancomycin-, ampicillin-, aminoglycoside-resistant *Enterococcus faecium* bacteremia in an adult oncology unit. *Antimicrob Agents Chemother* 1994;38:1363–1367.

45. Norden C. A critical review of antibiotic prophylaxis in orthopedic surgery. *Rev Infect Dis* 1983;5:928–932.

46. Heydemann JS, Nelson CL. Short-term preventive antibiotics. *Clin Orthop* 1986;205:184–187.

47. Page CP, Bohnen JMA, Fletcher JR, et al. Antimicrobial prophylaxis for surgical wounds: guidelines for clinical care. *Arch Surg* 1993;128:79–88.

48. Brause BD. Infectious disease perspectives on musculoskeletal sepsis. In: Esterhai JL Jr, Gristina AG, Poss R, eds. *Musculoskeletal infection.* Park Ridge, IL: American Academy of Orthopaedic Surgeons, 1992:35–48.

49. Cioffi GA, Terezhalmy GT, Taybos GM. Total joint replacement: a consideration for antimicrobial prophylaxis. *Oral Surg Oral Med Oral Pathol* 1988;66:124–129.

50. Hanssen AD, Osmon DR, Nelson CL. Prevention of deep periprosthetic joint infection. *J Bone Joint Surg Am* 1996;78:458–471.

51. Advisory statement. Antibiotic prophylaxis for dental patients with total joint replacements. American Dental Association; American Academy of Orthopaedic Surgeons. *J Am Dental Assoc* 1997;128:1004–1008.

52. Abramowicz M. Antimicrobial prophylaxis in surgery. *Med Lett* 1995;41:75–79.

CHAPTER 113

Retention

Kevin L. Garvin and Joshua A. Urban

Total knee arthroplasty (TKA) continues to be successful in alleviating the painful arthritic joint and restoring function of the knee. This procedure has resulted in high levels of patient satisfaction, which, when coupled with the excellent longevity reported for it, has made TKA one of the most successful orthopedic interventions to date. Crucial to the success of TKA is the avoidance of periprosthetic infection, which continues to be the most dreaded complication of this procedure (1,2). Although successful eradication of the infection can be achieved in a majority of cases, the functional outcome is commonly inferior to that of uncomplicated primary TKA (3–5). In a patient population that is generally older and that commonly has comorbid medical conditions, the multiple extensive surgeries and prolonged hospitalization that are often required for treatment also increase the morbidity and mortality of this complication (6–9). Fortunately, with the enlistment of prophylactic techniques, the rate of infection after TKA has decreased from early rates as high as 15% (10) to the current incidence of 1% to 2%.

The primary goals in the treatment of TKA infections are the relief of pain, maintenance of a functional lower extremity, and eradication of the infection. Meeting these goals requires a prolonged antibiotic regimen combined with surgical intervention. The various surgical techniques that have been proposed in the treatment of periprosthetic infections of the knee include: (a) retention, (b) one-stage reimplantation, (c) two-stage reimplantation, (d) arthrodesis, and (e) amputation. Currently, two-stage reimplantation is the most consistently successful surgical option, as success rates as high as 77% to 100% have been frequently reported (11–19). The two-stage reimplantation technique involves resection of all components at an initial surgical setting, followed by an interval during which parenteral antibiotics are administered, and finally a second surgical procedure to reimplant new components if the infection has been eradicated. Despite the high success rates using the two-stage technique, it has been associated with several complications, including

extensor lag (20), late rupture of the extensor mechanism (9,21), and loss of bone stock (18).

Retention of the prosthetic components offers an attractive alternative to two-stage reimplantation. With retention, the surgical procedures are less extensive as bone stock is preserved. Furthermore, the prolonged interval between surgeries in the two-stage technique that is characterized by a resection arthroplasty is avoided. This interval, during which the ipsilateral lower extremity is minimally functional, may contribute to the decreased functional results seen with two-stage reimplantation TKAs in comparison with primary TKAs (4,6,9,20).

Retention of the components can be achieved by any of the following methods: (a) open irrigation and débridement, (b) arthroscopic débridement, (c) use of long-term suppressive antibiotics only, and (d) multiple aspirations and antibiotic administration (Table 1). Although acceptable success rates have been achieved with the use of some of these techniques, predictable results are less common than with two-stage reimplantation. Adherence to the strict indications listed below optimizes the chance for success when these retention techniques are used.

OPEN IRRIGATION AND DÉBRIDEMENT

Open irrigation and débridement are the most commonly reported methods of component retention. This technique consists of an open arthrotomy, usually through the previous arthroplasty incision, with complete synovectomy and copious irrigation of the joint. The débridement of all infected tissue must be meticulous and thorough. Parenteral antibiotics do not compensate for inadequate surgical technique. The modular prosthetic components that can be removed (polyethylene tibial liner) without violating the bone-cement, cement-prosthesis, or bone-prosthesis interfaces are exchanged (Fig. 1).

TABLE 1. *Treatment methods and indications in periprosthetic knee infections*

Treatment	Success rate (%)	Indications	Comments
Open débridement and retention[a]	60–83	Duration of infection <2–4 wk. Antibiotic-susceptible, low-virulence organism. Absence of prolonged drainage or sinus tract. Well-fixed components. Absence of osteolysis.	Most consistently effective retention technique. Low success rates if indications not followed. Polyethylene insert should be exchanged.
Arthroscopic débridement and retention[b]	16–38	Patient's medical condition precludes open débridement.	Very few reports in the literature. Less effective than open débridement and retention. Difficult to perform a complete synovectomy. Unable to débride between the tibial tray and polyethylene.
Long-term suppressive antibiotics	21–45	Patient's medical condition precludes any surgical procedure. Patient refuses further surgery. Antibiotic-susceptible, low-virulence organism. Oral antibiotics must be effective with minimal side effects.	Will not eradicate the infection. Potential complication of emergence of resistant bacteria.
Multiple aspirations	10–15	Same as for long-term suppressive antibiotics.	Very few reports in the literature. Least invasive of the surgical retention techniques.

[a]Studies adhering to the indications.
[b]Does not include case reports or smaller series.

Historically, treatment with retention of the prosthetic components has been, at best, controversial, as several studies reported low rates of success using this technique. Woods et al. (22) reported the successful treatment of only 3 of 27 infected knees (11%) after TKA. In patients followed for a mean of 4 years, Burger et al. (23) reported a 17.9% success rate, as 7 of 39 periprosthetic knee infections were eradicated. In a multicenter study, Bengston and Knutson (6) reported success in 37 of 154 infected TKA cases (24%). When the results of multiple series in the literature are combined, 110 of 377 knees (29%) were successfully treated (24).

A closer evaluation of these reports reveals subgroups of patients who can, in fact, be treated with prosthesis retention and still achieve consistently high success rates. It has been shown that the most important factor influencing successful treatment with this technique is the duration of infection before treatment (7,21,25,26). An upper limit of 2 to 4 weeks has been suggested based on several reports that show improved success rates in patients treated with open irrigation and débridement with retention within this time period. It is difficult, however, to determine accurately the onset of infection and, therefore, its duration, unless it is in the early postoperative period. In these cases, it is assumed that the infection occurred at the time of index arthroplasty or shortly thereafter, and as a result, the time from index arthroplasty becomes the "duration of infection."

Several studies have examined the effectiveness of open débridement and retention in the treatment of acute infections with duration defined by the time from index arthroplasty. Borden and Gearen (25) successfully treated five of six knees (83%) that underwent open débridement and retention for infection that developed within 2 weeks of the index TKA. For the five knees that had chronic symptoms (longer than 2 weeks), retention treatment failed in all five knees. Teeny et al. (21) successfully treated three of five cases (60%) that became infected

within 2 weeks of the index TKA, but only 3 of 16 (19%) infected longer than 2 weeks after the index TKA.

Those TKA infections that do not occur in the postoperative period but rather become apparent months to years after the index arthroplasty often present a challenge in determining when the infection actually began. These acute hematogenous infections occasionally can be linked to a bacteremic event that preceded the onset of symptoms. In other cases of acute hematogenous infection, no source of the infection can be identified (3,7,27). In these instances, the duration of symptoms is used as an objective method to quantify the duration of infection.

Several studies have reported results with the use of open débridement and retention in acute TKA infections as defined by the duration of symptoms. Wasielewski et al. (26) reported successful treatment of TKA infections symptomatic for less than 2 weeks in six of eight (75%) cases. In TKA infections of more than 2 weeks in duration, only one of two cases (50%) was successfully treated. Likewise, Hartman et al. (7), in their overall group of 33 TKA infections, achieved success in only 13 cases (39%). However, in the subgroup of patients who were treated within 4 weeks of developing symptoms, 7 of 11 TKA infections (64%) were successfully treated.

Using the duration of symptoms as an indicator of the duration of infection can be problematic, as it is difficult to determine whether the development of symptoms results from an acute infection that has just established itself or from a subacute indolent infection that has just become symptomatic despite being present for several weeks to months. Higher success rates with shorter duration of symptoms would be expected in the former, but not the latter. In a group of 33 TKA infections treated by open débridement and retention, Hartman et al. (7) reported success in 13 knees (39%). No correlation was found between successful eradication of the infection and the duration of symptoms. The majority of knees (30 of 33 knees, 91%) had

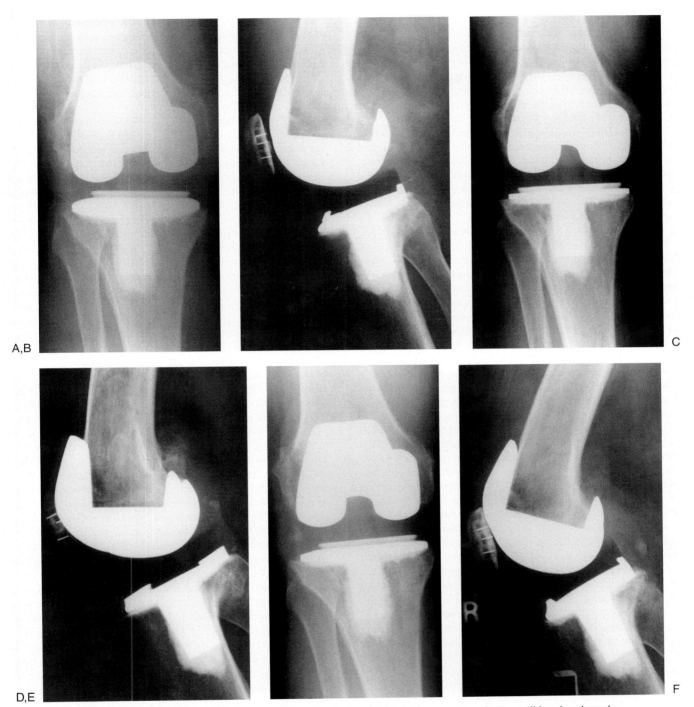

FIG. 1. A 76-year-old man was doing very well after a right total knee arthroplasty until he developed a sudden onset of right knee pain with erythema and swelling. Examination of knee aspirate revealed a highly antibiotic-susceptible group G *Streptococcus*. **A, B:** Radiographs of right knee immediately after the index arthroplasty. **C, D:** Radiographs taken within 48 hours of development of symptoms demonstrate the absence of progressive radiolucent lines, loosening, and osteolysis. The patient underwent open irrigation and débridement with polyethylene exchange and retention of the metallic components. **E, F:** Postoperative radiographs taken 4 years after open débridement showing no radiographic evidence of infection.

been symptomatic for less than 4 weeks. In the 13 treatment successes, the average duration of symptoms was 18.6 days, whereas in the treatment failures, the average duration of symptoms was 10.5 days. Instead of duration of symptoms, a correlation was found between successful treatment and time from index TKA. Successful eradication occurred in 7 of 11 TKA cases (64%) treated with open débridement and retention less than 4 weeks after the index arthroplasty. In contrast, only 6 of 22 TKA infections were successfully treated more than 4 weeks from the index surgery. The findings of Mont et al. (3) support the results reported by Hartman and coworkers. In their report, ten of ten postoperative infections (100%) occurring less than 4 weeks from the index arthroplasty were successfully treated. In contrast, 10 of 14 acute hematogenous infections (71%) were successfully treated.

The increased efficacy of open débridement and retention performed within a short time after the onset of infection has been linked to the ability of certain microorganisms to produce a biofilm or glycocalyx (28). The glycocalyx is a polysaccharide film synthesized by certain bacteria that envelops and sequesters the bacteria from host defenses and antibiotics and thereby prevents the eradication of the infection. It has been postulated that the success of component retention early in the course of the infection is due to the relatively short time that the infecting bacteria have to establish this glycocalyx. In the absence of a glycocalyx, mechanical débridement and antibiotic treatment are more effective at eradicating the offending organisms. The longer an infection has been present, the greater the possibility of glycocalyx formation and the more formidable the task of eradicating the bacteria.

In addition to the timing of treatment, other factors have been identified that also predict success with retention of the prosthetic components (23): (a) infection with an antibiotic-susceptible, low-virulence organism, (b) absence of a sinus tract or drainage, (c) absence of radiographic or intraoperative evidence of component loosening, and (d) absence of radiographic evidence of infection (signs of osteolysis or osteomyelitis).

Infection with an antibiotic-susceptible organism of low virulence increases the likelihood that treatment with retention of the components will succeed (19,23,29). Burger et al. (23) reported on 5 of 39 (13%) TKA infections successfully treated with open débridement and retention. In all five successes, the offending organism was an antibiotic-sensitive Gram-positive bacterium, whereas in 47% of the failures the infectious agent was a Gram-negative or antibiotic-resistant bacterium. In this age of increasing antibiotic resistance (30), the number of periprosthetic knee infections meeting the prerequisite of infection by antibiotic-sensitive organisms may diminish in the future.

A history of prolonged drainage or the presence of a sinus tract is indicative of a compromised soft-tissue envelope about the knee and is a contraindication to open débridement with retention of the components. In this setting, retention of the components has a high likelihood of failure. Burger et al. (23), in their report of 39 TKA infections, reported successful treatment in five cases (13%) using open débridement and retention alone. In none of these five cases was there a history of prolonged postoperative drainage (longer than 2 weeks). In the remaining 34 treatment failures, however, 24 knees (71%) had a history of prolonged drainage, difficulty with primary wound healing, or the development of a sinus tract.

The absence of both progressive radiolucent lines and intraoperative evidence of component loosening are also prerequisites

for treatment by component retention. Borden and Gearen (25) identified progressive radiolucent lines in 4 of 21 knees infected after TKA. In each case, retention of the components failed. Loosening of prosthetic components may expose the deep interfaces to the infecting organism. This renders débridement and retention ineffective, as this technique is incapable of reaching these interfaces. If loosening is present, and the patient can survive the procedure, two-stage reimplantation should be performed.

The presence of osteomyelitis is a contraindication to débridement and retention as it has been shown to result in high failure rates. This phenomenon is generally either manifested by periprosthetic osteolysis apparent radiographically or identified by pathologic inspection of specimens obtained at the time of surgery. Osteomyelitis associated with a periprosthetic infection indicates an infectious process of increased duration and involvement that requires extensive bony débridement for eradication. Mont et al. (3) reported successful treatment in 20 of 24 TKA infections (83%) with the use of débridement and retention. In all four cases in which treatment failed, chronic osteomyelitis was identified after surgery during pathologic inspection. Kramhoft et al. (8) reported successful eradication of 4 of 27 TKA infections (15%) with open débridement and retention. No radiographic evidence of osteomyelitis was present in the four successfully treated knees, whereas osteomyelitis was present in 12 of the 23 knees for which treatment failed (52%). Likewise, of the 5 of 39 successfully treated TKA infections reported by Burger et al. (23), none showed radiographic evidence of infection; however, 14 of the 34 knees (41%) in which treatment failed did show such evidence.

Although not as critical as the aforementioned criteria, additional factors that may influence the success of treatment are the age of the patient at the time of treatment and the type of prosthesis that is involved in the TKA infection. Schoifet and Morrey (19), in their experience with 31 TKA infections, were able to achieve success with prosthetic retention in seven knees. The average age for these patients was 50 years, compared with an average age of 62 years for the 24 cases in which open débridement and retention was ineffective (p <.01). Additional studies have supported this correlation (31,32), whereas others have refuted it (7,29).

The presence of an infection about a highly constrained prosthesis has also been linked to increased failure rates with open débridement and retention (8,19,23). The sheer bulk of foreign material associated with highly constrained prostheses may decrease the chance for eradication. As a result, resection arthroplasty with or without eventual reimplantation may be the treatment of choice in these cases. Other authors have found no association between the use of infected hinged prostheses and higher failure rates when infection is treated with open débridement and retention (29).

In addition to strict adherence to the aforementioned criteria, repeated open débridements may be necessary to optimize the chance of success when using this retention technique. Multiple débridements serve to decrease the infectious load and thereby increase the effectiveness of the concomitant antibiotic regimen. In the study by Mont et al. (3), which reported the highest success rate using open débridement and retention, 20 of 24 TKA infections (83%) were treated successfully using this method. In ten of these successfully treated knees, repeat open irrigation and débridement was necessary. If the investigators had stopped after only one procedure, success would have been achieved in only 10 of 24 cases

(41%). Surgeons are therefore cautioned not to abandon this retention technique if failure occurs after the initial débridement. As long as the aforementioned criteria are still observed, repeated open irrigation and débridement has a significant chance of success.

It is controversial whether the failure of open débridement and retention compromises the results of subsequent treatment methods. Teeny et al. were able to successfully treat all of seven TKA infections with two-stage reimplantation after the initial treatment with débridement and retention had failed (21). Likewise, other authors (3,7,26) have reported successful salvage of failed open irrigation and débridement with arthrodesis or two-stage reimplantation. To the contrary, yet other authors have found that failure of open débridement and retention has led to inferior results with subsequent treatment modalities, including two-stage reimplantation (23).

ARTHROSCOPIC IRRIGATION AND DÉBRIDEMENT

In the technique of arthroscopic irrigation and débridement, arthroscopic portals are made at the knee to facilitate inspection and irrigation of the joint (using at least 10 L) with the débridement of all infected and necrotic tissue. As complete a synovectomy as the arthroscopic technique affords should be attempted. All the prosthetic components are left *in situ*. The advantages of this technique include its minimal invasiveness and decreased likelihood of significant functional loss from arthrotomy (33).

Treatment of periprosthetic knee infections by arthroscopic irrigation and débridement has been infrequently reported in the literature. In the largest series to date, Waldman et al. (27) reviewed their experience with this technique in the treatment of 16 TKA infections at a mean follow-up of 64 months. Only 6 of 16 (38%) of these periprosthetic knee infections were eradicated. All 16 patients in this study had fewer than 28 days of symptoms before diagnosis and treatment. It also seems that repeated arthroscopic débridement is less effective than repeated open débridement, as only one of seven patients (14%) who underwent a repeat arthroscopic irrigation and débridement was successfully treated. This is in sharp contrast to the report by Mont et al. (3) in which repeated *open* irrigation and débridement procedures with prosthesis retention resulted in success in 10 of 12 TKA infections.

The remainder of the studies of arthroscopic treatment for TKA infections consists of case reports or small numbers of patients in larger series of infection cases (26,33,34). Flood and Kolarik (33) reported successful treatment in two of two TKA infections using this technique. In each case, the patient presented within 24 hours of the onset of symptoms, an antibiotic-sensitive infecting organism was present, and there were no radiographic signs of loosening or infection. Grogan et al. (34), reporting on a total of 14 TKA infections, documented successful treatment in two of three cases (67%) in which the arthroscopic retention technique was used. Wasielewski et al. (26), describing a series of 76 TKA infections, reported a successful outcome in the only case treated using the arthroscopic technique.

In summary, the limited reports to date have shown that the arthroscopic method is an inferior retention technique compared to open débridement. The disadvantages of this technique compared to open débridement and retention include the inability to perform a complete synovectomy and to exchange the polyethylene tibial component. Modular polyethylene exchange affords exposure of the posterior aspect of the joint as well as the space between the metal tibial tray and the polyethylene—areas in which residual bacteria could be sequestered from arthroscopic techniques. It is recommended that this technique be reserved for those cases in which the medical condition of the patient dictates a less invasive approach (i.e., patients with a coagulopathy). Patients who are medically ill might be better served with arthroscopy rather than waiting the extra time necessary for medical improvement.

LONG-TERM ANTIBIOTIC SUPPRESSION

Long-term antibiotic treatment without surgical intervention has been used to treat TKA infection. The goal of this technique is to inhibit the growth and proliferation of the offending bacteria, as antibiotic treatment alone will not completely eradicate the infection. Long-term antibiotic suppression is most commonly used when the patient's medical condition precludes further surgery, or when the patient refuses further surgical intervention. The offending organism must be identified and must be sensitive to oral antibiotics with minimal side effects (35). A potential complication of this prolonged antibiotic treatment is the emergence of resistant organisms.

The success rates reported with chronic suppressive antibiotic therapy have been disappointing. In a Swedish multicenter study (6), antibiotic suppression was successful in 47 of 225 cases (21%) of periprosthetic infection. If the experiences of several other studies using this method are combined (11,20,22,29,34,36), successful eradication is seen to have occurred in only 37 of 83 cases (45%). As a result of these poor success rates, the use of antibiotic suppression is recommended only if the aforementioned criteria are met (Table 1).

Some have proposed that the treatment of periprosthetic knee infections with use of long-term suppressive antibiotics may compromise later surgical treatment (37). Other authors, however, have not encountered any deleterious effect of a period of prolonged systemic antibiotic therapy on subsequent surgical treatment (6).

MULTIPLE ASPIRATIONS

As its name implies, the technique of multiple aspirations involves repeated attempts at withdrawing aspirate from the infected periprosthetic knee environment. The goal is to decrease the bacterial load enough to optimize the bactericidal activity of intravenously administered antibiotics, whose use must always accompany this technique. Reports of the use of this technique are uncommon, and eradication rates using aspiration have been low, often around 10% to 15% (38). Aspiration probably is best considered as a form of suppression, as it is relatively ineffective at irrigating the joint and does not provide the opportunity for synovectomy. The indications for use of this technique are similar to those cited for the use of long-term suppressive antibiotics earlier.

CONCLUSION

In the treatment of TKA infections, component retention and successful outcomes are not mutually exclusive (Table 2).

TABLE 2. *Highlight points and technical pearls*

Highlight points

Of the reported retention techniques, open irrigation and débridement with polyethylene exchange (if possible) and metallic component retention has been the most successful.

Strict adherence to recommended indications is essential to optimize the chances of successful eradication of periprosthetic knee infections with the use of retention techniques.

Open débridement with retention as a treatment for periprosthetic knee infections should be considered only if the following indications are met:

> The infection is <2–4 wk in duration.
> The infecting organism is of low virulence.
> There is no sinus tract or wound drainage.
> The components are well-fixed.
> No radiographic evidence of infection is seen.

Arthroscopic débridement and retention is inferior to open retention techniques due to its inability to ensure a complete synovectomy or to allow exchange of the polyethylene tibial component. Its use should be limited to cases in which the medical condition of the patient dictates a less invasive approach.

Long-term antibiotic suppression has demonstrated poor success rates. This technique should be considered only in patients who refuse surgery or are too medically unstable for the use of any surgical technique. The bacterium must be identified and must be sensitive to oral antibiotics with minimal side effects.

Multiple aspirations are best considered as a form of long-term antibiotic suppression and should be used as the primary treatment only when the criteria for use of suppressive antibiotics are met.

Technical pearls

As long as the aforementioned indications still exist, repeated open débridement and retention retains a high degree of success after failure of the initial retention procedure.

Although no agreement exists in the literature, several reports have shown no compromise of the final result in cases in which retention efforts fail and the patient undergoes two-stage reimplantation.

Infections occurring in the early postoperative period may be more amenable to treatment with open débridement and retention than infections that occur months to years after the index arthroplasty.

Although retention techniques are of limited application, retention of the components preserve bone stock and may result in an improved functional outcome in comparison to what is currently considered the gold standard in the treatment of TKA infections—two-stage reimplantation. The most successful of the retention techniques is open irrigation and débridement in which a thorough synovectomy is performed, with the removal of all necrotic and infected tissue and the exchange of the modular polyethylene component (if possible). Although the overall results of all of the retention techniques have historically been poor, if specific criteria are adhered to, success rates as high as 83% can be achieved with use of the open débridement method. Chief among these criteria is short duration of infection before treatment. An upper limit of 2 to 4 weeks has been suggested based on improved success rates when the technique is used within this time period. Less favorable results have been reported for this technique if the infection has been present for longer than 2 to 4 weeks. Early postoperative infections (infections that present within 4 weeks of the index TKA) appear to be more easily eradicated than acute hematogenous infections (infections that occur months to years after the index arthroplasty but have been symptomatic for fewer than 4 weeks).

In addition to short duration of infection, other recommended criteria for the use of open débridement and retention include (a) infection with an antibiotic-susceptible, low-virulence organism, (b) absence of a sinus tract or drainage, (3) absence of radiographic or intraoperative evidence of component loosening, and (d) absence of radiographic evidence of infection (signs of osteolysis or osteomyelitis). If all of these criteria are present, retention of the components with open irrigation and débridement can be highly successful.

The other retention techniques (arthroscopic débridement, long-term antibiotic suppression, multiple aspirations) have resulted in inferior eradication rates and should be used only in the patient who cannot withstand open débridement.

REFERENCES

1. Glynn MK, Sheehan JM. An analysis of the causes of deep infection after hip and knee arthroplasties. *Clin Orthop* 1983;178:202–206.
2. Stern SH, Insall JN. Total knee arthroplasty in obese patients. *J Bone Joint Surg Am* 1990;72:1400–1404.
3. Mont MA, Waldman B, Banerjee C, et al. Multiple irrigation, debridement, and retention of compartments in infected total knee arthroplasty. *J Arthroplasty* 1997;12:426–433.
4. Walker RH, Schurman DJ. Management of infected total knee arthroplasties. *Clin Orthop* 1984;186:81–89.
5. Windsor RE, Insall JN, Urs WK, et al. Two-stage reimplantation for the salvage of total knee arthroplasty complicated by infection: further follow-up and refinement of indications. *J Bone Joint Surg Am* 1990;72:272–278.
6. Bengston S, Knutson K. The infected knee arthroplasty: a six year follow-up of 357 cases. *Acta Orthop Scand* 1991;62:301–311.
7. Hartman MB, Fehring TK, Jordan L, et al. Periprosthetic knee sepsis: the role of irrigation and débridement. *Clin Orthop* 1991;273:113–118.
8. Kramhoft M, Bodtker S, Carlsen A. Outcome of infected total knee arthroplasty. *J Arthroplasty* 1994;9:617–621.
9. Rand JA, Bryan RS. Reimplantation for the salvage of an infected total knee arthroplasty. *J Bone Joint Surg Am* 1983;65:1081–1086.
10. Rand JA, Chao EYS, Stauffer RN. Kinematic rotating hinge total knee arthroplasty. *J Bone Joint Surg Am* 1987;69:489–497.
11. Bengston S, Knutson K, Lidgren L. Treatment of infected knee arthroplasty. *Clin Orthop* 1989;245:173–178.
12. Bliss DG, McBride GG. Infected total knee arthroplasties. *Clin Orthop* 1985;199:207–214.
13. Brodersen MP, Fitzgerald RH, Peterson LFA, et al. Arthrodesis of the knee following failed total knee arthroplasty. *J Bone Joint Surg Am* 1979;61:181–185.
14. Figgie HE, Brody GA, Inglis AE, et al. Knee arthrodesis following total knee arthroplasty in rheumatoid arthritis. *Clin Orthop* 1987;224:237–243.
15. Knutson K, Lindstrand A, Lidgren L. Arthrodesis for failed knee arthroplasty. *J Bone Joint Surg Br* 1985;67:47–52.
16. Nichols SJ, Landon GC, Tullos HS. Arthrodesis with dual plates after total knee arthroplasty. *J Bone Joint Surg Am* 1991;73:1020–1024.
17. Rand JA, Bryan RS, Chao EYS. Failed total knee arthroplasty treated by arthrodesis of the knee using the Ace-Fischer apparatus. *J Bone Joint Surg Am* 1987;69:39–45.
18. Rand JA, Bryan RS, Morrey BF, et al. Management of infected total knee arthroplasty. *Clin Orthop* 1986;205:75–85.
19. Schoifet SD, Morrey BF. Persistent infection after successful arthrodesis for infected total knee arthroplasty. *J Arthroplasty* 1990;5:277–279.
20. Insall JN, Thompson FM, Brause BD. Two-stage reimplantation for

the salvage of infected total knee arthroplasty. *J Bone Joint Surg Am* 1983;65:1087–1098.

21. Teeny SM, Dorr L, Murata G, et al. Treatment of infected total knee arthroplasty. *J Arthroplasty* 1990;5:35–39.

22. Woods GW, Lionberger DR, Tullos HS. Failed total knee arthroplasty. *Clin Orthop* 1983;173:184–190.

23. Burger RR, Basch T, Hopson CN. Implant salvage in infected total knee arthroplasty. *Clin Orthop* 1991;273:105–112.

24. Rand JA. Alternatives to reimplantation for salvage of the total knee arthroplasty complicated by infection. *J Bone Joint Surg Am* 1993;75:282–289.

25. Borden LS, Gearen PF. Infected total knee arthroplasty: a protocol for management. *J Arthroplasty* 1987;2:27–36.

26. Wasielewski RC, Barden RM, Rosenberg AG. Results of different surgical procedures on total knee arthroplasty infections. *J Arthroplasty* 1996;11:931–938.

27. Waldman BJ, Hostin E, Mont MA, et al. Infected total knee arthroplasty treated by arthroscopic irrigation and débridement. *J Arthroplasty* 2000;15(4):430–436.

28. Gristina AG, Barth E, Webb LX. Microbial adhesion and the pathogenesis of biomaterial centered infections. In: Gustillo R, ed. *Orthopaedic infection, diagnosis and treatment.* Philadelphia: WB Saunders, 1989:3–25.

29. Wilson MG, Kelley K, Thornhill TS. Infection as a complication of total knee-replacement arthroplasty: risk factors and treatment in sixty-seven cases. *J Bone Joint Surg Am* 1990;72:878–883.

30. Garvin KL, Hinrichs SH, Urban JA. Emerging antibiotic-resistant bacteria. Their treatment in total joint arthroplasty. *Clin Orthop* 1999;369:110–123.

31. Hood RW, Insall JN. Infected total knee joint replacement arthroplasties. In: Evarts CM, ed. *Surgery of the musculoskeletal system.* New York: Churchill Livingstone, 1983:173–195.

32. Nelson CL. Prevention of sepsis. *Clin Orthop* 1987;222:66–72.

33. Flood JN, Kolarik, DB. Arthroscopic irrigation and débridement of infected total knee arthroplasty: report of two cases. *Arthroscopy* 1988;4(3):182–186.

34. Grogan TJ, Dorey F, Rollins J, et al. Deep sepsis following total knee arthroplasty: ten-year experience at the University of California at Los Angeles Medical Center. *J Bone Joint Surg Am* 1986;68:226–234.

35. Brause BD. Infected total knee replacement. *Orthop Clin North Am* 1982;13:245–249.

36. Johnson DP, Bannister GC. The outcome of infected arthroplasty of the knee. *J Bone Joint Surg Br* 1986;68:289–291.

37. Thornhill TS, Maguire JH. Infected total knee arthroplasty. In: Scoot WN, ed. *Total knee revision arthroplasty.* Orlando, FL: Grune and Stratton, 1987:79–98.

38. Mulvey TJ, Thornhill TS, Kelly MA, et al. Complications associated with total knee arthroplasty. In: Pellicci PM, Tria AJ, Garvin KL, et al., eds. *Orthopaedic knowledge update. Hip and knee reconstruction 2.* Rosemont, IL: American Academy of Orthopaedic Surgeons, 2000:323–329.

CHAPTER 114

Reimplantation for Infection after Total Knee Arthroplasty

Arlen D. Hanssen

Deep infection after knee arthroplasty remains one of the most dreaded complications of this highly successful surgical procedure. Fortunately the incidence of infection has decreased over the past several decades and improved treatment methods have enhanced clinical outcomes (1). It is important to remember that the treatment goals of the infected knee arthroplasty include successful eradication of infection, reduction of pain, and continuance of maximal patient function. Variables to be considered before initiating treatment are shown in Table 1 (2). Incorporation of these variables into an infection classification system also helps guide selection of the appropriate treatment approach (Table 2) (3).

The primary treatment decision to be made when evaluating these treatment variables and this classification system is whether or not removal of the prosthesis is required. Most situations require prosthesis removal to eradicate the infection (1). It is also likely that failed débridement attempts or delay of prosthesis removal adversely affects the eventual outcome of subsequent reimplantation efforts (2). In general, there are six basic options for treatment of an infected total knee arthroplasty, shown in Table 3 (2). Successful treatment requires careful assessment of treatment variables and skilled implementation of the appropriate treatment plan. Excluding long-term antibiotic suppression, which does not eliminate infection, the cornerstone of treatment in these options is a thorough surgical débridement combined with the appropriate use of antibiotics.

Clearly, reimplantation is the preferred treatment method for many patients. However, the opportunity for improved functional outcome with a new prosthesis must be balanced with the inherently higher risk of reinfection associated with reimplanta-

tion compared with other treatment alternatives such as arthrodesis. Generally accepted contraindications for reimplantation include the presence of persistent infection, medical conditions that prevent the use of multiple reconstructive procedures, extensor mechanism disruption, and poor soft tissue coverage of the knee joint (1).

The primary treatment controversies when the decision is to proceed with reimplantation include the proper duration of antibiotic therapy, use of direct-exchange techniques versus delayed reimplantation, use versus nonuse of antibiotic-loaded spacers or blocks, and method of prosthesis fixation used at reimplantation. This chapter addresses these controversies by outlining the treatment principles, describing aspects of the surgical technique, and discussing the reported clinical results of reimplantation for periprosthetic infection. The diagnosis of infection after knee arthroplasty and surgical treatment alternatives other than reimplantation are detailed elsewhere.

PREOPERATIVE SETTING

The expected activity requirements and the personal expectations of the patient regarding the different treatment approaches must be assessed and fully discussed. Patients and their families are often afraid or angry about the presence or causes of the infection, and treatment decision discussions are often prolonged and emotional. The treating physician must also assess whether his or her abilities and the available facilities provide the level of care necessary for a successful outcome. Success is most probable when the first treatment method is appropriately

TABLE 1. *Treatment variables determining treatment approach*

Depth of infection (superficial vs. deep)
Time interval between arthroplasty and diagnosis of infection
Host factors potentially affecting treatment adversely
Status of the soft tissue envelope, particularly the extensor mechanism
Status of implant fixation (loose or well fixed)
Identity of the pathogenic organism(s)
Physician's ability to provide the proper level of care
Patient expectations and functional requirements

selected and properly performed. Secondary treatment attempts are often affected adversely by progressive scarring, soft tissue devitalization, and continued bone loss (4). Patients with infected knees after revision arthroplasty have a poorer prognosis than those with infected knees after primary replacement (5). The final outcome of a reimplantation is highly correlated with the functional class of the patient as determined preoperatively (6). When possible, high-risk hosts with suppressed immune systems or malnourishment should undergo treatment to optimize physical status before surgery (1).

Evaluation should include documentation of range of motion, knee stability, neurovascular status, and status of the soft tissue envelope, particularly extensor mechanism integrity. Radiographic observation of staples or other fixation devices used for patellar tendon reattachment may suggest potential extensor mechanism difficulties. The soft tissues must be viable enough to permit several surgical procedures, and the presence of multiple prior incisions predisposes toward wound healing problems. When possible, the need for soft tissue coverage procedures should be anticipated at the initial evaluation, as these procedures are optimally performed at implant removal

TABLE 2. *Classification of deep periprosthetic infection*

Infection type	Characteristics	Treatment
I	Positive results on culture specimens obtained during revision surgery	Course of intravenous antibiotics followed by possible long-term oral antibiotic suppressive therapy
II	Early postoperative infection diagnosed within the first month after arthroplasty	Débridement with retention of prosthesis and antibiotic therapy
III	Acute hematogenous seeding of an otherwise well-functioning prosthesis	Débridement with retention of prosthesis and antibiotic therapy
IV	Chronic periprosthetic infection, including infections diagnosed more than 1 month after arthroplasty	Prosthesis removal and antibiotic therapy followed by selected treatment approach such as reimplantation

TABLE 3. *Treatment options for the infected total knee replacement*

Prosthesis retained
    Long-term suppressive therapy with antibiotics
    Débridement with prosthesis retention
Prosthesis removed
    Resection arthroplasty
    Arthrodesis
    Amputation
    Reinsertion of another prosthesis (reimplantation)

rather than at reimplantation. Performing soft tissue coverage procedures at reimplantation often delays efforts to proceed with aggressive range-of-motion exercises (7). If soft tissue coverage procedures are deemed necessary, the use of alternative salvage methods rather than reimplantation should be carefully considered.

Erythrocyte sedimentation rate and C-reactive protein levels are commonly used to monitor response to therapy, but their usefulness is not clearly defined (1). Many patients with a periprosthetic knee infection are anemic, and the vast majority require blood transfusions in the perioperative setting (8). Preoperative aspiration for culture and antibiotic sensitivity testing is extremely helpful to direct the initial postoperative antibiotic regimen until final culture results from specimens obtained at débridement are obtained (9). Cultures of sinus tract or wound drainage specimens are discouraged. To aid in identifying the microorganisms by culture and sensitivity testing, all antibiotics are discontinued for 10 to 14 days before aspiration or implant removal. If the patient has a history of systemic sepsis with discontinuation of antibiotics or has other joint replacements present, the time interval for discontinuation of antibiotics should be empirically shortened or discontinuance should be avoided, with recognition that culture testing may be adversely affected.

ADMINISTRATION OF ANTIBIOTICS

The optimal duration and route of antibiotic delivery for treatment of the infected knee after arthroplasty has not been clearly determined. Adherence to a 6-week course of intravenous antibiotic administration before reimplantation has provided excellent success rates, and this time frame represents the most commonly accepted clinical standard (10,11). It is important to note that there are no published trials that directly compare different durations of antibiotic treatment. In addition, most of the studies using the 6-week intravenous regimen did not routinely use adjunctive methods of antibiotic delivery such as antibiotic-impregnated cement spacers or antibiotic-impregnated cement for prosthesis fixation (10–12). The use of these adjunctive antibiotic delivery methods is discussed later in this chapter.

Excellent success rates with a shorter duration of intravenous antibiotic treatment have been reported, with good results in 10 of 11 patients after 3 weeks of antibiotic therapy (13). Others have administered intravenous antibiotics for an average of 4.2 weeks (14). It is important to note that antibiotic-impregnated cement was used for prosthesis fixation at the time of reimplantation in both of these studies. In a retrospective analysis of 89 infected knees in arthroplasty patients, no difference could be determined between the patients treated with intravenous antibiotics for 4

tion but without the use of antibiotic-impregnated beads or spacers was successful in 93% of cases, whereas delayed reimplantation using antibiotic-impregnated cement for beads or spacers and for prosthesis fixation was successful in 91%. It should be noted that any beneficial local effect of the use of antibiotic-impregnated spacers or beads is not readily apparent, and some investigators remain concerned about the potential deleterious effects of leaving foreign material in a heavily contaminated wound (7). It would appear that both an adequate time delay before reimplantation and the use of antibiotic-impregnated cement for prosthesis fixation are the important treatment variables improving success rates.

SURGICAL TECHNIQUE

Débridement

Fundamental requirements include adequate exposure and thorough débridement of all infected and necrotic tissue with complete removal of all foreign material. The implementation of these steps is difficult to assess in a quantitative manner but almost certainly means the difference between success and failure for many patients. Careful placement of the incision is crucial, and when multiple incisions are present, use of the most longitudinal midline incision is recommended. If a choice must be made between parallel midline incisions, use of the lateral incision is reasonable. Sinus tracts within the incision should be elliptically excised as a part of the skin incision. Incisions with inverted skin edges or those with wide scarring should be excised back to healthy tissue if this permits eventual wound closure without undue skin tension. Elevation of subcutaneous tissue flaps should be minimized or avoided if at all possible.

Arthrotomy is usually performed through a medial parapatellar capsulotomy unless old nonabsorbable sutures are visible, and then every effort should be made to use the prior capsular incision, which minimizes the creation of extensor mechanism necrosis and facilitates removal of all old sutures. It is often necessary to excise or incise the edges of the arthrotomy to expose hidden sutures. An extremely effective technique to increase exposure in these knees is the quadriceps-snip surgical approach. Subperiosteal release of the deep medial collateral ligament allows anterolateral tibial subluxation, which greatly facilitates exposure. Removal of modular tibial polyethylene inserts during this portion of the exposure is also usually very helpful. In knees with extensive scarring and stiffness, continuation of the subperiosteal tibial exposure includes release of the semimembranosus insertion and posterior cruciate ligament.

Eversion of the patella during exposure of the infected total knee replacement can be very difficult and is unnecessary. When the tibia is translated anterolaterally, the extensor mechanism easily dislocates laterally, and this combined maneuver obviates the need for a lateral retinacular release or partial removal of the patellar ligament insertion. When the sequence of surgical exposures described earlier is used, it is extremely uncommon for specialized exposure techniques to be required. Use of a formal V-Y quadriceps turndown should be avoided because of the potential for extensor mechanism necrosis, which is disastrous in the setting of deep infection. Tibial tubercle osteotomy at the time of implant removal is also avoided due to the need for internal fixation of the osteotomy site. If additional surgical exposure is required, the medial femoral peel technique is generally sufficient for adequate exposure.

The prosthesis is removed carefully to preserve bone stock, and care is taken to remove any cement fragments during implant removal to avoid leaving any cement fragments in the depths of the wound. Patellar component removal is easily performed with the knee extended. This position minimizes patellar ligament insertion tension compared to removal during knee flexion and patellar eversion.

Implants should be extracted so as to minimize loss of bone stock; however, areas of necrotic bone should be removed. If the knee implant has cemented stems, it is helpful to identify the prosthesis type when planning implant removal. Many currently used cemented stem systems are designed to facilitate easy removal by simple disimpaction. Cemented long stems that are curved or porous are extremely difficult to remove, and under these circumstances the author prefers the following technique.

A cortical window is created in the anterior aspect of the distal femur or the anteromedial aspect of the tibia at the junction of the diaphysis and metaphyseal flare. The stem is then transected with a high-speed cutting burr and the intraarticular portion of the prosthesis is removed. The remaining stem is then exposed by removing cement around the stem with osteotomes or a pencil-tipped burr. Once the stem is removed, the remaining cement is extracted with cement-removal tools as in a hip revision procedure. The author prefers the use of ultrasonic cement removal.

After implant removal, open tibial or femoral canals are packed with sponges to prevent the introduction of errant debris into the canals. Although preservation of bone stock is a desirable goal, isolated islands of bone between areas of osteolysis or prominent small spikes of bone are excised, as these areas are typically avascular and are not essential for subsequent implant support.

Thorough débridement of the femoral and tibial canals is required when the removed implant has stems, however, extension of the infectious process into the medullary canals even in the absence of stems is quite common (7). Screw tracts and serpiginous areas of osteolysis are débrided with a high-speed burr. Careful identification and removal of all cement is essential. An area in which cement frequently is retained is the region where drill holes were prepared for intrusion of cement into a sclerotic medial tibial plateau. Additional hiding places include femoral component lug holes, the posterior femoral condyles, any drill holes used with knee instrumentation systems, and lug holes in the patella.

The final step is a complete synovectomy of the suprapatellar pouch, medial and lateral gutters, and posterior capsular region. It is preferable to perform the synovectomy as the last débridement step to ensure the removal of cement fragments that may have fallen into these areas during implant and cement removal. The posterior capsular region is a difficult region for confident débridement due to the proximity of the neurovascular structures; however, it is in this territory that fragments of polyethylene or large accumulations of foreign body response often reside. The volume of globular foreign material retrieved from the popliteal fossa region is often astonishing.

Representative tissue samples should be obtained throughout the débridement process for culture and sensitivity testing. Specimens are obtained from the intercondylar notch, the prosthesis-bone interface of the femur and tibia, any suspicious areas of abscess formation in the suprapatellar pouch or gutters, and any extension of the infectious process into the medullary canals. Three to five samples are usually adequate and are prepared for aerobic and anaerobic testing. If testing for fungi or mycobacteria is desirable, only one or two samples are submitted for these cumbersome and expensive tests. Antibiotics are then administered, and the antibiotic choice is based on test results obtained from the preoperative aspiration. If there are no culture results available, a cephalosporin is usually used while final culture results are awaited.

Irrespective of the method of staged revision, the knee is typically closed in the following fashion. The tourniquet is deflated to allow for hemostasis and influx of antibiotics, and then the tourniquet is reinflated to minimize blood loss and prevent excessive hematoma formation during wound closure. The knee joint is copiously irrigated and then antibiotic spacers are inserted just before wound closure. Capsular closure is accomplished over two deep drains with a large running absorbable monofilament suture, as the use of braided sutures is avoided. The skin and subcutaneous tissues are closed with large No. 2 monofilament retention sutures and smaller interrupted skin sutures. This closure method minimizes the overall number of sutures in the deep tissues and probably decreases the rate of marginal wound necrosis compared with a subcuticular skin closure. It cannot be overemphasized how important it is to obtain perfect epidermal apposition to facilitate primary wound healing. A compressive dressing is then applied to the limb, and the tourniquet is deflated.

The issue of how many times to débride the wound before final wound closure has not been determined. Occasionally more than one débridement is judged to be important due to the presence of severe soft tissue necrosis, which may require a second look to adequately assess tissue viability. The chronically infected knee joint is unlike the zone of injury associated with severe open fractures, which presents an evolving pattern of tissue necrosis and therefore requires multiple assessments and débridements. The use of multiple anesthetics for these débridements also increases the cost and morbidity of treatment, and repeated débridements have the potential disadvantage of allowing entry of nosocomial organisms. It is extremely rare, in our opinion, for more than one débridement to be required in the management of an infected total knee replacement.

Insertion of Spacer Blocks

Spacer blocks were introduced in the 1980s as a method to treat an infected knee replacement between the time of removal of the infected prosthesis and eventual reinsertion of another prosthesis (22,23). Over the past decade, many characteristics of these block spacers have evolved, but there has been no definitive study demonstrating the treatment superiority of using these spacers. Use of these spacers has facilitated reimplantation for both the surgeon and patient. The primary functions of block spacers are delivery of local antimicrobial agents and maintenance of collateral ligament length. Potential disadvantages of block spacers include the presence of a foreign body and bone loss incurred while awaiting reimplantation.

Essentially, the different types of block spacers include a simple tibiofemoral block, the molded arthrodesis block, articulating mobile spacers, and medullary dowels. The simple tibiofemoral block (Fig. 1) was the original spacer block. It was preformed and then inserted into the tibiofemoral space after the cement had polymerized. These blocks were shaped as simple

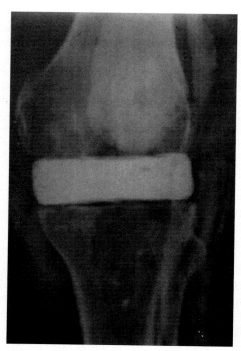

FIG. 1. Anteroposterior radiograph of a simple tibiofemoral block fabricated from antibiotic-impregnated bone cement.

"hockey pucks" inserted into the tibiofemoral space, and additional antibiotic beads or thin discs were often placed into the suprapatellar pouch or lateral gutters. Difficulties with this type of block spacer include the inability to match the surfaces of the block with the irregular surfaces of the distal femur and proximal tibia. Patients occasionally experience subluxation of the bony surfaces off the surface of the spacer, and instances of extensor mechanism necrosis, wound breakdown, and progressive bone loss have been observed (24).

The molded arthrodesis block was developed due to the difficulties encountered with preformed spacer blocks. These spacers are fabricated so that the cement is polymerized within the knee; this allows the cement to conform to the irregular contour of the femur and tibia (Fig. 2). This macrointerdigitation of the cement into bone defects and the intercondylar notch, and extension into the medullary canals and suprapatellar pouch create a cement arthrodesis of the knee joint. This stability is helpful for patient comfort and prevents the difficulties of spacer migration and progressive bone erosion. Removal of these spacers requires fragmentation of the spacer into several large pieces with an osteotome at the time of reimplantation.

The mobile articulating spacer allows the patient to place the knee through a range of motion during the time between prosthesis removal and insertion of the new prosthesis. These spacers, originally facsimiles of antibiotic-impregnated cement shaped into femoral and tibial components, allowed knee motion through articulation of the acrylic cement surfaces (25). Eventually, a system of molds was developed to incorporate small metal runners and polyethylene tibial trays so that cement surfaces were not articulating against each other (25). One alternative has been to sterilize the prosthesis just removed and then incorporate the femoral component and tibial tray into the antibiotic-loaded spacer (Fig. 3) (26). The theoretic advantages

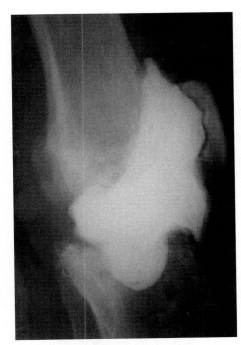

FIG. 2. Lateral radiograph of molded arthrodesis block that fills the tibiofemoral space and the space between the anterior femur and patellar remnant. The spacer is irregular in shape to accommodate areas of bone loss, and this increases the stability of the knee joint.

of mobile articulating spacers include the potential for improved functional outcomes and better range of motion. To date, these benefits have not been realized, but use of these mobile spacers does simplify the surgical exposure at reimplantation and is particularly helpful for patients requiring simultaneous removal of bilateral infected knee prostheses.

Insertion of antibiotic-impregnated medullary dowels is a reasonable measure, as even in infected knee replacements without stems there is extension of the infectious process into the medullary canals of the femur or tibia in roughly one-third of cases (7). Antibiotic beads inserted into the medullary canals may be extremely difficult to remove at reimplantation. A tapered

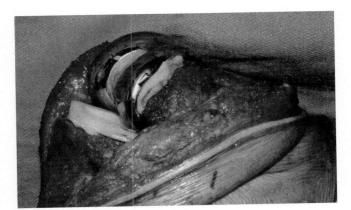

FIG. 3. Articulating spacer made from the old prosthesis, which was sterilized and reinserted with antibiotic-impregnated cement interdigitated into the surfaces of the femur and tibia.

cement dowel fashioned from the nozzle of a cement gun is of excellent size and shape to be inserted into the medullary canal (Fig. 4). The smooth taper of the dowel facilitates removal at reimplantation.

Combining two antibiotics in bone cement improves elution of both antibiotics. The two most commonly used antibiotics in clinical practice are vancomycin hydrochloride and tobramycin (1). The use of at least 3.6 g of tobramycin and 1 g of vancomycin per package of bone cement is recommended. Several technical tips are helpful when mixing these high-dose antibiotic-loaded cement spacers. Mix the polymethyl methacrylate monomer and powder together to form liquid cement before adding the antibiotic powder to prevent mixing difficulties. Vancomycin powder is crystalline, and leaving the large crystals intact enhances the volume of antibiotic eluted from the final composite. In contrast, when mixing vancomycin into cement being used for prosthesis fixation, completely pulverize all crystals, as these crystal defects significantly weaken the cement. Creating surface patterns in the cement to produce an increased surface area facilitates antibiotic elution. Producing micromotion of the cement spacer during curing creates macrointerdigitation into the irregular bony contours but prevents integration of the cement into the cancellous bone. Avoid overdistraction of the tibiofemoral space with these cement spacers; otherwise, flexion and extension space balancing may be difficult at reimplantation.

Interval Resection Arthroplasty

The effect of the time delay between resection arthroplasty and reimplantation on functional outcome has not been clearly established. Scarring and joint stiffness worsen with extended time delays. The use of spacer blocks maintains the collateral ligament and extensor mechanism length, and facilitates reimplantation. Additional potential benefits of spacer blocks include patient comfort and mobility during the interval after resection arthroplasty, and this seems particularly true of mobile articulating spacers. There have been no significant differences in knee scores, functional scores, or range of motion when knees were analyzed according to the length of delay, type of knee prosthesis used at reimplantation, and the use of a block cement spacer (15).

Despite the lack of evidence for improved functional outcomes with the use of spacers, the advantages of mechanical stability for the patient and the reduction of difficulty with surgical exposure at reimplantation have led to common acceptance and use of these spacers. Spacer blocks should be supplemented by external immobilization, such as with a brace or cast, as the patient awaits the reimplantation. In the author's opinion, casting is preferable, as patients can be partially weightbearing and the wound, which is protected, heals more effectively. Patients with mobile articulating spacers are encouraged to perform range-of-motion exercises and are allowed up to 50% partial weightbearing (25). The motion permitted by mobile articulating spacers particularly helps patients who have undergone removal of bilateral infected knees.

Patients undergoing delayed reimplantation are typically anemic, and 88% require allogeneic blood transfusions, particularly because the two surgeries are temporally close (8). The presence of infection precludes traditional alternatives such as reinfusion or autologous blood donation; thus, novel blood management prac-

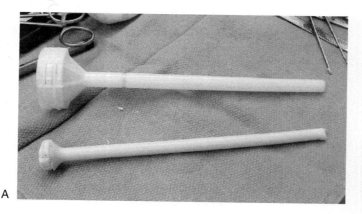

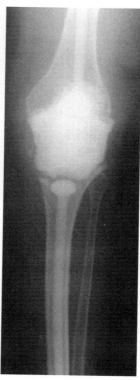

FIG. 4. A: Medullary dowel adjacent to cement gun nozzle. **B:** Anteroposterior radiograph of a knee joint with a molded arthrodesis spacer block and medullary dowels inserted into the tibia and femur.

tices are required in this patient population. Thirty-nine consecutively treated patients undergoing two-stage reimplantation were enrolled in a prospective study to determine whether the use of recombinant human erythropoietin could lower allogeneic transfusion requirements (27). Compared with a group of 81 patients not receiving recombinant human erythropoietin, the requirement for transfusion was found to be significantly lower in the group given erythropoietin ($p <.001$). In patients receiving recombinant human erythropoietin, 52% avoided transfusion for the entire period encompassing both stages of reimplantation.

One of the most important issues for both patient and surgeon is the determination of when it is safe and appropriate to proceed with reimplantation. In just 4 or 6 weeks, erythrocyte sedimentation rates would not be expected to normalize; however, the trend should suggest that the values obtained just before reimplantation show improvement (1). The C-reactive protein levels typically normalize by the twenty-first day after surgery. If the levels remain elevated, this may suggest the presence of persistent infection (1). Open biopsy or aspiration for culture and sensitivity testing has been suggested before proceeding with reimplantation, but these maneuvers have not been beneficial in our practice, and we prefer the use of an intraoperative decision process (empiric reimplantation) based on the appearance of the knee joint supplemented by analysis of frozen sections (15). It is important to recognize that this method requires considerable experience on the part of the surgeon and the pathologist, and the presence of spacers or beads may alter the appearance of the tissues at reimplantation. In one study, analysis of frozen sections at reimplantation to determine the presence of infection had a sensitivity of 25%, a specificity of 98%, a positive predictive value of 50%, a negative predictive value of 95%, and an accuracy of 94% (28). If there is concern about the presence of persistent infection, it is prudent to perform another débride-

ment, insert new spacers, close the wound, and await the results of culture and sensitivity testing.

Reimplantation Procedure

The surgical approach is typically more difficult at reimplantation than at implant removal, particularly if the delay before reimplantation is more than 6 to 8 weeks. Exposure at reimplantation is generally easier in patients with an articulating spacer who have performed range-of-motion exercises than in patients in whom the knee was immobilized during the interval after resection arthroplasty.

In reimplantation knee arthroplasty, the surgeon often encounters bone deficiencies and occasionally attendant ligamentous insufficiency, which requires the use of more constrained prosthetic designs to achieve knee stability. In the setting of minimal bone loss and an intact posterior cruciate ligament, it has not been demonstrated that either cruciate-retaining or cruciate-substituting prostheses are preferable. Currently, the majority of prostheses used for reimplantation at our institution are posterior stabilized prostheses fixed with antibiotic-impregnated cement (Fig. 5).

Stemmed prosthetic components are typically used for reimplantation to augment prosthetic fixation. Although the use of stemmed cemented implants provides excellent fixation, the extraction of these prostheses is more difficult should reinfection occur. When possible, fluted press-fit stems are used with cementation of the distal femur and proximal tibia, and if reinfection should occur, these implants are easier to remove than cemented stems. The use of hinged constrained prostheses should be avoided if at all possible (29).

Although the use of bone graft at reimplantation has been reported, there are no comparative studies evaluating the effect of

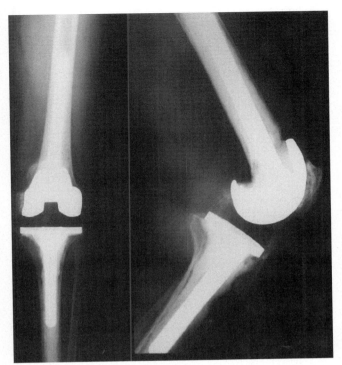

FIG. 5. Anteroposterior and lateral radiographs of a reimplantation posterior stabilized prosthesis with stem fixated using antibiotic-impregnated bone cement.

bone grafting on the incidence of recurrent infection. Soaking of bone graft in antibiotic solution is an alternative means of providing local antibiotic delivery, particularly when uncemented implants are used. In a series of 33 patients treated with interval antibiotic-loaded beads, 6 weeks of intravenous antibiotics, and an uncemented prosthesis augmented with antibiotic-soaked bone graft, there was only one reinfection, for an infection cure rate of 97% (30). Unless one chooses to use an uncemented implant, bone graft is rarely required for the reimplantation arthroplasty. This avoidance of bone graft is accomplished by using other alternatives such as modular wedges or filling of bone defects with bone cement.

Postoperative Management

Antibiotics are generally administered for 5 days until results are available from culture and sensitivity testing of intraoperative tissue samples obtained at reimplantation. If there are positive culture results showing the same organism that was identified at the time of implant removal, an additional course of intravenous antibiotics is administered for 28 days. Then the need for prolonged oral antibiotic suppression is individually assessed with the consultation of an infectious disease specialist. If the organism in a positive culture result is determined to be a contaminant because of growth in broth only or a different organism is recovered from only one tissue sample, antibiotics are discontinued. Otherwise, all antibiotics are discontinued on the fifth postoperative day. Postoperative rehabilitation is similar to that for aseptic revision knee surgery. Patients are then followed with examination, radiographs, and determination of

erythrocyte sedimentation rate and C-reactive protein levels on an annual basis.

FAILURE OF REIMPLANTATION

Although reimplantation has become a commonly accepted treatment modality for the infected knee prosthesis, the poor outcome of patients who develop reinfection after reimplantation has not been fully appreciated. For 24 knees treated for reinfection after reimplantation, the final outcome included 10 knees undergoing a successful knee arthrodesis, five patients who were maintained on suppressive oral antibiotics, four cases of above-the-knee amputation, three knees with persistent pseudarthrosis, 1 resection arthroplasty, and one uninfected total knee prosthesis (31). A poor prognosis was associated with the use of a hinged-knee design, as three of the four amputations were for failed hinge-knee prostheses. A successful arthrodesis on the initial attempt using an external fixation device was more likely for patients with unstemmed prostheses (75%) than for those with cemented stemmed prostheses (40%). Long intramedullary arthrodesis was successful in all three attempts. A second attempt at reimplantation was successful in only one (33%) of three attempts.

A study of 12 patients who acquired another infection in the reimplanted knee reported different findings (32). Three knees were treated by arthrodesis, whereas nine knees underwent another salvage attempt with implant removal, débridement, 6 weeks of parenteral antibiotics, and reimplantation. At an average of 31 months of follow-up, the mean Knee Society knee score was 79 and the mean functional score was 73; no instance of recurrent infection occurred. Despite these contrasting findings, the difficulties encountered in achieving wound healing, successful knee arthrodesis, and successful eradication of infection with nonprosthetic salvage procedures after a failed reimplantation are considerable. The morbidity and increased likelihood of amputation associated with reinfection must be carefully considered and presented to the patient before proceeding with reimplantation for treatment of the infected total knee replacement.

COST ISSUES

It has been documented that treating an infected knee replacement incurs an estimated net loss of approximately $15,000, and this loss is doubled for the Medicare patient (33). These procedures are associated with increased operative times, longer hospital stays, increased number of hospitalizations, increased number of surgical procedures, and increased blood loss compared with aseptic revision knee surgery. These issues need to be considered in health care reimbursement schemes. Preoperative planning and arrangements for postoperative care, proper patient selection, preoperative identification of the offending microorganism, close collaboration with an infectious disease expert, minimization of the number of débridements after implant removal, use of empiric reimplantation, avoidance of bone graft and modular augments when possible by using cement fill, and treatment referral to experienced and interested surgeons help minimize the cost of treatment for these patients. This is particularly true if the first attempt to treat an infected knee replacement is successful.

REFERENCES

1. Hanssen AD, Rand JA. Evaluation and treatment of infection at the site of a total hip or knee arthroplasty. *J Bone Joint Surg Am* 1998;80:910–922.
2. Hanssen AD. Management of the infected total knee arthroplasty. In: Engh GA, Rorabeck CH, eds. *Revision total knee arthroplasty.* Baltimore: Williams and Wilkins, 1997:371–393.
3. Segawa H, Tsukayama DT, Kyle RF, et al. Infection after total knee arthroplasty. A retrospective study of the treatment of eighty-one infections. *J Bone Joint Surg Am* 1999;81(10):1434–1445.
4. Kramhoft M, Bodtker S, Carlsen A. Outcome of infected total knee arthroplasty. *J Arthroplasty* 1994;9(6):617–621.
5. Hirakawa K, Stulberg BN, Wilde AH, et al. Results of 2-stage reimplantation for infected total knee arthroplasty. *J Arthroplasty* 1998;13(1):22–28.
6. Wasielewski RC, Barden RM, Rosenberg AG. Results of different surgical procedures on total knee arthroplasty infections. *J Arthroplasty* 1996;11(8):931–938.
7. McPherson EJ, Patzakis MJ, Gross JE, et al. Infected total knee arthroplasty. Two-stage reimplantation with a gastrocnemius rotational flap. *Clin Orthop* 1997;341:73–81.
8. Pagnano M, Cushner FD, Hanssen A, et al. Blood management in two-stage revision knee arthroplasty for deep prosthetic infection. *Clin Orthop* 1999;367:238–242.
9. Barrack RL, Jennings RW, Wolfe MW, et al. The Coventry Award. The value of preoperative aspiration before total knee revision. *Clin Orthop* 1997;345:8–16.
10. Insall JN, Thompson FM, Brause BD. Two-stage reimplantation for the salvage of infected total knee arthroplasty. *J Bone Joint Surg Am* 1983;65(8):1087–1098.
11. Windsor RE, Insall JN, Urs WK, et al. Two-stage reimplantation for the salvage of total knee arthroplasty complicated by infection. Further follow-up and refinement of indications. *J Bone Joint Surg Am* 1990;72(2):272–278.
12. Goldman RT, Scuderi GR, Insall JN. Two-stage reimplantation for infected total knee replacement. *Clin Orthop* 1996;331:118–124.
13. Borden LS, Gearen PF. Infected total knee arthroplasty. A protocol for management. *J Arthroplasty* 1987;2(1):27–36.
14. Wilde AH, Ruth JT. Two-stage reimplantation in infected total knee arthroplasty. *Clin Orthop* 1988;236:23–35.
15. Hanssen AD, Rand JA, Osmon DR. Treatment of the infected total knee arthroplasty with insertion of another prosthesis. The effect of antibiotic-impregnated bone cement. *Clin Orthop* 1994;309:44–55.
16. Buechel FF. Primary exchange revision arthroplasty using antibiotic-impregnated cement for infected total knee replacement. *Orthop Rev* 1990;19:83–88.
17. Goksan SB, Freeman MA. One-stage reimplantation for infected total knee arthroplasty. *J Bone Joint Surg Br* 1992;74(1):78–82.
18. Scott IR, Stockley I, Getty CJ. Exchange arthroplasty for infected knee replacements. A new two-stage method. *J Bone Joint Surg Br* 1993;75(1):28–31.
19. Rand JA, Bryan RS. Reimplantation for the salvage of an infected total knee arthroplasty. *J Bone Joint Surg Am* 1983;65(8):1081–1086.
20. Cadambi A, Jones RE, Maale GE. A protocol for staged revision of infected total hip and knee arthroplasties: the use of antibiotic-cement-implant composites. *Orthop Int* 1995;3:133–145.
21. Wilson MG, Kelly K, Thornhill TS. Infection as a complication of total knee replacement arthroplasty. Risk factors and treatment in sixty-seven cases. *J Bone Joint Surg Am* 1990;72:878–883.
22. Booth RE Jr, Lotke PA. The results of spacer block technique in revision of infected total knee arthroplasty. *Clin Orthop* 1989;248:57–60.
23. Cohen J, Hosack W, Cuckler J, et al. Two stage reimplantation using an antibiotic PMMA spacer block. *J Arthroplasty* 1988;3:369–377.
24. Calton TF, Fehring TK, Griffin WL. Bone loss associated with the use of spacer blocks in infected total knee arthroplasty. *Clin Orthop* 1997;345:148–154.
25. Masri BA, Kendall RW, Duncan CP, et al. Two-stage exchange arthroplasty using a functional antibiotic-loaded spacer in the treatment of the infected knee replacement: the Vancouver experience. *Semin Arthroplasty* 1994;5(3):122–136.
26. Hofmann AA, Kane KR, Tkach TK, et al. Treatment of infected total knee arthroplasty using an articulating spacer. *Clin Orthop* 1995;321:45–54.
27. Cushner FD, Barrack RL, Hanssen AD, et al. The use of EPO in two stage exchange TKA for infection. Paper presented at: Interim Meeting of the Knee Society; September 14–16, 2000; Boston, MA.
28. Della Valle CJ, Bogner E, Desai P, et al. Analysis of frozen sections of intraoperative specimens obtained at the time of reoperation after hip or knee resection arthroplasty for the treatment of infection. *J Bone Joint Surg Am* 1999;81(5):684–689.
29. Isiklar ZU, Landon GC, Tullos HS. Amputation after failed total knee arthroplasty. *Clin Orthop* 1994;299:173–178.
30. Whiteside LA. Treatment of infected total knee arthroplasty. *Clin Orthop* 1994;299:169–172.
31. Hanssen AD, Trousdale RT, Osmon DR. Patient outcome with reinfection following reimplantation for the infected total knee arthroplasty. *Clin Orthop* 1995;321:55–67.
32. Backe HA Jr, Wolff DA, Windsor RE. Total knee replacement infection after 2-stage reimplantation: results of subsequent 2-stage reimplantation. *Clin Orthop* 1996;331:125–131.
33. Hebert CK, Williams RE, Levy RS, et al. Cost of treating an infected total knee replacement. *Clin Orthop* 1996;331:140–145.
34. Bengtson S, Knutson K. The infected knee arthroplasty. A 6-year follow-up of 357 cases. *Acta Orthop Scand* 1991;62(4):301–311.
35. Bliss DG, McBride GG. Infected total knee arthroplasties. *Clin Orthop* 1985;199:207–214.
36. Bose WJ, Gearen PF, Randall JC, et al. Long-term outcome of 42 knees with chronic infection after total knee arthroplasty. *Clin Orthop* 1995;319:285–296.
37. Freeman MAR, Sudlow RA, Casewell MW, et al. The management of infected total knee replacement. *J Bone Joint Surg Br* 1985;67:764–768.
38. Gacon G, Laurencon M, Van de Velde D, et al. Two stage reimplantation for infection after knee arthroplasty. Apropos of a series of 29 cases [in French]. *Rev Chir Orthop Reparatrice Appar Mot* 1997;83(4):313–323.
39. Grogan TJ, Dorey F, Rollins J, et al. Deep sepsis following total knee arthroplasty. Ten year experience at the University of California at Los Angelos medical center. *J Bone Joint Surg Am* 1986;68:226–234.
40. Ivey FM, Hicks CA, Calhoun JH, et al. Treatment options for infected knee arthroplasties. *Rev Infect Dis* 1990;12(3):468–478.
41. Jacobs MA, Hungerford DS, Krackow KA, et al. Revision of septic total knee arthroplasty. *Clin Orthop* 1989;238:159.
42. Johnson DP, Bannister GC. The outcome of infected arthroplasty of the knee. *J Bone Joint Surg Br* 1986;68(2):289–291.
43. Rosenberg AG, Haas B, Barden R, et al. Salvage of infected total knee arthroplasty. *Clin Orthop* 1988;226:29–33.
44. Teeny SM, Dorr L, Murata G, et al. Treatment of infected total knee arthroplasty. Irrigation and debridement versus two-stage reimplantation. *J Arthroplasty* 1990;5(1):35–39.
45. von Foerster G, Kluber D, Kabler U. Mid- to long-term results after treatment of 118 cases of periprosthetic infections after knee joint replacement using one-stage exchange surgery [in German]. *Orthopade* 1991;20:244–252.
46. Walker RH, Schurman DJ. Management of infected total knee arthroplasties. *Clin Orthop* 1984;186:81–89.
47. Woods GW, Lionberger DR, Tullos HS. Failed total knee arthroplasty. *Clin Orthop* 1983;173:184–190.

CHAPTER 115

Knee Arthrodesis and Resection

James B. Stiehl

Knee arthrodesis remains an important salvage technique for complex problems of the knee such as severe trauma, chronic infection, or failed total joint arthroplasty. Technical advances with intramedullary fixation have dramatically increased fusion rates to the extent that resection arthroplasty has been eliminated as a long-term solution for chronic problems. Patients undergoing simple resection have significant instability, and the knee must be splinted or braced indefinitely. However, two-stage débridement and reconstruction for chronic knee infection remain a reason for a temporary resection. Although late reconstruction with total knee arthroplasty is successful in over 90% of cases, fusion may be required in certain patients. This chapter explores the indications, surgical technique, and results of knee arthrodesis.

INDICATIONS

Primary Arthrodesis

With the evolutionary success of total knee arthroplasty, primary arthrodesis of the arthritic knee has become an unusual operation; however, there are several settings in which primary fusion remains an attractive or at least a reasonable option. The first is that of a young patient with severe extremity trauma to the knee joint complicated by chronic sepsis and extensor mechanism loss. In this instance, the consideration is to prevent the possible long-term problem of a potentially functional young person who becomes depressed, divorced, and destitute with marginal long-term prospects. Knee arthrodesis has been shown by numerous authors to be durable in the long term even if interposing grafts are needed. Wolf et al. followed patients undergoing arthrodesis after tumor limb salvage and found independent ambulation in

86%. At a mean follow-up of 17 years, the majority continued to have satisfactory function (1). Benson et al. compared arthrodesis after failed knee arthroplasty with primary total knee arthroplasty and found nearly identical Short-Form 36 scores. Physical mobility was better with knee arthroplasty, but pain control was better with arthrodesis (2).

The second indication is a neuropathic Charcot joint in which the limb may be asensate and the patient has very poor control of knee function due to severe spinal cord involvement or has a myelopathic process. Other indications include primary malignant bone tumors, which may be treated with primary arthrodesis using augments such as autologous grafts or vascularized fibular transplants, or situations in which there is inadequate motor function for maintenance of stability in extension, such as in chronic poliomyelitis syndrome. For virtually all other circumstances, primary arthrodesis has been displaced by total knee arthroplasty. The functional outcome is significantly inferior with arthrodesis; most older patients require ambulatory aids such as a cane or crutches, and lifestyle compromise for some may be severe.

Secondary Arthrodesis

The most common current circumstance for use of arthrodesis is chronic sepsis after total knee arthroplasty in a patient who is not a candidate for reimplantation. This is typically a type B or C host, in whom the risk of infection recurrence is high, especially when extensor mechanism problems such as patellar tendon rupture are also present. Type B hosts have significant local and systemic factors that impair the normal immune processes. Local factors include chronic lymphedema, major vessel disease, venous stasis, extensive scarring, and radiation fibrosis. Systemic problems include malnutrition, malignancy, extremes of age, hepatic or renal failure, diabetes mellitus, and alcohol abuse. Type C hosts are sufficiently fragile that undertaking aggressive treatment could endanger the patient. We are particularly concerned about patients who have evidence of chronic malnutrition with depressed levels of serum albumin and protein; become infected from a chronic source such as a stoma, urine, or diverticulum; have infection with multiple organisms; have chronic infections that respond poorly to débridements and antibiotic therapy with persistent signs of inflammation; or have life-threatening infections with methicillin-resistant *Staphylococcus aureus* or vancomycin-resistant *Enterococcus*. One study has shown that infection which recurs following two-stage débridement and reimplantation after chronic sepsis has at least a 50% chance of recurring a second time. Careful judgment is needed for each patient, and close consultation with an infectious disease specialist is required to balance the risk of long-term antibiotic treatment or suppressive antibiotic therapy against the surgical choices of fibrous resection arthroplasty, total knee reimplantation, arthrodesis, and occasionally amputation.

TECHNIQUE

External Fixation

One publication has reported 100% solid fusion using an anterior unilateral frame for arthrodesis (3,4). This contrasts with the 40% to 80% failure rate of earlier methods that attempted something near the Charnley compression technique. Inadequate stability probably explained the large failure rates. The author would hesitate to recommend the use of external fixators, particularly in older patients with soft osteopenic bone. The most sound construct is a double-frame technique in which two or three threaded pin groups are applied proximally and distally in sound cortical bone of the femur and tibia. Optimum apposition with a degree of compression is desired. Careful pin site care is desired, and chronic bone osteomyelitis is a risk of long-term pin use. Patients are best kept non-weightbearing for extended periods of 3 to 5 months (Fig. 1).

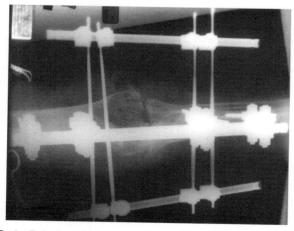

FIG. 1. Failed total knee arthroplasty after chronic sepsis and extensor mechanism loss treated with a double-plane external fixation device.

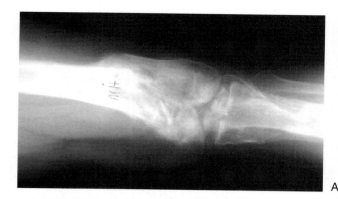

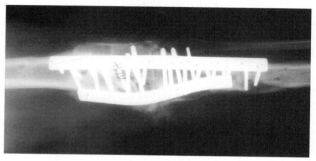

FIG. 2. A: Healed intraarticular distal femoral and proximal tibial type 3C open fracture complicated with extensor mechanism loss and chronic sepsis in a 22-year-old male factory worker. **B:** Successful double-plate fixation after failed attempt at external fixation.

Double-Plate Fixation

The double-plate fixation technique first described by Nichols (13) uses two broad atlantooccipital dynamic compression plates with 10 to 18 holes (average, 12 holes) (5). Bone cuts are made such that the normal femorotibial valgus of 7 degrees is restored. One plate is placed anteromedial, whereas the other is positioned anterolateral. Careful contouring of the plates is usually needed. The patella may be osteotomized and applied to the anterior surface of the femur and tibia as a graft. Sepsis requires a two-stage technique, with fusion performed after 8 weeks of antibiotic therapy. Postoperative management includes use of a long leg cast until the fusion is ascertained to be solid (average, 5.6 months; range, 3 to 10 months) (Fig. 2).

Intramedullary Nail Fixation

Küntscher Nail

Several different rod configurations have been developed, with particular advantages noted for each (6). The author's original experience was with a simple Küntscher nail that was inserted anterograde through a separate incision with the use of a medial ten-hole dynamic compression plate. This technique is particularly valuable if a long interposing allograft is required, as rigid fixation of the graft is essential for union. The patient is placed supine on a radiopative table with a 45-degree bump under the affected buttock. The pelvis and lower extremity are

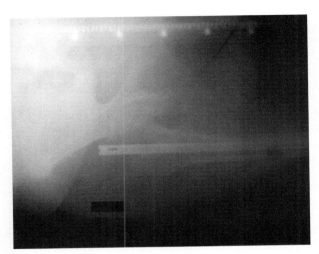

FIG. 3. Prominent and symptomatic intramedullary nail inserted 2 cm above the tip of the greater trochanter; the nail required removal.

draped so that proximal hip exposure allows entry, and reaming of the femur anterograde is done under fluoroscopic view. It is important to have the image machine placed so that one can follow the nail insertion all the way down the leg, especially distally, as rods have passed out of the soft distal tibia. A sterile tourniquet is used to minimize blood loss. The fusion site is entered with a longitudinal anterior knee incision. The knee implant is removed, or the previously débrided infected knee is assessed, and the fusion site is prepared. Next, an incision is made over the greater trochanter with split of the gluteus medius muscle to expose the pyriformis fossa. The proximal

femoral canal is entered as for a femoral fracture, and a guidewire is passed down to the knee joint. At this point, the surfaces may be cut using the axis of the guide pin to create maximally abutting surfaces. Anterograde reaming is done over the guidewire. Generally, this can be done to 12 or 13 mm, which is the nominal size of the tibial reaming and accommodates a suitable nail size for strength. The guide pin is passed down the tibia, and fluoroscopic control is used to make certain that the center of the ankle joint is reached. Depending on the nail used, one may overream 0.5 mm on the tibial side and 1 mm on the femoral side. Nail dimension is determined on the tibial size. The length of the nail is based on guide pin measurement from the tip of the greater trochanter to a point 2 cm above the ankle joint. The bowed fusion nail is then carefully inserted over the guide pin down to the knee joint and passed across to the tibia with an assistant holding the fusion site opposed. The anterior bow of the femoral shaft determines the position of the nail and tends to direct the nail out the very anterior cortex of the distal femur. One must carefully assess insertion distally into the tibia to prevent perforation and to ensure distal positioning approximately 2 cm above the ankle joint. The proximal end of the nail should be within 1 cm of the tip of the greater trochanter (Fig. 3). At this point, adjunct fixation may be considered. This may include a ten-hole medial neutralization plate, crossed cancellous screws, or proximal and distal locking screws in the nail. Additional bone graft and enhancing substances may be added to the fusion site. Closure of the wound may be problematic because of the shortening of the leg and chronic scar tissue, which is a reason to avoid the use of additional plates. Postoperatively, no external splints or casts are needed, but the patient must be non-weightbearing for 6 to 10 weeks, depending on the progression of healing (Fig. 4).

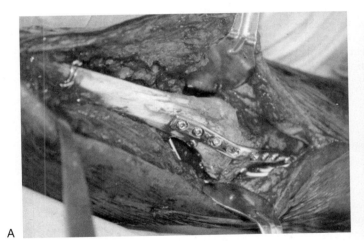

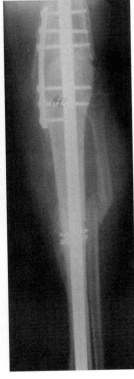

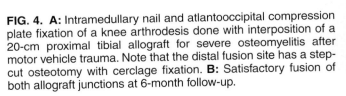

FIG. 4. A: Intramedullary nail and atlantooccipital compression plate fixation of a knee arthrodesis done with interposition of a 20-cm proximal tibial allograft for severe osteomyelitis after motor vehicle trauma. Note that the distal fusion site has a step-cut osteotomy with cerclage fixation. **B:** Satisfactory fusion of both allograft junctions at 6-month follow-up.

TABLE 1. *Results after knee arthrodesis*

Study	No. of patients	Rate of fusion (%)	Peroneal palsy (N)	Stress fracture (N)	Technique
Arroyo et al. (7)	21	90	3	3	Neff (titanium) nail
Cheng and Gross (12)	2	100	?	?	Short intramedullary nail
Donley (15)	20	85	0	0	Intramedullary nail
Hak et al. (5)	19	58	?	?	Single-plane external fixation
Hak et al. (5)	17	61	?	?	Double-plane external fixation
Hessmann et al. (6)	19	100	?	?	External fixation
Nichols et al. (13)	11	100	0	1	Double plate
Rasmussen et al. (14)	13	92	1	0	Intramedullary rod, vascularized fibula
Stiehl and Hanel (11)	8	100	1	0	Intramedullary rod, plate

Titanium Nail

The titanium modular nail was developed for insertion retrograde of the femoral side with anterograde insertion of the tibial side (7). The implant comes in sizes of 11, 13, and 15 mm with a bowed segment on the femoral side and straight rod on the tibial side. The rods are locked with a conical tapered locking mechanism supplemented with small engaging screws that add additional compression and prevent separation if the nail becomes disengaged. The nail is fluted and is designed to engage the isthmus segments of the tibia and femur and then extend 4 to 6 cm beyond this region. The rods may be cut off intraoperatively to provide the appropriate length. Finally, preparation requires reaming of 1.5 mm over the nominal size to be used. With slight rotation of the femoral side, a valgus alignment of the femur can be developed. The particular advantages of this nail system are that it can be inserted through the knee joint, allows different sizes of nails to be applied to the femur and tibia, avoids the hip joint if concurrent hip arthroplasty is required, and currently has shown extremely successful results at the hands of the developing surgeons. Use with segmental allografts has been reported with the addition of supplemental plates. The nail has never required removal in the experience of the developers but may require the use of a high-speed burr to transect the implant for removal.

Wichita Nail

The Wichita nail has relatively short femoral and tibial segments that are fixed with interlocking screws at each end. Reaming is done using fixed-dimension reamers. Adjustment of tibial placement allows for eventual engagement of a locking segment that can be screwed together, creating longitudinal compression. The particular advantage of this system is that excellent compression of the fusion site is possible, and blood loss, which can be a problem if intramedullary reaming is needed, is minimal.

RESULTS

Although the report of Hessmann et al. demonstrated 100% fusion with anterior external frames, the report of Hak et al. noted a success rate of 58% with unilateral frames and 61% with double frames (5,6). The other problems with this approach include pin tract infections and stress fractures through old hole sites. Reports of intramedullary fixation and double-plate fixation have revealed healing rates of 85% to 100% in virtually all cases, including patients with severe bone loss requiring allografts or vascularized fibular transplants (Table 1).

A literature review indicates that complications include delayed union, recurrence of infection, wound healing problems, stress fracture, reflex dystrophy, and partial peroneal palsy. Complication rates have ranged from 38% to 50% in selected series (3–8). Partial peroneal palsy has been noted by multiple authors, and no obvious explanation is offered other than stretching of the nerve from positioning of the knee during the operative procedure. Most of the cases mentioned resolved in time, and there were no cases in which direct surgical trauma has been described. Treatment of recurrent sepsis has included débridement of the site and eventual nail removal in certain cases. The author personally has an anecdotal case in which the proximal femur fractured on insertion of a special interlocking nail designed for arthrodesis. The proximal femur shattered, which created an intertrochanteric-subtrochanteric fracture that was successfully treated using a custom nail for the arthrodesis that allowed proximal screw insertion into the femoral neck and reconstruction by wiring the proximal femur together.

Authors have discussed the possibility of late takedown of fusions after failed total knee arthroplasty. In general, patients have been satisfied with this approach, with the majority stating that they would consider having the operation again if offered. All series have reported very high complication rates exceeding 50%, however, and for this reason, patients must be selected carefully with realistic expectations of failure (8–10).

The greatest disadvantage of knee arthrodesis is the resultant complete stiffness. If the knee is fused in extension, walking is effective and generally smooth. Unfortunately, sitting is inconvenient, and attendance in social settings with crowded seating such a movies, sporting events, church, and so on can be particularly difficult. Stiehl and Hanel noted that an optimal amount of shortening for clearance of the shoe on gait swing through ambulation was 1.5 to 2.5 cm. Patients would choose shoe lift adjustments to this level. Most older patients required a cane or walker for community ambulation (11).

Green et al. carefully assessed a group of patients after successful knee arthrodesis. Automobile driving did not prove any problem, particularly if the car had automatic transmission. Most patients avoided theater seats unless an aisle seat could be reserved. Performance of household chores posed special problems, but most patients could bend to the floor due to stretching of the hamstrings and hypermobility of the lumbar spine. Patients were capable of engaging in virtually every type of sport or recreational activity, including tennis, golf, bowling, baseball, handball, and even horseback riding. However, no patient was known to have attempted snow skiing (4).

DISCUSSION

The use of intramedullary nail techniques appears to offer an extremely satisfactory solution to difficult problems after sepsis and bone loss in failed total knee arthroplasty. With chronic sepsis after total knee arthroplasty, a staged reconstruction seems appropriate with a delay of 6 to 8 weeks, combined with appropriate adjunctive antibiotic therapy. The choice of nail does not seem to affect fusion rates, but certain advantages accrue with each particular nail type. The simple bowed femoral nail allows straightforward anterograde insertion but carries the possibility of migration, bone perforation, and proximal femoral fracture if reaming is inadequate. Adjunct fixation such as crossed cancellous screws or a neutralization bone plate may be needed at the fusion site. The addition of interlocking screws can add rotational stability at the fusion site. The availability of the Wichita nail is a significant improvement over older methods. This nail is inserted at the fusion site, has an excellent external jig for insertion of interlocking screws, and has an articulating turnbuckle that assembles at the fusion site. Compression at the fusion site is optimal with the turnbuckle, and early experience has been excellent. In addition, the nail may be taken apart at a later date.

REFERENCES

1. Wolf RE, Scarborough MT, Enneking WF. Long-term followup of patients with autogenous resection arthrodesis of the knee. *Clin Orthop* 1999;358:36–40.
2. Benson ER, Resine ST, Lewis CG. Functional outcome of arthrodesis for failed total knee arthroplasty. *Orthopedics* 1998;21:875–879.
3. Deldycke J, Rommens P, Reynders P, et al. Primary arthrodesis of the injured knee: still a solution in 1994? Case Report. *J Trauma* 1994;37:862–866.
4. Green DP, Parkes JC, Stinchfield FE. Arthrodesis of the knee. A follow-up study. *J Bone Joint Surg Am* 1967;49:1065–1074.
5. Hak DJ, Lieberman JR, Finerman GA. Single plane and biplane external fixators for knee arthrodesis. *Clin Orthop* 1995;316:134–144.
6. Hessmann M, Gotzen L, Boumgaertal F. Knee arthrodesis with a unilateral external fixator. *Acta Chir Belg* 1996;96:123–127.
7. Arroyo JS, Garvin KL, Neff JR. Arthrodesis of the knee with a modular titanium intramedullary nail. *J Bone Joint Surg Am* 1997;79:26–35.
8. Henkel TR, Boldt JG, Drobny TK, et al. Total knee arthroplasty after formal knee fusion using unconstrained and semiconstrained components: a report of 7 cases. *J Arthroplasty* 2001;16:768–776.
9. Cameron HU. Results of total knee arthroplasty following takedown of formal knee fusion. *J Arthroplasty* 1996;11:732–737.
10. Kim JH, Kim JS, Cho SH. Total knee arthroplasty after spontaneous osseous ankylosis and takedown of formal knee fusion. *J Arthroplasty* 2000;15:453–460.
11. Stiehl JB, Hanel DP. Knee arthrodesis using combined intramedullary rod and plate fixation. *Clin Orthop* 1993;294:238–241.
12. Cheng SL, Gross AE. Knee arthrodesis using a short locked intramedullary nail. A new technique. *Am J Knee Surg* 1995;8:56–59.
13. Nichols SJ, Landon GC, Tullos HS. Arthrodesis with dual plates after failed total knee arthroplasty. *J Bone Joint Surg Am* 1991;73:1020–1024.
14. Rasmussen MR, Bishop AT, Wood MB. Arthrodesis of the knee with a vascularized fibular rotatory graft. *J Bone Joint Surg Am* 1995;77:751–759.
15. Donley BG, Matthews LS, Kaufer H. Arthrodesis of the knee with an intramedullary nail. *J Bone Joint Surg* 1991;73A:907–913.

CHAPTER 116

Total Knee Replacement—Future Perspectives

Jorge O. Galante

Total knee replacement has become one of the most successful procedures in orthopedic surgery. Developed after total hip replacement was already established, it plays a major role in the management of the patient with joint disabilities today. Although some of the basic principles of joint replacement are common to both the hip and the knee, many issues considered are different.

Since the inception of total knee replacement in the early 1970s (1), the devices have evolved from conceptually simplistic designs to more complex and more functional designs that in many instances attempt to replicate the anatomical features of the normal knee joint. In addition, instrumentation has been developed that allows reproducible limb alignment and precise component positioning. These innovations have resulted in prosthetic devices capable of providing reliable and reproducible functional performance, very satisfactory patient outcomes, and excellent survivorship (2–12).

Do we need new designs of total knee prostheses? There are a number of reasons to introduce a new design or to modify an existing one. They include market pressures, unmet functional needs, and design flaws in current implants that may limit the survival or the functional performance of a prosthetic device. Market pressures often constitute a powerful reason to induce a manufacturer to engage in the introduction of a new design. Although these pressures cannot be ignored (they are at the core of our economic system), design initiatives must address real needs and must incorporate sound, scientifically based principles and innovations.

There are a number of unresolved issues that require a legitimate effort in research toward the development of new and improved prosthetic devices. Thus, design concepts are still evolving in an attempt to address needs such as faster and easier postoperative rehabilitation, functional performance adequate for an active lifestyle, a larger range of motion in flexion, improved wear resistance, and long-term survival in the young and active patient. Achieving some of these goals is not an effort limited to the design of the prosthesis. It is often the result of the patient selection criteria, the surgical technique, and the rehabilitation process, in addition to the prosthetic design chosen.

For example, achieving consistently a high range of flexion (beyond 130 degrees) is a desirable outcome that might require some specific design features in the femoral and tibial component. A number of manufacturers have introduced or are in the process of developing such designs. Regardless of the prosthesis used, however, the preoperative range of motion is a variable that currently has an overwhelming influence on postoperative flexion. A patient with a limited preoperative range of flexion is likely to have a limited range of flexion postoperatively. Innovations in the surgical procedure are also important. For example, the operation should routinely include an extensive débridement of the posterior aspect of the femoral condyles and sometimes of the upper tibia. If that is thoroughly carried out, it is possible to significantly improve postoperative flexion using a conventional prosthesis. Finally, the postoperative rehabilitation regime can play an important role as well. Thus, prosthetic design is just one feature to be taken into account in achieving the goals of surgical reconstruction.

A requirement that has some bearing in the design of the prosthesis, the surgical instruments, and the surgical procedure is that of early hospital discharge and early rehabilitation. These are issues particularly attractive to the younger patient populations. The concept of minimally invasive surgery, a principle of increasing popularity in all surgical fields, has some definite application in this context. It has been introduced in unicompartmental arthroplasty. It will evolve as well into the area of tricompartmental replacement with the need to incorporate related new developments in prosthetic design and instrumentation.

A number of controversies have evolved and have resulted in a series of different concepts in the design and use of total knee replacements. These controversies are at the core of the future perspectives in the field. They include, among others, issues related to indications, fixation, the role of the posterior cruciate ligament, the patellofemoral joint, wear and the shape of the articular surfaces, modularity, and the relative advantages of mobile bearings.

INDICATIONS

Total knee replacement is indicated in patients with pain or disability, or both, resulting from major structural alteration of the knee joint (13). This includes conditions such as osteoarthritis, rheumatoid arthritis, posttraumatic arthritis, other arthritic conditions, chondrocalcinosis, some benign and malignant tumors, certain complex supracondylar or intracondylar fractures, and any other condition that results in a major destruction of the joint structures.

Active infection still constitutes an absolute contraindication. Although a total knee replacement is possible in a patient with a history of a previous knee infection, a sterile environment must be obtained before implantation to provide the best chances for a successful result (14).

Major skin loss or alterations in the local skin due to scars and other systemic or local conditions that would preclude primary healing of the wound are also relative contraindications. Appropriate grafting procedures, such as muscle pedicle grafts or vascularized skin flaps, can in the proper circumstances provide adequate skin cover and thus make the replacement feasible.

A successful total knee arthroplasty requires a functional quadriceps mechanism, and unless it can be restored, a knee replacement is contraindicated. Ligament instability per se is not a contraindication to a total knee replacement. Prosthetic devices incorporating various degrees of constraint depending on the type and degree of instability, from a posterior stabilized prosthesis to a constrained condylar device or a hinge, can provide the stability required for a satisfactory functional outcome.

Young age and a high level of physical activity have in the past been relative contraindications for the procedure. At the present time we have limited long-term prosthesis survival data in the young and active patient populations (15), although common sense would indicate that failure rates may be higher than in older, more sedentary patients. Furthermore, in contrast to total hip replacement, limited advances have been made in the last few years in understanding wear mechanisms in total knees, a major potential cause of long-term failure. Regardless of these considerations, there is a growing trend to implant total knee prostheses in younger and more active patients. This trend will continue to increase, as people in general become more active and as surgeons address the needs of younger patients. Prosthetic devices will need to be able to withstand increased functional demands. The development and introduction of wear-resistant surfaces, in addition to design innovations, are critical steps in this context to assure extended service lifetimes.

In the last few years, there has been a renewed interest in use of the unicompartmental prosthesis as a conservative approach to total knee arthroplasty for the more active patient with unicompartmental disease (16–31). It is often seen as an alternative to a high tibial osteotomy, with the expectation that, after some years of functional restoration, the conversion to a tricompartmental arthroplasty might be a relatively simple procedure with no additional potential complications (32). In this manner, the indications for replacement surgery are being extended today to a more active patient population.

FIXATION

Since the introduction of total hip replacement by Sir John Charnley in the 1960s (33), acrylic cement has played a fundamental role in the fixation of prosthetic components. It remains the most frequently used method of fixation in total knee replacement today.

Because of the real or perceived problems associated with the use of cement, a number of investigators developed cementless techniques of fixation (6,34–43). The basic principle is that laying a porous coating on the implant allows bone ingrowth into the open pore structure of the material, which provides biologic fixation and is capable of remodeling over time. Several porous composites have been developed and used clinically in knee replacements, with the largest experience available with those made from sintered cobalt-chromium beads, plasma-sprayed titanium, and sintered titanium fibers.

In the late 1960s, we developed a sintered fiber titanium composite made from unalloyed titanium wires (44). This material has interconnecting porosity, can be bonded to a solid metallic substrate, has desirable mechanical properties and excellent biocompatibility, and has proven to be an excellent substrate for bone ingrowth.

Given the ideal environment of close proximity to a living bone surface and minimal micromotion (45), bone formation within the open pore structure will begin within days. The bone will mature, will remodel, and can provide a superior method of biologic fixation for a prosthetic device (46,47).

There has been extensive experience with the use of this porous composite in total knee replacement. Autopsy retrievals of tibial components have shown reproducible bone ingrowth (48). Extensive bone ingrowth can be obtained on the femoral side as well.

The average extent of bone ingrowth in the tibia (49) was 35% with a characteristic distribution. The histologic appearance was typified by the presence of areas of bony ingrowth and areas in which infiltration by fibrous and granulation tissue was observed. In some cases, the granulation tissue appeared to progress from the periphery of the implant, but in many instances, granulation tissue advanced along the screws that had been used for initial fixation of the device.

Mechanical testing of the cementless tibial specimens revealed excellent stability, in the same range as that obtained when retrieved cemented prosthesis were tested using the same experimental protocol.

In spite of these encouraging laboratory and autopsy retrieval findings, our clinical experience with cementless fixation in total knee replacement using an early design (Miller-Galante I) was not as satisfactory (50). A tibial loosening rate of 8% and a 12% incidence of small osteolytic tibial lesions at a mean follow-up of 11 years were noted. Other investigators have reported mixed results with cementless fixation (40,41,51–57).

The use of acrylic cement, on the other hand, provides reliable and reproducible fixation both early and late, and today it is the method of choice in our institution. On the tibial side, excellent results have been reported with the use of cement, with an incidence of loosening of less than 2% (5,7,8,58). In our experience using a metal-backed modular prosthesis with four short pegs, the survivorship at 10 years with tibial loosening as an end point was 100% (59).

On the femoral side, loosening is a rare event with either cement or cementless techniques. If revision becomes necessary, however, the removal of a well-fixed cementless femoral component can result in appreciable bone loss on the femoral side, as a consequence of the severe osteoporosis that develops underneath an ingrown femoral component. When cement is used, this is not the case, which makes potential revision of a cemented femoral component an easier and safer undertaking.

On the patellar side, cement should be used routinely, as cementing an all-polyethylene patella represents, today, the best alternative.

The use of cementless fixation in total knee replacements is still of interest to many surgeons and may well increase in the future. Designs that do not use screws for initial fixation would be desirable, as this would eliminate potential pathways for transfer of particles from the joint to the bone interface. Nonmodular designs can have some advantages in this context, and porous nonmodular tibial components are available. Of course, with this approach, the advantages of modularity are lost, and I believe that modularity is an important feature, in particular for the young patient, in whom biologic fixation might be considered.

The addition to the porous surface of bioactive coatings capable of enhancing the phenomena of bone ingrowth is another strategy that may have an impact on future practices.

POSTERIOR CRUCIATE LIGAMENT

One area of controversy in total knee replacement relates to the preservation or substitution of the posterior cruciate ligament and its impact on prosthetic design, implantation procedures, and functional performance. In spite of the various arguments put forward for either preservation or substitution, however, reported intermediate and long-term clinical results are similar with both approaches (5,10,41,60).

It has been argued that retention of the posterior cruciate ligament results in improved knee kinematics, improved quadriceps strength, better stair-climbing ability, better stability, and probably the retention of some degree of proprioception (61).

From a practical viewpoint, an important consideration is that retaining the posterior cruciate ligament allows the surgeon to preserve additional bone stock. In the femur, bone is saved in the intercondylar notch; in the upper end of the tibia, bone can be preserved with the use of a tibial tray with short pegs, without a central stem. We have had extensive experience with that type of design in a cemented application, with excellent long-term prosthesis survival.

The posterior cruciate ligament is one of the important anatomical structures influencing the kinematics of the human knee. It affects femoral rollback, one of the critical parameters of knee function. The posterior displacement of the femoral condyles during flexion increases the lever arm of the quadriceps mechanism and thus improves its mechanical efficiency. This effect is most important in stair climbing and other similar activities of daily living (62).

The critical issue in posterior cruciate ligament retention is to maintain adequate tension. If the ligament is too tense, the result may be limited flexion, posterior polyethylene wear, a rocking force on the tibia, and high fixation stresses with a potential for eventual component loosening. If the ligament is too lax, there could be anterior posterior instability leading to an unsatisfactory clinical result. Appropriate ligament tension is a function of both prosthetic design and surgical technique.

There are some elements of component design that are critical to allow appropriate tension and function of the posterior cruciate ligament. Restoration of the anteroposterior dimensions of the femur is one essential requirement. Thus the prosthetic system must provide adequate femoral sizes to restore normal kinematics. Given the size distribution in a normal population, a minimum of nine different femoral component sizes are probably required to provide for adequate reproduction of the anteroposterior dimensions of the femur. This then allows an accurate restoration of the flexion space, one of the key elements.

The femoral rollback is asymmetric; that is to say, the lateral femoral condyle displaces further than the medial condyle. In addition to the influence of the posterior cruciate ligament, the difference in radius between the medial and lateral condyles makes possible this asymmetric rollback. The medial condyle has a smaller radius than the lateral condyle, another important element in prosthetic design.

Because of the need for rollback and rotation, excessive constraint and conformity are not desirable in a cruciate-retaining prosthesis. A large radius of curvature on the articular surfaces of both the tibia and the femur, in the sagittal and in the frontal planes, is desirable to allow the displacement required for restoration of good kinematics. For the same reasons, a posterior slope in the tibial cut of 7 to 10 degrees is preferable to avoid a progressive increase in ligament tension as the knee goes into flexion.

Use of a prosthesis adhering to these design principles, coupled with the appropriate surgical technique, allows the surgeon to preserve the posterior cruciate ligament with its appropriate tension and, thus, its appropriate function in the vast majority of patients. The implication from a prosthetic design viewpoint is that the replication of the anatomical features of the normal human knee with the purpose of replicating the normal kinematics is an intrinsic element of most current and future cruciate-retaining prosthetic designs.

Similar considerations may be applied to some of the criteria used for the design of posterior cruciate–substituting devices. In this instance, however, increased constraint and conformity can be incorporated, as these designs do not require or do not allow the reproduction of normal kinematics.

There are some patients who are poor candidates for cruciate-retaining designs. The posterior cruciate ligament is difficult to balance in severely deformed knees, in those with a significant flexion contracture, or in knees with severe varus deformity. It is also difficult to preserve in those patients who have a valgus deformity with an incompetent medial collateral ligament.

PATELLAR REPLACEMENT

Should the patella routinely be replaced in total knee arthroplasty? Many surgeons have adopted the principle of not replacing the patella, based on the high incidence of patellofemoral complications that characterized some of the earlier prosthetic designs. These problems were related to a number of variables that have been addressed, to a large extent, by most contemporary designs and by the currently accepted principles of surgical technique (63–65).

Metal backing, a design feature that led to delamination of the polyethylene and eventual failure (66,67), has been abandoned, for the most part, in exchange for the routine used of a cemented all-polyethylene implant. The shape of the femoral component must replicate the anatomical features of the normal femur to restore the kinematics of the patellofemoral joint and allow the patella to track along a normal path (64). Contemporary femoral designs should incorporate those features in the trochlear groove profile. In the frontal plane, the femoral trochlea should allow for the mediolateral translation of the patella that takes place in the course of flexion-extension motion. In the sagittal plane, the patella tracks backward, and hence an adequate resection of bone from the anterior femoral condyles is required to allow for the appropriate shape of the femoral prosthesis.

Appropriate external rotation of the femoral component is now an accepted principle of surgical technique and a critical method of ensuring appropriate patellar tracking (68,69). Adherence to the proper surgical technique and the incorporation of the key design features referred to earlier have led today to a minimal incidence of patellofemoral complications.

Patients without a patellar replacement may experience more pain, particularly in stair climbing and some other complex activities of daily living other than walking, and may exhibit less strength in their quadriceps compared to patients in whom the patella was replaced. For these reasons, the author believes that patellar replacement should be routinely performed using a prosthetic device that replicates normal anatomical structures, a practice that will continue to prevail in the future.

WEAR

Wear of the polyethylene insert and the resulting biologic complications, granuloma formation, and periprosthetic osteolysis are considered to be the most devastating long-term events in total joint arthroplasty. This is certainly true for the hip, in which osteolysis is a serious limiting complication, particularly in the young (and therefore active) patient population.

Severe wear, osteolysis, and subsequent loosening have been infrequently reported in total knee arthroplasty (52,53,55,56, 58,70–74). These phenomena have been associated with some design features and with specific ultrahigh molecular weight polyethylene resins, manufacturing methods, or sterilization techniques. In contrast to hip prostheses, the magnitude and the mechanism of wear in total knee prostheses are still a matter of considerable discussion (75–82). At the present time, in vitro wear testing of total knee prostheses has some significant limitations. Although most wear tests replicate the type of motion and loads seen in level walking, the knee is exposed to different demands and conditions during function, including higher degrees of flexion and varying rotations under changing muscle and weightbearing-generated loads. Thus in vitro wear tests should incorporate these kinematic events to provide a more realistic evaluation of the in vivo mechanism of wear.

Even in the more semiconstrained designs in total knee devices, the degree of congruity between the articulating surfaces is relative. A combination of rolling and sliding dominates the relative types of motion between these surfaces (83), and surface fatigue consequently plays a dominant role. This is in contrast to hip prostheses, in which an adhesive-abrasive wear mechanism is prevalent.

The most commonly seen types of surface damage are dimensional change, pitting, and delamination (76,78,79,84–86).

Dimensional change may be a product of creep or of actual material loss (87,88), but this is difficult to elucidate in radiologic or retrieval studies. Pitting and delamination produce relatively larger wear particles than those seen in total hip replacements (77). These particles are less biologically active and are less likely to be phagocytized. They have lesser capacity to induce cell activation, granuloma formation, and bone resorption.

Cruciate-retaining designs require less constraint at the articular surfaces. This allows for asymmetric femoral rollback and other more complex motions imposed by the presence of the posterior cruciate ligament, the shape of the articular surfaces, and the effect of agonist and antagonist muscle activity. Thus, large radii of curvature and somewhat flatter tibial surfaces are desirable. In contrast, in posterior cruciate–substituting designs, a higher degree of constraint and congruence is possible.

The assumption that higher congruence and thus a larger contact area with a corresponding decrease in contact stresses will decrease wear may not be valid (89,90). Although retrieval studies show less surface delamination in more constrained designs, other types of surface damage are more prevalent, including pitting, edge loading, and damage at the stabilizing peg, which may produce a larger degree of material loss from the surface. The method of fabrication, type of resin used, method of sterilization, and surgical factors such as malrotation of the prosthetic components may be variables of more importance than the shape of the articular surfaces in the generation and severity of the wear process (75,79,82).

Another potential source of wear debris is the nonarticular surface in modular designs (91,92). Motion at this interface is capable of creating very small wear particles with high potential for granuloma formation and production of osteolysis. Thus, an important consideration in present and future prosthetic design is the creation of stability and lack of relative motion at modular interfaces.

An alternative is the implantation of nonmodular devices. Although their use is appealing from a theoretical viewpoint, the advantages of modularity are such that the author believes it will remain an intrinsic feature of tibial designs. It is an advantage for the surgeon, as it allows versatility in the operative procedure. It is an advantage for the patient, as it makes possible an exchange of the articular surface without the need for a complete revision should the surface wear. It is an advantage for the hospital and for the manufacturer as it decreases the size of the required inventory.

Highly cross-linked ultrahigh molecular weight resin is now used in total hip replacements and has been introduced as an improved articulating wear-resistant surface in total knee prostheses. Although the preliminary laboratory wear data are encouraging, the mechanical environment is very different in the knee than in the hip, and we do not yet have enough clinical information to ascertain its advantages in practical use. Unfortunately, several years will be required before longer term clinical information becomes available.

The potential for a highly wear-resistant surface is intriguing, as a change in indications becomes more reasonable, which makes implantation possible in younger and more active individuals with considerably higher functional demands.

MOBILE BEARINGS

The premise leading to the development and introduction of mobile bearings in total knee prostheses was the potential for decreasing wear and providing improvements in functional performance. It is not clear that at the present time mobile bearings fulfill either of these two objectives.

At best, mobile bearings or rotating platforms exhibit survivorship levels and functional performance that are comparable to those seen in fixed bearings (2,6,17,25,93–96). In addition, a number of complications are possible, including dislocation and failure of the mobile part (97). From a theoretical viewpoint, a large surface area with near total congruence can be obtained. Thus the assumption was made that substantial improvements in wear resistance can be derived (89). These very conforming surface features, however, may lead to an adhesive-abrasive mechanism of wear capable of generating very small, biologically reactive wear particles at either one of the two articulating surfaces. Thus the potential for biologic wear–related failure modes, such as osteolysis, may well be enhanced in the long term. The author's own perception is that at the present time mobile bearings do not offer enough distinct advantages to overcome their potential drawbacks.

CONCLUSION

Total knee replacement has evolved over the last three decades into a reliable and reproducible reconstruction method for patients with knee joint disability. Excellent survival times have been reported with a very satisfactory functional performance for a number of prosthetic systems.

The patient selection criteria have progressively changed, and younger, more active patients are being considered as candidates for the procedure. These patients have higher expectations and are eager in many instances to resume a normal lifestyle, including participation in recreational activities such as running, jumping, cycling, and a number of other sports. Higher functional demands are expected from this patient population, and thus new requirements are being placed on the prosthetic devices. The goals at hand include a faster and easier postoperative rehabilitation process, functional performance adequate for an active lifestyle, and long-term prosthesis survivorship in the young and active patient.

Improved wear resistance, the ability to reproduce the normal kinematics through a full range of motion, and the possibility of using a simpler, less invasive surgical procedure are necessary to achieve those goals. Thus, we witness the introduction of highly cross-linked ultrahigh molecular weight polyethylene as a wear-resistant articular surface. Prosthetic designs increasingly incorporate the morphologic features of the normal knee to allow for the interactions between prosthesis, ligaments, and muscles that are necessary to replicate normal kinematics and obtain the highest degree of satisfactory functional performance. In addition, the development of surgical techniques, instrumentation, and modified prosthetic devices will make possible the incorporation of minimally invasive approaches in total knee replacement as a means of decreasing morbidity and expediting the rehabilitation process.

REFERENCES

1. Gunston PH. Polycentric knee arthroplasty: prosthetic simulation of normal knee movement. *J Bone Joint Surg Am* 1979;53:272–275.
2. Buechel FF, Pappas MJ. Long-term survivorship analysis of cruciate-sparing versus cruciate-sacrificing knee prostheses using meniscal bearings. *Clin Orthop* 1990;260:162–169.
3. Callaghan JJ, Squire MW, Goetz DD, et al. Cemented rotating-platform total knee replacement: a nine to twelve-year follow-up study. *J Bone Joint Surg Am* 1995;77:1713–1720.
4. Dennis DA, Clayton ML, O'Donnell S, et al. Posterior cruciate condylar total knee arthroplasty: average 11 year follow-up. *Clin Orthop* 1992;281:168–176.
5. Font-Rodriguez DE, Scuderi GR, Insall JN. Survivorship of cemented total knee arthroplasty. *Clin Orthop* 1997;345:79–86.
6. Jordan LR, Olivo JL, Voorhorst PE. Survivorship analysis of cementless meniscal bearing total knee arthroplasty. *Clin Orthop* 1997;338:119–123.
7. Malkani AL, Rand JA, Bryan RS, et al. Total knee arthroplasty with the kinematic condylar prosthesis. *J Bone Joint Surg Am* 1995;77:423–431.
8. Ranawat CS, Flynn WF, Saddler S, et al. Long term results of the total condylar knee arthroplasty: a 15 year survivorship study. *Clin Orthop* 1993;286:94–102.
9. Ritter MA, Campbell E, Farris PM, et al. Long term survival analysis of the posterior cruciate condylar total knee arthroplasty: 10 year evaluation. *J Arthroplasty* 1989;4:293–296.
10. Schai PA, Thornhill TS, Scott RD. Total knee arthroplasty with the PFC system: results at a minimum of ten years and survivorship analysis. *J Bone Joint Surg Br* 1998;80:850–858.
11. Stern SH, Insall JN. Posterior stabilized prosthesis: results after follow-up of nine to twelve years. *J Bone Joint Surg Am* 1992;74:980–986.
12. Vince KG, Insall JN, Kelly MA. The total condylar prosthesis: 10–12 year results of a cemented knee replacement. *J Bone Joint Surg Br* 1989;71:793–797.
13. Insall JN. Total knee replacement. In: Insall JN, ed. *Surgery of the knee.* New York: Churchill Livingstone, 1993:719–721.
14. Backe HA, Wolff DA, Windsor RE. Total knee replacement after 2-stage reimplantation. *Clin Orthop* 1996;331:125–131.
15. Diduch DR, Insall JN, Scott WN, et al. Total knee replacement in young, active patients: long-term follow-up and functional outcome. *J Bone Joint Surg Am* 1997;79:575–582.
16. Capra SWI, Fehring TK. Unicondylar arthroplasty: a survivorship analysis. *J Arthroplasty* 1992;7:247–251.
17. Carr A, Keyes G, Miller R, et al. Medial unicompartmental arthroplasty. A survival study of the Oxford meniscal knee. *Clin Orthop* 1993;295:205–213.
18. Cartier P, Sanouiller JL. Marmor unicompartmental knee arthroplasty. In: Cartier P, ed. *Unicompartmental knee arthroplasty.* Paris: Expansion Scientifique Française, 1997:167–173.
19. Chassin EP, Mikosz RP, Andriacchi TP, et al. Functional analysis of cemented medial unicompartmental knee arthroplasty. *J Arthroplasty* 1996;11:553–559.
20. Christensen NO. Unicompartmental prosthesis for gonarthrosis. A nine-year series of 575 knees from a Swedish hospital. *Clin Orthop* 1991;273:165–169.
21. Deshmukh RV, Scott RD. Unicompartmental knee arthroplasty: long-term results. *Clin Orthop* 2001;392:272–278.
22. Heck DA, Marmor L, Gibson A, et al. Unicompartmental knee arthroplasty. A multicenter investigation with long-term follow up evaluation. *Clin Orthop* 1993;286:154–159.
23. Kozinn SC, Scott RD. Current concepts review: unicondylar knee arthroplasty. *J Bone Joint Surg Am* 1989;71:145–150.
24. Laurencin CT, Zelicof SB, Scott RD, et al. Unicompartmental versus total knee arthroplasty in the same patient: a comparative study. *Clin Orthop* 1991;273:151–156.
25. Lewold S, Goodman S, Knutson K, et al. Oxford meniscal bearing knee versus the Marmor knee in unicompartmental arthroplasty for arthrosis: a Swedish multicenter survival study. *J Arthroplasty* 1995;10:722–731.
26. Marmor L. Unicompartmental knee arthroplasty. 10 to 13 year follow up study. *Clin Orthop* 1988;226:14–20.
27. Murray DW, Goodfellow JW, O'Connor JJ. The Oxford medial unicompartmental arthroplasty: a ten year survival study. *J Bone Joint Surg Br* 1998;80:983–989.
28. Scott RD, Cobb AG, McQueary FG, et al. Unicompartmental knee arthroplasty. Eight- to 12-year followup evaluation with survivorship analysis. *Clin Orthop* 1991;271:96–100.
29. Stenstrom A, Lindstrand A, Lewold S. Unicompartmental knee arthroplasty with special reference to the Swedish Knee Arthroplasty Register. In: Cartier P, ed. *Unicompartmental knee arthroplasty.* Paris: Expansion Scientifique Française, 1997:159–162.

30. Thornhill TS, Scott RD. Unicompartmental knee arthroplasty. *Orthop Clin North Am* 1989;20:245–256.

31. Weale AE, Murray DW, Crawford R, et al. Does arthritis progress in the retained compartments after "Oxford" medial unicompartmental arthroplasty? A clinical and radiological study with a minimum ten-year follow-up. *J Bone Joint Surg Br* 1999;81:783–789.

32. Jackson M, Sarangi PP, Newman JH. Revision total knee arthroplasty. Comparison of outcome following primary proximal tibial osteotomy or unicompartmental arthroplasty. *J Arthroplasty* 1994;9:539–542.

33. Charnley J. *Low friction arthroplasty of the hip—theory and practices.* New York: Springer-Verlag, 1979.

34. Dodd CAF, Hungerfold DS, Krackow KA. Total knee arthroplasty fixation: comparison of the early results of paired cemented versus uncemented porous coated anatomic knee prostheses. *Clin Orthop* 1990;260:66–70.

35. Joseph J, Kaufman EE. Preliminary results of Miller-Galante uncemented total knee arthroplasty. *Orthopedics* 1990;13:511–516.

36. Kim YH. Knee arthroplasty using a cementless PCA prosthesis with a porous coated central tibial stem. *J Bone Joint Surg Br* 1990;72:412–417.

37. Landon GC, Galante JO, Maley MM. Noncemented total knee arthroplasty. *Clin Orthop* 1986;205:49–57.

38. Miura H, Whiteside LA, Easley JC, et al. Effects of screws and sleeve on initial fixation in uncemented total knee tibial components. *Clin Orthop* 1990;259:160–168.

39. Moran CG, Pinder IM, Lees TA, et al. Survivorship analysis of the uncemented porous-coated anatomic knee replacement. *J Bone Joint Surg Am* 1991;73:848–857.

40. Rand JA. Cement or cementless fixation in total knee arthroplasty? *Clin Orthop* 1991;273:52–62.

41. Rorabeck CH, Bourne RB, Lewis PL, et al. The Miller-Galante knee prosthesis for the treatment of osteoarthrosis: a comparison of the results of partial fixation with cement and fixation without any cement. *J Bone Joint Surg Am* 1993;75:402–408.

42. Rosenberg AG, Galante JO. Cementless total knee arthroplasty. In: Insall JN, ed. *Surgery of the knee.* New York: Churchill Livingstone, 1993:869–890.

43. Whiteside LA. Four screws for fixation of the tibial component in cementless total knee arthroplasty. *Clin Orthop* 1994;299:72–76.

44. Galante JO, Rostoker W, Lueck R, et al. Sintered fiber metal composites as a basis for attachment of implants to bone. *J Bone Joint Surg Am* 1971;53:101–114.

45. Pilliar RM, Lee JM, Maniatopoulos C. Observations on the effect of movement on bone ingrowth into porous surfaced implants. *Clin Orthop* 1986;208:108–113.

46. Turner TM, Urban RM, Sumner DR, et al. Bone ingrowth in the tibial component of a canine total condylar knee replacement prosthesis. *J Orthop Res* 1989;7:893–901.

47. Volz RG, Nisbet JK, Lee RW, et al. The mechanical stability of various noncemented tibial components. *Clin Orthop* 1988;226:38–42.

48. Jacobs JJ, Sumner DR, Urban RM, et al. Retrieval of successful uncemented implants. In: Morrey BF, ed. *Biological, material and mechanical considerations of joint replacement.* New York: Raven Press, 1993:185–196.

49. Sapienza CI, Urban RM, Jacobs JJ, et al. Patterns of bone ingrowth and osteolysis in cementless total knee replacement tibial components retrieved at autopsy. *Orthop Trans* 1997;21:57–58.

50. Berger RA, Lyon JH, Jacobs JJ, et al. Problems with cementless total knee arthroplasty at 11 years follow up. *Clin Orthop* 2001;392:196–207.

51. Collins DN, Heim SA, Nelson CL, et al. Porous coated anatomic total knee arthroplasty: a prospective analysis comparing cemented and cementless fixation. *Clin Orthop* 1991;267:128–136.

52. Han C, Choe W, Yoo J. Effect of polyethylene wear on osteolysis in cementless primary total hip arthroplasty: minimal 5-year follow-up study. *J Arthroplasty* 1999;14:714–723.

53. Lewonowske K, Dorr LD. Revision of cementless total knee arthroplasty with massive osteolytic lesions. *J Arthroplasty* 1994;9:661–663.

54. Nafei A, Nielson S, Kristensen O, et al. The press-fit Kinemax knee arthroplasty: high failure of noncemented implants. *J Bone Joint Surg Br* 1992;74:243–246.

55. Nolan JF, Bucknill TM. Aggressive granulomatosis from polyethylene failure in an uncemented knee replacement. *J Bone Joint Surg Br* 1992;74:23–24.

56. Peters PC, Engh GA, Dwyer KA, et al. Osteolysis after total knee arthroplasty without cement. *J Bone Joint Surg Am* 1992;74:864–876.

57. Rorabeck CH, Bourne RB, Nott L. The cemented Kinematic-II and the non-cemented porous coated anatomic prosthesis for total knee replacement. *J Bone Joint Surg Am* 1988;70:483–490.

58. Colizza WA, Insall JN, Scuderi GR. The posterior stabilized total knee prosthesis: assessment of polyethylene damage and osteolysis after a ten year minimum follow-up. *J Bone Joint Surg Am* 1995;77:1713–1720.

59. Berger RA, Rosenberg A, Barden R, et al. Long term followup of the MG total knee arthroplasty. *Clin Orthop* 2001;388:58–67.

60. Clark CR, Rorabeck CH, MacDonald S, et al. Posterior-stabilized and cruciate-retaining total knee replacement: a randomized study. *Clin Orthop* 2001;392:208–212.

61. Brugioni DJ, Andriacchi TP, Galante JO. A functional and radiographic analysis of the total condylar knee arthroplasty. *J Arthroplasty* 1990;5:173–180.

62. Andriacchi TP, Galante JO, Fermier RW. The influence of total knee replacement design on walking and stair climbing. *J Bone Joint Surg Am* 1982;64:1328–1335.

63. Abraham W, Buchanan JR, Daubert H, et al. Should the patella be resurfaced in total knee arthroplasty? Efficacy of patella resurfacing. *Clin Orthop* 1988;236:128–134.

64. Andriacchi TP, Yoder D, Conley A, et al. Patellofemoral design influences function following total knee arthroplasty. *J Arthroplasty* 1997;12:243–249.

65. Barrack RL, Wolfe MW, Waldman DA, et al. Resurfacing of the patella in total knee arthroplasty. A prospective, randomized, double-blind study. *J Bone Joint Surg Am* 1997;79:1121–1131.

66. Rosenberg AG, Andriacchi TP, Barden R, et al. Patellar component failure in cementless total knee arthroplasty. *Clin Orthop* 1988;236:106–114.

67. Stulberg SD, Stulberg BN, Hamati Y, et al. Failure mechanisms of metal-backed patellar components. *Clin Orthop* 1988; 236:88–105.

68. Griffin FM, Math K, Scuderi GR, et al. Anatomy of the epicondyles of the distal femur: MRI analysis of normal knees. *J Arthroplasty* 2000;15:354–359.

69. Miller M, Berger R, Petrella A, et al. Optimizing femoral component rotation in total knee arthroplasty. *Clin Orthop* 2001;392:38–45.

70. Cadambi A, Engh GA, Dwyer KA, et al. Osteolysis of the distal femur after total knee arthroplasty. *J Arthroplasty* 1994;9:579–594.

71. Engh G, Dwyer K, Hanes C. Polyethylene wear of metal backed tibial components in total and unicompartmental knee prostheses. *J Bone Joint Surg Br* 1992;74:9–17.

72. Gross TP, Lennox DW. Osteolytic cyst-like area associated with polyethylene and metallic debris after total knee replacement with uncemented vitallium prosthesis. *J Bone Joint Surg Am* 1992;74:1096–1101.

73. Gustafson A, Clark IC, Saha S. Catastrophic peri-implant bone loss caused by polyethylene and metallic wear in total knees. *J Long Term Eff Med Implants* 1993;3:91–104.

74. Knezevich S, Vaughn BK, Lombardi AW, et al. Failure of polyethylene tibial component of a TKR associated with aseptic loosening secondary to polyethylene and metallic wear debris. *Orthopedics* 1993;16:1136–1140.

75. Benjamin J, Szivek J, Dersam G, et al. Linear and volumetric wear of tibial inserts in posterior cruciate-retaining knee arthroplasties. *Clin Orthop* 2001;392:131–138.

76. Collier J, Mayor M, McNamara J, et al. Analysis of the failure of 122 polyethylene inserts from uncemented tibial knee components. *Clin Orthop* 1991;273:232–242.

77. Hirakawa K, Bauer T, Yamaguchi M, et al. Relationship between wear debris particles and polyethylene surface damage in primary total knee arthroplasty. *J Arthroplasty* 1999;13:165–171.

78. Hood RW, Wright TM, Burnstein AH. Retrieval analysis of total knee prosthesis: a method and application to 48 total condylar prostheses. *J Biomed Mater Res* 1983;17:829–842.

79. Landy M, Walker P. Wear of ultra-high-molecular-weight polyethylene components of 90 retrieved knee prostheses. *J Arthroplasty* 1988;3[Suppl]:73–85.

80. Lavernia C, Guzman J, Kabo M, et al. Polyethylene wear in autopsy retrieved fully functional total knee replacement. In: *Proceedings of*

the Sixtieth Meeting of the American Academy of Orthopaedic Surgeons. Rosemont, IL: American Academy of Orthopaedic Surgeons, 1993:273.

81. Lewis P, Rorabeck C, Bourne R, et al. Posteromedial tibial polyethylene failure in total knee replacements. *Clin Orthop* 1994;299:11–17.

82. Wasielewski F, Galante J, Leithty R, et al. Wear patterns on retrieved polyethylene tibial inserts and their relationship to technical considerations during total knee arthroplasty. *Clin Orthop* 1994;299:31–43.

83. Blunn G, Walker P, Atul J, et al. The dominance of cyclic sliding in producing wear in total knee replacements. *Clin Orthop* 1991;273:253–260.

84. Hoshino A, Fukuoka Y, Ishida A. Accurate in-vivo measurement of polyethylene wear in total knee arthroplasty. In: *Proceedings of the Sixty-seventh Meeting of the American Academy of Orthopaedic Surgeons*. Rosemont, IL: American Academy of Orthopaedic Surgeons, 2000:362.

85. Jones S, Pinder I, Moran C, et al. Polyethylene wear in uncemented knee replacements. *J Bone Joint Surg Br* 1992;74:18–22.

86. Wright T, Rimnac C, Stulberg D, et al. Wear of polyethylene in total joint replacement: observations from retrieved PCA knee implants. *Clin Orthop* 1992;276:126–134.

87. Edidin A, Pruitt L, Jewett C, et al. Plasticity-induced damage layer is a precursor to wear in radiation-cross-linked UHMWPE acetabular components for total hip replacement. *J Arthroplasty* 1999;14:616–627.

88. Sychterz C, Engh CA, Yang A, et al. Analysis of temporal wear patterns of porous-coated acetabular components: distinguishing between true wear and so-called bedding-in. *J Bone Joint Surg Am* 1999;81:821–830.

89. Psychoyios V, Crawford RW, O'Connor JJ, et al. Wear of congruent meniscal bearings in unicompartmental knee arthroplasty: a retrieval study of 16 specimens. *J Bone Joint Surg Br* 1998;80:976–982.

90. Ritter M, Worland R, Saliske J, et al. Flat on flat, non-constrained compression molded polyethylene total knee replacement. *Clin Orthop* 1995;321:79–85.

91. Parks NL, Engh GA, Topoleski LD, et al. Modular tibial insert micromotion: a concern with contemporary knee implants. *Clin Orthop* 1998;356:10–15.

92. Shepard M, Lieberman J, Kabo M. Ultra-high molecular weight polyethylene wear: an in-vitro comparison of acetabular metal types and polished surfaces. *J Arthroplasty* 1999;14:860–866.

93. Callaghan JJ. Mobile-bearing knee replacement: clinical results. A review of the literature. *Clin Orthop* 2001;392:221–225.

94. Callaghan JJ, Insall JN, Greenwald AS, et al. Mobile-bearing knee replacement: concepts and results. *J Bone Joint Surg Am* 2000;82:1020–1041.

95. Kim YH, Kook HK, Kim JS. Comparison of fixed-bearing and mobile-bearing total knee arthroplasties. *Clin Orthop* 2001;392:101–115.

96. Sorrells RB. The rotating platform mobile-bearing TKA. *Orthopedics* 1996;19:793–796.

97. Weaver JK, Derkash RS, Greenwald AS. Difficulties with bearing dislocation and breakage using a movable bearing total knee replacement system. *Clin Orthop* 1993;290:244–252.

CHAPTER 117

Management of Knee Ligament Injuries— Future Perspectives

Bertram Zarins

Concepts regarding the treatment of torn knee ligaments that have come and gone in the past 50 years include cast immobilization of acutely injured knees, dynamic operations to stabilize knees (whereby muscles or tendons were transferred to substitute for torn ligaments), primary surgical repair of torn medial collateral ligaments, extraarticular reconstruction of torn anterior cruciate ligaments, primary suturing of torn anterior cruciate ligaments, "olecranization" of the tibia to correct posterior knee instability, temporary transarticular skeletal fixation of dislocated knees after repair, classification of rotatory instabilities, and use of xenografts, synthetic prosthetic ligaments, scaffolds for ingrowth of ligaments, ligament augmentation devices, operating arthroscopes, needle arthroscopes, and wide notchplasty.

More recently developed concepts that have so far withstood the test of time include early motion after knee injury or surgery, continuous passive motion, accelerated postoperative rehabilitation, nonoperative treatment of torn medial collateral ligaments, arthroscopically assisted anterior and posterior cruciate ligament replacement, interference screw fixation, biodegradable fixation devices, use of allografts, partial meniscectomy, meniscus repairs, and emphasis on performing anatomically and biomechanically correct ligament operations (rather than functional procedures).

The long-term efficacy of several procedures currently in use is either controversial or undetermined. These include lateral retinacular release, autologous chondrocyte implantation, allograft meniscus transplantation, laser and heat ablation chondroplasty, other applications of heat and radio-frequency devices, and thermal shrinkage of torn or stretched anterior cruciate ligaments.

The evolution of arthroscopic operative techniques has endangered open knee surgery and the survival of the requisite surgical skills. Recently trained surgeons have not performed many knee arthrotomies. This problem is compounded by the reduced emphasis on anatomy in medical schools today compared with the past. Therefore, many young orthopedic surgeons today have a deficit in knowledge of surgical anatomy and open operative procedures.

The dizzying changes in concepts regarding the treatment of knee ligament injuries that occurred from the 1970s through the early 1990s have given way to a period of relative calm. Not much new information is being added now, but recently developed ideas are being refined. It is hard to imagine that the next 25 years will bring as much new knowledge as did the 25 years that have just passed. One can look at what is on the horizon today, however, and speculate as to what we might be doing in the future.

DIAGNOSIS AND IMAGING

Imaging techniques such as magnetic resonance imaging (MRI) and computerized tomography as well as arthroscopy have greatly increased our knowledge of knee anatomy, physiology, and pathology. Current MRI scanners have the capabilities for displaying normal cruciate and collateral ligaments in all patients and can usually aid in the accurate discrimination of partial ligament tears from complete ruptures. Associated lesions are routinely identified, including focal articular cartilage defects and occult bone contusions or unsuspected fractures in patients who have negative findings on radiographs. Further advances in MRI technology will improve our ability to evaluate knee function. Kinematic MRI can show real-time movements in ligaments, menisci, and osseous structures, and allow computer modeling of joint motion in preparation for ligament reconstruction. In the future, dedicated extremity scanners in orthopedic offices may have the same capabilities of high-resolution imaging as current high-field scanners.

COMPUTER-ASSISTED SURGERY

Three-dimensional reconstruction of computed tomographic images and real-time fluoroscopy can be used in the operating room to aid in surgery (1). There are other applications of virtual reality that could be used in orthopedics. Combined with robotics, these will probably change the way we operate (2).

Arthroscopic simulators are being developed that will be similar to flight simulators currently used to train airplane pilots. The American Academy of Orthopaedic Surgeons has an ad hoc Committee on Virtual Reality that is working with industry to promote the development of an arthroscopic knee simulator (3). The simulator will be used to train residents in the skills of arthroscopy and to measure the skills that are learned.

Teleimmersion is a new telecommunications medium that combines virtual reality with video conferencing. It creates the illusion that users in different physical spaces are in the same location. Teleimmersion will change the way we attend conferences, communicate with each other, and teach (4).

TISSUE ENGINEERING

Tissue engineering integrates life sciences such as cell biology, biochemistry, and bioengineering with surgery to assemble regenerative musculoskeletal tissue. The three basic components of tissue engineering are the cells, the extracellular matrix or scaffold, and the signaling system or growth factors. Inductive bioactive factors (such as proteins or genes) influence the direction and sequence of the regenerative process (5–8).

The potential benefits of tissue engineering are accelerated healing of acute injuries, predictable restoration of normal structure and function, and regeneration of absent or injured tissues (9). Methods that are being studied to promote ligament and tendon healing include use of growth factors, gene therapy, and cell transplants; use of matrix guides for repair, remodeling, and structural stability; and mechanical loading.

The future direction of tissue engineering for meniscal regeneration will probably be a combination of a biomechanically functional scaffold with either pluripotential or committed cells and inductive agents (10).

The use of molecular genetics to study genes related to skeletal disease, also termed the orthopedic genome, is progressing rapidly. A clinical trial conducted by Dr. James Herndon and his co-workers in Pittsburgh has shown for the first time that gene therapy may be of use in orthopedics. Researchers were able to deliver antiarthritic genes into the hands of patients who had severe rheumatoid arthritis (11). This new technology undoubtedly will eventually be used to study knee ligaments.

A study has explored the efficacy of small intestine submucosa as a scaffold for tissue-engineered rotator cuff tendons in dogs (12). The theory was that the submucosal implant would

act as a biologic scaffold to induce the regeneration of resected rotator cuff tendons. Clinical studies have not been done, but further research will be forthcoming. The track record of xenograft tissue in the past, however, has not been good.

Bone morphogenic proteins (BMPs) have been shown to elicit bone formation in ectopic sites and to heal segmental bone defects in animals. Some of the cellular and molecular mechanisms of BMPs have been elucidated (13). The BMPs bind to the mesenchymal cell surface receptors. The expression of the genes leads to the synthesis of macromolecules involved in cartilage and bone formation. The mesenchymal cell thus becomes a chondrocyte or an osteoblast. It is possible that similar substances will be found for ligaments (8). There has been a report that enhanced cartilage-derived morphogenic protein 2 (CDMP-2), or BMP-13, improves healing in a transected rat Achilles tendon (14).

In the field of cell therapy, only one product has been approved by the U.S. Food and Drug Administration for use in the United States: autologous chondrocyte implantation (15). Approval was gained by taking advantage of the regulation on "minimal manipulation." A patient's cells were removed, multiplied outside the body, and then returned to the same patient.

Dunn et al. in 1992 reported successful replacement of the anterior cruciate ligament in rabbits by a cross-linked collagen prosthesis (16). It is possible that this is one direction for the development of a bioengineered human ligament replacement in the future (8).

An experimental bioengineered anterior cruciate ligament has been developed *in vitro* by seeding human ligament fibroblasts in a hydrated collagen matrix. The bioengineered anterior cruciate ligament contains living fibroblasts and is produced without chemical cross-linking agents and synthetic material. It is anchored with two bones (8). In the future, if a bioengineered ligament or tendon could be started in a laboratory and reach completion in the body, the need to take autogenous grafts could be eliminated.

Research is being conducted in isolating various stem cells from autologous or allogenic sources (including fetal tissue). Stem cells seem to elicit no immune response.

MECHANISMS OF INJURY

Dr. Robert Johnson and co-workers in Vermont analyzed video recordings of skiers falling and tearing knee ligaments. These data have led to recommendations on how to prevent tearing of the anterior cruciate ligament while skiing. As video recordings of sports become more common and the ability to study the digital images improves, we will be better able to understand exactly what forces caused the injuries.

The current epidemic of anterior cruciate ligament injuries in skiing may be abated by developing better ski boots and release mechanisms that will spare anterior cruciate ligaments when skiers fall. Similar advances in prevention of injuries can be expected from studies that are currently being carried out on shoe-surface interfaces.

KNEE DOCUMENTATION

Comparing the results of various treatments of knee instabilities is difficult because of the lack of standardized methods of gathering data. The International Knee Documentation Committee is a committee of international knee experts that has developed a knee-specific, rather than disease-specific, measure of symptoms, knee function, and sports activity (17). The form the committee developed has been validated, and if it becomes widely adopted, it will permit comparisons of outcomes across groups of patients who have different knee lesions.

The whole subject of outcome assessment is gaining in importance and will play a major role in future clinical studies (18). Computer-based patient databases will be important (19,20).

ARTHROSCOPY

Arthroscopy revolutionized the treatment of knee ligament injuries. Most anterior cruciate ligament replacement surgery is now performed with the aid of the arthroscope. Similar advancements are currently being made in posterior cruciate ligament surgery. Techniques to perform autologous chondrocyte implantation arthroscopically may be developed. Research is being conducted to develop meniscus scaffolds that could be implanted with arthroscopic assistance.

New techniques that are currently on the horizon include thermal energy applications, articular cartilage regeneration techniques, and tissue engineering. New meniscus repair techniques are also evolving (21).

The needle arthroscope is making a comeback as an instrument for diagnostic arthroscopy in an office setting.

ANTERIOR CRUCIATE LIGAMENT

The anterior cruciate ligament was regarded as a relatively unimportant knee-stabilizing structure as late as the 1960s. In the past 25 years, its stature has grown to such a level that more publications seem to have appeared on the treatment of torn anterior cruciate ligaments in the sports medicine literature than on treatment of all other knee ligaments combined.

Accumulation of new information on the treatment of the torn anterior cruciate ligament has plateaued. For the time being, the anterior cruciate ligament problem appears to have been "solved." Current debates will focus on refining existing concepts, unless a bioengineered anterior cruciate ligament can be developed.

In the foreseeable future, debates will probably be on the merits of hamstring versus patellar tendon autografts. A survey of orthopedic surgeons in the United States revealed that 93% use midthird patellar tendon autografts, 6% use hamstring grafts, and 1% use allografts (22). An informal survey of National Football League team physicians in 1999 showed that 29 used patellar tendon autografts and only one used hamstring tendon grafts to replace torn anterior cruciate ligaments in professional football players. These percentages may change if fixation of hamstring grafts into bone tunnels can be improved.

Reoperation on knees that have had anterior cruciate ligament replacement grafts remains a problem. The failure rate of revision surgery is high. Improvements will undoubtedly come in this field, possibly in the area of biologic fixation devices.

MEDIAL COLLATERAL LIGAMENT

Acute surgical repair of torn medial collateral ligaments, once regarded as important, has slipped into obscurity. A relatively relaxed attitude has developed toward treatment of torn medial

collateral ligaments because there are relatively few long-term problems from excess laxity due to valgus stress. Tissue engineering has the potential to develop ligaments in vitro that could be used to treat chronic laxity in knees.

POSTERIOR CRUCIATE LIGAMENT AND POSTEROLATERAL ROTATORY INSTABILITY

The same gains that have been achieved in treating anterior cruciate ligament injuries have not been made in treating injuries to the posterior cruciate ligament. Although torn posterior cruciate ligaments can be replaced using autogenous or, more commonly, allograft tissues, results are not as good as those of similar operations for anterior cruciate ligaments (23). Research is being done to improve techniques (24). Perhaps inlay grafts to the posterior tibia will be more successful (24). Use of two strands of graft tissue passed through two femoral tunnels (double-tunnel technique) rather than one may improve postoperative stability.

Arthroscopic repair of acute posterior cruciate ligament avulsions from the tibia has been shown to be feasible (25). Although technically difficult, this method is evolving.

One type of instability taken from the classification of rotatory instability that is still considered important is posterolateral rotatory instability. A satisfactory operation to correct this instability, especially when it is not combined with posterior cruciate ligament injury, has not been found. Clarification of the pathomechanics of posterolateral rotatory instability may aid in arriving at a satisfactory surgical solution for this instability (26).

GENDER

Knee injuries in men and women have been treated in similar manners. Gender differences are coming to be recognized, however, especially in terms of risk factors for injury. Knee braces are now being marketed for women. Further knowledge of differences may result in different training techniques and in management of knee ligament injuries based on gender.

OTHER POSSIBLE DEVELOPMENTS

Shortening of collagenous tissue (such as in shrinkage capsulorraphy) by applying heat or radiofrequency waves is being used widely. In fact, market penetration of radiofrequency devices has been more rapid than that of any orthopedic device in history (21). Various forms of energy, such as heat, laser, and other types of radiofrequency, have been used. There is insufficient basic scientific evidence or long-term follow-up to know what will be the role of this treatment modality in the future.

Welding of tissues by applying heat has also been used. Meniscal repairs and articular cartilage chondroplasties (e.g., to try to make smooth fibrillated hyaline cartilage) have been attempted. Heat severely degrades the collagen and ground substance, and causes tissue necrosis. It is possible that radiofrequency waves are more effective and safe.

Photodynamic therapy, in which collagen tissues are coated with a photosensitive dye and exposed to light, is a potential method to join collagen fibrils. Rather than denaturing the collagen fibrils and surrounding ground substance and killing the cells, the treatment causes chemical bonds to be formed. If this method proves to be effective, it may have application to the treatment of torn or repaired ligaments and tendons. Another potential application of photodynamic therapy may be in the treatment of chronic tendinoses, such as lateral epicondylitis of the elbow.

There is interest in research on growth factors that could speed healing of fractures and promote the growth of bone (27,28). It may be possible in the future to inject growth factors into sites that need new bone. If this is effective, a similar approach could be developed for collagenous tissues, such as ligaments and tendons.

A great deal of interest is currently centered on attempts to regenerate articular cartilage. A commonly accepted classification system is needed to allow comparison of the results of various treatments. The natural history of untreated chondral injury needs to be elucidated to be sure new treatments improve on the natural processes. Enhanced MRI assessments, evaluation with indentation probes, and use of biochemical markers may add objectivity to the analyses of end results.

Autologous chondrocyte transplantation and osteochondral autograft transplantation are currently being performed. These methods may or may not survive the test of time, but will probably lead to new ways to regenerate articular cartilage. Articular cartilage may eventually be regrown using pharmacologic means. Perhaps the matrix or chondrocytes can be stimulated using genetic engineering or growth factors such as transforming growth factor or insulin-like growth factor. There may be a role for use of a scaffolding. Rather than enhancing regeneration, ways may be found to inhibit degeneration of articular cartilage.

Dramatic advances have been made in all aspects of the diagnosis and treatment of knee ligament injuries. The greatest current deficiencies lie in the management of posterior cruciate ligament injuries and posterolateral rotatory instability, as well as meniscal and chondral repair.

REFERENCES

1. Kahler D. Applications of computer assisted orthopaedic surgery for orthopaedic trauma. In: *Proceedings of the 68th Annual Meeting of the American Academy of Orthopaedic Surgeons*, vol 2. Rosemont, IL: American Academy of Orthopaedic Surgeons, 2001:87–88.
2. Petermann J. Computer and robot assisted ACL reconstruction with Caspar System. In: *Proceedings of the 68th Annual Meeting of the American Academy of Orthopaedic Surgeons*, vol 2. Rosemont, IL: American Academy of Orthopaedic Surgeons, 2001:533.
3. Poss R, Mabrey JD, Gillogly SD, et al. Development of a virtual reality arthroscopic knee simulator. *J Bone Joint Surg Am* 2000;82:1495–1502.
4. Lanier J. Virtually there. *Sci Am* 2001;284:66–75.
5. Caplan A, Goldberg V. Principles of tissue engineered regeneration of skeletal tissues. *Clin Orthop* 1999;367[Suppl]:12–16.
6. Jackson D, Simon T. Tissue engineering principles in orthopaedic surgery. *Clin Orthop* 1999;367[Suppl]:31–45.
7. Goldberg V. Introduction and overview of tissue engineering. In: *Proceedings of the 68th Annual Meeting of the American Academy of Orthopaedic Surgeons*, vol 2. Rosemont, IL: American Academy of Orthopaedic Surgeons, 2001:11.
8. Goulet F, Rancourt D, Cloutier R, et al. Tendons and ligaments. In: Lanza RP, Langer R, Vacanti J, eds. *Principles of tissue engineering*, 2nd ed. San Diego: Academic Press, 2000:711–722.
9. Buckwalter J. Promoting ligament and tendon healing: what does tissue engineering have to offer. In: *Proceedings of the 68th Annual Meeting of the American Academy of Orthopaedic Surgeons*, vol 2. Rosemont, IL: American Academy of Orthopaedic Surgeons, 2001:14–15.
10. Goldberg V. Tissue engineering approaches to meniscal regeneration. In: *Proceedings of the 68th Annual Meeting of the American Academy of Orthopaedic Surgeons*, vol 2. Rosemont, IL: American Academy of Orthopaedic Surgeons, 2001:16–17.
11. Evans CH, Ghivizzani SC, Kang R, et al. Gene therapy for rheumatic diseases. *Arthritis Rheum* 1999;42:1–16.
12. Dejardin LM, Arnoczky SP, Ewers BJ, et al. Tissue-engineered rotator cuff tendon using porcine small intestine submucosa. Histologic and mechanical evaluation in dogs. *Am J Sports Med* 2001;29:175–184.
13. Reddi A. Bone morphogenetic proteins: from basic science to clinical applications. *J Bone Joint Surg Am* 2001;83[Suppl 1, Pt 1]:S1-1-S6-6.
14. Forslund C, Aspenberg P. Tendon healing stimulated by injected CDMP-2. *Med Sci Sports Exerc* 2001;33:685–687.
15. Brittberg M, Lindahl A, Nilsson A, et al. Treatment of deep cartilage defects in the knee with autologous chondrocyte transplantations. *N Engl J Med* 1994;33:889–895.
16. Dunn MG, Tria AJ, Kato YP, et al. Anterior cruciate ligament reconstruction using a composite collagenous prosthesis: a biomechanical and histologic study in rabbits. *Am J Sports Med* 1992;20:507–515.
17. Irrgang J. Development and validation of the new International Knee Documentation Committee (IKDC) subjective knee form. In: *Proceedings of the 68th Annual Meeting of the American Academy of Orthopaedic Surgeons*, vol 2. Rosemont, IL: American Academy of Orthopaedic Surgeons, 2001:563.
18. Swiontkowski MF, Buckwalter JA, Keller RB, et al. The outcomes movement in orthopaedic surgery. *J Bone Joint Surg Am* 1999;81:732–740.
19. Johnston RC. Implementation of a computer-based patient record and outcomes data-collection system at the Department of Orthopaedic Surgery, University of Iowa. *J Bone Joint Surg Am* 2000;82:1502–1505.
20. Harrast JJ, Poss R. The value and promise of patient databases in orthopaedic surgery. *J Bone Joint Surg Am* 2000;82:1506–1509.
21. Twentieth Annual Meeting of the Arthroscopy Association of North America; April 19–22, 2001; Seattle, WA. Abst 515–528.
22. Delay B, Smolinski R, Nicoletta R, et al. Current trends in anterior cruciate ligament reconstruction: results of a survey. In: *Proceedings of the 68th Annual Meeting of the American Academy of Orthopaedic Surgeons*, vol 2. Rosemont, IL: American Academy of Orthopaedic Surgeons, 2001:366–367.
23. Bergfeld JA, McAllister DR, Parker RD, et al. Biomechanical comparison of posterior cruciate ligament reconstruction techniques. *Am J Sports Med* 2001;29:129–136.
24. Berg EE. Posterior cruciate ligament tibial inlay reconstruction. *Arthroscopy* 1995;11:69–76.
25. Kim SJ, Shin SJ, Choi NH, et al. Arthroscopically assisted treatment of avulsion fractures of the posterior cruciate ligament from the tibia. *J Bone Joint Surg Am* 2001;83:698–708.
26. Covey DC. Injuries of the posterolateral corner of the knee. *J Bone Joint Surg Am* 2001;83:106–118.
27. Einhorn T. Genetic engineering in the future of fracture care. In: *Proceedings of the 68th Annual Meeting of the American Academy of Orthopaedic Surgeons*, vol 2. Rosemont, IL: American Academy of Orthopaedic Surgeons, 2001:89–90.
28. Bauer T. Cell therapy in your operating room today: tissue engineering principles and the use of bone marrow derived cells for bone grafting. In: *Proceedings of the 68th Annual Meeting of the American Academy of Orthopaedic Surgeons*, vol 2. Rosemont, IL: American Academy of Orthopaedic Surgeons, 2001:26–27.

Index

Page numbers followed by *f* refer to figures; those followed by *t* refer to tables.